Practical Nephrology

Practical Nephrology

Editor: Adriana Jones

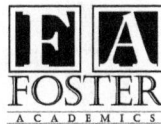

FOSTER
ACADEMICS

www.fosteracademics.com

www.fosteracademics.com

FA
FOSTER
A C A D E M I C S

Cataloging-in-Publication Data

Practical nephrology / edited by Adriana Jones.
    p. cm.
Includes bibliographical references and index.
ISBN 978-1-63242-708-3
1. Nephrology. 2. Kidneys--Diseases. I. Jones, Adriana.
RC902 .P73 2019
616.61--dc23

Foster Academics,
118-35 Queens Blvd., Suite 400,
Forest Hills, NY 11375, USA

ISBN 978-1-63242-708-3 (Hardback)

Contents

Preface

Nephrology is the study of the kidney function and the diseases associated with them. It also involves the diagnosis, prevention and the treatment of kidney diseases. The assessment of the blood pressure and the condition of the heart, lungs, abdomen and joints is required for diagnosing kidney diseases. Examination of the urine is the most common and direct way to assess kidney problems. In some cases, blood tests for checking the concentration of hemoglobin, platelets, calcium, urea or creatinine in the blood are also used to assess kidney problems. Imaging techniques like ultrasonography, computed axial tomography (CT) and magnetic resonance imaging (MRI) are also used to diagnose the structural abnormalities in the kidneys. The various advancements in nephrology are glanced at in this book and their applications as well as ramifications are looked at in detail. Different approaches, evaluations, methodologies and advanced studies on nephrology have also been included in it. This book is an essential guide for both academicians and those who wish to pursue this discipline further.

The information shared in this book is based on empirical researches made by veterans in this field of study. The elaborative information provided in this book will help the readers further their scope of knowledge leading to advancements in this field.

Finally, I would like to thank my fellow researchers who gave constructive feedback and my family members who supported me at every step of my research.

Editor

Prognosis of Acute Kidney Injury and Hepatorenal Syndrome in Patients with Cirrhosis

Andrew S. Allegretti,[1] Guillermo Ortiz,[1] Julia Wenger,[1] Joseph J. Deferio,[1]
Joshua Wibecan,[1] Sahir Kalim,[1] Hector Tamez,[2] Raymond T. Chung,[3]
S. Ananth Karumanchi,[4] and Ravi I. Thadhani[1]

[1]*Division of Nephrology, Department of Medicine, Massachusetts General Hospital, Boston, MA 02114, USA*
[2]*Division of Cardiology, Department of Medicine, Beth Israel Deaconess Medical Center, Boston, MA 02114, USA*
[3]*Liver Center and Gastrointestinal Division, Department of Medicine, Massachusetts General Hospital, Boston, MA 02114, USA*
[4]*Division of Nephrology, Department of Medicine, Beth Israel Deaconess Medical Center, Boston, MA 02215, USA*

Correspondence should be addressed to Andrew S. Allegretti; aallegretti@partners.org

Academic Editor: Suresh C. Tiwari

Background/Aims. Acute kidney injury is a common problem for patients with cirrhosis and is associated with poor survival. We aimed to examine the association between type of acute kidney injury and 90-day mortality. *Methods.* Prospective cohort study at a major US liver transplant center. A nephrologist's review of the urinary sediment was used in conjunction with the 2007 Ascites Club Criteria to stratify acute kidney injury into four groups: prerenal azotemia, hepatorenal syndrome, acute tubular necrosis, or other. *Results.* 120 participants with cirrhosis and acute kidney injury were analyzed. Ninety-day mortality was 14/40 (35%) with prerenal azotemia, 20/35 (57%) with hepatorenal syndrome, 21/36 (58%) with acute tubular necrosis, and 1/9 (11%) with other ($p = 0.04$ overall). Mortality was the same in hepatorenal syndrome compared to acute tubular necrosis ($p = 0.99$). Mortality was lower in prerenal azotemia compared to hepatorenal syndrome ($p = 0.05$) and acute tubular necrosis ($p = 0.04$). Ten participants (22%) were reclassified from hepatorenal syndrome to acute tubular necrosis because of granular casts on urinary sediment. *Conclusions.* Hepatorenal syndrome and acute tubular necrosis result in similar 90-day mortality. Review of urinary sediment may add important diagnostic information to this population. Multicenter studies are needed to validate these findings and better guide management.

1. Introduction

Acute kidney injury (AKI) is a common and life-threatening problem for patients with cirrhosis [1–3]. The differential diagnosis for AKI in this population is large. The most common etiologies are prerenal azotemia (PRA), acute tubular necrosis (ATN), and hepatorenal syndrome (HRS), but other causes such as glomerulonephritis, medication toxicity, and abdominal compartment syndrome from tense ascites occur as well [3, 4]. Regardless of etiology, AKI is associated with reduced survival [5–7]. Measures of renal function (i.e., serum creatinine) are factored prominently into prognostic scores such as the Model for End-Stage Liver Disease (MELD) and Chronic Liver Failure-Sequential Organ Failure Assessment (CLIF-SOFA) and have major implications for liver transplant allocation [8–10].

One cause of AKI unique to liver disease is HRS. Hepatorenal syndrome is thought to be due to splanchnic vasodilation causing hormonal imbalances that ultimately result in renal vasoconstriction and impaired renal function [4, 11]. Several studies suggest that HRS is associated with the highest mortality of all types of AKI [12–14]. As such, a diagnosis of HRS-related AKI is felt to have greater clinical significance over other types of AKI. Despite this, there is no definitive test for HRS, which remains a challenging diagnosis for clinicians.

Over the last several years, consensus guidelines have evolved to aid in the diagnosis of AKI in cirrhosis. The diagnostic criteria for HRS have been updated several times, most recently in 2007 [14, 15]. The definition of AKI itself has been debated as well, as some of the older definitions of AKI that used a doubling of serum creatinine or a preset threshold value had limited sensitivity to detect AKI in patients with cirrhosis [16, 17]. Recent studies support using the Acute Kidney Injury Network (AKIN) definition of AKI, which correlates closely with mortality in cirrhosis [17–23]. We sought to evaluate whether the type of AKI influenced the 90-day mortality of hospitalized patients with cirrhosis. We hypothesized that those with HRS would have the worst 90-day mortality.

2. Methods

2.1. Study Population and Setting. Between January 2013 and December 2014, consenting adult patients (age 18 years or older) who were hospitalized at Massachusetts General Hospital with cirrhosis and AKI (see "Definitions") were enrolled in this prospective study. Massachusetts General Hospital is a 1008-bed academic tertiary care center with an active liver transplant program. Potential participants were excluded from this study if they previously received a renal transplant, if they were on renal replacement therapy at the time of admission, or if they were pregnant or nursing. Participants were followed during their inpatient admission and subsequently as outpatients after discharge.

2.2. Definitions

2.2.1. Cirrhosis. The diagnosis of cirrhosis was based on clinical evaluation by a hepatologist using laboratory values, liver imaging, endoscopy, and (when available) liver biopsy.

2.2.2. Acute Kidney Injury. The AKIN criteria were used to diagnose AKI, which required an absolute increase in serum creatinine of 0.3 mg/dL (26.4 μmol/L) above baseline or an increase of serum creatinine to 150% of baseline within 48 hours [21]. The AKIN criterion for decline in urine output was not used in the initial diagnosis of AKI as it was felt to be unreliable in patients with ascites and without a bladder catheter.

2.2.3. Classification of AKI. Participants were classified as having one of four types of AKI: (1) prerenal azotemia (PRA), (2) hepatorenal syndrome (HRS), (3) acute tubular necrosis (ATN), and (4) other causes. Participants were classified as having HRS based on the 2007 Ascites Club Criteria [14]. These include the following: (1) presence of cirrhosis and ascites, (2) serum creatinine greater than 1.5 mg/dL, (3) failure of improvement in serum creatinine below 1.5 mg/dL after administration of albumin and withdrawal of diuretics for 48 hours, (4) absence of nephrotoxic drugs, (5) absence of shock, and (6) absence of parenchymal renal disease. Parenchymal renal disease was defined as presence of abnormal kidneys on ultrasound, >500 mg proteinuria per day, presence of >50 RBCs per high-powered field of urinary sediment, or presence of granular casts on a nephrologist's review of the urinary sediment. Participants were classified as having PRA if they presented with AKI, a clinical history consistent with a prerenal state (such as bleeding or GI fluid losses), and their serum creatinine improved following the administration of volume and withdrawal of diuretics. Participants were diagnosed with ATN if they failed to meet criteria for PRA and HRS and had a clinical history consistent with tubular/parenchymal kidney injury. Participants were diagnosed with "other" causes of AKI if they had evidence of another process on serology or renal biopsy, such as glomerulonephritis.

Diagnoses of AKI were reviewed and confirmed independently by two study investigators. If a discrepancy in diagnosis was found, a third investigator reviewed the medical record and provided a tie-breaking diagnosis.

2.3. Data Collection and Management. All data was registered as part of the routine clinical care and collected from review of the electronic medical record. This included demographics, laboratory findings, radiology, procedural findings (including microscopic examination of urine sediment by a nephrologist), medical history, and medications. MELD and CLIF-SOFA scores were taken from the time of admission. The reference laboratory at the study site reported the lowest cutoff of urine sodium as "less than 10 mmol/L," so this variable was dichotomized for analysis at this value. All values reported are taken from the time of enrollment unless otherwise noted. Study data were collected and managed using REDCap electronic data capture tools hosted at the Harvard Clinical and Translational Science Center [24]. Each participant also provided serum, plasma, and urine samples on enrollment and on days 5 and 30 after enrollment (as available) to create a biorepository for future evaluation of markers of kidney and liver injury.

Participants were treated as per local standard of care by the managing internists, hepatologists, and nephrologists on service. Members of the study team did not intervene in patient care. Management of AKI was done using guidelines and evidenced-based medicine at the discretion of treating clinicians, including (1) withdrawal of potential offending agents, such as diuretics, (2) empiric and culture based treatment of infections, (3) administration of volume, (4) reversal of underlying insults, such as endoscopic treatment of bleeding, (5) treatment of suspected HRS using albumin and midodrine/octreotide or vasopressors, and (6) use of intermittent hemodialysis or continuous venovenous hemofiltration for AKI refractory to medical management. Participants diagnosed with spontaneous bacterial peritonitis were given 1.5 g/kg albumin on day of diagnosis and 1 g/kg albumin 48 hours later along with antibiotics [25].

2.4. Statistical Analysis. Demographic and clinical characteristics of participants are presented as medians (quartile 1, quartile 3) or number (percentage) and compared between the four subgroups of AKI by one-way analysis of variance tests or Fisher's exact tests. These variables were also compared between those alive and those who died at 90 days using Mann-Whitney U tests for continuous variables and Fisher's exact test for categorical variables. Additional outcomes (need for dialysis, recovery from dialysis, creatinine at 90 days, and liver transplantation after enrollment) were analyzed by type of AKI in a similar fashion. Pairwise testing was also performed to compare outcomes between participants with HRS versus ATN.

Differences in the primary outcome of death by 90 days by type of AKI were visualized using a Kaplan-Meier curve and compared using a log-rank test. Cox proportional hazard models were used to create a multivariable model to predict death by 90 days by type of AKI. The subgroup of "other causes" of AKI was not analyzed in the multivariable model to better highlight the three subgroups affected by altered hemodynamics (PRA, HRS, and ATN). Because of sample size limitations, two prespecified models were selected for analysis using type of AKI, age, and either MELD or CLIF-SOFA score as predictors. The assumption of proportional hazards was tested for all models. Results of Cox proportional hazard models are summarized with hazard ratios and Wald asymptotic 95% confidence intervals. Four sensitivity analyses were performed: (1) excluding four participants who had previously received a liver transplant, (2) using a composite endpoint of death or liver transplant by 90 days, (3) reclassifying 10 participants with granular casts on sediment as having HRS if all other criteria were met, and (4) including infection as a subgroup of AKI (AKI with infection compared to three subgroups [PRA, HRS, and HRS] without infection). SAS version 9.4 (Gary, NC) was used for all analyses. Two-tailed p values < 0.05 were considered to indicate statistical significance.

2.5. Ethics Statement. This study was approved by the site's institutional review board and abides by the guidelines set forth by the Declaration of Helsinki. No donor organs were obtained from executed prisoners or other institutionalized persons at this liver transplant center. All participants (or their health care designee) provided written informed consent.

3. Results

3.1. General Demographics. One hundred twenty participants with cirrhosis and AKI were analyzed in this study. Forty (33%) had PRA, 35 (29%) had HRS, 36 (30%) had ATN, and 9 (8%) had other causes of AKI (Figure 1). Of the other causes of AKI, 5 (56%) had evidence of glomerulonephritis. Ten participants who met all inclusion criteria for HRS (22%) were reclassified to acute tubular necrosis because of the presence of granular casts on urinary sediment.

Median (quartile 1, quartile 3) age of the entire cohort was 58 (50, 65) years. The majority of participants were male (71%), white race (93%), and of non-Hispanic ethnicity (87%). Median length of hospital admission was 16 (9, 24) days. Median time from admission to enrollment was 4 (3, 10) days. Median MELD score was 24 (18, 30) and median CLIF-SOFA score was 9 (6, 10). The most common etiologies of cirrhosis were alcoholic (30%), multifactorial (27%), and hepatitis C (20%). Eleven participants (9%) had stage I AKI, 23 participants (19%) had stage II AKI, and 86 participants (72%) had stage III AKI. Ninety-four participants (78%) received nephrology consultation. Thirty-eight participants (32%) required renal replacement therapy. Twenty-one participants (18%) went on to receive liver transplantation. Forty-nine participants (41%) received vasopressors while being hospitalized in the intensive care unit. Thirty-one participants with HRS (89%) were treated with midodrine and

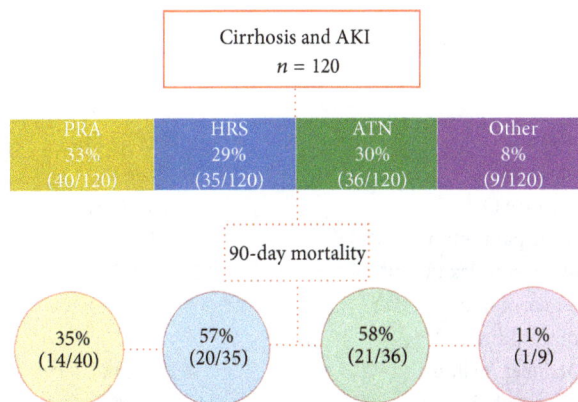

FIGURE 1: Distribution of participants and 90-day mortality. AKI (acute kidney injury), PRA (prerenal azotemia), HRS (hepatorenal syndrome), and ATN (acute tubular necrosis).

octreotide. Characteristics of all participants by type of AKI are presented in Table 1.

Across the entire cohort, 56 (47%) participants died by day 90 after enrollment. Participants who died had a significantly higher MELD score, CLIF-SOFA score, serum creatinine on enrollment, peak creatinine during their admission, INR, and total bilirubin and had a lower urine output and mean arterial pressure. Participants who died were more likely to receive nephrology consultation, receive dialysis, receive intravenous albumin, or be treated with midodrine, octreotide, or intravenous vasopressors (Table 2).

Among those with HRS, 13/15 (87%) who survived and 18/20 (90%) who died were treated with midodrine and octreotide ($p = 1.00$). Intravenous vasopressors were given to 6/15 (40%) who survived and 10/20 (50%) who died ($p = 0.73$).

3.2. Outcomes by Type of AKI. The primary and secondary outcomes were analyzed across all four types of AKI (PRA, HRS, ATN, and other) and in pairwise analysis between those with HRS and ATN (Table 3). There was a significant difference in death by 90 days across all four subgroups ($p = 0.02$) but not between HRS and ATN (20/35 [57%] versus 21/36 [58%]; $p = 1.00$). There was no significant difference in the need for dialysis ($p = 0.13$), recovery from dialysis (among survivors to 90 days; $p = 0.16$), and new liver transplant ($p = 0.44$). Among those who were alive and did not require dialysis, participants with HRS had a higher serum creatinine at 90 days than those with ATN (1.5 [1.2, 2.0] mg/dL versus 1.0 [0.8, 1.5] mg/dL; $p = 0.01$).

Overall, MELD score was significantly different across all four groups for all participants ($p = 0.04$), but not between HRS and ATN (24 [21, 31] versus 26 [20, 34]; $p = 0.67$). Among those who died, there was no significant difference in MELD score across all four groups ($p = 0.90$). CLIF-SOFA score was significantly different across all four groups for all participants ($p = 0.01$), but not between HRS and ATN (9 [8, 10] versus 10 [7, 12]; $p = 0.17$). Similarly, there was no significant difference in CLIF-SOFA scores among participants

TABLE 1: Demographics and clinical characteristics.

	PRA (n = 40)	HRS (n = 35)	ATN (n = 36)	Other (n = 9)	p value
Age (years)	58 (49.5, 66)	57 (49, 65)	60 (51, 63)	57 (51, 62)	0.80
Male sex (%)	26 (65%)	25 (71%)	26 (72%)	8 (89%)	0.60
White race (%)	34 (85%)	34 (97%)	34 (94%)	9 (100%)	0.49
Non-Hispanic ethnicity (%)	31 (78%)	30 (86%)	34 (94%)	9 (100%)	0.23
Body mass index (kg/m^2)	28.8 (26.5, 34.6)	28.3 (23.7, 32.0)	27.4 (22.5, 32.8)	26.9 (25.1, 31.0)	0.38
Presence of infection (%)	15 (38%)	11 (31%)	18 (50%)	1 (11%)	0.14
Comorbidities (%)					
Diabetes mellitus	11 (29%)	10 (29%)	11 (31%)	4 (8%)	0.81
Chronic kidney disease	7 (18%)	14 (41%)	10 (28%)	7 (78%)	0.01
Cardiovascular disease	8 (20%)	6 (17%)	7 (19%)	3 (33%)	0.73
Hypertension	17 (43%)	14 (40%)	14 (40%)	3 (33%)	0.99
Etiology of cirrhosis (%)					0.24
Hepatitis C	11 (28%)	4 (11%)	7 (19%)	2 (22%)	
Alcohol	12 (30%)	12 (35%)	12 (33%)	0 (0%)	
Nonalcoholic steatohepatitis	3 (8%)	4 (11%)	5 (14%)	1 (11%)	
Multifactorial	12 (30%)	11 (31%)	6 (17%)	3 (33%)	
Other	2 (5%)	4 (11%)	6 (17%)	3 (33%)	
Prior complications of cirrhosis (%)					
Ascites requiring prior paracentesis	14 (36%)	27 (82%)	12 (33%)	4 (44%)	<0.001
Encephalopathy	14 (35%)	20 (57%)	12 (33%)	3 (33%)	0.15
Gastrointestinal bleeding	7 (18%)	8 (23%)	6 (17%)	0 (0%)	0.52
Spontaneous bacterial peritonitis	4 (10%)	7 (20%)	3 (8%)	0 (0%)	0.35
Portosystemic shunt	3 (8%)	2 (6%)	4 (11%)	2 (22%)	0.42
Prior liver transplantation (%)	2 (5%)	1 (3%)	0 (0%)	1 (11%)	0.57
MELD score (admission)	19 (17, 28)	24 (21, 31)	26 (20, 34)	20 (18, 21)	0.04
CLIF-SOFA score (admission)	8 (6, 9)	9 (8, 10)	10 (7, 12)	6 (5, 7)	0.01
Nephrologist consulted (%)	23 (58%)	31 (89%)	33 (92%)	6 (67%)	<0.001
AKI stage I or II (%)/stage III (%)	15 (38%)/25 (63%)	9 (26%)/26 (75%)	7 (19%)/29 (81%)	3 (33%)/6 (67%)	0.34
Medications received (%)					
Intravenous albumin	28 (70%)	34 (97%)[*]	29 (81%)	4 (44%)	<0.001
Midodrine	15 (38%)	31 (89%)	25 (69%)	2 (22%)	<0.001
Octreotide	21 (53%)	31 (89%)	24 (67%)	1 (11%)	<0.001
Intravenous vasopressor	13 (33%)	15 (43%)	19 (53%)	2 (22%)	0.21
Laboratory values/vital signs					
Mean arterial pressure (mmHg)	78 (73, 85)	74 (69, 80)	73 (68, 80)	86 (79, 88)	0.07
Urine output (mL/24 hours)[**]	763 (475, 1125)	488 (325, 750)	625 (300, 1095)	873 (525, 1450)	0.23
Enrollment creatinine (mg/dL)	1.4 (1.2, 1.8)	2.7 (2.0, 3.0)	2.3 (1.9, 3.6)	2.3 (2.0, 3.7)	<0.001
Peak creatinine (mg/dL)	1.9 (1.6, 2.6)	3.4 (2.7, 4.7)	3.5 (2.5, 6.8)	4.1 (2.3, 4.5)	<0.001
Sodium (mEq/L)	133 (130, 137)	131 (128, 136)	136 (132, 141)	136 (129, 140)	0.10
White blood count (K/uL)	7.2 (4.3, 10.6)	7.0 (4.8, 10.6)	9.1 (5.5, 15.7)	6.4 (4.1, 8.8)	0.10
Hemoglobin (g/dL)	8.3 (8.0, 9.5)	9.0 (7.9, 10.0)	8.6 (7.9, 9.4)	8.9 (8.4, 11.1)	0.44
Platelets (K/uL)	89 (57, 124)	77 (58, 101)	64 (47, 125)	93 (77, 143)	0.50
Albumin (g/dL)	2.9 (2.5, 3.6)	3.5 (3.2, 3.7)	2.8 (2.7, 3.2)	2.8 (2.5, 4.1)	0.01
International normalized ratio (INR)	1.7 (1.3, 2.0)	1.8 (1.5, 2.1)	1.9 (1.5, 2.3)	1.4 (1.2, 1.5)	0.01
Total bilirubin (mg/dL)	3.8 (1.7, 8.2)	5.0 (2.2, 11.0)	9.6 (2.5, 22.2)	2.0 (1.1, 3.8)	0.06
Urine sodium <10 mmol/L (%)[***]	9 (43%)	21 (75%)	5 (26%)	2 (33%)	<0.001

All values were taken at time of study enrollment unless otherwise noted. Continuous variables presented as median (quartile 1, quartile 3).
PRA: prerenal azotemia, HRS: hepatorenal syndrome, and ATN: acute tubular necrosis.
[*] One participant received red blood cell transfusion instead of albumin.
[**] n = 36 for PRA, n = 34 for HRS, n = 30 for ATN, and n = 8 for other.
[***] n = 21 for PRA, n = 28 for HRS, n = 19 for ATN, and n = 6 for other.

TABLE 2: Relationship of variables to death at 90 days for all participants[*].

	Alive (n = 64)	Died (n = 56)	p value
Age (years)	58 (48, 64)	59 (53, 66)	0.12
Male sex (%)	43 (69%)	41 (73%)	0.69
White race (%)	58 (91%)	53 (95%)	0.44
Non-Hispanic ethnicity (%)	53 (82%)	51 (91%)	0.34
Body mass index (kg/m^2)	27.2 (23.6, 33.2)	29.0 (25.5, 32.2)	0.47
Presence of infection (%)	20 (31%)	25 (45%)	0.14
Other medical problems (%)			
Diabetes mellitus	19 (31%)	17 (31%)	1.00
Chronic kidney disease	23 (37%)	15 (27%)	0.33
Cardiovascular disease	14 (22%)	10 (18%)	0.65
Hypertension	27 (43%)	21 (38%)	0.58
Etiology of cirrhosis[**]	—	—	0.46
Prior complications of cirrhosis (%)			
Any ascites	41 (64%)	33 (59%)	0.58
Ascites requiring paracentesis	28 (45%)	29 (53%)	0.46
Encephalopathy	27 (42%)	22 (39%)	0.85
Gastrointestinal bleeding	8 (13%)	13 (23%)	0.15
Spontaneous bacterial peritonitis	8 (13%)	6 (11%)	0.78
Portosystemic shunt	7 (11%)	4 (8%)	0.54
MELD score (admission)	23 (18, 29)	29 (23, 36)	<0.001
CLIF-SOFA score (admission)	8 (5, 10)	9 (8, 11)	0.01
Nephrologist consulted (%)	42 (66%)	51 (91%)	<0.001
AKI stage I or II (%)/stage III (%)	23 (36%)/41 (64%)	11 (20%)/45 (80%)	0.07
Required dialysis (%)	14 (22%)	24 (43%)	0.02
Medications received (%)			
Intravenous albumin	45 (70%)	50 (89%)	0.01
Midodrine	28 (44%)	45 (80%)	<0.001
Octreotide	32 (50%)	45 (80%)	<0.001
Intravenous vasopressor	20 (31%)	30 (54%)	0.02
Laboratory values/vital signs			
Mean arterial pressure (mmHg)	78 (71, 84)	74 (68, 80)	0.03
Urine output (mL/24 hours)[***]	850 (500, 1200)	450 (275, 750)	<0.001
Enrollment creatinine (mg/dL)	1.8 (1.3, 2.4)	2.6 (1.9, 3.5)	<0.001
Peak creatinine (mg/dL)	2.3 (1.8, 3.9)	3.4 (2.8, 4.7)	<0.001
Sodium (mEq/L)	133 (129, 137)	134 (130, 139)	0.41
White blood count (K/uL)	10.1 (6.9, 16.9)	8.2 (5.3, 13.5)	0.09
Hemoglobin (g/dL)	8.3 (7.8, 9.5)	8.9 (8.1, 10.1)	0.09
Platelets (K/uL)	88 (59, 124)	72 (48, 104)	0.20
Albumin (g/dL)	2.9 (2.5, 3.5)	3.3 (2.8, 3.6)	0.06
International normalized ratio (INR)	1.6 (1.3, 2.0)	1.9 (1.5, 2.1)	0.02
Total bilirubin (mg/dL)	3.7 (1.5, 8.7)	7.1 (3.0, 19.9)	0.001
Urine sodium < 10 mmol/L (%)[****]	15 (39%)	22 (61%)	0.10

All values were taken at time of study enrollment unless otherwise noted. Continuous variables presented as median (quartile 1, quartile 3).
AKI: acute kidney injury.
[*]Three participants who were lost to follow-up were included in the alive category.
[**]Subcategories the same as Table 1 (hepatitis C, alcohol, nonalcoholic steatohepatitis, multifactorial, other).
[***]n = 108 total.
[****]n = 74 total.

TABLE 3: Outcomes and variables by type of acute kidney injury.

	PRA $n = 40$	HRS $n = 35$	ATN $n = 36$	Other $n = 9$	p value (overall)	p value (HRS versus ATN)
Death by 90 days (%)	14 (35%)	20 (57%)	21 (58%)	1 (11%)	0.02	1.00
Required dialysis (%)	8 (20%)	12 (34%)	16 (44%)	2 (22%)	0.13	0.47
Recovered from dialysis (%)*	4 (44%)	1 (8%)	3 (19%)	1 (50%)	0.16	0.61
Creatinine at 90 days (mg/dL)**	1.0 (0.8, 1.3)	1.5 (1.2, 2.0)	1.0 (0.8, 1.5)	1.6 (1.2, 2.1)	0.01	0.02
Received liver transplant (%)	6 (15%)	9 (26%)	5 (15%)	1 (11%)	0.44	0.24

Continuous variables presented as median (quartile 1, quartile 3).
PRA: prerenal azotemia, HRS: hepatorenal syndrome, ATN: acute tubular necrosis, MELD: Model for End-Stage Liver Disease, and CLIF-SOFA: Chronic Liver Failure-Sequential Organ Failure Assessment.
*Among those who required dialysis ($n = 9$ for PRA, $n = 12$ for HRS, $n = 16$ for ATN, and $n = 2$ for other).
**Among those who were alive and were not requiring dialysis at 90 days ($n = 24$ for PRA, $n = 13$ for HRS, $n = 10$ for ATN, and $n = 6$ for other).

who died across all four subgroups ($p = 0.84$). Those with HRS were more likely to have a urine sodium less than 10 mmol/L compared to those with ATN (21/28 [75%] versus 5/19 [26%]; $p = 0.01$).

A Kaplan-Meier curve depicts survival through 90 days by type of AKI (PRA, HRS, and ATN) in Figure 2. Overall, there was a significant difference in survival between the three subgroups ($p = 0.04$). However, there was no difference in survival between HRS and ATN ($p = 0.99$). Mortality was significantly lower in PRA compared to HRS and ATN ($p = 0.05$ and $p = 0.04$, resp.).

In a sensitivity analysis using a combined composite endpoint of death or liver transplant by 90 days, results were similar to the primary outcome, with a significant difference across all three subgroups ($p < 0.001$), but not between HRS and ATN ($p = 0.41$). When examining those with AKI and infection, there was no difference in 90-day mortality between groups with infection and those without infection ($p = 0.09$ between all groups; $p = 0.06$ for AKI with infection versus PRA without infection; $p = 0.39$ for AKI with infection versus HRS without infection; $p = 0.97$ for AKI with infection versus ATN without infection).

Because 10 participants met HRS criteria but were classified as having ATN due to granular casts on urinary sediment, a sensitivity analysis was performed including them in the HRS subgroup. This resulted in 45 participants being classified as having HRS and reduced the number of those with ATN to 26. There was no change in the 90-day survival in this sensitivity analysis ($p = 0.03$ overall and $p = 0.63$ for HRS versus ATN).

In multivariable Cox proportional hazard models containing terms for type of AKI, age, and a prognostic score (either MELD score [Model 1] or CLIF-SOFA score [Model 2]), there was a trend towards lower risk of death with a diagnosis of PRA compared to ATN (Model 1 HR: 0.52, 95% CI [0.25–1.07]; $p = 0.08$, and Model 2 HR: 0.55, 95% CI [0.27–1.14]; $p = 0.11$) while risk of death for HRS did not differ from ATN (Model 1 HR: 0.97, 95% CI [0.52–1.79]; $p = 0.91$, and Model 2 HR: 1.03, 95% CI [0.55–1.93]; $p = 0.93$). Age was associated with increased risk of death (Model 1 HR: 1.05, 95% CI [1.02–1.09]; $p = 0.01$, and Model 2 HR: 1.05, 95% CI [1.02–1.09]; $p = 0.001$). Higher MELD or CLIF-SOFA scores were associated with increased risk of death (Model 1 HR: 1.04, 95%

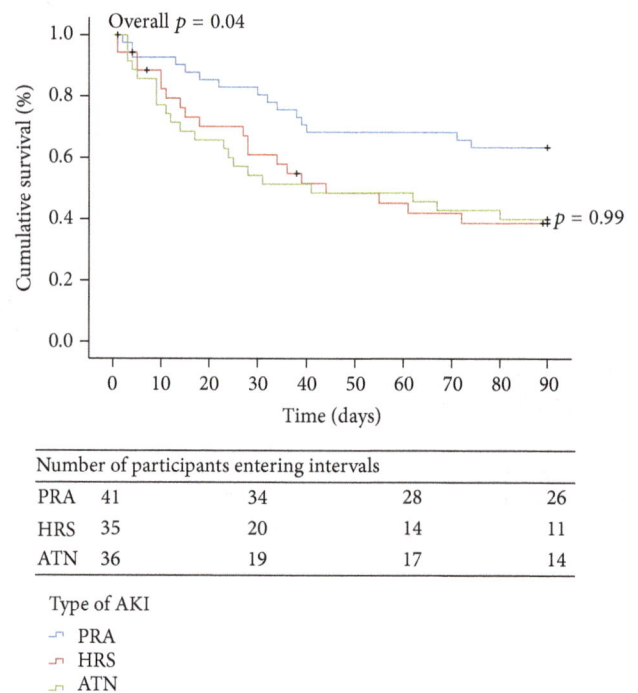

Number of participants entering intervals			
PRA	41	34	28	26
HRS	35	20	14	11
ATN	36	19	17	14

Type of AKI
⌐ PRA
⌐ HRS
⌐ ATN

FIGURE 2: Ninety-day probability of survival of participants with cirrhosis by type of acute kidney injury. PRA (prerenal azotemia), HRS (hepatorenal syndrome), and ATN (acute tubular necrosis).

CI [1.01–1.08]; $p = 0.04$, and Model 2 HR: 1.15, 95% CI [1.02–1.30]; $p = 0.02$).

3.3. Hepatorenal Syndrome Diagnostic Criteria. Each of the six components of the Ascites Club Criteria was analyzed in the PRA, ATN, and "other" AKI subgroups to determine how each participant failed to meet diagnostic criteria for HRS (Figure 3). In the ATN subgroup, participants most commonly had evidence of parenchymal renal disease (55%) or shock (33%). In the PRA subgroup, participants most commonly had a serum creatinine lower than 1.5 mg/dL (20%), had a reduction of creatinine below 1.5 mg/dL with albumin and holding diuretics (55%), or had shock (20%). In the subgroup of "other" causes of AKI, participants most commonly

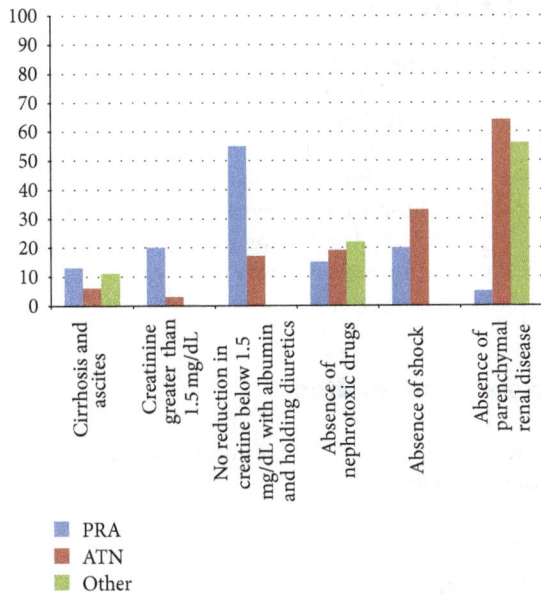

FIGURE 3: Percentage of participants with acute kidney injury who failed to satisfy Ascites Club Criteria for hepatorenal syndrome. PRA (prerenal azotemia), ATN (acute tubular necrosis).

had evidence of parenchymal renal disease (56%) or exposure to nephrotoxic drugs (22%).

4. Discussion

Our results suggest that, among those with cirrhosis and AKI, 90-day mortality is the same between those with HRS and ATN in crude analysis and after adjusting for age and a cirrhosis-specific prognostic assessment (MELD or CLIF-SOFA score). Those with PRA have a better 90-day mortality rate compared to HRS and ATN. In univariate analysis, several factors related to liver and kidney function were associated with mortality, including serum creatinine, need for dialysis, urine output, international normalized ratio, and total bilirubin. Many of these factors are reflected in widely used risk scores [8, 9, 26, 27], thus highlighting their importance in prognosis and transplant allocation.

Interestingly, our results differ from the work done by Martin-Llahi and colleagues in a similar study [13]. In their single-center, prospective cohort study of inpatients with cirrhosis and AKI, these investigators found that 90-day mortality was highest in those with HRS. Those with parenchymal nephropathy had the lowest mortality, and those with hypovolemia-mediated AKI (i.e., PRA) fell in between these two groups. We do not believe that it is biologically plausible for those with PRA to have worse mortality than those with ATN. However, there may be several reasons for the differences between our studies. First, Martin-Llahi and colleagues originally classified AKI into four subgroups, including an additional category of those with AKI mediated by infection. Because infection can be a trigger of PRA (through volume depletion from fluid losses and decreased effective circulating volume), HRS (as can be the case with spontaneous bacterial

peritonitis) [25, 28], and ATN (through systemic inflammation or shock) [29], we elected to include those with infection within a PRA/HRS/ATN scheme. An analysis of 90-day mortality that stratified AKI by presence of infection did not show a significant difference between groups in our cohort. Nevertheless, it may be useful to consider infection as an independent risk factor for mortality with AKI in cirrhosis [13, 30]. Second, there are likely variations in populations between our two studies, potentially due to differences in patient demographics and local practice patterns (e.g., terlipressin, an approved treatment for HRS, is not available in the United States but is commonly employed in Europe) or in the definition of HRS and AKI (the most recent Ascites Club Criteria and AKIN definition of AKI were not available at the time of Martin-Llahi et al.'s study recruitment). These differences are highlighted in HRS incidences (29% in our study versus 51% in their cohort) as well as overall 90-day mortality (47% versus 70%, resp.). These differences, along with variable incidence and survival rates in the literature, suggest a critical need for a multicenter study to better describe the importance of type of AKI in cirrhosis.

One important area of AKI in cirrhosis is the role of the nephrologist, though to our knowledge no prior studies have examined this aspect of care. In our sample, 78% of participants received a nephrology consultation. The nephrologist can offer careful examination of the urine sediment. Coarse pigmented granular casts are a hallmark of ATN; their absence has an excellent negative predictive value in distinguishing prerenal disease (such as PRA and HRS) from intrinsic renal insults [31]. Although one criterion for HRS is the "absence of parenchymal renal injury," only significant proteinuria, hematuria, and ultrasonographic abnormalities are listed as examples [14]. The presence of granular casts is a by-product of the pathophysiology of parenchymal injury, yet it has not been listed in the diagnostic algorithm for HRS for two iterations (it was listed as "minor criteria" in the 1979 Sassari criteria) [15]. We believe that the presence of granular casts on a nephrologist's review of sediment should be considered in the diagnosis of HRS as a tool to guide therapeutic approach to this population.

While we consider HRS a diagnosis of exclusion, it remains possible that overlap between the clinical syndromes of HRS and ATN partially explains their similar mortality rates in this study. Increasingly, clinicians are recognizing the presence of bilirubin nephropathy (sometimes referred to as cholemic nephrosis) as a consequence of advanced cirrhosis. The pathophysiology of bilirubin nephropathy is similar to that of myoglobinuria or rhabdomyolysis, where high serum bilirubin levels are directly toxic to renal tubules when filtered, resulting in a clinical picture consistent with ATN [32]. In an autopsy series in patients with jaundice, van Slambrouck et al. noted that 11/13 of those with a clinical diagnosis of HRS had evidence of tubular bile casts on histologic examination of the kidney [33]. Our current understanding of HRS suggests that it is a hemodynamically driven process without intrinsic renal damage; thus it is possible that some patients with HRS have a secondary insult of ATN. The absence of a diagnostic test linked to the biology of disease and nonspecific clinical criteria do not allow the clinician to simultaneously diagnose a patient with ATN and HRS, even though it is possible that multiple insults may explain a patient's clinical status. Martin-Llahi et al. excluded 8% of their cohort from final analysis due to a mixed etiology of AKI, which further supports this idea [13].

Regardless of the nuances in diagnostic differences between HRS and ATN, our results confirm that those with cirrhosis and AKI represent a critically ill population. Instead of debating the current framework on which we diagnose HRS, it is more important for the clinician to determine whether there is a rapidly reversible, volume-responsive injury (such as PRA) or an insult like HRS or ATN that requires close supportive care. Small trials suggest that vasoconstrictors, albumin, and (in certain circumstances) transjugular intrahepatic shunt placement may be beneficial in HRS [34–41]. Increase in mean arterial pressure (via midodrine, octreotide, or vasopressors) has been linked to improved outcomes in HRS. Maintaining acceptable blood pressure and euvolemic volume status is within the guidelines of managing ATN as well [29]. Empiric use of available therapies, along with early and appropriate use of dialysis as a bridge to transplantation, remains the cornerstone of care for all those with AKI that is not responsive to volume repletion.

Our study should be interpreted within the context of its limitations. This was a single-center trial and may not be generalizable to the experience at other liver transplant centers. However, no multicenter studies have been published examining this subject; thus we believe that our results represent an important contribution to the literature. Similarly, our cohort was predominantly male, white race, and of non-Hispanic ethnicity, limiting generalizability. However, prior studies on cirrhosis and AKI either are similarly homogenous or do not report these patient characteristics, and our results describe the first American cohort in this area. This study was unable to use urine output as part of the AKIN criteria due to unreliable recorded data, a limitation that is commonly reported across many different clinical and research settings. Given our sample size, we were limited in methods of constructing a multivariable model to explain 90-day mortality and were unable to perform a model building process that allowed for screening or selection of a list of candidate variables. However, we feel that our model reflects a pragmatic scientific approach, as age and prognostic assessments like MELD and CLIF-SOFA scores have been well established as important contributors to mortality.

5. Conclusions

We present one of the only studies of US cohort examining implications of the etiology of AKI in cirrhosis. We showed a similar 90-day mortality rate between individuals with HRS and ATN, which was higher compared to the mortality in those with PRA. While there may be some differences in patient characteristics or in the diagnostic approach to HRS from center to center, it remains clear that AKI in cirrhosis portends a high mortality. Further study and multicenter clinical trials are needed to help clinicians better diagnose and improve outcomes in this critically ill group of patients.

List of Abbreviations

AKI: Acute kidney injury
PRA: Prerenal azotemia
ATN: Acute tubular necrosis
HRS: Hepatorenal syndrome
MELD: Model for End-Stage Liver Disease
CLIF-SOFA: Chronic Liver Failure-Sequential Organ
              Failure Assessment
AKIN: Acute Kidney Injury Network.

Authors' Contribution

Andrew S. Allegretti and Guillermo Ortiz are equally contributing first authors.

Acknowledgments

Andrew S. Allegretti is supported by NIH Grant 5T32DK007540-29. Sahir Kalim is supported by NIH Award KL2TR001100. Raymond T. Chung is supported by NIH Grant K24DK078772. S. Ananth Karumanchi is an investigator of the Howard Hughes Medical Institute.

References

[1] P. Ginès and R. W. Schrier, "Renal failure in cirrhosis," *The New England Journal of Medicine*, vol. 361, no. 13, pp. 1279–1290, 2009.

[2] P. Ginès, M. Guevara, V. Arroyo, and J. Rodés, "Hepatorenal syndrome," *The Lancet*, vol. 362, no. 9398, pp. 1819–1827, 2003.

[3] G. Garcia-Tsao, C. R. Parikh, and A. Viola, "Acute kidney injury in cirrhosis," *Hepatology*, vol. 48, no. 6, pp. 2064–2077, 2008.

[4] H. M. Wadei, M. L. Mai, N. Ahsan, and T. A. Gonwa, "Hepatorenal syndrome: pathophysiology and management," *Clinical Journal of the American Society of Nephrology*, vol. 1, no. 5, pp. 1066–1079, 2006.

[5] D. du Cheyron, B. Bouchet, J.-J. Parienti, M. Ramakers, and P. Charbonneau, "The attributable mortality of acute renal failure in critically ill patients with liver cirrhosis," *Intensive Care Medicine*, vol. 31, no. 12, pp. 1693–1699, 2005.

[6] E. Cholongitas, M. Senzolo, D. Patch, S. Shaw, J. O'Beirne, and A. K. Burroughs, "Cirrhotics admitted to intensive care unit: the impact of acute renal failure on mortality," *European Journal of Gastroenterology and Hepatology*, vol. 21, no. 7, pp. 744–750, 2009.

[7] C. D. Tsien, R. Rabie, and F. Wong, "Acute kidney injury in decompensated cirrhosis," *Gut*, vol. 62, no. 1, pp. 131–137, 2013.

[8] R. Wiesner, E. Edwards, R. Freeman et al., "Model for end-stage liver disease (MELD) and allocation of donor livers," *Gastroenterology*, vol. 124, no. 1, pp. 91–96, 2003.

[9] R. Moreau, R. Jalan, P. Gines et al., "Acute-on-chronic liver failure is a distinct syndrome that develops in patients with acute decompensation of cirrhosis," *Gastroenterology*, vol. 144, no. 7, pp. 1426.e9–1437.e9, 2013.

[10] M. Lee, J.-H. Lee, S. Oh et al., "CLIF-SOFA scoring system accurately predicts short-term mortality in acutely decompensated patients with alcoholic cirrhosis: a retrospective analysis," *Liver International*, vol. 35, no. 1, pp. 46–57, 2015.

[11] A. Ginès, A. Escorsell, P. Ginès et al., "Incidence, predictive factors, and prognosis of the hepatorenal syndrome in cirrhosis with ascites," *Gastroenterology*, vol. 105, no. 1, pp. 229–236, 1993.

[12] C. Alessandria, O. Ozdogan, M. Guevara et al., "MELD score and clinical type predict prognosis in hepatorenal syndrome: relevance to liver transplantation," *Hepatology*, vol. 41, no. 6, pp. 1282–1289, 2005.

[13] M. Martin-Llahi, M. Guevara, A. Torre et al., "Prognostic importance of the cause of renal failure in patients with cirrhosis," *Gastroenterology*, vol. 140, no. 2, pp. 488.e4–496.e4, 2011.

[14] F. Salerno, A. Gerbes, P. Ginès, F. Wong, and V. Arroyo, "Diagnosis, prevention and treatment of hepatorenal syndrome in cirrhosis," *Gut*, vol. 56, no. 9, pp. 1310–1318, 2007.

[15] V. Arroyo, P. Ginès, A. L. Gerbes et al., "Definition and diagnostic criteria of refractory ascites and hepatorenal syndrome in cirrhosis," *Hepatology*, vol. 23, no. 1, pp. 164–176, 1996.

[16] C. Francoz, D. Prié, W. AbdelRazek et al., "Inaccuracies of creatinine and creatinine-based equations in candidates for liver transplantation with low creatinine: impact on the model for end-stage liver disease score," *Liver Transplantation*, vol. 16, no. 10, pp. 1169–1177, 2010.

[17] F. Wong, M. K. Nadim, J. A. Kellum et al., "Working Party proposal for a revised classification system of renal dysfunction in patients with cirrhosis," *Gut*, vol. 60, no. 5, pp. 702–709, 2011.

[18] F. Wong, J. G. O'Leary, K. R. Reddy et al., "New consensus definition of acute kidney injury accurately predicts 30-day mortality in patients with cirrhosis and infection," *Gastroenterology*, vol. 145, no. 6, pp. 1280.e1–1288.e1, 2013.

[19] J. M. Belcher, G. Garcia-Tsao, A. J. Sanyal et al., "Association of AKI with mortality and complications in hospitalized patients with cirrhosis," *Hepatology*, vol. 57, no. 2, pp. 753–762, 2013.

[20] A. de Araujo and M. R. Alvares-da-Silva, "Akin criteria as a predictor of mortality in cirrhotic patients after spontaneous bacterial peritonitis," *Annals of Hepatology*, vol. 13, no. 3, pp. 390–395, 2014.

[21] "Section 2: AKI definition," *Kidney International Supplements*, vol. 2, no. 1, pp. 19–36, 2011.

[22] J. Altamirano, C. Fagundes, M. Dominguez et al., "Acute kidney injury is an early predictor of mortality for patients with alcoholic hepatitis," *Clinical Gastroenterology and Hepatology*, vol. 10, no. 1, pp. 65.e3–71.e3, 2012.

[23] C. Fagundes, R. Barreto, M. Guevara et al., "A modified acute kidney injury classification for diagnosis and risk stratification of impairment of kidney function in cirrhosis," *Journal of Hepatology*, vol. 59, no. 3, pp. 474–481, 2013.

[24] P. A. Harris, R. Taylor, R. Thielke, J. Payne, N. Gonzalez, and J. G. Conde, "Research electronic data capture (REDCap)— a metadata-driven methodology and workflow process for providing translational research informatics support," *Journal of Biomedical Informatics*, vol. 42, no. 2, pp. 377–381, 2009.

[25] P. Sort, M. Navasa, V. Arroyo et al., "Effect of intravenous albumin on renal impairment and mortality in patients with cirrhosis and spontaneous bacterial peritonitis," *The New England Journal of Medicine*, vol. 341, no. 6, pp. 403–409, 1999.

[26] K.-H. Tu, C.-C. Jenq, M.-H. Tsai et al., "Outcome scoring systems for short-term prognosis in critically ill cirrhotic patients," *Shock*, vol. 36, no. 5, pp. 445–450, 2011.

[27] H.-C. Pan, C.-C. Jenq, M.-H. Tsai et al., "Risk models and scoring systems for predicting the prognosis in critically ill cirrhotic patients with acute kidney injury: a prospective validation study," *PLoS ONE*, vol. 7, no. 12, Article ID e51094, 2012.

[28] A. Follo, J. M. Llovet, M. Navasa et al., "Renal impairment after spontaneous bacterial peritonitis in cirrhosis: incidence, clinical course, predictive factors and prognosis," *Hepatology*, vol. 20, no. 6, pp. 1495–1501, 1994.

[29] J. G. Abuelo, "Normotensive ischemic acute renal failure," *The New England Journal of Medicine*, vol. 357, no. 8, pp. 797–805, 2007.

[30] R. Barreto, C. Fagundes, M. Guevara et al., "Type-1 hepatorenal syndrome associated with infections in cirrhosis: natural history, outcome of kidney function, and survival," *Hepatology*, vol. 59, no. 4, pp. 1505–1513, 2014.

[31] M. A. Perazella, S. G. Coca, M. Kanbay, U. C. Brewster, and C. R. Parikh, "Diagnostic value of urine microscopy for differential diagnosis of acute kidney injury in hospitalized patients," *Clinical Journal of the American Society of Nephrology*, vol. 3, no. 6, pp. 1615–1619, 2008.

[32] M. G. H. Betjes and I. Bajema, "The pathology of jaundice-related renal insufficiency: cholemic nephrosis revisited," *Journal of Nephrology*, vol. 19, no. 2, pp. 229–233, 2006.

[33] C. M. van Slambrouck, F. Salem, S. M. Meehan, and A. Chang, "Bile cast nephropathy is a common pathologic finding for kidney injury associated with severe liver dysfunction," *Kidney International*, vol. 84, no. 1, pp. 192–197, 2013.

[34] M. Rössle and A. L. Gerbes, "TIPS for the treatment of refractory ascites, hepatorenal syndrome and hepatic hydrothorax: a critical update," *Gut*, vol. 59, no. 7, pp. 988–1000, 2010.

[35] L. L. Gluud, K. Christensen, E. Christensen, and A. Krag, "Terlipressin for hepatorenal syndrome," *Cochrane Database of Systematic Reviews*, vol. 9, Article ID CD005162, 2012.

[36] M. Martín-Llahí, M.-N. Pépin, M. Guevara et al., "Terlipressin and albumin vs albumin in patients with cirrhosis and hepatorenal syndrome: a randomized study," *Gastroenterology*, vol. 134, no. 5, pp. 1352–1359, 2008.

[37] J. C. Q. Velez and P. J. Nietert, "Therapeutic response to vasoconstrictors in hepatorenal syndrome parallels increase in mean arterial pressure: a pooled analysis of clinical trials," *The American Journal of Kidney Diseases*, vol. 58, no. 6, pp. 928–938, 2011.

[38] S. Ghosh, N. S. Choudhary, A. K. Sharma et al., "Noradrenaline vs terlipressin in the treatment of type 2 hepatorenal syndrome: a randomized pilot study," *Liver International*, vol. 33, no. 8, pp. 1187–1193, 2013.

[39] E. Esrailian, E. R. Pantangco, N. L. Kyulo, K.-Q. Hu, and B. A. Runyon, "Octreotide/midodrine therapy significantly improves renal function and 30-day survival in patients with type 1 hepatorenal syndrome," *Digestive Diseases and Sciences*, vol. 52, no. 3, pp. 742–748, 2007.

[40] E. T. Schroeder, G. H. Anderson Jr., and H. Smulyan, "Effects of a portacaval or peritoneovenous shunt on renin in the hepatorenal syndrome," *Kidney International*, vol. 15, no. 1, pp. 54–61, 1979.

[41] A. Castells, J. Saló, R. Planas et al., "Impact of shunt surgery for variceal bleeding in the natural history of ascites in cirrhosis: a retrospective study," *Hepatology*, vol. 20, no. 3, pp. 584–591, 1994.

R229Q Polymorphism of NPHS2 Gene in Group of Iraqi Children with Steroid-Resistant Nephrotic Syndrome

Shatha Hussain Ali,[1] Rasha Kasim Mohammed,[2] Hussein Ali Saheb,[3] and Ban A. Abdulmajeed[1]

[1]College of Medicine, Al-Nahrain University, Baghdad, Iraq
[2]Al-Imamein Al-Kadhimein Medical City, Baghdad, Iraq
[3]College of Pharmacy, University of Al Qadisiyah, Diwaniyah, Iraq

Correspondence should be addressed to Shatha Hussain Ali; shatha6ali@yahoo.com

Academic Editor: Alessandro Amore

Background. The polymorphism R229Q is one of the most commonly reported podocin sequence variations among steroid-resistant nephrotic syndromes (SRNS). *Aim of the Study.* We investigated the frequency and risk of this polymorphism among a group of Iraqi children with SRNS and steroid-sensitive nephrotic syndrome (SSNS). *Patients and Methods.* A prospective case control study which was conducted in Al-Imamein Al-Kadhimein Medical City, spanning the period from the 1st of April 2015 to 30th of November 2015. Study sample consisted of 54 children having NS, divided into 2 groups: patients group consisted of 27 children with SRNS, and control group involved 27 children with SSNS. Both were screened by real time polymerase chain reaction for R229Q in exon 5 of NPHS2 gene. *Results.* Molecular study showed R229Q polymorphism in 96.3% of SRNS and 100% of SSNS. There were no phenotypic or histologic characteristics of patients bearing homozygous R229Q polymorphism and the patients with heterozygous R229Q polymorphism. *Conclusion.* Polymorphism R229Q of NPHS2 gene is prevalent in Iraqi children with SRNS and SSNS. Further study needs to be done, for other exons and polymorphism of NPHS2 gene in those patients.

1. Introduction

Positional cloning identified NPHS2, encoding podocin, as a causative gene in autosomal recessive SRNS, including focal segmental glomerulosclerosis (FSGS) [1, 2]. NPHS2 is the predominant mutation found in children over the age of 1 year [3, 4]. NPHS2 expression is restricted to the podocyte as shown by in situ hybridization studies. About 50 NPHS2 gene mutations and variants and/or nonsilent polymorphisms have been reported and recognized as potentially being involved in proteinuria. The polymorphism R229Q is one of the most commonly reported podocin sequence variations [5–7]. A functional polymorphism of NPHS2 gene, R229Q, was associated with a late-onset nephrotic syndrome and also with an increased risk of microalbuminuria in the general population [8, 9]. FSGS associated with NPHS2 mutation is uniformly steroid resistant and generally shows poor response to cyclosporine as well [10].

2. Aim of the Study

The aim of this study is to determine the frequency of R229Q polymorphic site of the NPHS2 gene in children with SRNS in comparison with SSNS, to study the relation of this polymorphic site to important demographics and clinical characteristics, and to determine the risk of having SRNS in relation to R229Q polymorphism.

3. Patients and Methods

This was a prospective case control study which was conducted in Al-Imamein Al-Kadhimein Medical City, spanning

TABLE 1: Distribution of the study group according to demographic data.

Data	SRNS		SSNS		P value
	Number	%	Number	%	
Sex					
Male	20	74.1%	17	63.0%	0.379
Female	7	25.9%	10	37.0%	0.379
Age					
1–6 years	7	25.9%	10	37.0%	0.379
6–12 years	13	48.1%	17	63.0%	0.273
12–18 years	7	25.9%	0	0.0%	0.005
Age at diagnosis					
1–6 years	17	63.0%	18	66.7%	0.776
6–12 years	6	22.2%	9	33.3%	0.362
12–18 years	4	14.8%	0	0.0%	0.038
Family history					
Positive	4	14.8%	4	14.8%	0.444
Consanguinity					
Positive	23	85.2%	16	59.3%	0.033

the period from the 1st of April 2015 to 30th of November 2015. Study sample consisted of 54 children having NS. Study sample was categorized into 2 groups: patients group consisted of 27 children with SRNS. Control group involved 27 children with SSNS.

Steroid responsive NS was regarded as complete remission achieved with steroid therapy. Steroid-resistant NS was regarded as failure to achieve remission following 4-week prednisone 60 mg/m^2 followed by three methylprednisolone pulses [1, 2].

3.1. Data Collected.
The data collected were gender, age, age of onset of NS, steroid responsiveness, family history of NS, consanguinity, and renal biopsy if done and its report. The following laboratory investigations were performed for all children: urinalysis, plasma albumin, blood urea, and serum creatinine.

Normal values of blood urea were as follows: 1-2 y = 1.8–5.4 mmol/l; >2 y = 2.9–7.1 mmol/l. Normal values of serum creatinine were as follows: child = 27–62 mmol/l; adolescent = 44–88 mmol/l [4].

Renal insufficiency was explained by 5 stages of chronic kidney disease by estimated GFR based on serum creatinine using Schwartz formula [5].

The data about hypertension and renal insufficiency are at the last follow-up time.

Each child donated 3 ml of venous blood, collected in an EDTA-containing blood collection tube. Samples were transferred to the molecular Pathology Laboratory, Department of Pathology, College of Medicine, Al-Nahrain University.

Genetic methods included DNA extraction and TaqMan real time PCR genotyping.

3.2. Statistical Analysis.
The SPSS version 21 was employed in this research. Chi-square test was used for comparison of frequencies and t tests were used for comparing means. Odd ratio was used to discriminate between alleles in patients and control.

4. Results

Table 1 shows the demographic characteristics of both patients and control groups. Mean age of patients was 5.253 ± 4.80 years for SRNS (range from 2 to 17) and 7.7037 ± 2.829 for SSNS (age range from 2 to 15 years), while mean age at diagnosis was 5.420 ± 4.114 years for SRNS and 4.666 ± 2.650 years for SSNS. Three age groups for age of presentation and age of diagnosis are shown in Table 1.

Older age group (12–18 years) were all SRNS at time of presentation and time of diagnosis with no SSNS children (P value = 0.005 and 0.038, resp.).

Correlation between gender and family history of NS of the two groups was statistically nonsignificant. The patients and control groups were compared according to their clinical data and laboratory investigations as shown in Table 2. The difference was statistically significant regarding hypertension, hematuria, renal insufficiency, mean of blood urea, and mean s. creatinine level, while no significant correlation was found with serum albumin.

Renal biopsy was performed for 21 patients; results are shown in Table 3.

5. Genetic Results

In Table 4, genetic results were put in form of G allele (VIC labeled) representing the wild type and A allele (FAM labeled) representing the polymorphism, and comparison between patients and control has been done.

The wild type allele was found in 16 (59.3%) and the polymorphic allele (FAM) was found in 26 (96.3%) of SRNS

TABLE 2: Patient distribution according to clinical data and laboratory investigations.

Data	SRNS		SSNS		P value
	Number	%	Number	%	
Hypertension					
Hypertensive	16	59.3	2	7.4	0.000
Normotensive	11	40.7	25	92.6	
Hematuria					
Hematuria	9	33.3	1	3.7	0.005
No hematuria	18	66.7	26	96.3	
Renal insufficiency					
RI	8	29.6	0.00	0.00	0.002
No RI	19	70.4	27	100	
Mean s. albumin, g/L (mean ± SD)					
2.400 ± 0.889			2.525 ± 0.867		0.601
Mean blood urea, mmol/L (mean ± SD)					
6.499 ± 3.491			4.149 ± 1.405		0.002
Mean s. creatinine, mmol/L (mean ± SD)					
79.518 ± 73.150			47.696 ± 14.904		0.031

TABLE 3: Renal biopsy results of 21 patients.

	Steroid responsiveness	
	Steroid-sensitive	Steroid-resistant
Minimal change disease	3 (75.0%)	8 (47.0%)
Focal segmental glomerulosclerosis	1 (25.0%)	7 (41.1%)
Mesangioproliferative	0 (0.0%)	2 (11.7%)
Total	4	17

patients. In the control group, the wild allele was found in 11 (40.7%) and the polymorphic allele was found in 27 (100%). The difference between these readings was nonsignificant P value.

The genotype was divided into homozygous wild gene (G/G), homozygous polymorphic gene (A/A), and heterozygous gene (G/A). No significant statistical difference was found between the two groups regarding the 3 genotypes.

In Table 5, clinical data and disease progression of 53 children with heterozygous and homozygous polymorphic R229Q were compared. No significant correlation was found regarding mean ages at diagnosis, gender, consanguinity, family history of NS, hypertension, steroid responsiveness, renal insufficiency, and renal biopsy results.

6. Discussion

In the present study, males predominated in both patients (SRNS) group and control (SSNS) group with slight difference. This is similar to many other studies from different regions [11–16]. Consanguinity was found in high percentage in both groups, which is expected in this community because of social traditions. This is important to be surveyed in all nephrotic children to relate this disease to its associated genes and the type of inheritance.

Coming to the genetic results found in this study, the polymorphism R229Q was found in 26 (96.3%) of 27 children

with SRNS in both heterozygous and homozygous genotypes. A lower percent of this polymorphism was found by many studies [11, 13, 15, 16]. In addition, several other studies did not report any polymorphism in SRNS [7, 8, 12, 16, 17]. The polymorphism R229Q was found 100% among SSNS group in both homozygous and heterozygous genotype, which is much less than its frequency in Landau et al. [14], who did not find any, as well as Lahdenkari et al. [18] and Caridi et al. [19].

The present results are important, because the frequency of R229Q polymorphism of NPHS2 mutation among Iraqi children is largely unknown. This is because a small number of founding individuals and a high rate of consanguineous and endogamous marriages, typical of small communities, increase genetic homogeneity and highlight susceptibility genes.

In this study, obvious genotype/phenotype correlation regarding age at diagnosis, sex, consanguinity, family history, hypertension, renal insufficiency, and renal histology in both homozygous and heterozygous patients were not observed.

Such findings were similarly mentioned by several studies [13, 17, 20, 21]. While Phelan et al. found that R229Q polymorphism was associated with early onset childhood SRNS [22], Sadowski et al. found FSGS in 68% of R229Q polymorphism [23] and Tsukaguchi et al. found R229Q polymorphism associated with late-onset SRNS [24].

This polymorphism is prevalent among Czech (12%), Spanish (3.1%), French (4.5%), Brazilian (3.1%), and Italian

TABLE 4: The frequency of genotyping in patients and control groups.

Alleles	SRNS		SSNS		P value
	Number	%	Number	%	
G (VIC)	16	59.3	11	40.7	0.174
A (FAM)	26	96.3	27	100	0.313
Genotype					
G/G	1	3.7	0	0.0	0.313
G/A	15	55.6	11	40.7	0.267
A/A	11	40.7	16	59.3	0.174

TABLE 5: The clinical data and disease progression of 53 children with heterozygous and homozygous polymorphic R229Q.

Parameter	Heterozygous GA ($n = 26$)	Homozygous AA ($n = 27$)	P value
Age at diagnosis (year ± SD)	4.853 ± 3.777	5.079 ± 3.144	0.814*
Male/female	16/10	20/7	0.328*
Consanguinity	21	18	0.244*
Family history	5	2	0.204*
Hypertension	9	8	0.697*
Renal insufficiency	5	3	0.409*
Response to steroids			
SRNS	15	11	0.217*
SSNS	11	16	
Renal biopsy			
MC	6	5	
FSGS	5	3	0.920*
MP	1	1	

*: NS.

(3.2) [16, 25]. The highest frequency of R229Q, after Czech population, has been reported in Chileans and Argentineans (7.3%) [26]. The R229Q polymorphism has a lower frequency among Africans, African-Americans, and Asians (zero to 1.5%) [16, 27]. Tryggvason and colleagues proposed that R229Q, which is present in around 4% of European populations, is associated with an increased risk of microalbuminuria [28]. Pereira and colleagues found that p.R229Q was associated with a 2.77-fold increased risk of microalbuminuria [29].

Both SRNS and SSNS in the present study did not show a significant difference regarding the polymorphism. It seems that at least one polymorphic allele of R229Q may participate in their nephrotic process, and by this a conclusive role in steroid resistance was not reached. In order to reach a conclusive decision about the role of R229Q in the pathogenicity of nephrotic syndrome, its association with other exon mutations of the NPHS2 gene must be searched for in the same study groups. Its exact frequency in the Iraqi population needs to be determined as well, by studying the frequency of this polymorphism in normal nonnephrotic children and comparing the findings with those of affected ones. Studying other exon mutations including the most

reported pathologic ones like mutations in exons 7 and 8 of the same gene is necessary to unravel the pathogenesis of SRNS in Iraqi children. Of no less importance is studying other nephrotic syndrome genes. These topics are put into consideration as future perspectives of the present work.

References

[1] P. Niaudet and O. Boyer, "Idiopathic nephrotic syndrome in children: clinical aspects," in *Pediatric Nephrology*, E. D. Avner, W. E. Harmon, P. Niaudet, N. Yoshikawa, F. Emma, and L. S. Goldstein, Eds., pp. 839–869, Lippincott Williams & amp; Wilkins, Philadelphia, Pa, USA, 7th edition, 2016.

[2] J. Floege and J. Feehally, "Introduction to glome-rular disease: clinical presentations," in *Comprehensive Clinical Nephrology*, R. J. Johnson, J. Feehally, and Floege J., Eds., pp. 184–197, Mosby, Philadelphia, Pa, USA, 5th edition, 2015.

[3] T. J. Stephen and N. Alexander et al., "NPHS2 variation in focal and segmental glomerulosclerosis," *BMC Nephrology*, vol. 9 Article 13, 2008.

[4] J. Sharma and A. Vasudevan, "Normal reference values of blood and urine chemistries," in *Manual of Pediatric Nephrology*, K.

Phadke, P. Goodyer, and M. Bitzan, Eds., pp. 533–610, Springer, London, UK, 2014.

[5] C. S. Wong and R. H. Mak, "Chronic kidney disease," in *Clinical Pediatric Nephrology*, K. K. H. Kher, S. H. W. William, and S. P. Makker, Eds., pp. 339–352, Informa Ltd, London, UK, 2nd edition, 2007.

[6] G. Chernin, S. F. Heeringa, R. Gbadegesin et al., "Low prevalence of NPHS2 mutations in African American children with steroid-resistant nephrotic syndrome," *Pediatric Nephrology*, vol. 23, no. 9, pp. 1455–1460, 2008.

[7] D. Rachmadi, A. Melani, and L. Monnens et al., "NPHS2 gene mutation and polymorphisms in indonesian children with steroid-resistant nephrotic syndrome," *Open Journal of Pediatrics*, vol. 5, no. 1, pp. 27–33, 2015.

[8] Z. B. Özçakar, F. B. Cengiz, N. Çakar et al., "Analysis of NPHS2 mutations in Turkish steroid-resistant nephrotic syndrome patients," *Pediatric Nephrology*, vol. 21, no. 8, pp. 1093–1096, 2006.

[9] N. Franceschini, K. E. North, J. B. Kopp, L. Mckenzie, and C. Winkler, "NPHS2 gene, nephrotic syndrome and focal segmental glomerulosclerosis: a HuGE review," *Genetics in Medicine*, vol. 8, no. 2, pp. 63–75, 2006.

[10] R. G. Ruf, A. Lichtenberger, S. M. Karle et al., "Patients with mutations in NPHS2 (podocin) do not respond to standard steroid treatment of nephrotic syndrome," *Journal of the American Society of Nephrology*, vol. 15, no. 3, pp. 722–732, 2004.

[11] R. Gbadegesin, B. Bartkowiak, and P. J. Lavin et al., "Exclusion of homozygous PLCE1 (NPHS3) mutations in 69 families with idiopathic and hereditary FSGS," *Pediatric Nephrology*, vol. 24, no. 2, pp. 281–285, 2009.

[12] D. N. Feng, Y. H. Yang, D. J. Wang et al., "Mutational analysis of podocyte genes in children with sporadic steroid-resistant nephrotic syndrome," *Genetics and Molecular Research*, vol. 13, no. 4, pp. 9514–9522, 2014.

[13] A. Berdeli, S. Mir, O. Yavascan et al., "NPHS2 (podicin) mutations in Turkish children with idiopathic nephrotic syndrome," *Pediatric Nephrology*, vol. 22, no. 12, pp. 2031–2040, 2007.

[14] D. Landau, T. Oved, D. Geiger, L. Abizov, H. Shalev, and R. Parvari, "Familial steroid-sensitive nephrotic syndrome in Southern Israel: clinical and genetic observations," *Pediatric Nephrology*, vol. 22, no. 5, pp. 661–669, 2007.

[15] G. Chernin, S. F. Heeringa, and V. Vega-Warner et al., "Adequate use of allele frequencies in Hispanics–a problem elucidated in nephrotic syndrome," *Pediatric Nephrology*, vol. 25, no. 2, pp. 261–266, 2010.

[16] J. Reiterova, H. Safrankova, and L. Obeidova et al., "Mutational analysis of the NPHS2 gene in Czech patients with idiopathic nephrotic syndrome," *Folia Biol (Praha)*, vol. 58, pp. 64–68, 2012.

[17] K. Ismaili, K. M. Wissing, F. Janssen, and M. Hall, "Genetic forms of nephrotic syndrome: a single-center experience in Brussels," *Pediatric Nephrology*, vol. 24, no. 2, pp. 287–294, 2009.

[18] A.-T. Lahdenkari, M. Suvanto, E. Kajantie, O. Koskimies, M. Kestilä, and H. Jalanko, "Clinical features and outcome of childhood minimal change nephrotic syndrome: is genetics involved?" *Pediatric Nephrology*, vol. 20, no. 8, pp. 1073–1080, 2005.

[19] G. Caridi, M. Gigante, P. Ravani et al., "Clinical features and long-term outcome of nephrotic syndrome associated with heterozygous NPHS1 and NPHS2 mutations," *Clinical Journal of the American Society of Nephrology*, vol. 4, no. 6, pp. 1065–1072, 2009.

[20] M. Schultheiss, R. G. Ruf, B. E. Mucha et al., "No evidence for genotype/phenotype correlation in NPHS1 and NPHS2 mutations," *Pediatric Nephrology*, vol. 19, no. 12, pp. 1340–1348, 2004.

[21] K. Tory, D. K. Menyhárd, S. Woerner et al., "Mutation-dependent recessive inheritance of NPHS2-associated steroid-resistant nephrotic syndrome," *Nature Genetics*, vol. 46, no. 3, pp. 299–304, 2014.

[22] P. J. Phelan, G. Hall, D. Wigfall et al., "Variability in phenotype induced by the podocin variant R229Q plus a single pathogenic mutation," *Clinical Kidney Journal*, vol. 8, no. 5, pp. 538–542, 2015.

[23] C. E. Sadowski, S. Lovric, and S. Ashraf et al., "A single-gene cause in 29.5% of cases of steroid-resistant nephrotic syndrome," *J Am Soc Nephrol*, vol. 26, pp. 1279–1289, 2015.

[24] H. Tsukaguchi, A. Sudhakar, T. C. Le et al., "NPHS2 mutations in late-onset focal segmental glomerulosclerosis: R229Q is a common disease-associated allele," *Journal of Clinical Investigation*, vol. 110, no. 11, pp. 1659–1666, 2002.

[25] Z. Yu, J. Ding, J. Huang et al., "Mutations in NPHS2 in sporadic steroid-resistant nephrotic syndrome in Chinese children," *Nephrology Dialysis Transplantation*, vol. 20, no. 5, pp. 902–908, 2005.

[26] E. Machuca, A. Hummel, F. Nevo et al., "Clinical and epidemiological assessment of steroid-resistant nephrotic syndrome associated with the NPHS2 R229Q variant," *Kidney International*, vol. 75, no. 7, pp. 727–735, 2009.

[27] S. Santín, B. Tazón-Vega, I. Silva et al., "Clinical value of *NPHS2* analysis in early- and adult-onset steroid-resistant nephrotic syndrome," *Clinical Journal of the American Society of Nephrology*, vol. 6, no. 2, pp. 344–354, 2011.

[28] K. Tryggvason, J. Patrakka, and J. Wartiovaara, "Hereditary proteinuria syndromes and mechanisms of proteinuria," *The New England Journal of Medicine*, vol. 354, no. 13, pp. 1387–1401, 2006.

[29] A. C. Pereira, A. B. Pereira, G. F. Mota et al., "NPHS2 R229Q functional variant is associated with microalbuminuria in the general population," *Kidney International*, vol. 65, no. 3, pp. 1026–1030, 2004.

3

The Effects of Simvastatin on Proteinuria and Renal Function in Patients with Chronic Kidney Disease

Bancha Satirapoj, Anan Promrattanakun, Ouppatham Supasyndh, and Panbuppa Choovichian

Division of Nephrology, Department of Medicine, Phramongkutklao Hospital and College of Medicine, Bangkok 10400, Thailand

Correspondence should be addressed to Bancha Satirapoj; satirapoj@yahoo.com

Academic Editor: Jochen Reiser

Current data suggests that statins might have beneficial effects on renal outcomes. Beneficial effects of statin treatment on renal progression in advanced chronic kidney disease (CKD) are obviously controversial. In a retrospective, controlled study, the authors have evaluated the effects of 53-week treatment with simvastatin, versus no treatment on proteinuria and renal function among 51 patients with CKD stages III-IV. By the end of the 53-week treatment, urine protein excretion decreased from 0.96 (IQR 0.54, 2.9) to 0.48 (IQR 0.18, 0.79) g/g creatinine ($P < 0.001$) in patients treated with simvastatin in addition to ACEI and ARBs, while no change was observed among the untreated patients. Moreover, a significantly greater decrease in urine protein excretion was observed in the simvastatin group as compared with the untreated group. The mean changes of serum creatinine and eGFR did not significantly differ in both groups. A significantly greater decrease in total cholesterol and LDL-cholesterol was found in the simvastatin group than in the untreated group. In summary, apart from lipid lowering among CKD patients, ingesting simvastatin was associated with a decrease in proteinuria. These statin effects may become important for supportive therapy in renal damage in the future.

1. Introduction

Chronic kidney disease (CKD) is a common condition and its prevalence is increasing worldwide [1]. According to data from the health information on subjects at the Armed Forces Research Institute of Medical Sciences, Thailand, the overall prevalence of patients with CKD is 7.5% [2]. The importance of understanding modifiable risk factors serves as a basis for devising treatment strategies to prevent the development and progression of CKD [3]. CKD patients frequently manifest dyslipidemia, such as hypercholesterolemia, as well as hypertension [4]. Extensive knowledge about abnormal lipid patterns among patients with advanced CKD and elevated total cholesterol, high non-HDL cholesterol, a high ratio of total cholesterol/HDL, and low HDL in particular was significantly associated with an increased risk of developing renal dysfunction [5]. Hyperlipidemia has been hypothesized to play an important role in the progression of renal injury [6].

Use of statins is beneficial for most patients with CKD who are at high cardiovascular risk [7], although research is needed to ascertain how to best prevent kidney injury. Experimental evidence suggests that statin can prevent the progression of kidney injury [3]. However, studies among humans on the subject are scarce. In meta-analysis, claims of improved renal outcomes have been made, encouraging broader adoption of statins among patients with predialysis CKD [8, 9]. Renoprotective effects of statins remain uncertain because of relatively sparse data and possible outcome reporting bias [10]. The aim of our study was to evaluate the efficacy and safety of statins for renal outcomes in advanced stages of proteinuric CKD.

2. Materials and Methods

2.1. Subjects and Study Design. The research employed a retrospective cohort-based design that randomly used medical records from April 2012 to March 2013 on CKD patients who routinely visited an outpatient facility including stable blood pressure and blood glucose within 3 months. Inclusion criteria of the study included age, 18 years or older, proteinuric CKD > 300 mg/day, and urinary protein creatinine ratio (UPCR) test before and after initiating simvastatin for 53 weeks. Treatment group of patients received simvastatin 10–40 mg daily. The other patients in the normal care group were treated according to their physician's standard of care. Normal care included life style changes, such as low fat diet, weight loss, and exercise, in addition to all necessary drug treatment without statins. Exclusion criteria included active malignancy, severe heart, lung, or liver disease, stroke, chronic infection, for example, tuberculosis, within one year of starting the study, and any immunological or inflammatory disorders.

2.2. Data Collection.

From their clinical data, we determined the effects of statins on renal parameters after a 53-week period. At the time of entry, all patients were also taking standard antihypertensive agents including angiotensin receptor blockers, angiotensin converting enzyme inhibitors, calcium channel blocker, beta-blockers, alpha-blockers, and diuretics. A complete medical history was taken and physical examination was performed on all subjects. All subjects fasted for at least 12 hours overnight before all blood drawing. Complete blood counts, blood urea nitrogen, serum creatinine, and comprehensive serum chemistries were measured. The serum concentration of creatinine using the enzymatic method was determined with reagents from Roche Diagnostics (Mannheim, Germany) and the calibrator was IDMS standarized. Glomerular filtration rate (GFR) was estimated from calibrated serum creatinine with the 2009 CKD-EPI creatinine equation [11]. Random urine samples were collected from patients. Urinary protein and creatinine concentrations were measured and expressed as the UPCR. The study was approved by the Institutional Review Board of the Royal Thai Army Medical Department, Bangkok, Thailand. All participants gave their written informed consent.

2.3. Statistical Analysis.

Results are expressed as the mean ± SD, as medians with interquartile ranges, or as a percentage in categorical variables. Differences between groups mean or median values were evaluated using the independent Student's t-test or Mann-Whitney test. In the case of continuous variables measured at the baseline and the end of study, differences within the group were analyzed by paired t-test or Wilcoxon Signed ranks test. Statistical significance was defined as $P < 0.05$. All analyses were performed with SPSS Software (SPSS, Inc., Chicago, IL, USA, Version 17).

3. Results

3.1. Patient Characteristics.

Patient characteristics are shown in Table 1. Blood pressure was fairly well controlled and most patients were taking renin angiotensin system (RAS) inhibitors (68-69%). Diuretics were prescribed for 14 patients, alpha blockers were prescribed for 14 patients, and calcium channel blockers were prescribed for 12 patients. The mean

simvastatin dose was 28 mg/day. Average estimated GFR was 40.10 ± 26.55 mL/min/1.73 m^2 and average UPCR was 1.92 ± 1.95 g/g creatinine. Kidney diseases among 51 of the study patients comprised glomerular diseases ($N = 20$) and chronic tubulointerstitium disease ($N = 1$) and the remaining 30 patients were not well characterized. Underlying disease of type 2 diabetes was significantly higher among patients treated with simvastatin (68%) than in patients with nonsimvastatin group (30.8%). Age, sex, body weight, systolic blood pressure, diastolic blood pressure, BUN, serum creatinine, estimated GFR, UACR, cholesterol, low density lipoprotein (LDL) cholesterol, high density lipoprotein (HDL) cholesterol, and triglycerides did not differ at baseline between the simvastatin and nonsimvastatin groups (Table 1).

3.2. Effect of Simvastatin Use on Metabolic Profiles.

Both systolic and diastolic blood pressure remain unaltered during the observation period. However, lipid profiles improved after 53 weeks of simvastatin treatment. Mean changes of total cholesterol (-52.44 ± 106.05 versus -6.65 ± 36.88 mg/dL, $P = 0.045$), (LDL-C -41.28 ± 79.96 versus -3.81 ± 25.44 mg/dL, $P = 0.033$), and non-HDL-C (-56.04 ± 111.34 versus -8.50 ± 29.78 mg/dL, $P = 0.049$) were significantly reduced in the simvastatin group when compared with the nonsimvastatin group (Table 2).

3.3. Effect of Simvastatin Use on Renal Outcomes.

Renal function did not significantly change in both groups. Finally, mean changes of serum creatinine (0.1 ± 0.62 versus 0.1 ± 0.68 mg/dL, $P = 0.308$) and mean changes of estimated GFR (-1.2 ± 7.2 versus -3.3 ± 11.9 mL/min/1.73 m^2, $P = 0.458$) did not significantly differ in the simvastatin and nonsimvastatin groups.

Individual CKD patients with proteinuria >300 mg/day receiving simvastatin had a statistically significant decreased UPCR from 0.96 (IQR 0.54, 2.9) to 0.48 (IQR 0.18, 0.79) g/g creatinine ($P < 0.001$) at 53 weeks after treatment, but no significant change was observed in the nonsimvastatin group (1.41 (IQR 0.66, 2.41) to 1.21 (IQR 0.19, 1.56) g/g creatinine). Moreover, mean change of UPCR also significantly differed in the simvastatin and nonsimvastatin groups (Table 3).

3.4. Safety.

No unexpected safety concerns were identified and similar incidences of adverse events were experienced in each of the treatment groups. No serious adverse effects such as persistent elevations in liver function enzymes and creatine phosphokinase values were observed in those using simvastatin.

4. Discussion

The present study reported that simvastatin was associated with lipid lowering and antiproteinuric benefits in patients with moderate to advanced CKD. They seemed to be safe with CKD, with respect to the risk of hepatotoxicity. However, the present study could not clearly confirm evidence of any renoprotective effect of statins in patients with CKD,

TABLE 1: Patients' characteristics.

	Simvastatin (N = 25)	Nonsimvastatin (N = 26)	P value
Male (%)	17 (68%)	20 (76.9%)	0.556
Age (year)	62 ± 19.86	60.04 ± 21.31	0.735
Weight (kg)	67.80 ± 13.92	63.34 ± 13.80	0.256
Primary renal diseases, N (%)			0.612
Glomerular diseases	11	9	
CTIN	—	1	
Unknown	14	16	
Diabetes mellitus (%)	17 (68%)	8 (30.8%)	0.012
Hypertension (%)	21 (84%)	17 (65.4%)	0.199
Atherosclerosis (%)	6 (24.0%)	5 (19.2%)	0.743
Current antihypertensive agents (%)			
ACEI/ARB	17 (68.0%)	18 (69.2%)	0.572
Diuretics	9 (36.0%)	5 (19.2%)	0.220
Alpha-blockers	9 (36.0%)	5 (19.2%)	0.220
Beta-blockers	5 (20.0%)	3 (11.5%)	0.171
CCB	7 (28.0%)	5 (19.2%)	0.258
SBP (mmHg)	139.08 ± 17.24	137.38 ± 17.88	0.732
DBP (mmHg)	79.44 ± 14.22	77.27 ± 13.26	0.575
UPCR (g/g creatinine)	0.96 (0.54, 2.9)	1.41 (0.66, 2.41)	0.445
GFR (mL/min/1.73 m^2)	41.12 ± 28.97	39.77 ± 23.55	0.856
BUN (mg/dL)	27.75 ± 12.68	30.60 ± 15.16	0.472
Serum creatinine (mg/dL)	1.97 ± 0.72	1.97 ± 0.73	0.995
Cholesterol (mg/dL)	211.72 ± 123.80	185.62 ± 57.15	0.335
Triglyceride (mg/dL)	158.48 ± 154.03	143.04 ± 112.93	0.684
HDL (mg/dL)	52.24 ± 15.05	57.19 ± 27.02	0.425
LDL (mg/dL)	134.04 ± 93.90	109.00 ± 42.80	0.232
Non-HDL (mg/dL)	157.56 ± 126.09	122.27 ± 55.55	0.199
AST (mg/dL)	24.80 ± 11.39	23.69 ± 10.88	0.724
ALT (mg/dL)	23.44 ± 19.07	21.04 ± 13.36	0.604

Values expressed as mean ± SD or median with interquartile ranges, ACEI: angiotensin converting enzyme inhibitor; ARB: angiotensin type 1 receptor blocker; ALT: alanine aminotransferase; AST: aspartate aminotransferase; BUN: blood urea nitrogen; CCB: calcium channel blockers; DBP: diastolic blood pressure; HDL: high density lipoprotein; LDL: low density lipoprotein; GFR: glomerular filtration rate; SBP: systolic blood pressure; UPCR: urine protein creatinine ratio.

TABLE 2: Changes of metabolic profiles after 53 weeks of statin treatment.

Variables	Mean changes		P value
	Simvastatin	Nonsimvastatin	
SBP (mmHg)	−5.72 ± 21.88	−0.77 ± 20.19	0.405
DBP (mmHg)	−1.84 ± 13.89	−4.50 ± 13.64	0.493
Cholesterol (mg/dL)	−52.44 ± 106.05	−6.65 ± 36.88	0.045
Triglyceride (mg/dL)	−34.68 ± 140.77	−15.81 ± 83.44	0.561
HDL (mg/dL)	0.36 ± 15.95	1.65 ± 20.31	0.802
LDL (mg/dL)	−41.28 ± 79.96	−3.81 ± 25.44	0.033
Non-HDL (mg/dL)	−56.04 ± 111.34	−8.50 ± 29.78	0.049
AST (U/L)	−2.12 ± 7.57	5.15 ± 18.83	0.079
ALT (U/L)	3.36 ± 28.03	10.96 ± 44.41	0.470

Data are expressed as mean changes of 53 weeks ± SD; ALT: alanine aminotransferase; AST: aspartate aminotransferase; DBP: diastolic blood pressure; HDL: high density lipoprotein; LDL: low density lipoprotein; SBP: systolic blood pressure.

as indicated by no difference found in GFR and serum creatinine between simvastatin and control groups.

Patients with higher levels of proteinuria have an increased risk of severe CKD and as a predictor of future decline in GFR [12], but limited therapeutic options are available to decrease proteinuria. In the PLANET I study among patients with diabetic nephropathy and the PLANET II study among patients without diabetic nephropathy, atorvastatin significantly reduced proteinuria by 15% to 23.8%. Recent meta-analyses of randomized, placebo-controlled trials among patients have suggested that statins were associated with reductions in high levels of proteinuria [9]. As was consistent with our study, statins produced a beneficial effect on pathologic proteinuria in CKD populations. However, the reduction of proteinuria in our study might be the effect of decreasing renal function in the simvastatin treated group.

The beneficial effect of statins on proteinuria seen in our study may be potentially explained by cholesterol dependent effects and cholesterol independent effects. Experimental

TABLE 3: Renal outcomes after 53 weeks of statin treatment.

Variables	Simvastatin (N = 25)			Nonsimvastatin (N = 26)			P value between groups[&]
	Baseline	At 53 weeks	Mean differences	P value[#]	Baseline	At 53 weeks	Mean differences	P value[#]	
Mean UPCR (g/g creatinine)	2.26 ± 2.99	0.83 ± 0.95	−1.4 ± 2.8	0.019	1.79 ± 1.47	1.77 ± 2.68	−0.02 ± 2.4	0.969	0.049
Median UPCR (g/g creatinine)	0.96 (0.54, 2.9)	0.48 (0.18, 0.79)		<0.001	1.41 (0.66, 2.41)	1.21 (0.19, 1.56)		0.485	
GFR (mL/min/1.73 m^2)	41.12 ± 28.97	39.88 ± 29.74	−1.2 ± 7.2	0.396	39.77 ± 23.55	36.46 ± 18.82	−3.3 ± 11.9	0.168	0.458
Serum creatinine (mg/dL)	1.97 ± 0.73	2.06 ± 0.72	0.1 ± 0.62	0.315	1.97 ± 0.72	2.07 ± 0.67	0.1 ± 0.68	0.458	0.308

Values expressed as mean ± SD or median with interquartile ranges; GFR: glomerular filtration rate; UPCR: urine protein creatinine ratio; (#) comparisons within groups; (&) comparisons between groups.

studies have documented that dyslipidemia contributes to glomerular and interstitial injury and the severity of the hypercholesterolemia correlates with proteinuria [13]. In addition to the beneficial effects of lowering lipids, statins also influence important intracellular pathways that are involved in the inflammatory and fibrogenic responses, the main pathway of progressive renal injury [14, 15]. Moreover, the reasons to favor the use of statins in CKD include beneficial effects on endothelial function, suppressing monocyte recruitment, mesangial cell proliferation and mesangial matrix accumulation, antifibrotic effects, and antioxidation and anti-inflammatory cytokines [13, 16].

Our findings are consistent with a recent study, reporting that urinary protein losses had fallen, but renal function was stable among CKD patients at the end of one year of therapy with intensified lipid-lowering statin [17]. Intensified lipid-lowering therapy did not appear to have any GFR effect. Another meta-analysis also showed that statins significantly reduced total cholesterol but did not improve GFR [10]. However, data from several small studies and subgroup analysis from main studies suggest that statins might slow CKD progression. The secondary coronary heart disease prevention GREACE study suggested that dose titration with atorvastatin prevented creatinine clearance decline and significantly improved renal function among patients with coronary heart disease and normal GFR [18]. A post hoc analysis of the Cholesterol and Recurrent Events (CARE) trial reported slow renal function loss with the use of pravastatin in patients with previous myocardial infarction and moderate to severe CKD, especially among those with proteinuria [19]. The published heart protection study (HPS) subgroup analysis for participants with diabetes mellitus also showed that simvastatin significantly decreased the rise in serum creatinine in patients with and without diabetes mellitus [20]. All previous subgroup analyses suggested that statin was associated with a significantly smaller fall in the estimated GFR compared with the placebo group. In addition, as a post hoc analysis, using estimates of renal function, some limitations were observed in interpreting these data, so a small proportion of patients, who had advanced CKD, were included in this analysis, whereas our findings in the simvastatin group revealed estimated GFR did not improve, but no significant decline was observed among advanced CKD subjects. Therefore, the available data on statin with GFR in CKD patients are still conflicting, because of possible outcome reporting bias.

One possible explanation of estimated GFR improvement in previous studies may be related to the intensity of statin therapy. Improvement in estimated GFR occurred with low-dosage atorvastatin (10 mg/day), but high-dosage atorvastatin (80 mg/day) demonstrated significantly greater improvement in estimated GFR than that achieved by low-dosage atorvastatin [21]. Previous studies with moderate to high doses of statins demonstrated a slowing in renal function decline [17, 19, 20]. Mild to moderate doses of simvastatin were used in our study, and, therefore, they might have produced a negative GFR effect of simvastatin in proteinuric CKD patients.

Our study had limitations that should be considered. First, this was a retrospective controlled study, and the limitations of it are well described. Thus, other confounding factors and change of metabolic parameters might have affected the proteinuria in the simvastatin group during the follow-up period. Although a significant reduction of urinary protein excretion in the statin treated group and mean changes of urine protein between the statin treated and nonstatin treated groups were observed, differences in baseline data of comorbid diseases included type 2 diabetes, hypertension, and medications between both groups. Second, renal outcomes in the current study were estimated using the CKD-EPI-GFR formula and UPCR, which are less accurate than nuclear isotope estimates of GFR and 24-hour urine protein. Finally, this study enrolled a small sample size and had a short duration of follow-up. However, our study revealed that individuals with moderate to severe kidney disease may derive clinically relevant proteinuric benefits from the use of simvastatin, especially those with proteinuria. These findings should be confirmed by a large randomized trial conducted specifically among this patient population.

5. Conclusion

This study has showed that treatment with statins in addition to a regimen with ACE inhibitors or ARBs can reduce proteinuria in patients with proteinuric CKD and hyperlipidemia. The benefits appear to occur in addition to those treated with standard CKD management.

Acknowledgment

This work was supported by a grant from the Department of Medicine, Phramongkutklao Hospital and College of Medicine, Bangkok, Thailand.

References

[1] M. T. James, B. R. Hemmelgarn, and M. Tonelli, "Early recognition and prevention of chronic kidney disease," The Lancet, vol. 375, no. 9722, pp. 1296–1309, 2010.

[2] B. Satirapoj, O. Supasyndh, N. Mayteedol et al., "Obesity and its relation to chronic kidney disease: a population-based, cross-sectional study of a Thai army population and relatives," Nephrology, vol. 18, no. 3, pp. 229–234, 2013.

[3] V. M. Campese, "Dyslipidemia and progression of kidney disease: role of lipid-lowering drugs," Clinical and Experimental Nephrology, vol. 18, no. 2, pp. 291–295, 2014.

[4] B. Satirapoj, O. Supasyndh, N. Mayteedol, A. Chaiprasert, and P. Choovichian, "Metabolic syndrome and its relation to chronic kidney disease in a Southeast Asian population," Southeast Asian Journal of Tropical Medicine and Public Health, vol. 42, no. 1, pp. 176–183, 2011.

[5] E. S. Schaeffner, T. Kurth, G. C. Curhan et al., "Cholesterol and the risk of renal dysfunction in apparently healthy men," *Journal of the American Society of Nephrology*, vol. 14, no. 8, pp. 2084–2091, 2003.

[6] B. Satirapoj, K. W. Bruhn, C. C. Nast et al., "Oxidized low-density lipoprotein antigen transport induces autoimmunity in the renal tubulointerstitium," *American Journal of Nephrology*, vol. 35, no. 6, pp. 520–530, 2012.

[7] T. W. Dasari, D. J. Cohen, N. S. Kleiman et al., "Statin therapy in patients with chronic kidney disease undergoing percutaneous coronary intervention (from the evaluation of drug eluting stents and ischemic events registry)," *American Journal of Cardiology*, vol. 113, no. 4, pp. 621–625, 2014.

[8] S. Sandhu, N. Wiebe, L. F. Fried, and M. Tonelli, "Statins for improving renal outcomes: a meta-analysis," *Journal of the American Society of Nephrology*, vol. 17, no. 7, pp. 2006–2016, 2006.

[9] K. Douglas, P. G. O'Malley, and J. L. Jackson, "Meta-analysis: the effect of statins on albuminuria," *Annals of Internal Medicine*, vol. 145, no. 2, pp. 117–124, 2006.

[10] G. F. M. Strippoli, S. D. Navaneethan, D. W. Johnson et al., "Effects of statins in patients with chronic kidney disease: meta-analysis and meta-regression of randomised controlled trials," *British Medical Journal*, vol. 336, no. 7645, pp. 645–651, 2008.

[11] Kidney Disease: Improving Global Outcomes (KDIGO) CKD Work Group, "KDIGO 2012 clinical practice guideline for the evaluation and management of chronic kidney disease," *Kidney International Supplements*, vol. 3, pp. 136–150, 2013.

[12] P. Cravedi and G. Remuzzi, "Pathophysiology of proteinuria and its value as an outcome measure in chronic kidney disease," *British Journal of Clinical Pharmacology*, vol. 76, no. 4, pp. 516–523, 2013.

[13] W. F. Keane, "The role of lipids in renal disease: future challenges," *Kidney International, Supplement*, vol. 57, no. 75, pp. S27–S31, 2000.

[14] C. K. Abrass, "Cellular lipid metabolism and the role of lipids in progressive renal disease," *American Journal of Nephrology*, vol. 24, no. 1, pp. 46–53, 2004.

[15] H. Oda and W. F. Keane, "Recent advances in statins and the kidney," *Kidney International Supplements*, vol. 56, no. 71, pp. S2–S5, 1999.

[16] V. M. Campese, M. K. Nadim, and M. Epstein, "Are 3-hydroxy-3-methylglutaryl-CoA reductase inhibitors renoprotective?" *Journal of the American Society of Nephrology*, vol. 16, no. 3, supplement 1, pp. S11–S17, 2005.

[17] S. Bianchi, R. Bigazzi, A. Caiazza, and V. M. Campese, "A controlled, prospective study of the effects of atorvastatin on proteinuria and progression of kidney disease," *American Journal of Kidney Diseases*, vol. 41, no. 3, pp. 565–570, 2003.

[18] V. G. Athyros, D. P. Mikhailidis, A. A. Papageorgiou et al., "The effect of statins versus untreated dyslipidaemia on renal function in patients with coronary heart disease. A subgroup analysis of the Greek atorvastatin and coronary heart disease evaluation (GREACE) study," *Journal of Clinical Pathology*, vol. 57, no. 7, pp. 728–734, 2004.

[19] M. Tonelli, L. Moyé, F. M. Sacks, T. Cole, and G. C. Curhan, "Effect of pravastatin on loss of renal function in people with moderate chronic renal insufficiency and cardiovascular disease," *Journal of the American Society of Nephrology*, vol. 14, no. 6, pp. 1605–1613, 2003.

[20] Heart Protection Study Collaborative Group, "MRC/BHF Heart Protection Study of cholesterol-lowering with simvastatin in 5963 people with diabetes: a randomised placebo-controlled trial," *The Lancet*, vol. 361, no. 9374, pp. 2005–2016, 2003.

[21] J. Shepherd, J. J. P. Kastelein, V. Bittner et al., "Effect of intensive lipid lowering with atorvastatin on renal function in patients with coronary heart disease: the Treating to New Targets (TNT) study," *Clinical Journal of the American Society of Nephrology*, vol. 2, no. 6, pp. 1131–1139, 2007.

4

Peritoneal Dialysis as a First versus Second Option after Previous Haemodialysis: A Very Long-Term Assessment

Roberto José Barone, María Inés Cámpora, Nélida Susana Gimenez, Liliana Ramirez, Sergio Alberto Panese, and Mónica Santopietro

Peritoneal Dialysis Program, Hurlingham Renal Therapy Services, 1431 Buenos Aires, Argentina

Correspondence should be addressed to Roberto José Barone; 3.barone@gmail.com

Academic Editor: Laszlo Rosivall

For renal replacement therapy, overall survival is more important than the choice of currently available individual therapy. *Objectives.* To compare patients and technique survival on peritoneal dialysis as first treatment (PDF) versus after previous haemodialysis (HDPD) and other indicators of follow-up. *Methods.* We prospectively studied 110 incident patients, during the period from August 4, 1993, to June 30, 2012, for patients and technique survival (Kaplan-Meier) (log rank $P < 0.05$). *Results.* Groups: (A) PDF: 37 patients, 24 females, age: 52.2 ± 14.9 years old, time at risk: 2123 patient-months (p/m), mean: 57 ± 42 months; (B) HDPD: 73 patients, 42 females, age: 52.45 ± 14.7 years old, time in haemodialysis: 3569.2 (p/m), range: 3–216 months, mean: 49 ± 45 months, time at risk in PD: 3700 (p/m), mean: 51 ± 49 months. Patients' survival: (A) PDF: 100%, 76.6%, 65.6%, and 19.7%; (B) HDPD: 95.4%, 65.6%, 43%, and 43% at 12, 60, 120, and 144 months, respectively, $P = 0.34$. Technique: (A) PDF: 100%, 90%, 59.8%, and 24%; (B) HDPD: 94%, 75%, 32%, and 32% at 12, 60, 120, and 144 months, respectively, $P = 0.40$. *Conclusions.* Comparable patient and technique survival were observed. Peritoneal dialysis enables a greater extension of renal replacement therapy for patients with serious difficulties continuing with haemodialysis.

1. Introduction

Since the beginning of the chronic renal substitutive therapy, many advances have been made regarding medical and technological aspects that have undoubtedly contributed to the quality of life and survival of the patients [1–4]. Too much time was previously spent by nephrologists attempting to understand that the treatments that are currently available—haemodialysis, peritoneal dialysis, and renal transplantation—are part of a group of options enabling patients to live their life; the challenge for the nephrologist must be continuing with advances in the replacement therapy area and renal prevention avoiding meaningless confrontations among them concerning the treatments [5, 6].

From the early years of the peritoneal dialysis, countless articles have been published comparing peritoneal dialysis versus haemodialysis in many aspects of the replacement therapy like anaemia, adequacy, residual renal function impact, quality of life, patient satisfaction, cost of treatment,

reimbursement, and so on, but patient survival is undoubtedly the most important index that stresses the effectiveness of a therapy. Likewise, in this aspect, technique survival is another important indicator that is often cited as information that is "required" of the peritoneal dialysis performance; however, papers showing technique survival in haemodialysis are lacking.

In PD, comparisons among diabetic and nondiabetic and anuric patients and patients with residual renal function are frequent, but comparisons between patients undergoing PD as first option versus PD as a second option after haemodialysis are scarce [7–10].

In this work, we showed our experience in very long-term treatment, comparing technique, catheter, and patient survival, as well as other indices of those patients who initiated peritoneal dialysis as a first option versus patients who initiated substitutive therapy in haemodialysis and were transferred to peritoneal dialysis as a second option for different reasons.

2. Methods

We prospectively evaluated 110 patients who had been undergoing continuous ambulatory peritoneal dialysis (CAPD) or automated PD (APD) for at least three months during the period August 4, 1993, to June 30, 2012. We established two groups: (A) all incident patients who initiated renal substitutive therapy in peritoneal dialysis as a first option (PDF) and (B) patients who were first treated in haemodialysis for more than three months and then switched to PD as a second option (HDPD) for different reasons. Patients with 24 hr urine volumes at the start of PD lower than 100 mL/day were considered anuric.

We used the Kaplan-Meier product-limit estimation method to calculate patients and technique survival as "intention-to-treat survival" and catheter survival. For patients' survival, death was considered the endpoint. For technique survival, transfer to haemodialysis or death related to PD therapy was considered the endpoint. Patients who were transplanted or lost to follow-up or who achieved partial recovery of renal function were censored. Furthermore, patients and technique survivals between PDF patients and anuric patients of the HDPD group were compared. For catheter survival, catheter removal was considered the endpoint; patients whose only reason for catheter extraction was transplantation, elective transfer to haemodialysis, or death from concurrent disease with functioning catheter were censored at time of that event.

The Kaplan-Meier curve comparisons mentioned previously between both groups of patients were performed using the log-rank method. Cumulative peritonitis rate (CPR) in both groups was measured.

Overall admission rates and hospital days per patient year per group were calculated and compared (unpaired t-test) during the study period. In our peritoneal dialysis program, the patients were not hospitalised for training in dialysis. Hospitalisation for the first peritoneal catheter placement was not considered in the morbidity evaluation. The chi-square test was used to analyse the proportion of patients hospitalised per group and number of diabetic patients per group. Relative risk (RR) for mortality was used to determine the impact of diabetes as morbid risk factor.

Adequacy studies were performed every 3 to 6 months; weekly total urea clearance (Kt/V) and weekly total creatinine clearance/1.73 m^2 were calculated. We measured total body water (TBW) according to the Watson formulas [11] and body surface area (BSA) was calculated according to D. D. Bois and E. F. D. Bois [12].

For women, TBW $= -2.097 + (0.1069 \cdot$ Height$) + (0.2466 \cdot$ Weight$)$.

For men, TBW $= 2.447 - (0.09156 \cdot$ Age$) + (0.1074 \cdot$ Height$) + (0.3362 \cdot$ Weight$)$.

BSA (m^2) $= 0.007184 \cdot$ Height (cm) $0.725 \cdot$ Weight (kg) 0.425.

The normalized protein catabolic rate (nPCR) was calculated by the Randerson formula:

TABLE 1: Patients characteristic.

Variables	Group A-PDF ($n = 37$)	Group B-HDPD ($n = 73$)
Age (years)	52.2 ± 14.9	52.45 ± 14.7
Age range (years)	16–75	22–80
Sex (male-female)	13–24	31–42
Time at risk on PD (p/m)	2123 57 ± 42	3700 51 ± 49
Time at risk on hemodialysis (p/m)	—	3569.2 49 ± 45
Diabetes (n)	10 (27%)	11 (15%)
Peritonitis rate	0.34	0.36

p/m: patient-months. Data are expressed as mean ± SD.

nPCR $= 10.76$ (Gun $+ 1.46)/V$, where Gun is urea nitrogen generation rate (mg/min) and V is volume of urea distribution [13].

Mean comparisons of the following indices were performed during the study period (unpaired t-test): weekly Kt/V, total weekly creatinine clearance, weekly peritoneal urea clearance, weekly renal urea clearance, BSA, TBW, nPCR, total daily drainage volume, and total daily drainage volume/m^2 BSA. The data were collected prospectively from our database. Continuous variables are expressed as mean ± standard deviation; categorical data are expressed as frequencies and percentages. A P value of 0.05 or less was considered statistically significant. The statistical analysis was performed with SPSS 15 (SPSS Inc., Chicago, IL, EEUU).

3. Results

Our study enrolled 110 patients, who were divided into two groups: (A) PDF: there were 37 patients, 24 females (64.8%) and 13 males; the mean age was 52.2 ± 14.9 years old and the age range when they started PD was 16–75 years; the time at risk was 2123 patient-months, mean: 57 ± 42 months; 14 patients (37.84%) switched from CAPD to APD; the percentage of diabetic patients was 27% and the cumulative peritonitis rate was 0.34, (B) HDPD: it included 73 patients, 42 females (57.53%) and 31 males; mean age was 52.45 ± 14.7 years old and the age range when patients initiated PD was 22–80 years; the time at risk in PD was 3700 patient-months, mean: 51 ± 49 months; 33 patients (45%) switched from CAPD to APD; the percentage of diabetic patients was 15%; 48 patients (65.7%) were anuric and the cumulative peritonitis rate was 0.36. In the latter group of patients, the time at risk in haemodialysis was 3569.2 patient-months, mean: 49 ± 45 months and range: 3 to 216 months. Furthermore, in this group, 43 patients (58.9%) were shifted from haemodialysis to peritoneal dialysis due to multiple vascular access failure; 32 (74.4%) of these patients were women; 32.8% switched by personal choice; 6.85% switched due to cardiovascular disorders and 1.37% due to living a long distance from the dialysis centre. No statistical significance was observed in the number of diabetic patients per group ($P = 0.21$). Patients' characteristics are shown in Table 1.

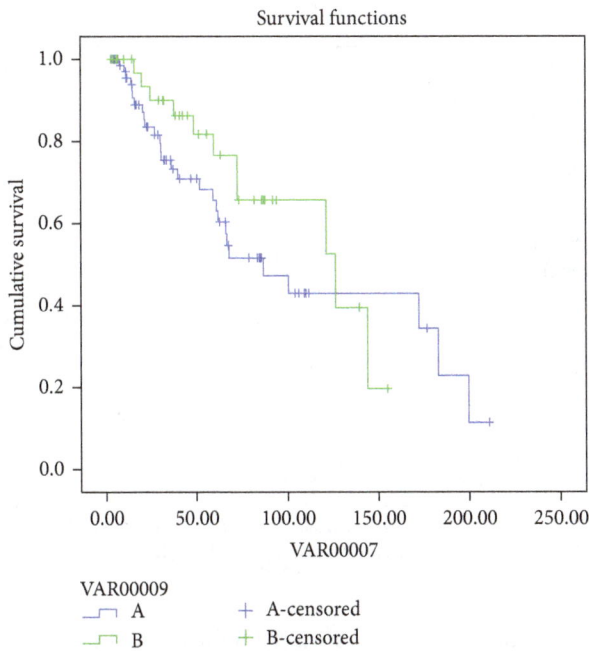

FIGURE 1: Patients survival PDF (green) and HDPD (blue) (log rank P = 0.33).

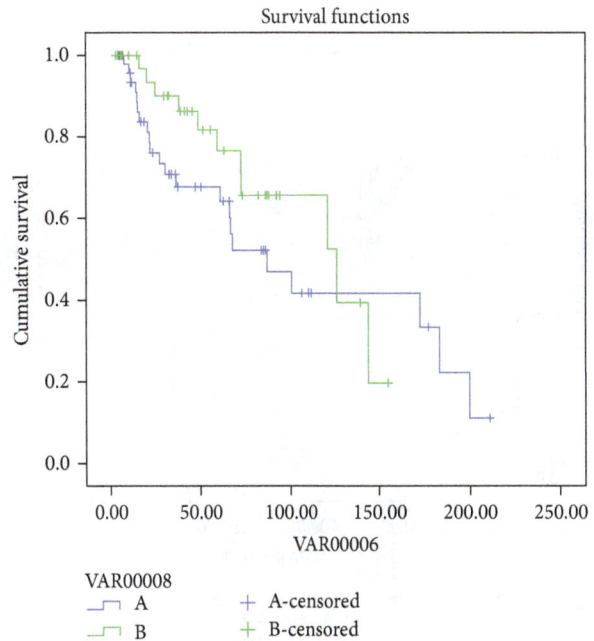

FIGURE 2: Technique survival PDF (green) and HDPD (blue) (log rank P = 0.20).

It is important to point out that 35 (47.9%) out of 73 patients in the second group moved onto our peritoneal dialysis program from other dialysis clinics because peritoneal dialysis was not practiced in those units.

The probability of patient's survival in group (A) PDF at 12, 36, 60, 84, 120, and 144 months was 100%, 90%, 76.6%, 65.6%, 65.6%, and 19.7%, respectively, and, in group (B) HDPD, at 12, 36, 60, 84, 120, 144, and 180 months, it was 95.4%, 75.5%, 65.6%, 51.5%, 43%, 43%, and 34%, respectively (log rank P = 0.33) (Figure 1).

The estimation of technique survival was 100%, 96%, 90%, 76%, 59.8%, and 24% at 12, 36, 60, 84, 120, and 144 months, respectively, in group A, and 94%, 83%, 75%, 57%, 32%, 32%, and 24% at 12, 36, 60, 84, 120, 144, and 180 months, respectively, in group B (log rank P = 0.20) (Figure 2).

No statistical significance was observed when patient and technique survival were compared between patients of group A (all patients started PD with residual renal function) and the anuric patients of the HDPD group (log rank P = 0.31 and P = 0.48, resp.) (Figures 3 and 4).

Forty-seven catheters (35 swan neck and 12 Tenckhöff ones) were placed in the PDF group (1.27 catheters per patient) and 85 (62 swan neck and 23 Tenckhöff) in the HDPD group (1.16 catheters per patient) during the period of study. The observation of the catheters survival in group A at 12, 36, 60, 84, and 144 months was 95%, 80%, 76%, 56%, and 37%, respectively, and in group B, at 12, 36, 60, 84, 144, and 180 months, it was 93%, 84%, 72%, 47%, 32%, and 22%, respectively (log rank P = 0.62) (Figure 5).

Unadjusted hospitalisation rates were similar for the groups. During the study period there were forty-five admissions (16% of cardiovascular cause, 26.6% due to peritonitis)

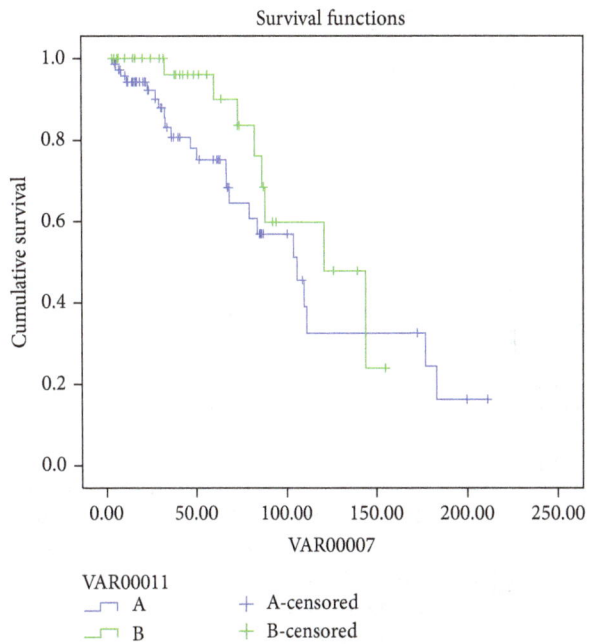

FIGURE 3: Patients survival PDF (green) and HDPD (anuric) (blue) (log rank P = 0.31).

in 21 out of 37 patients of the PDF group, which equates to 0.25 admissions per patient/year, and the numbers of hospital days were 1.95 per patient/year. In the HDPD group, there were 98 admissions (27.5% of them due to cardiovascular disorders and 17.5% for peritonitis) in forty-nine out of 73 patients in the time at risk, which equates to 0.32 admissions per patient/year, and the number of days of hospitalisation

Survival functions

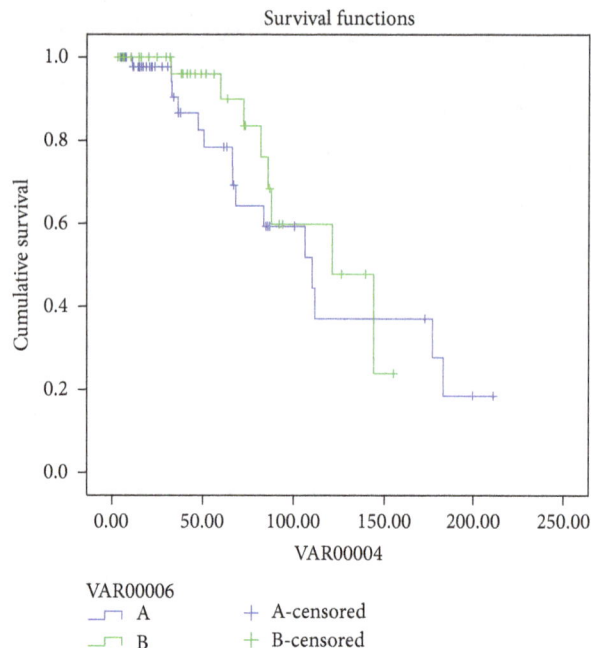

VAR00006

A	+ A-censored
B	+ B-censored

FIGURE 4: Technique survival PDF (green) and HDPD (anuric) (blue) (log rank $P = 0.48$).

Survival functions

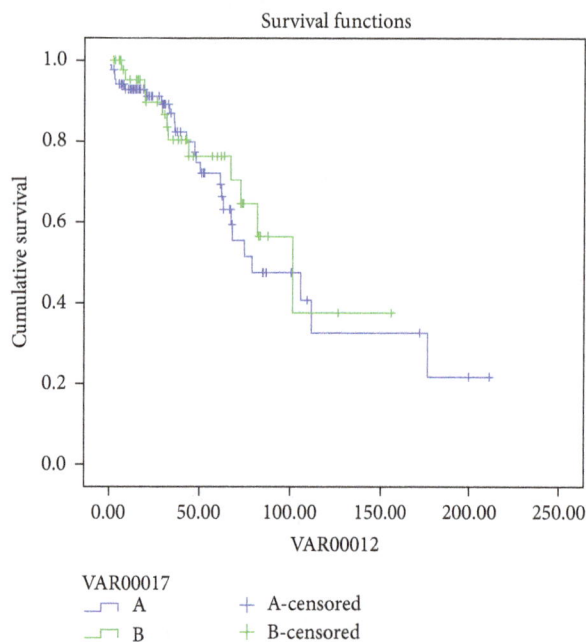

VAR00017

A	+ A-censored
B	+ B-censored

FIGURE 5: Catheters survival PDF (green) and HDPD (blue) (log rank $P = 0.62$).

per patient/year was 1.88. There were no statistical differences in the proportion of patients hospitalised or the proportion of admissions due to cardiovascular disorders ($P = 0.28$ and $P = 0.29$, resp.), in neither the number of admissions nor the duration of hospitalisations (unpaired t-test) ($P = 0.55$ and $P = 0.62$, resp.). Furthermore, the number of admissions per

TABLE 2: Adequacy indices.

Variables	PDF	HDPD	P value
Total Kt/V (week)	2.26 ± 0.44	2.24 ± 0.56	NS
Total C. Cr (week)	71.97 ± 25.41	62.35 ± 18.7	NS
TBW	33.07 ± 6.91	33.8 ± 5.74	NS
BSA	1.68 ± 0.2	1.71 ± 0.17	NS
Peritoneal urea clearance (week)	54.83 ± 13.7	66.03 ± 11.79	$P < 0.05$
Renal urea clearance (week)	19.17 ± 18.7	6.39 ± 10.9	$P < 0.05$
nPCR	1.03 ± 0.2	1.06 ± 0.26	NS
Total daily drainage volume	8.98 ± 2.4	10.95 ± 1.67	$P < 0.05$
Total daily drainage volume/m^2 BSA	5.34 ± 1.23	6.42 ± 0.94	$P < 0.05$

Total body water (TBW), body surface area (BSA), and normalised protein catabolic rate (nPCR). Data are expressed as mean $\pm$ SD.

patient/year for peritonitis was 0.06 for the first group and 0.07 for HDPD patients ($P = 0.41$).

The RR for diabetes was 0.60 and 0.67 in the PDF and HDPD groups, respectively. Body surface area and total body water were comparable between the groups; the observation of the mean adequacy indices (Kt/V and total weekly creatinine clearance) and nPCR did not show statistical significance, but the mean values of peritoneal and renal urea clearances and total daily drainage volume were statistically significant (Table 2).

4. Discussion

There are innumerable publications that have shown the attributes of the peritoneal dialysis as substitutive renal therapy. In the decades of the eighties and nineties, researchers published comparisons between peritoneal dialysis and haemodialysis regarding patient and technique survival with dissimilar results [14–34]. Nowadays, patient survival and the relationship between modality of dialysis and mortality are an unsolved debate. van Biesen and coworkers introduced the concept of integrative care of end stage renal disease patients using both modalities of treatment according to individual needs [35, 36]. In the last few years, the concept "PD first" has deeply impacted the nephrologists' circle; however, this impact was not translated into the growth of this treatment worldwide [37]. Chaudhary et al., among others, described the advantages of peritoneal dialysis as the first modality and the reasons of underutilisation [14]. Some studies show the outcome of patients transferred from peritoneal dialysis to haemodialysis, but long-term studies analysing the outcome of patients transferred from haemodialysis to peritoneal dialysis are sparse [7–10].

In Argentina, the relation haemodialysis/peritoneal dialysis patients is about 96%/4%, respectively; thus, peritoneal dialysis population is too scarce. Our paper shows comparisons of some of the most important indices of follow-up of patients undergoing peritoneal dialysis on the very long term, with those patients who initiated peritoneal dialysis as first option compared to those transferred from haemodialysis to peritoneal dialysis. We believed that the sample of patients in this aspect is acceptable due to such a long time of follow-up. It is important to point out that many patients moved from other clinics to our peritoneal dialysis program after having been exposed to between two and thirty-three procedures of vascular access among native and prosthetic fistulas in arms and transitory or permanents catheters in veins subclavia, jugular and femoral before starting peritoneal dialysis.

Patient and technique survival are some of the most important indices in the assessment of the substitutive therapies; in our study, the comparison between both groups did not show statistical differences. Similar findings were observed by Zhang and coworkers [10]. Residual renal function plays an important role in the solute clearance and in fluids balance in the dialysis population; Heaf et al. inferred that preservation of the RRF in peritoneal dialysis could be a cause of better survival in the first 2 years of dialysis treatment regarding HD [38]. Some studies support that the diminution of urine volume is a predictor of technique failure and a cause of mortality [39–42]. In contrast, in the NECOSAD study, the authors considered anuric peritoneal dialysis patients to have acceptable patient and technique survival, and the risk factors for death were the same as in the dialysis population as a whole [43]; similar conclusions were found in the EAPOS study in anuric patients on APD [44] and in anuric patients with high body surface area [45]. Lobo and coworkers performed a nationwide study of 739 patients but did not find any differences between survival rates between patients with and patients without previous haemodialysis or in anuric or residual renal function patients [46]. As expected in our study, many patients from the second group were anuric (65.7%); however, we also did not observe statistical differences on the very long term when comparing these anuric patients versusPDF patients (Figures 3 and 4).

Residual renal function contributes to achieving adequacy targets; however, due to the fact that diuresis declines during the course of treatment, the dialysis prescription must be modified to maintain the adequacy level, especially for patients with high body weight [45, 47]. In our study, targets of small solute clearance were achieved in both groups of patients [48]. Although the participation of RRF is obvious in the first group, in the HDPD group, the target was reached relying heavily on peritoneal clearance, with the largest peritoneal fluid delivery as well; this was also observed by Bammens et al. [49] (Table 2). Many patients who started CAPD in both groups were transferred to APD to improve adequacy levels and meet target recommendations through optimisation of the transport characteristics of peritoneal membrane or to increase the UF volume. On the other hand, other reasons for transferring to APD were often linked to social situations, job or study possibilities, the needs of a partner, lifestyle, back pain, and so on.

A twenty-four-hour daily volume of ultrafiltration is very important in order to satisfy the individual negative daily balance requirements; Ateş et al. warned about the importance of the total fluid removal in the survival of the patients [50]. On the other hand, in many cases in which

patients start PD as the first therapy, their urine output is important; if their blood pressure is under control, it is probable that it was not initially essential to get a negative fluid balance in excess of individual necessities; thus high glucose concentration solutions could be avoided. In our study, statistical differences observed between the groups regarding total daily drainage volume are linked to a smaller peritoneal volume prescribed at the beginning of PD due to the contribution of the RRF, which was mainly seen in the first group. The condition of diabetes surprisingly did not have impact as a risk factor of mortality in both groups of patients; nevertheless, there is an atypical prevalence of diabetic and nondiabetic patients' relation and its impact as risk factor observed in our study, in this distribution of patients, might have a bias because the sample was not taken at random.

Technique survival often depends on catheter-related problems; our catheter survival evaluation showed a satisfactory outcome in such a long-term follow-up regarding published data [51–53].

Hospitalisation is a very important indicator of morbidity in assessment of the peritoneal dialysis program, such as in haemodialysis. There are many publications comparing hospitalisations between PD and HD, but there are few and small studies in this aspect between patients who started PD as a substitutive therapy and patients treated sequentially with haemodialysis and peritoneal dialysis [54–56]. In our study period, we did not observe any statistical differences in admissions nor number of hospitalizations days per patients/year between both groups. Moreover, the results showed an overall low admission rate and very low rate regarding admissions for peritonitis [57, 58].

5. Conclusion

The outcome on the very long term of a medical therapy, in a way, discloses its effectiveness; the assessment of the recognised indicators for the replacement therapies of the end stage renal disease patients observed in our study shows that peritoneal dialysis as a first option and continuing haemodialysis are both highly reliable; also, the concept of integrative care is clear, allowing the life of patients to be prolonged. Therefore, it would be very positive to avoid risky vascular access procedures in excess for patients in conditions requiring peritoneal dialysis.

References

[1] D. N. Churchill, D. W. Taylor, S. I. Vas et al., "Peritonitis in continuous ambulatory peritoneal dialysis (CAPD): a multi-centre randomized clinical trial comparing the Y connector disinfectant system to standard systems," *Peritoneal Dialysis International*, vol. 9, no. 3, pp. 159–163, 1989.

[2] N. W. Boyce, N. M. Thomson, and R. C. Atkins, "Management of peritonitis complicating continuous ambulatory peritoneal

dialysis: an Australian perspective," *Peritoneal Dialysis Bulletin*, vol. 7, no. 2, pp. 93–97, 1987.

[3] U. Buoncristiani, "The Y set with disinfectant is here to stay," *Peritoneal Dialysis International*, vol. 9, no. 3, pp. 149–150, 1989.

[4] R. Maiorca, G. C. Cancarini, A. Cantaluppi et al., "Prospective controlled trial of a Y-connector and disinfectant to prevent peritonitis in continuous ambulatory peritoneal dialysis," *The Lancet*, vol. 2, no. 8351, pp. 642–644, 1983.

[5] R. Gokal and A. Hutchison, "Dialysis therapies for end-stage renal disease," *Seminars in Dialysis*, vol. 15, no. 4, pp. 220–226, 2002.

[6] N. Lameire and W. van Biesen, "Epidemiology of peritoneal dialysis: a story of believers and nonbelievers," *Nature Reviews Nephrology*, vol. 6, no. 2, pp. 75–83, 2010.

[7] W. van Biesen, C. Dequidt, D. Vijt, R. Vanholder, and N. Lameire, "Analysis of the reasons for transfers between hemodialysis and peritoneal dialysis and their effect on survivals," *Advances in Peritoneal Dialysis*, vol. 14, pp. 90–94, 1998.

[8] S. J. Nessim, J. M. Bargman, S. V. Jassal, M. J. Oliver, Y. Na, and J. Perl, "The impact of transfer from hemodialysis on peritoneal dialysis technique survival," *Peritoneal Dialysis International*, 2013.

[9] X. Zhang, F. Han, Q. He et al., "Outcomes and risk factors for mortality after transfer from hemodialysis to peritoneal dialysis in uremic patients," *Peritoneal Dialysis International*, vol. 28, no. 3, pp. 313–314, 2008.

[10] L. Zhang, T. Cao, Z. Li et al., "Clinical outcomes of peritoneal dialysis patients transferred from hemodialysis: a matched case-control study," *Peritoneal Dialysis International*, vol. 33, no. 3, pp. 259–266, 2013.

[11] P. E. Watson, I. D. Watson, and R. D. Batt, "Total body water volumes for adult males and females estimated from simple anthropometric measurements," *The American Journal of Clinical Nutrition*, vol. 33, no. 1, pp. 27–39, 1980.

[12] D. D. Bois and E. F. D. Bois, "A formula to estimate the approximate surface area if height and weight be known," *Archives of Internal Medicine*, vol. 17, no. 6, pp. 863–871, 1916.

[13] D. H. Randerson, G. V. Chapman, and P. C. Farrell, "Amino acid and dietary status in CAPD patients," in *Peritoneal Dialysis*, R. C. Atkins, P. C. Farrell, and N. M. Thomson, Eds., pp. 171–191, Churchill Livingstone, Edinburgh, UK, 1981.

[14] K. Chaudhary, H. Sangha, and R. Khanna, "Peritoneal dialysis first: rationale," *Clinical Journal of the American Society of Nephrology*, vol. 6, no. 2, pp. 447–456, 2011.

[15] R. Maiorca, E. Vonesh, G. Cancarini et al., "A six-year comparison of patient and technique survivals in CAPD and HD," *Kidney International*, vol. 34, no. 4, pp. 518–524, 1988.

[16] R. Maiorca, G. C. Cancarini, C. Camerini et al., "Is CAPD competitive with haemodialysis for long-term treatment of uraemic patients?" *Nephrology Dialysis Transplantation*, vol. 4, no. 4, pp. 244–253, 1989.

[17] R. Maiorca, G. C. Cancarini, G. Brunori, C. Camerini, and L. Manili, "Morbidity and mortality of CAPD and hemodialysis," *Kidney International, Supplement*, vol. 40, pp. S4–S15, 1993.

[18] R. Maiorca, G. C. Cancarini, R. Zubani et al., "CAPD viability: a long-term comparison with hemodialysis," *Peritoneal Dialysis International*, vol. 16, no. 3, pp. 276–287, 1996.

[19] K. D. Serkes, C. R. Blagg, K. D. Nolph, E. F. Vonesh, and F. Shapiro, "Comparison of patient and technique survival in continuous ambulatory peritoneal dialysis (CAPD) and hemodialysis: a multicenter study," *Peritoneal Dialysis International*, vol. 10, no. 1, pp. 15–19, 1990.

[20] R. Gokal, J. King, S. Bogle et al., "Outcome in patients on continuous ambulatory peritoneal dialysis and haemodialysis: 4-year analysis of a prospective multicentre study," *The Lancet*, vol. 2, no. 8568, pp. 1105–1109, 1987.

[21] J. F. Marichal, B. Cordier, B. Faller, and P. Brignon, "Continuous ambulatory peritoneal dialysis (CAPD) or center hemodialysis? Retrospective evaluation of the success of both methods," *Peritoneal Dialysis International*, vol. 10, no. 3, pp. 205–208, 1990.

[22] R. Gokal, R. Baillod, S. Bogle et al., "Multi-centre study on outcome of treatment in patients on continuous ambulatory peritoneal dialysis and haemodialysis," *Nephrology Dialysis Transplantation*, vol. 2, no. 3, pp. 172–178, 1987.

[23] A. Lupo, R. Tarchini, G. Cancarini et al., "Long-term outcome in continuous ambulatory peritoneal dialysis: a 10-year survey by the Italian Cooperative Peritoneal Dialysis Study Group," *American Journal of Kidney Diseases*, vol. 24, no. 5, pp. 826–837, 1994.

[24] S. S. A. Fenton, D. E. Schaubel, M. Desmeules et al., "Hemodialysis versus peritoneal dialysis: a comparison of adjusted mortality rates," *American Journal of Kidney Diseases*, vol. 30, no. 3, pp. 334–342, 1997.

[25] E. F. Vonesh, J. J. Snyder, R. N. Foley, and A. J. Collins, "The differential impact of risk factors on mortality in hemodialysis and peritoneal dialysis," *Kidney International*, vol. 66, no. 6, pp. 2389–2401, 2004.

[26] B. G. Jaar, J. Coresh, L. C. Plantinga et al., "Comparing the risk for death with peritoneal dialysis and hemodialysis in a national cohort of patients with chronic kidney disease," *Annals of Internal Medicine*, vol. 143, no. 3, pp. 174–183, 2005.

[27] S. P. McDonald, M. R. Marshall, D. W. Johnson, and K. R. Polkinghorne, "Relationship between dialysis modality and mortality," *Journal of the American Society of Nephrology*, vol. 20, no. 1, pp. 155–163, 2009.

[28] H. R. Rubin, N. E. Fink, L. C. Plantinga, J. H. Sadler, A. S. Kliger, and N. R. Powe, "Patient ratings of dialysis care with peritoneal dialysis vs hemodialysis," *The Journal of the American Medical Association*, vol. 291, no. 6, pp. 697–703, 2004.

[29] E. D. Weinhandl, R. N. Foley, D. T. Gilbertson, T. J. Arneson, J. J. Snyder, and A. J. Collins, "Propensity-matched mortality comparison of incident hemodialysis and peritoneal dialysis patients," *Journal of the American Society of Nephrology*, vol. 21, no. 3, pp. 499–506, 2010.

[30] W. E. Bloembergen, F. K. Port, A. Mauger, and R. A. Wolfe, "A comparison of mortality between patients treated with hemodialysis and peritoneal dialysis," *Journal of the American Society of Nephrology*, vol. 6, no. 2, pp. 177–183, 1995.

[31] E. F. Vonesh and J. Moran, "Mortality in end-stage renal disease: a reassessment of differences between patients treated with hemodialysis and peritoneal dialysis," *Journal of the American Society of Nephrology*, vol. 10, no. 2, pp. 354–365, 1999.

[32] R. Mehrotra, Y.-W. Chiu, K. Kalantar-Zadeh, J. Bargman, and E. Vonesh, "Similar outcomes with hemodialysis and peritoneal dialysis in patients with end-stage renal disease," *Archives of Internal Medicine*, vol. 171, no. 2, pp. 110–118, 2011.

[33] B. G. Jaar, L. C. Plantinga, D. C. Crews et al., "Timing, causes, predictors and prognosis of switching from peritoneal dialysis to hemodialysis: a prospective study," *BMC Nephrology*, vol. 10, no. 1, article 3, 2009.

[34] R. N. Foley, P. S. Parfrey, J. D. Harnett et al., "Mode of dialysis therapy and mortality in end-stage renal disease," *Journal of the American Society of Nephrology*, vol. 9, no. 2, pp. 267–276, 1998.

[35] W. van Biesen, R. C. Vanholder, N. Veys, A. Dhondt, and N. H. Lameire, "An evaluation of an integrative care approach for end-stage renal disease patients," *Journal of the American Society of Nephrology*, vol. 11, no. 1, pp. 116–125, 2000.

[36] N. Lameire, W. van Biesen, and R. Vanholder, "The role of peritoneal dialysis as first modality in an integrative approach to patients with end-stage renal disease," *Peritoneal Dialysis International*, vol. 20, no. 2, pp. S134–S141, 2000.

[37] O. Khawar, K. Kalantar-Zadeh, W. K. Lo, D. Johnson, and R. Mehrotra, "Is the declining use of long-term peritoneal dialysis justified by outcome data?" *Clinical Journal of the American Society of Nephrology*, vol. 2, no. 6, pp. 1317–1328, 2007.

[38] J. G. Heaf, H. Løkkegaard, and M. Madsen, "Initial survival advantage of peritoneal dialysis relative to haemodialysis," *Nephrology Dialysis Transplantation*, vol. 17, no. 1, pp. 112–117, 2002.

[39] K. J. Jager, M. P. Merkus, F. W. Dekker et al., "Mortality and technique failure in patients starting chronic peritoneal dialysis: results of the Netherlands Cooperative Study on the Adequacy of Dialysis," *Kidney International*, vol. 55, no. 4, pp. 1476–1485, 1999.

[40] C.-T. Liao, Y.-M. Chen, C.-C. Shiao et al., "Rate of decline of residual renal function is associated with all-cause mortality and technique failure in patients on long-term peritoneal dialysis," *Nephrology Dialysis Transplantation*, vol. 24, no. 9, pp. 2909–2914, 2009.

[41] J. Perl and J. M. Bargman, "The importance of residual kidney function for patients on dialysis: a critical review," *American Journal of Kidney Diseases*, vol. 53, no. 6, pp. 1068–1081, 2009.

[42] A. Y. Wang, J. Woo, M. Wang et al., "Important differentiation of factors that predict outcome in peritoneal dialysis patients with different degrees of residual renal function," *Nephrology Dialysis Transplantation*, vol. 20, no. 2, pp. 396–403, 2005.

[43] M. A. Jansen, F. Termorshuizen, J. C. Korevaar, F. W. Dekker, E. Boeschoten, and R. T. Krediet, "Predictors of survival in anuric peritoneal dialysis patients," *Kidney International*, vol. 68, no. 3, pp. 1199–1205, 2005.

[44] E. A. Brown, S. J. Davies, P. Rutherford et al., "Survival of functionally anuric patients on automated peritoneal dialysis: the European APD Outcome Study," *Journal of the American Society of Nephrology*, vol. 14, no. 11, pp. 2948–2957, 2003.

[45] R. J. Barone, M. I. Cámpora, N. S. Gimenez, L. Ramirez, M. Santopietro, and S. A. Panese, "Body surface area, adequacy and technique failure in chronic peritoneal dialysis," *Advances in Peritoneal Dialysis*, vol. 26, pp. 105–109, 2010.

[46] J. Lobo, J. Schargorodsky, M. A. Quiroga, I. Hendel, C. Vallvé, and R. Barone, "Peritoneal dialysis in Argentina. A nationwide study," *Peritoneal Dialysis International*, vol. 31, no. 1, pp. 19–26, 2011.

[47] K. D. Nolph, R. A. Jensen, R. Khanna, and Z. J. Twardowski, "Weight limitations for weekly urea clearances using various exchange volumes in continuous ambulatory peritoneal dialysis," *Peritoneal Dialysis International*, vol. 14, no. 3, pp. 261–266, 1994.

[48] W. K. Lo, J. M. Bargman, J. Burkart et al., "Guideline on targets for solute and fluid removal in adult patients on chronic peritoneal dialysis," *Peritoneal Dialysis International*, vol. 26, no. 5, pp. 520–522, 2006.

[49] B. Bammens, P. Evenepoel, K. Verbeke, and Y. Vanrenterghem, "Time profiles of peritoneal and renal clearances of different uremic solutes in incident peritoneal dialysis patients," *The American Journal of Kidney Diseases*, vol. 46, no. 3, pp. 512–519, 2005.

[50] K. Ateş, G. Nergizoğlu, K. Keven et al., "Effect of fluid and sodium removal on mortality in peritoneal dialysis patients," *Kidney International*, vol. 60, no. 2, pp. 767–776, 2001.

[51] J. M. Burkart, "Strategies for optimizing peritoneal dialysis catheter outcomes: catheter implantation issues," *Journal of the American Society of Nephrology*, vol. 9, no. 12, pp. S130–S136, 1998.

[52] N. Singh, I. Davidson, A. Minhajuddin, S. Gieser, M. Nurenberg, and R. Saxena, "Risk factors associated with peritoneal dialysis catheter survival: a 9-year single-center study in 315 patients," *The Journal of Vascular Access*, vol. 11, no. 4, pp. 316–322, 2010.

[53] S. M. Hagen, J. A. Lafranca, J. N. M. Ijzermans, and F. J. M. F. Dor, "A systematic review and meta-analysis of the influence of peritoneal dialysis catheter type on complication rate and catheter survival," *Kidney International*, vol. 85, no. 4, pp. 920–932, 2014.

[54] G. Morduchowicz, J. Winkler, and G. Boner, "CAPD versus haemodialysis: a comparison in the same patients," *International Urology and Nephrology*, vol. 24, no. 5, pp. 575–579, 1992.

[55] S. Singh, J. Yium, E. Macon, E. Clark, D. Schaffer, and P. Teschan, "Multicenter study of change in dialysis therapy-maintenance hemodialysis to continuous ambulatory peritoneal dialysis," *American Journal of Kidney Diseases*, vol. 19, no. 3, pp. 246–251, 1992.

[56] M. Adeniyi, H. Kassam, E. I. Agaba et al., "Hospitalizations in patients treated sequentially by chronic hemodialysis and continuous peritoneal dialysis," *Advances in Peritoneal Dialysis*, vol. 25, pp. 72–75, 2009.

[57] L. Fried, S. Abidi, J. Bernardini, J. R. Johnston, and B. Piraino, "Hospitalization in peritoneal dialysis patients," *The American Journal of Kidney Diseases*, vol. 33, no. 5, pp. 927–933, 1999.

[58] R. Paniagua, D. Amato, E. Vonesh et al., "Effects of increased peritoneal clearances on mortality rates in peritoneal dialysis: ADEMEX, a prospective, randomized, controlled trial," *Journal of the American Society of Nephrology*, vol. 13, no. 5, pp. 1307–1320, 2002.

5

Expression of uPAR in Urinary Podocytes of Patients with Fabry Disease

Hernán Trimarchi,[1] Romina Canzonieri,[2] Amalia Schiel,[2] Juan Politei,[3]
Cristian Costales-Collaguazo,[4] Aníbal Stern,[2] Matías Paulero,[1]
Tatiana Rengel,[1] Lara Valiño-Rivas,[5] Mariano Forrester,[1] Fernando Lombi,[1]
Vanesa Pomeranz,[1] Romina Iriarte,[1] Alexis Muryan,[2] Alberto Ortiz,[5,6]
María Dolores Sanchez-Niño,[5,6] and Elsa Zotta[4]

[1]*Nephrology Service, Hospital Británico de Buenos Aires, Buenos Aires, Argentina*
[2]*Central Laboratory, Hospital Británico de Buenos Aires, Buenos Aires, Argentina*
[3]*Neurology Department, Laboratorio de Neuroquímica Dr. Nestor Chamoles, Buenos Aires, Argentina*
[4]*IFIBIO Houssay, CONICET, Physiopathology, Pharmacy and Biochemistry Faculty, Universidad de Buenos Aires,*
Buenos Aires, Argentina
[5]*IIS-Fundación Jimenez Diaz, School of Medicine, UAM, Madrid, Spain*
[6]*REDINREN, Madrid, Spain*

Correspondence should be addressed to Hernán Trimarchi; htrimarchi@hotmail.com

Academic Editor: Jochen Reiser

Background. Despite enzyme replacement therapy, Fabry nephropathy still progresses. Podocyturia is an irreversible event that antedates proteinuria and leads to chronic renal failure. We evaluated a potential mechanism of podocyte detachment via the expression of the urokinase-type Plasminogen Activator Receptor (uPAR) in urinary podocytes of Fabry patients. *Methods*. This is a cross-sectional study that included controls ($n = 20$) and Fabry patients ($n = 44$) either untreated ($n = 23$) or treated with agalsidase-β ($n = 21$). *Variables*. Variables are estimated glomerular filtration rate (eGFR), urinary protein : creatinine ratio, and urinary uPAR+ podocyte : creatinine ratio. uPAR mRNA expression in response to lyso-Gb3, a bioactive glycolipid accumulated in Fabry disease, was studied in cultured human podocytes. *Results*. Controls and Fabry patients had similar age, gender, and renal function. Urinary uPAR+ podocytes were higher in patients than in controls. Untreated patients were significantly younger; had more females, and presented lower urinary protein : creatinine ratios and significantly higher urinary uPAR+ podocytes than treated subjects. In treated patients, urinary uPAR+ podocytes correlated with urinary protein : creatinine ratio ($\rho = 0.5$; $p = 0.02$). Lyso-Gb3 at concentrations found in the circulation of Fabry patients increased uPAR expression in cultured podocytes. *Conclusions*. Urinary podocytes expressing uPAR are increased in Fabry patients, especially in untreated patients. The potential contribution of uPAR expression to podocyte detachment merits further studies.

1. Introduction

Fabry disease is an X-linked storage disease due to mutations in the GLA gene encoding the lysosomal enzyme α-galactosidase A, leading to the accumulation of enzyme substrates, namely, globotriaosylceramide (Gb3), lyso-globotriaosylceramide (lyso-Gb3), and galabiosylceramide [1].

The overload of these glycosphingolipids disturbs the morphology of affected cells and leads to cell dysfunction [2–4]. However, the exact mechanisms by which these metabolites lead to cell dysfunction remain elusive. It has been speculated that mechanical overload either inside or outside lysosomes or the interaction of glycosphingolipids with ion channels or transporters may contribute to tissue damage [5, 6]. Within

TABLE 1: General characteristics of controls and Fabry patients.

Variables	Controls (n: 20)	Fabry (n: 44)	p value
Age (years)	30 (20–48)	31 (11–86)	0.92
Gender (males)	10 (50%)	17 (38.6%)	0.59
Hypertension	0 (0%)	6 (14%)	**0.001**
eGFR (ml/min/1.73 m^2)	110 (86–141)	120.5 (60–165)	0.10
UPCR (g/g)	0.03 (0.02–0.27)	0.06 (0.02–5.68)	**0.01**
Urinary uPAR+ podocytes/creatininuria (cells/g)	0 (0–73.99)	28.88 (0–284.46)	**<0.001**

the kidney, podocytes are a major albeit not exclusive target in Fabry disease, since they do not proliferate and henceforth accumulate glycosphingolipids throughout their very long lifespan, until they detach and are washed away into urine, rendering a denuded area of glomerular basement membrane [7–9]. During the initial phases, other podocytes may cover the denuded glomerular area. However, when the podocyte number becomes critically low, the glomerulus is eventually obliterated [9]. Irreversible podocytopenia may underlie the observation that enzyme replacement therapy (ERT) may slow but not stop progression of Fabry nephropathy to end-stage renal disease once a certain degree of kidney injury has already occurred [10].

We have recently reported that untreated Fabry individuals with preserved glomerular filtration rate (GFR) and physiological values of proteinuria already present significantly higher levels of podocyturia than Fabry treated subjects [11]. Podocyte attachment to the glomerular basement membrane involves interactions between integrins and specific matrix ligands [12]. In this respect, uPAR is a transmembrane receptor located at the basal side of the podocyte which interacts with integrin $\alpha V\beta 3$. uPAR-integrin coupling promotes activation of integrin-actin binding and podocyte contraction. However, persistent uPAR-integrin coupling leads to mechanical cellular stress and podocyte detachment [13, 14].

In this study, we explored the urinary excretion of uPAR expressing podocytes in patients with Fabry disease and the induction of uPAR expression by lyso-Gb, a bioactive lipid accumulated in Fabry disease.

2. Methods

This is a cross-sectional, observational study, which included 65 individuals. A group of 20 healthy subjects without known clinical morbidities or pharmacological treatment was recruited among potential kidney donors and subjects with normal laboratory results and clinical history. In addition, 44 Fabry patients were studied. Of them, 23 were not treated with enzyme replacement therapy (ERT), while 21 had received ERT for at least 12 months with agalsidase-β 1 mg/kg every fortnight (Fabrazyme, Genzyme Corp., Cambridge, MA, USA). Fabry disease was diagnosed in all cases by low enzymatic alpha galactosidase A activity in dried blood spots and peripheral blood leukocytes and confirmed by the identification of a GLA gene mutation. Criteria for ERT therapy included symptoms related to Fabry disease (acroparesthesia, pain crisis or neuropathic pain of any kind,

sensorineural loss, hypohidrosis, and bowel disturbances), cardiologic compromise as hypertrophic cardiomyopathy and/or arrhythmias and/or valve disease, cerebrovascular disease or kidney involvement as proteinuria, decreased renal function, and kidney biopsy consistent with Fabry disease. Patient characteristics are outlined in Table 1. The following variables were studied: age, gender, glomerular filtration rate estimated (eGFR) by the Chronic Kidney Disease-Epidemiology Collaboration (CKD-EPI) equation, urinary protein : creatinine ratio (UPCR), podocyturia adjusted per gram of creatininuria, and urinary uPAR positive podocyte/creatinine ratio.

2.1. Podocyturia. We have previously described the method to study podocyturia in detail [11, 15]. Briefly, a mid-stream freshly voided urine sample was collected on-site after a minimum of 3 hours without voiding; 20 ml of urine was centrifuged at 700 g for 5 min using a cytospin; the supernatant was discarded and the sediment was stored in 100 μl aliquots at room temperature mixed with a 1.5 ml solution of 40% formaldehyde diluted in phosphate-buffered saline (PBS) (pH 7.2–7.4) to reach a final 10% formaldehyde concentration. Cells were preincubated with rabbit nonimmune serum (PBS dilution 1 : 100) in humid chamber at room temperature for 1 hour. Thereafter, podocytes were identified by immunofluorescence using rabbit anti-synaptopodin as the primary antibody (1 : 100, Abcam, Cambridge, MA, USA) and also stained with mouse polyclonal anti-uPAR antibody (1 : 200, Abcam, Cambridge, MA, USA) in a humid chamber at 4°C overnight. Three five-minute rinses with PBS were made and the samples were incubated with the secondary antibodies: anti-rabbit IgG ALEXA Fluor 488® (1 : 100, Abcam, Cambridge, MA, USA) for synaptopodin and anti-mouse IgG Alexa Fluor 568 (1 : 100, Abcam, Cambridge, MA, USA) for uPAR in humid chamber for 2 hours at room temperature. Three 5-minute rinses were followed by 40,6-diamidino-2-phenylindole (DAPI) staining of nuclei. Samples were analyzed employing an epifluorescent Nikon Eclipse E200 microscope. Following our standardized technique, synaptopodin-uPAR costained podocytes were counted in 10 randomly chosen 20x fields and the average of the counted podocytes in the microscopy fields was considered as the final count for each subject (Figure 1). The results were corrected based on the levels of urinary creatinine found in each sample [11, 15]. For that, the value of urinary creatinine was calculated for the initial urinary volume of 20 ml employed for podocyte counting.

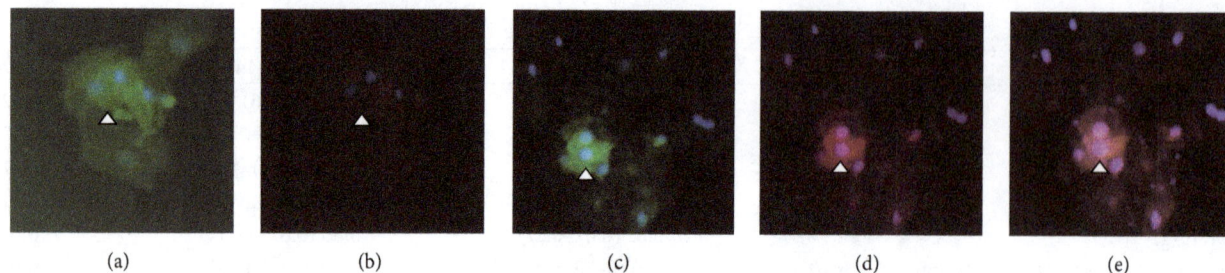

(a)   (b)   (c)   (d)   (e)

FIGURE 1: Expression of uPAR in urinary podocytes of patients with Fabry disease. (a) Synaptopodin negative cells (arrowhead). (b) uPAR negative cells (arrowhead). (c) Synaptopodin positive cells (arrowhead). (d) uPAR positive cells (white arrowhead). (e) Merge indicating the colocalization between synaptopodin and uPAR in Fabry podocytes (arrowhead). Magnification: ×200.

Serum creatinine was assessed the same week that the urine was collected for podocyte counting employing an enzymatic method. UPCR was measured from the specimen employed for podocyte assessment.

2.2. Cell Culture and Reagents. Human podocytes are an immortalized cell line transfected with a temperature-sensitive SV40 gene construct and a gene encoding the catalytic domain of human telomerase [16, 17]. At a permissive temperature of 33°C, cells remain in an undifferentiated proliferative state and divide. Raising the temperature to 37°C results in growth arrest and differentiation to the parental podocyte phenotype. Undifferentiated podocyte cultures were maintained at 33°C in RPMI 1640 medium with penicillin, streptomycin, ITS (insulin, transferrin, and selenite), and 10% FCS. Once cells reached 70 to 80% confluence, they were fully differentiated by culture at 37°C for at least 14 days [16, 17]. Cells were cultured in serum-free media 24 hours prior to the addition of stimuli and throughout the experiment. Lyso-Gb3 (Sigma, St. Louis, MO) was used at a concentration of 100 nM and tested negative for lipopolysaccharide. This concentration is clinically relevant, since circulating lyso-Gb3 has been reported to be in the 10–50 nM range for heterozygous females and above 100 nM in males [17]. Furthermore, this concentration was previously shown in dose-response studies to be bioactive in cultured human podocytes [16, 17].

2.3. Real-Time Reverse Transcription-Polymerase Chain Reaction. RNA was isolated using TRIzol reagent (Invitrogen, Paisley, UK). One μg RNA was reverse-transcribed with High Capacity cDNA Archive Kit (Applied Biosystems, Foster City, CA). Real-time PCR reactions were performed on the ABI Prism 7500 sequence detection PCR system (Applied Biosystems) according to the manufacturer's protocol using the DeltaDelta Ct method [16, 17]. Expression levels are given as ratios to GAPDH. Predeveloped primer and probe assays were from Applied Biosystems.

2.4. Western Blot Analysis. Cell samples were homogenized in lysis buffer [18] and then separated by 10% or 12% SDS-PAGE under reducing conditions and transferred to PVDF membranes (Millipore, Bedford, MA, USA), blocked with 5% skimmed milk in PBS/0.5% v/v Tween 20 for 1 h, and washed with PBS/Tween. Primary antibody was uPAR (1 : 500, Abcam). Antibody was diluted in 5% milk PBS/Tween. Blot was washed with PBS/Tween and subsequently incubated with appropriate horseradish peroxidase-conjugated secondary antibody (1 : 2000, GE Healthcare/Amersham, Aylesbury, UK). After washing, the blot was developed with the chemiluminescence method (ECL). Blot was then reprobed with monoclonal anti-mouse α-tubulin antibody (1 : 2000, Sigma, St. Louis, MO, USA) and levels of expression were corrected for minor differences in loading.

2.5. Statistical Analysis. Results are expressed as median and range. Variables were analyzed using the Wilcoxon-Mann-Whitney test. Correlations between variables were obtained with Spearman's correlation coefficient. Results were considered significant when $p < 0.05$. The statistical program employed was InfoStat 2016, Córdoba, Argentina.

2.6. Ethical Approval. The present protocol was approved by the Institutional Review Board of the Hospital Británico de Buenos Aires, Buenos Aires, Argentina. Informed consent was obtained from each study participant. All procedures performed in studies involving human participants were in accordance with the ethical standards of the institutional and/or national research committee and with the 1964 Declaration of Helsinki and its later amendments of comparable ethical standards.

3. Results

Controls and Fabry patients did not differ in age, gender, and renal function (Table 1). However, patients had significantly higher UPCR than controls. Moreover, urinary excretion of uPAR+ podocytes [28.88 (0–284.46) versus 0 (0–73.99) podocytes/g; $p < 0.001$] was higher in Fabry patients than in controls (Table 1).

Fabry patients were divided into natural history untreated Fabry patients and ERT-treated patients. Time on ERT for treated Fabry patients was 40 (34–50) months (Table 2).

As expected, Fabry patients not on ERT had less severe disease, since they were significantly younger and more frequently females (Table 2). In this regard, in untreated patients, the UPCR was lower [0.06 (0.02–2.35) versus 0.10 (0.02–5.68) g/g, $p = 0.04$] and eGFR was higher

TABLE 2: General characteristics of untreated (no ERT) and ERT-treated Fabry patients.

Variables	No ERT (n: 23)	ERT (n: 21)	p value
Age (years)	19 (11–75)	35.8 (17–86)	**0.03**
Gender (males)	4 (14%)	13 (59%)	**0.01**
Hypertension	1 (4.3%)	5 (24%)	**0.0001**
White matter ischaemia[*]	4 (17%)[**]	14 (68%)[**]	**0.003**
Myocardial hypertrophy	1 (4%)	5 (24%)	**0.001**
Time on ERT (months)	0	40 (34–50)	**<0.0001**
eGFR (ml/min/1.73 m^2)	141 (60–165)	131.5 (62–148)	**0.06**
UPCR (g/g)	0.06 (0.02–2.35)	0.10 (0.02–5.68)	**0.04**
Urinary uPAR+ podocytes/creatininuria (cells/g)	40.18 (9.51–284.46)	20.18 (0–191.26)	**0.009**
Mutations	D33G, L415P, R227X, A292T, N34D, C801, C326, C647A, C281, G640C	D33G, L415P, R227X, A292T, N34D, D264Y, D155H, L180F	

ERT, enzyme replacement therapy. [*]Diagnosed by magnetic resonance imaging; [**]asymptomatic cases, performed for screening purposes.

[141 (60–165) versus 131.5 (62–148) ml/min/1.73 m^2; $p = 0.06$] than in ERT Fabry patients. However, within Fabry patients, urinary podocytes stained for uPAR were significantly higher [40.18 (9.51–284.46) versus 20.18 (0–191.26) cells/g urinary creatinine; $p = 0.009$] in untreated patients than in ERT-treated patients (Table 2). Finally, more hypertensives were found in Fabry treated patients versus nontreated subjects (Table 2 and Figure 1).

There was a significant positive correlation between urinary excretion of uPAR+ podocytes and UPCR ($\rho = 0.5$; $p = 0.02$) in Fabry patients on ERT.

3.1. Lyso-Gb3 Increases uPAR Expression in Cultured Podocytes. Since uPAR+ podocytes were increased early in Fabry nephropathy, even in the group of patients with better preserved eGFR and lower albuminuria, we explored whether glycolipids accumulated in Fabry disease may increase uPAR expression in cultured human podocytes. We had previously shown that, at concentrations found in the circulation of Fabry disease patients, lyso-Gb3 increases the expression of diverse mediators of kidney injury in a dose-dependent fashion, with peak response observed at 100 nM, a concentration found in the circulation of Fabry patients [16, 17]. In human podocytes, lyso-Gb3 at the concentration of 100 nM induced an increase in the mRNA expression of uPAR which peaked at 3 hours (Figure 2(a)). Furthermore, lyso-Gb3 increased the protein expression of uPAR with the same time pattern (Figure 2(b)).

4. Discussion

In the present study, we have shown that in Fabry patients the urinary excretion of uPAR positive podocytes is higher than in controls and have confirmed the pathologically high podocyturia of Fabry nephropathy [11]. Interestingly, urinary excretion of uPAR positive podocytes was higher in untreated Fabry patients, despite their milder nonsignificant kidney

injury (Table 2) (Figure 1). This suggests that uPAR positivity is not secondary to more severe kidney injury. In this regard, we have identified glycolipid accumulation and, specifically, lyso-Gb3 accumulation as a driver of uPAR expression in podocytes (Figure 2).

Preservation of glomerular podocyte mass is critical for the preservation of a healthy glomerular filtration barrier. The initially silent urinary loss of podocytes heralds the loss of urinary proteins resulting from the disruption of the glomerular filtration barrier and the subsequent decline in renal function due to nephron loss [9]. Despite ERT, Fabry patients are at risk of progressive deterioration in renal function, especially if significant podocyte loss has already occurred as evidenced by the presence of proteinuria or glomerulosclerosis [10]. This may be influenced by many factors, including the genetic background, the existence of comorbidities, the age at which ERT is initiated, and the prescribed dose of ERT. Indeed, in index cases, ERT is usually initiated at more advanced disease stages [7, 10, 11]. In our population, hypertension could also be an additional factor of renal disease progression (Table 2). In this regard, an early intervention to prevent irreversible podocyte detachment and loss is mandatory [8]. Unraveling the mechanisms of podocyte detachment could lead to the design of novel pharmacological approaches aimed at preserving podocyte numbers by preventing detachment even in ERT-treated patients.

Podocyte adhesion to the glomerular basement membrane is mainly modulated by integrins. Integrins are heterodimeric transmembrane receptor proteins, consisting of α and β subunits, which mediate adhesion and interactions between cells and the extracellular matrix [8, 19]. Changes in the distribution and/or activity of integrins at the basal side of podocytes and of their ligands in the glomerular basement membrane may both reflect and cause podocyte stress and/or glomerular injury [8, 20]. The result is podocyte detachment, podocyturia, proteinuria, and chronic renal

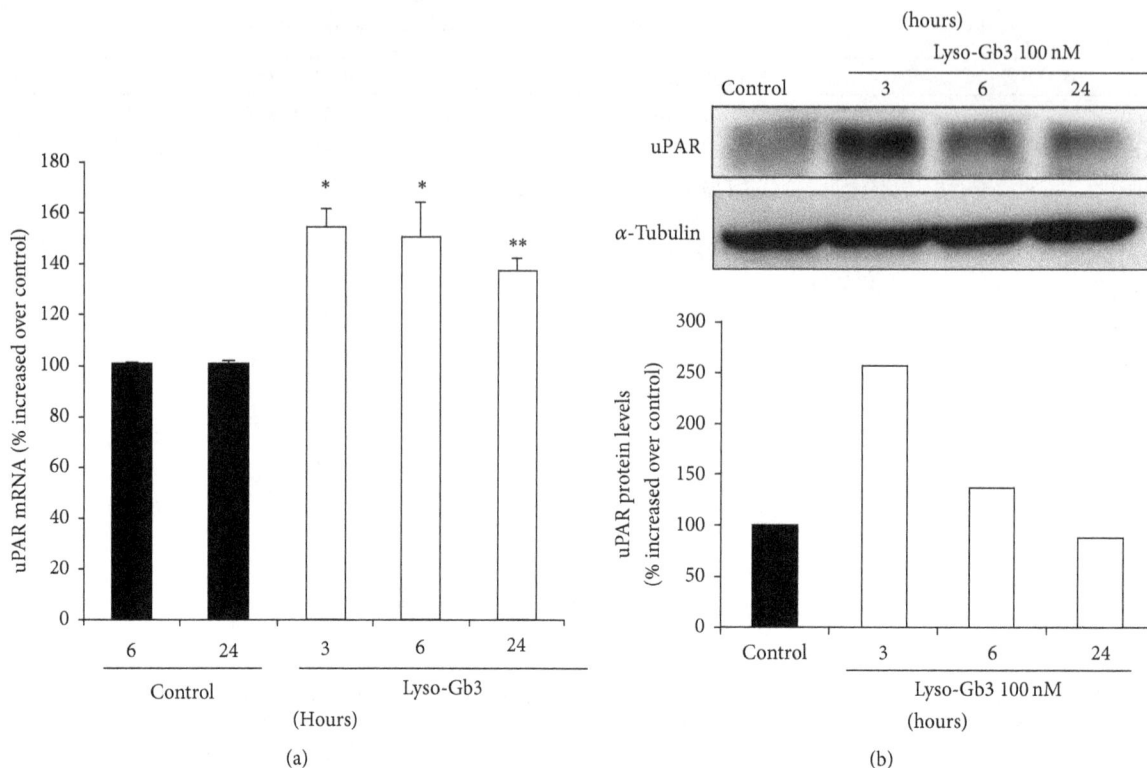

FIGURE 2: Lyso-Gb3 upregulates uPAR expression in podocytes. Cultured human podocytes were stimulated with 100 nM lyso-Gb3. (a) Time course of uPAR mRNA induction. $^*p < 0.002$ versus control; $^{**}p < 0.01$ versus control. Expression of mRNA was assessed by real-time RT-PCR. Mean ± SEM of four independent experiments. (b) Protein levels of uPAR assessed by Western blot. Representative image.

disease progression. Integrin $\alpha V\beta 3$ (the vitronectin receptor) was suggested to be involved in the pathogenesis of Fabry nephropathy. In Fabry patients, the urinary excretion of integrin $\alpha V\beta 3$ and the expression of the $\beta 3$ subunit in podocytes are increased, while the amount of vitronectin was moderately increased in kidneys from Fabry patients [21]. Some glycan phosphatidylinositol- (GPI-) linked proteins as uPAR can associate with specific integrins [22, 23]. Specifically, uPAR can associate with podocyte $\alpha V\beta 3$ [24, 25]. Interaction between uPAR and integrins is the best analyzed example of this type of complex interaction. Several recent reviews have highlighted the importance of the integrin-uPAR interaction for cell migration, tumor invasion, and host defense [23]. uPAR interaction with $\alpha V\beta 3$ integrin modulates its ligand-binding activities [13]. The complex of lipid raft-associated uPAR with $\beta 3$ integrin in podocytes results in integrin activation, leading to cell contraction, eventual detachment, and podocyturia [14]. Thus, the uPAR-$\alpha V\beta 3$ integrin interaction may be involved in podocyte detachment [11, 21]. Our study demonstrating uPAR expression in detached Fabry podocytes is in line with this hypothesis, although functional interventional studies are needed to prove the hypothesis. Interestingly, amiloride reduces uPAR expression in rat podocytes, and this was associated with decreased podocyte motility and decreased proteinuria. The antiproteinuric effect of amiloride may be at least partially related to inhibition of uPAR expression in podocytes [26].

In this regard, podocyturia was successfully decreased in one Fabry patient with the prescription of amiloride [27].

Lyso-Gb3 is a promising biomarker in Fabry disease. Circulating levels of lyso-Gb3 are related to the severity of the GLA mutation. In milder mutations, associated with late onset disease, circulating lyso-Gb3 is in the range of 3–18 nM, while severe mutations associated with classical Fabry disease (and earlier and more severe clinical disease) display lyso-Gb3 levels in the 80–300 nM range in males [28, 29]. This latter range is the one tested in the present study. Indeed, for genetic variants of unknown significance, lyso-Gb3 levels have been suggested to provide information on pathogenicity [30, 31]. Indeed, plasma lyso-Gb3 correlated to evidence of tissue injury, considering gender and age, and increased gradually as the subjects got older [28]. Finally, ERT decreases lyso-Gb3 levels in a dose-dependent manner [32]. Indeed, the lyso-Gb3 response has been associated with evidence of improved tissue injury [33]. There is a key difference between uPAR and lyso-Gb3. uPAR appears to be a marker of tissue injury, while lyso-Gb3 is a marker of glycolipid burden.

Our study presents certain limitations. It is a cross-sectional study and, thus, it cannot address cause-and-effect relationships, and the uPAR response to ERT in individual patients is not available. Furthermore, the number of patients is relatively low in absolute terms. Finally, the treated and untreated patients were not balanced for disease severity: as expected, untreated patients had less severe disease, and this was one of the reasons for not having started therapy yet. However, this lack of balance allowed excluding more severe, already established kidney disease as a nonspecific cause of higher urinary uPAR. Furthermore, this is a large study for Fabry disease standards, since Fabry is a rare disease. Assessment of podocyturia has not been standardized for clinical use, is time-consuming, and requires expertise [11]. Furthermore, synaptopodin negative podocyte subpopulations may have been missed by our experimental approach. Despite these limitations, the present study provides novel insights into the pathogenesis of podocyturia in Fabry disease which should be further explored by interventional in vivo studies. Thus, if a cause-and-effect relationship between uPAR expression and podocyturia is demonstrated, we may envision adjuvant therapeutic approaches targeted at uPAR, on top of ERT, to help preserve podocyte mass and prevent progression of Fabry nephropathy at least during the window period from ERT initiation to complete clearance of podocyte glycolipid deposits.

In conclusion, podocyturia in Fabry patients was associated with higher numbers of urinary uPAR positive podocytes. Interestingly, ERT was associated with lower uPAR expressing urinary podocytes. This observation is consistent with the increased expression of podocyte uPAR in response to lyso-Gb3 and suggests that glycolipid deposition may drive uPAR expression. The potential contribution of uPAR expression to podocyte detachment through interaction with integrin $\alpha V \beta 3$ merits further studies.

References

[1] R. O. Brady, A. E. Gal, R. M. Bradley, E. Martensson, A. L. Warshaw, and L. Laster, "Enzymatic defect in Fabry's disease. Ceramidetrihexosidase deficiency," *New England Journal of Medicine*, vol. 276, no. 21, pp. 1163–1167, 1967.

[2] A. Kanda, S. Nakao, S. Tsuyama, F. Murata, and T. Kanzaki, "Fabry disease: ultrastructural lectin histochemical analyses of lysosomal deposits," *Virchows Archiv*, vol. 436, no. 1, pp. 36–42, 2000.

[3] H. Askari, C. R. Kaneski, C. Semino-Mora et al., "Cellular and tissue localization of globotriaosylceramide in Fabry disease," *Virchows Archiv*, vol. 451, no. 4, pp. 823–834, 2007.

[4] R. J. Desnick and C. M. Eng, "α-Galactosidase A deficiency: Fabry disease," in *The Metabolic and Molecular Bases of Inherited Disease*, McGraw-Hill, 2001.

[5] E. Lloyd-Evans, D. Pelled, C. Riebeling et al., "Glucosylceramide and glucosylsphingosine modulate calcium mobilization from brain microsomes via different mechanisms," *Journal of Biological Chemistry*, vol. 278, no. 26, pp. 23594–23599, 2003.

[6] D. Pelled, S. Trajkovic-Bodennec, E. Lloyd-Evans, E. Sidransky, R. Schiffmann, and A. H. Futerman, "Enhanced calcium release in the acute neuronopathic form of Gaucher disease," *Neurobiology of Disease*, vol. 18, no. 1, pp. 83–88, 2005.

[7] D. P. Germain, S. Waldek, M. Banikazemi et al., "Sustained, long-term renal stabilization after 54 months of agalsidase β therapy in patients with Fabry disease," *Journal of the American Society of Nephrology*, vol. 18, no. 5, pp. 1547–1557, 2007.

[8] C. Tøndel, L. Bostad, K. K. Larsen et al., "Agalsidase benefits renal histology in young patients with Fabry disease," *Journal of the American Society of Nephrology*, vol. 24, no. 1, pp. 137–148, 2013.

[9] H. Trimarchi, "Podocyturia. What is in a name?" *Journal of Translational Internal Medicine*, vol. 3, pp. 51–56, 2015.

[10] A. Ortiz, B. Cianciaruso, M. Cizmarik et al., "End-stage renal disease in patients with Fabry disease: natural history data from the Fabry Registry," *Nephrology Dialysis Transplantation*, vol. 25, no. 3, pp. 769–775, 2010.

[11] H. Trimarchi, R. Canzonieri, A. Schiel et al., "Podocyturia is significantly elevated in untreated vs treated Fabry adult patients," *Journal of Nephrology*, vol. 29, no. 6, pp. 791–797, 2016.

[12] M. Nagata, "Podocyte injury and its consequences," *Kidney International*, vol. 89, no. 6, pp. 1221–1230, 2016.

[13] H. A. Chapman and Y. Wei, "Protease crosstalk with integrins: the urokinase receptor paradigm," *Thrombosis and Haemostasis*, vol. 86, no. 1, pp. 124–129, 2001.

[14] C. Wei, C. C. Möller, M. M. Altintas et al., "Modification of kidney barrier function by the urokinase receptor," *Nature Medicine*, vol. 14, no. 1, pp. 55–63, 2008.

[15] H. Trimarchi, R. Canzonieri, A. Schiel et al., "Increased urinary CD80 excretion and podocyturia in Fabry disease," *Journal of Translational Medicine*, vol. 14, article 289, 2016.

[16] M. D. Sanchez-Niño, D. Carpio, A. B. Sanz, M. Ruiz-Ortega, S. Mezzano, and A. Ortiz, "Lyso-Gb3 activates Notch1 in human podocytes," *Human Molecular Genetics*, vol. 24, no. 20, pp. 5720–5732, 2015.

[17] M. D. Sanchez-Niño, A. B. Sanz, S. Carrasco et al., "Globotriaosylsphingosine actions on human glomerular podocytes: implications for Fabry nephropathy," *Nephrology Dialysis Transplantation*, vol. 26, no. 6, pp. 1797–1802, 2011.

[18] A. Ortiz, H. Husi, L. Gonzalez-Lafuente et al., "Mitogen-activated protein kinase 14 promotes AKI," *Journal of the American Society of Nephrology*, vol. 28, no. 3, pp. 823–836, 2017.

[19] E. Ruoslahti, "Integrins," *The Journal of Clinical Investigation*, vol. 87, no. 1, pp. 1–5, 1991.

[20] S. Adler, "Integrin matrix receptors in renal injury," *Kidney International Supplements*, vol. 45, pp. S86–S89, 1994.

[21] K. Utsumi, K. Itoh, R. Kase et al., "Urinary excretion of the vitronectin receptor (integrin alpha V beta 3) in patients with Fabry disease," *Clinica Chimica Acta*, vol. 279, no. 1-2, pp. 55–68, 1999.

[22] A. Fornoni, S. Merscher, and J. B. Kopp, "Lipid biology of the podocyte-new perspectives offer new opportunities," *Nature Reviews Nephrology*, vol. 10, no. 7, pp. 379–388, 2014.

[23] K. T. Preissner, S. M. Kanse, and A. E. May, "Urokinase receptor: a molecular organizer in cellular communication," *Current Opinion in Cell Biology*, vol. 12, no. 5, pp. 621–628, 2000.

[24] E. J. Brown, "Integrin-associated proteins," *Current Opinion in Cell Biology*, vol. 14, no. 5, pp. 603–607, 2002.

[25] N. Sachs and A. Sonnenberg, "Cell-matrix adhesion of podocytes in physiology and disease," *Nature Reviews Nephrology*, vol. 9, no. 4, pp. 200–210, 2013.

[26] B. Zhang, S. Xie, W. Shi, and Y. Yang, "Amiloride off-target effect inhibits podocyte urokinase receptor expression and reduces proteinuria," *Nephrology Dialysis Transplantation*, vol. 27, no. 5, pp. 1746–1755, 2012.

[27] H. Trimarchi, M. Forrester, F. Lombi et al., "Amiloride as an alternate adjuvant antiproteinuric agent in Fabry disease: the potential roles of plasmin and uPAR," *Case Reports in Nephrology*, vol. 2014, Article ID 854521, 6 pages, 2014.

[28] H. C. Liao, Y. H. Huang, Y. J. Chen et al., "Plasma globotriaosyl-sphingosine (lysoGb3) could be a biomarker for Fabry disease with a Chinese hotspot late-onset mutation (IVS4+919G>A). Clin Chim Acta," in *doi*, pp. 426–114, 426, 114-120, 2013.

[29] J. M. Aerts, J. E. Groener, S. Kuiper et al., "Elevated globotriao-sylsphingosine is a hallmark of Fabry disease," *Proceedings of the National Academy of Sciences of the United States of America*, vol. 105, no. 8, pp. 2812–2817, 2008.

[30] B. E. Smid, L. Van Der Tol, F. Cecchi et al., "Uncertain diagnosis of Fabry disease: consensus recommendation on diagnosis in adults with left ventricular hypertrophy and genetic variants of unknown significance," *International Journal of Cardiology*, vol. 177, no. 2, pp. 400–408, 2014.

[31] M. Niemann, A. Rolfs, S. Störk et al., "Gene mutations versus clinically relevant phenotypes: lyso-gb3 defines Fabry disease," *Circulation: Cardiovascular Genetics*, vol. 7, no. 1, pp. 8–16, 2014.

[32] O. Goker-Alpan, M. J. Gambello, G. H. Maegawa et al., "Reduction of plasma globotriaosylsphingosine levels after switching from agalsidase alfa to agalsidase beta as enzyme replacement therapy for Fabry disease," *JIMD Reports*, vol. 25, pp. 95–106, 2016.

[33] K. H. Chen, Y. Chien, K. L. Wang et al., "Evaluation of pro-inflammatory prognostic biomarkers for fabry cardiomyopathy with enzyme replacement therapy," *Canadian Journal of Cardiology*, vol. 32, pp. 1221.e1–1221.e9, 2016.

6

Spot Urine Estimations Are Equivalent to 24-Hour Urine Assessments of Urine Protein Excretion for Predicting Clinical Outcomes

Boon Wee Teo,[1] Ping Tyug Loh,[1] Weng Kin Wong,[2] Peh Joo Ho,[3] Kwok Pui Choi,[3] Qi Chun Toh,[1] Hui Xu,[1] Sharon Saw,[4] Titus Lau,[5] Sunil Sethi,[6] and Evan J. C. Lee[1]

[1]Department of Medicine, Yong Loo Lin School of Medicine, National University of Singapore, 1E Kent Ridge Road, Level 10 NUHS Tower Block, Singapore 119228

[2]National University Health System, Singapore 119228

[3]Department of Statistics and Applied Probability, Faculty of Science, National University of Singapore, Singapore 119228

[4]Department of Laboratory Medicine, National University Health System, Singapore 119228

[5]Department of Medicine, National University Health System, Singapore 119228

[6]Department of Pathology, Yong Loo Lin School of Medicine, National University of Singapore, Singapore 119228

Correspondence should be addressed to Boon Wee Teo; mdctbw@nus.edu.sg

Academic Editor: Francesca Mallamaci

Background. The use of spot urine protein to creatinine ratios in estimating 24 hr urine protein excretion rates for diagnosing and managing chronic kidney disease (CKD) predated the standardization of creatinine assays. The comparative predictive performance of spot urine ratios and 24 hr urine collections (of albumin or protein) for the clinical outcomes of CKD progression, end-stage renal disease (ESRD), and mortality in Asians is unclear. We compared 4 methods of assessing urine protein excretion in a multiethnic population of CKD patients. *Methods.* Patients with CKD ($n = 232$) provided 24 hr urine collections followed by spot urine samples the next morning. We created multiple linear regression models to assess the factors associated with GFR decline (median follow-up: 37 months, IQR 26–41) and constructed Cox proportional-hazards models for predicting the combined outcome of ESRD and death. *Results.* The linear regression models showed that 24 hr urine protein excretion was most predictive of GFR decline but all other methods were similar. For the combined outcomes of ESRD and death, the proportional hazards models had similar predictive performance. *Conclusions.* We showed that all methods of assessments were comparable for clinical end-points, and any method can be used in clinical practice or research.

1. Background

The estimation of 24-hour urine protein excretion or 24-hour urine albumin excretion using urine protein to creatinine ratio (UPCR) and urine albumin to creatinine ratio (UACR), respectively, is well established in clinical practice and promulgated by practice guidelines [1]. The original studies were, however, performed prior to the standardization of creatinine assays [2–4]. The standardized creatinine values may differ by 5–20% from values obtained by methods not calibrated or traceable to the isotope dilution mass spectrometry (IDMS) standard [5]. As an example, if standardized creatinine is 20% higher than previously measured, UPCR or UACR may be

17% lower on estimation. Conversely if standardized creatinine is 10% lower, then UPCR or UACR may be 11% higher on estimation. Therefore, it is clear that creatinine standardization has important implications for the proteinuria estimation equations and their application in clinical practice. The measurement of proteinuria and albuminuria has not been standardized [6]. Moreover, the different assay methods may result in differences in the concentrations obtained. Research studies and clinical practice may favor UPCR over UACR for reason of cost, and there are no reliable methods to convert ratios [7]. However, the new iteration of the clinical practice guidelines for the identification and classification of chronic kidney disease incorporated urine albumin to creatinine ratio as part of risk stratification [8, 9]. In this study, we assessed the correlation of early morning spot urine tests to 24-hour urine protein and albumin excretion, provided conversion equations developed from a population of patients with a variety of chronic kidney disease, and compared their predictive effects for GFR decline, end-stage renal disease (ESRD), and mortality.

2. Methods

We used data from the Asian Kidney Disease Study as previously described [10]. Briefly, stable CKD patients were recruited from outpatient clinics for a study on glomerular filtration rates (GFR). They collected 24 hr urine collections and presented the next day for a GFR measurement and also provided early morning urine and blood samples. The 24 hr urine collection and early morning spot urine were tested for protein, albumin, and creatinine concentrations. We performed assays on the Siemens Advia 2400 (http://www.siemens.com/). Urine protein was measured using a pyrogallol-based assay calibrated to the manufacturer's internal standard. Urine albumin was measured using a PEG-enhanced immunoturbidimetric assay and was also calibrated to an internal standard. Creatinine was measured by an enzymatic method (creatininase) in a central laboratory accredited by the College of American Pathologists and the assay was calibrated with manufacturer-provided materials traceable to standardized creatinine (National Institute for Standards and Technology Standard Reference Material 967) measured by isotope dilution mass spectrometry (as recommended by the National Kidney Disease Education Program, http://www.nkdep.nih.gov/). To extract the last known serum creatinine, the hospital clinical laboratory database was reviewed. All participants were cross-referenced with our ESRD database for date of dialysis initiation or death. All longitudinal follow-up data for this study were correct till January 15, 2012. This study was approved by the National Healthcare Group, Domain-Specific Review Board (D/07/524 and 2007/00225).

3. Statistics

Where appropriate, variables were naturally Log-transformed before linear regression to correct for nonnormal distribution and nonconstant variability of observed points around the regression line. We used Bland-Altman analysis of agreement to assess UACR and UPCR in predicting 24 hr urine albumin excretion and 24 hr urine protein excretion, respectively. For comparisons with earlier studies, we used non-SI units in calculating the urine protein or albumin to creatinine ratios [3, 4]. Conversion equations between UACR, UPCR, 24 hr urine protein excretion, and 24 hr urine albumin excretion were developed. To assess these equations, an external dataset of 45 participants with similarly collected 24 hr urine sample followed by an early morning spot urine sample the next day was used as a validation test dataset. The predicted variable was compared to the measured values by Pearson correlation r and Wilcoxon signed rank test. Because clinical practice and research analysts commonly use UACR and UPCR to

estimate the respective 24 hr urine excretion rates above the clinically significant thresholds of albumin >300 mg/day and protein >0.5 g/day, we also analyzed the measured (main derivation dataset, $n = 232$) and equation-predicted UACR and UPCR (validation dataset, $n = 45$) for their predictive abilities in terms of sensitivity, specificity, positive predictive value (PPV), and negative predictive value (NPV) [11, 12].

We estimated GFR using the CKD-EPI equation [13]. To compare the predictive performance of each method of urine protein or albumin assessment with GFR decline, we developed models using linear regression. We used stepwise linear regression by P value threshold for entry or exit from the models in a mixed direction with no rules to select the variables for models predicting GFR decline. The initial variables screened were age, gender, ethnicity, initial serum creatinine, initial serum urea, smoking history, medical history of diabetes, hypertension, coronary artery disease, peripheral artery disease, systolic blood pressure, diastolic blood pressure, body mass index, serum albumin, UACR, UPCR, 24 hr urine protein excretion, and 24 hr urine albumin excretion. The urine estimation or measurement method in the best model was substituted in turn for three additional models for comparisons. Variables with P values $\leq$ 0.05 and ethnicity were included in the final models. We assessed the linear regression models by reviewing the R^2, AIC (Akaike information criterion), and BIC (Bayesian information criterion) [14, 15]. Since R^2 always will increase with an increasing number of predictor variables in a model, we select our model using the AIC and BIC which penalizes models for having large number of predictor variables. AIC might favor more complex models and overfit, while BIC may select a parsimonious model and underfit. For our model assessments, the lowest AIC and BIC criteria indicate the best model. Similarly, we also assessed the predictive performance of urine protein estimations for the combined end-point of ESRD and death using Cox-proportional hazards modeling. Analyses were performed on JMP 10 (Cary, NC, USA) and R (http://www.r-project.org/).

4. Results

There were 232 patients with characteristics as shown in Table 1. Four patients had 24-hour urine protein excretion >3.5 g. The correlation of spot urine estimation ratios (UPCR and UACR to 24 hr urine protein and albumin excretion, resp.) is shown in Figure 1. UACR appears to predict 24 hr urine albumin excretion better as the slope is closer to 1. The prediction equations are

Log 24 hr urine protein excretion (g)

$$= -0.617019 + 0.7150918 \times \text{Log UPCR (mg/mg)};$$

$$\left(R^2 = 0.64, P < 0.001 \right),$$

Log 24 hr urine albumin excretion (g)

$$= -0.800153 + 0.8257142 \times \text{Log UACR (mg/mg)};$$

$$\left(R^2 = 0.74, P < 0.001 \right).$$

$$(1)$$

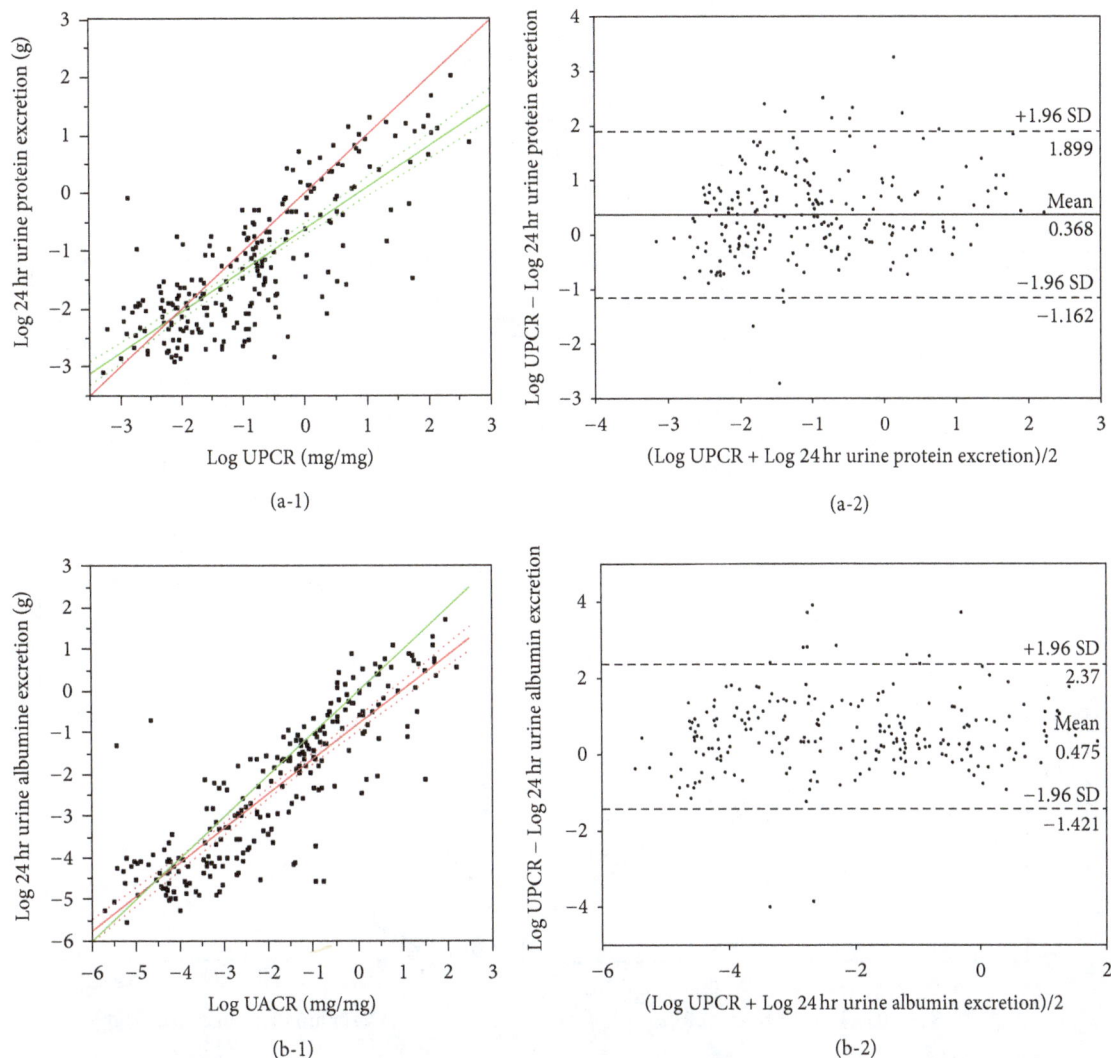

FIGURE 1: Distribution of urine estimation ratios to 24 hr urine measurements. (a-1) UPCR versus 24 hr urine protein excretion. Correlation $r = 0.79$, 95% CI 0.74–0.83. Bold line: line of identity; fine line: regression line; dotted lines: 95% CI of the regression line. (a-2) Limits of agreement of Log-transformed UPCR and 24 hr urine protein excretion. (b-1) UACR versus 24 hr urine albumin excretion. Correlation $r = 0.86$, 95% CI 0.82–0.89. Bold line: line of identity; fine line: regression line; dotted lines: 95% CI of the regression line. (b-2) Limits of agreement of Log-transformed UACR and 24 hr urine albumin excretion.

UPCR has poorer correlation to 24 hr urine protein excretion ($r = 0.80$, 95% CI 0.75–0.84) than UACR has to 24 hr urine albumin excretion ($r = 0.86$, 95% CI 0.82–0.89). UACR is highly correlated to UPCR ($r = 0.99$, 95% CI 0.99-0.99) (Figure 2). 24 hr urine albumin excretion is also highly correlated to 24 hr urine protein excretion ($r = 0.99$, 95% CI 0.99-0.99). UACR is less correlated with 24 hr urine protein excretion ($r = 0.78$, 95% CI 0.72–0.83) than UPCR is with 24 hr urine albumin excretion ($r = 0.81$, 95% CI 0.76–0.85). The sensitivity and specificity of UACR of between 30 and 300 mg/mg for predicting 24 hr urine albumin excretion of between 30 and 300 mg (microalbuminuria) are 0.69 and 0.77, respectively. The PPV and NPV are 0.63 and 0.81, respectively. The sensitivity and specificity of UACR of >300 mg/mg for predicting 24 hr urine albumin excretion of >300 mg (macroalbuminuria) are 0.94 and 0.84, respectively. The PPV and NPV are 0.70 and 0.97, respectively. The sensitivity and

specificity of UPCR of >0.5 mg/mg for predicting 24 hr urine protein excretion of >0.5 g/day are 0.90 and 0.81, respectively. The PPV and NPV are 0.66 and 0.95, respectively.

The various conversion equations derived from the main study data ($n = 232$) are in Table 2. Using the external validation dataset ($n = 45$) for assessing the performance of the conversion equations, predicted spot urine ratios were highly correlated but significantly differed from measured spot urine values. UPCR correlated with "predicted 24 hr urine protein excretion" ($r = 0.63$, 95% CI 0.41–0.78) better than UACR with "predicted 24 hr urine albumin excretion" ($r = 0.55$, 95% CI 0.31–0.73). The sensitivity and specificity of "predicted-UACR," calculated from UPCR, of >300 mg/mg for predicting 24 hr urine albumin excretion of >300 mg (macroalbuminuria) are 0.059 and 1.0, respectively. The PPV and NPV are 1.0 and 0.64, respectively. The sensitivity and specificity of "predicted-UACR," calculated from 24 hr urine

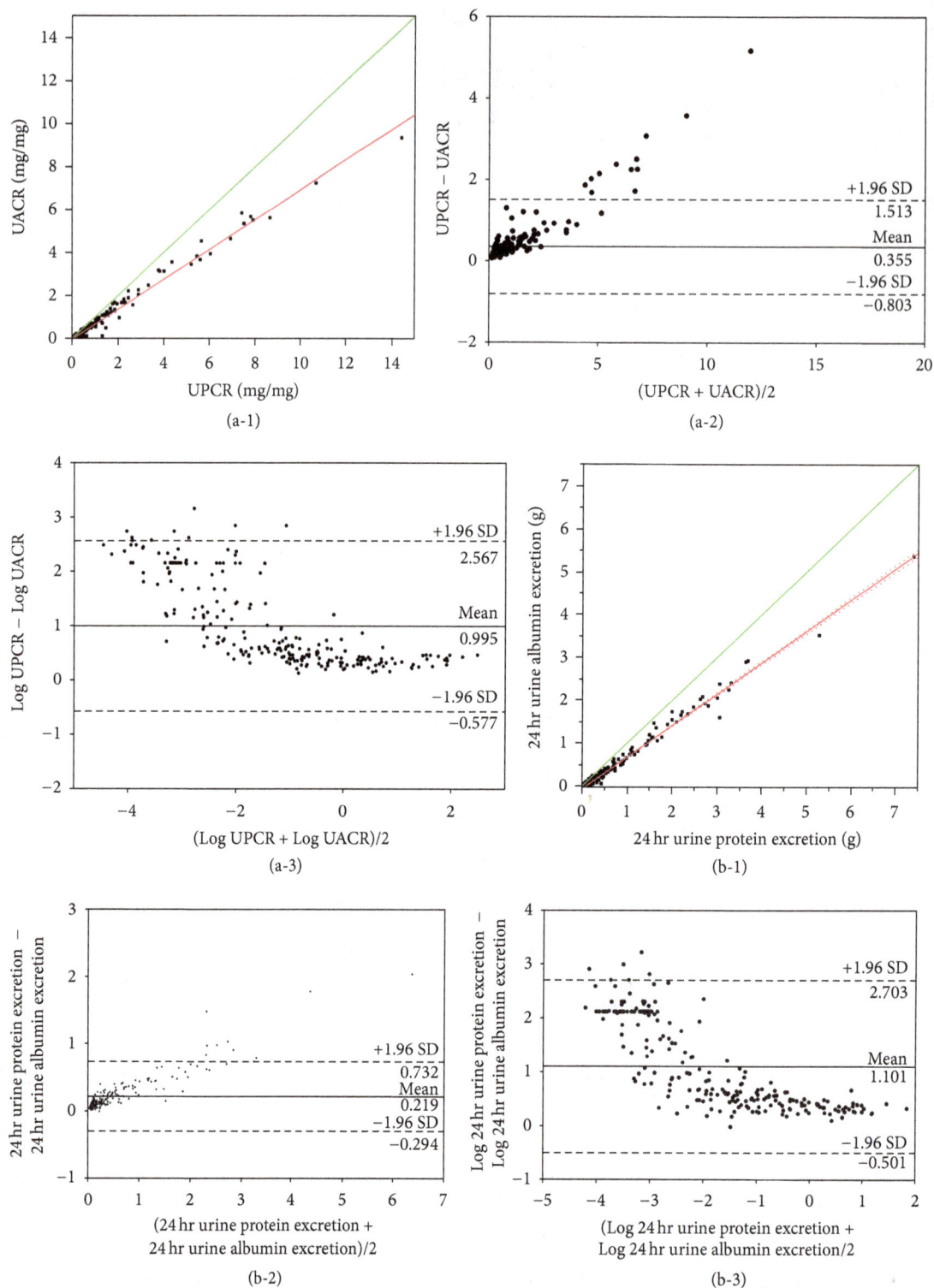

FIGURE 2: Urine albumin versus urine protein excretion. (a-1) UPCR versus UACR. Correlation $r = 0.99$, 95% CI 0.99-0.99. Bold line: line of identity; fine line: regression line; dotted lines: 95% CI of the regression line. (a-2) Limits of agreement of UPCR and UACR. (a-3) Limits of agreement of Log-transformed UPCR and UACR. (b-1) 24 hr urine protein excretion versus 24 hr urine albumin excretion. Correlation $r = 0.99$, 95% CI 0.99-0.99. Bold line: line of identity; fine line: regression line; dotted lines: 95% CI of the regression line. (b-2) Limits of agreement of 24 hr urine protein excretion and 24 hr urine albumin excretion. (b-3) Limits of agreement of Log-transformed 24 hr urine protein excretion and 24 hr urine albumin excretion.

TABLE 1: Characteristics of participants.

Age (years)	58.4 ± 12.8
Male (n, %)	120 (51.7)
Ethnicity (n, %)	
All	232 (100)
Chinese	94 (40.5)
Malay	74 (31.9)
Indian	56 (24.1)
Others	8 (0.03)
Height (m)	1.59 ± 0.09
Weight (kg)	70.3 ± 15.9
Body mass index (kg/m^2)	27.6 ± 5.5
Body surface area (m^2)	1.72 ± 0.21
Measured GFR (mL/min/1.73 m^2)	51.7 ± 27.5
Serum creatinine (μmol/L)	153 ± 92
Serum protein (g/L)	72.2 ± 5.7
Serum albumin (g/L)	41.8 ± 3.2
Serum urea (mmol/L)	8.35 ± 6.35
24 hr urine volume (L)	1.76 ± 0.78
24 hr urine protein (g)	0.6 ± 0.9
24 hr urine albumin (mg)	383.7 ± 685.9
24 hr urine creatinine (mmol)	8.2 ± 3.6
Spot urine protein (g/L)	0.64 ± 1.04
Spot urine albumin (mg/L)	413.3 ± 721.5
Spot urine creatinine (mmol/L)	6.9 ± 4.6
UPCR (mg/mg)	1.03 ± 1.87
UACR (mg/mg)	0.68 ± 1.3
Diabetes (n, %)	119 (51)
Hypertension (n, %)	192 (83)
Cause of CKD (n, %)	
Hypertension	115 (49.6)
Diabetic nephropathy	54 (23.3)
Glomerular disease	38 (16.4)
Polycystic kidney disease	6 (2.6)
Obstructive kidney disease	4 (1.7)
Other or unknown cause	15 (6.5)

Data shown as mean ± SD or frequency (percentage).

protein excretion, of >300 mg/mg for predicting 24 hr urine albumin excretion of >300 mg (macroalbuminuria) are 1.0 and 0.89, respectively. The PPV and NPV are 0.85 and 1.0, respectively. The sensitivity and specificity of "predicted-UPCR," calculated from UACR, of >0.5 mg/mg for predicting 24 hr urine protein excretion of >0.5 g/day are 0.1 and 1.0, respectively. The PPV and NPV are 1.0 and 0.58, respectively.

There were 225 patients with available follow-up serum creatinine to determine estimated GFR decline. By stepwise linear regression, we developed 4 final models to compare the performance of UACR, UPCR, and 24 hr urine protein or albumin excretion (Table 3). In all models, the method of urine protein or albumin assessment and the initial serum urea were significant. The model containing 24 hr urine protein excretion predicted GFR decline best. All the models had good predictive performance for GFR decline, with the best performance in the model that included 24 hr urine protein excretion, followed in order by 24 hr urine albumin excretion, UPCR, and UACR.

The median follow-up was 37 months (IQR 26–41). There were 19 patients who reached ESRD (9/19, 47% women) and 9 (3/9, 33% women) who died during the follow-up period (4 had ESRD before dying). Patients who reached ESRD were of similar age (59.8 ± 10.3 versus 58.8 ± 13.0 years) but had a higher serum creatinine (311 ± 113 versus 138 ± 75 μmol/L) and 24 hr urine albumin (1515 ± 1251 versus 283 ± 504 mg). We created 4 Cox proportional hazard models to compare the performance of the various proteinuria assessments for predicting the combined end-point of ESRD and death (Table 4). All models, which included the standard adjusters (age, gender, and ethnicity), were significant for all methods of proteinuria assessment (all $P < 0.001$) and Log- serum urea (all $P < 0.001$).

5. Discussion

This is the first prospective study of a multiethnic Asian population with a wide variety of CKD (diabetic and nondiabetic) patients that simultaneously evaluates early morning spot urine prediction ratios to 24 hr urine collections, while accounting for the standardization of the creatinine assay. Previous studies were retrospective and did not have simultaneous collection of spot urine and 24 hr urine collections [16]. Clinical practice and research involving CKD patients are highly dependent on the use of urine protein or albumin to creatinine ratios as estimates of their respective 24 hr urine excretions. Yet, many are unaware of the implications of the use of urine ratios [17, 18]. Fundamentally, the main questions that need to be answered are as follows. (1) Does UACR or UPCR predict 24 hr urine albumin or protein excretion? (2) Which spot urine ratio predicts 24 hr urine excretion better? (3) In our setting, how do the ratios relate to the 24 hr urine excretions? Especially, now that we have standardized creatinine assays but not for albumin and protein assays. And, of course, (4) which parameter (ratios or 24 hr urine excretions) predicts longitudinal outcomes data better (GFR declines, ESRD, or mortality in CKD patients)?

Our study shows that UACR is correlated to 24 hr urine albumin excretion better than UPCR. We did not find as high a correlation for UPCR as the earlier studies [3, 4]. This may be partly due to creatinine calibration which results in a systematically larger ratio. The clinical practice guideline for the identification and classification of CKD incorporates UACR in addition to estimated GFR for staging CKD. Our study derived the conversion equations for clinical research or practice needing spot or 24 hr urine albumin or protein excretions, specific to the assay methods. On average, predicted spot urine ratios were reasonably correlated but were significantly different from measured values. Many clinical and research databases contain both UACR and UPCR in the same patients; analysts often apply conversion equations for the purposes of analysis. But the sensitivity of "predicted UACR" or "predicted UPCR" for identifying clinically significant 24 hr urine excretion rates is poor. Therefore, we do not recommend using the conversion equations of

TABLE 2: Equations for converting spot estimates and 24 hr urine measurements.

(a) Conversion predicting equations

Equations	P value
Log 24 hr urine protein excretion (g) = −0.617019 + 0.7150918 × Log UPCR (mg/mg)	<0.001
Log 24 hr urine albumin excretion (g) = −0.800153 + 0.8257142 × Log UACR (mg/mg)	<0.001
Log UACR (mg/mg) = −0.656352 + 1.3881178 × Log UPCR (mg/mg)	<0.001
Log UPCR (mg/mg) = 0.3216439 + 0.6394674 × Log UACR (mg/mg)	<0.001
Log UACR (mg/mg) = −0.270587 + 1.2870223 × Log 24 hr urine protein excretion (g)	<0.001

(b) Performance of conversion equations using an external validation dataset ($n = 45$)

Predictor	Predicted variable	Predicted value	Measured value	P value	Correlation (95% CI)
UPCR (mg/mg)	24 hr urine protein excretion (g)	0.74 (0.67–0.82)	0.38 (0.14–0.92)	0.0051	0.63 (0.41–0.78)
UACR (mg/mg)	24 hr urine albumin excretion (g)	0.91 (0.87–0.94)	0.21 (0.02–0.58)	<0.001	0.55 (0.31–0.73)
UPCR (mg/mg)	UACR (mg/mg)	0.01 (0.00–0.03)	0.03 (0.00–0.08)	<0.001	0.97 (0.95–0.98)
UACR (mg/mg)	UPCR (mg/mg)	0.15 (0.04–0.29)	0.05 (0.02–0.13)	<0.001	0.95 (0.91–0.97)
24 hr urine protein excretion (g)	UACR (mg/mg)	0.22 (0.06–0.69)	0.03 (0.00–0.08)	<0.001	0.81 (0.68–0.89)

Reported as median (25th–75th percentile); P value of the difference between predicted and measured values; Pearson correlation r (95% confidence interval).

TABLE 3: Models predicting GFR decline*.

	R^2	95% CI	Estimate	Variables	P value	AIC	BIC
Model 1	0.10	0.028 to 0.172	−0.211	Log 24 hr urine protein excretion	<0.001	524.97	545.65
			0.311	Log serum urea	0.001		
Model 2	0.095	0.025 to 0.166	−0.127	Log 24 hr urine albumin excretion	<0.001	526.13	546.81
			0.291	Log serum urea	0.002		
Model 3	0.071	0.009 to 0.133	−0.148	Log UPCR	0.001	532.38	553.06
			0.289	Log serum urea	0.003		
Model 4	0.066	0.005 to 0.126	−0.092	Log UACR	0.002	533.65	554.33
			0.275	Log serum urea	0.0072		

*All models adjusted for ethnicity.

UACR to UPCR, and vice versa. However, the performance of "predicted-UACR" calculated from 24 hr urine protein excretion appears to be acceptable for identifying clinically significant proteinuria of >0.5 g/day. Nonetheless, in clinical practice, it is currently not recommended to interchangeably convert urine albumin and urine protein concentrations [11].

Contrary to the findings by Ruggenenti et al. in their cohort of only nondiabetic patients, we did not find that UPCR predicted GFR decline better than 24 hr urine protein excretion [4]. But, in all our models, all methods of assessing urine protein excretion rates were significant for predicting GFR decline, ESRD, and mortality. In our opinion, this supports the current practice of using spot urine tests as estimates of assessing 24 hr urine protein or albumin excretion [11, 16]. And all of the methods of assessments are significantly associated with predicting clinical outcomes in a multiethnic Asian population with different types of CKD, making our results more generalizable and supportive of clinical practice and research.

The strengths of our study include a fairly large multiethnic Asian population comprising of both diabetic and nondiabetic CKD, with systematically collected spot and 24 hr urine when compared to previous studies [3, 4]. We also used turbidimetry, a robust method for determining albumin concentrations, although some others advocate using nephelometry as the preferred albumin assay method [7]. Our study is also limited by fewer CKD patients with nephrotic-range proteinuria (24 hr urine protein excretion >3.5 g). However, it had been shown that spot urine estimates were less accurate at higher levels of proteinuria [3, 4]. The urine estimation to 24 hr measurements may be less accurate since the urine collections are self-directed. Conversely, others would also argue that the derived equations are more reflective of actual practice, and, therefore, prediction equations and longitudinal analyses will be more valid and generalizable to clinical practice. Moreover, in practice, we are generally interested in categories of proteinuria excretion, namely, <1 g/day, 1 to 3 g/day, and >3 g/day, and that, at higher levels, one should obtain a 24 hr urine collection to ascertain the parameters for initiating treatment of CKD. The sample size limits the accuracy of the multivariate regression models, and further definitive studies are required.

TABLE 4: Proportional hazards models predicting the combined end-point of ESRD and death.

	Model −Log likelihood	P value	Term	P value	Risk ratio	Lower 95% CI	Upper 95% CI
Model 1	−79.45	<0.001	Log 24 hr urine protein	<0.001	3.87	2.37	6.31
			Log serum urea	<0.001	17.62	6.27	49.54
			Age	0.225	0.97	0.93	1.02
			Gender	0.310	1.66	0.62	4.41
			Malay ethnicity	0.155	2.08	0.76	5.72
			Indian and others ethnicity	0.572	1.43	0.41	4.93
Model 2	−80.03	<0.001	Log 24 hr urine albumin	<0.001	2.90	1.87	4.51
			Log serum urea	<0.001	16.94	6.25	45.89
			Age	0.28	0.98	0.94	1.02
			Gender	0.31	1.65	0.62	4.40
			Malay ethnicity	0.16	2.07	0.75	5.69
			Indian and others ethnicity	0.63	1.36	0.39	4.72
Model 3	−77.30	<0.001	Log UPCR	<0.001	3.82	2.40	6.07
			Log serum urea	<0.001	23.52	7.60	72.85
			Age	0.07	0.96	0.92	1.00
			Gender	0.01	3.89	1.33	11.40
			Malay ethnicity	0.19	1.94	0.72	5.22
			Indian and others ethnicity	0.40	1.71	0.48	6.04
Model 4	−79.38	<0.001	Log UACR	<0.001	2.98	1.93	4.58
			Log serum urea	<0.001	20.67	7.09	60.23
			Age	0.12	0.97	0.92	1.01
			Gender	0.03	3.23	1.15	9.12
			Malay ethnicity	0.18	1.96	0.73	5.24
			Indian and others ethnicity	0.42	1.69	0.48	6.05

All models included the standard terms of age, gender, and ethnicity. Risk ratios for continuous variables are per unit change in the regressor, and for categorical variables: gender (men/women), with women being the reference level.

6. Conclusions

In summary, we appraised the use of urine spot ratios for assessing urine protein excretion rates and developed helpful conversion equations for both clinical research and practice. We showed that all methods of urine protein assessment were comparable for clinical end-points, and any method can be used in clinical practice or research.

Authors' Contribution

Boon Wee Teo, Ping Tyug Loh, and Evan J. C. Lee conceived, supervised, and conducted the study. Boon Wee Teo and Hui Xu recruited the participants and collected the data. Boon Wee Teo, Ping Tyug Loh, Peh Joo Ho, and Kwok Pui Choi analyzed the data. Sharon Saw, Sunil Sethi, Hui Xu, and Boon Wee Teo supervised the laboratory measurements of specimens. Weng Kin Wong, Boon Wee Teo, and Ping Tyug Loh wrote the initial draft of the paper. All authors reviewed and edited the paper.

Acknowledgments

Majority funding for the Asian Kidney Disease Study was awarded by the National University of Singapore Yong Loo Lin School of Medicine Faculty Research Committee, and it is funded in part by the National Medical Research Council (block vote) and the National Kidney Foundation of Singapore. Boon Wee Teo is a recipient of the NHG-NUS Clinical Leadership in Research Award 2007 and the NMRC Overseas Fellowship Award 2009 for research studies in kidney function. Sponsors had no role in the study design, data collection, analysis, and interpretation. Other coinvestigators of our study section include Dr. Jialiang Li, Dr. Borys Shuter, and Dr. Arvind Kumar Sinha. Dr. Li supervised the initial statistical analysis. Abstracts of this study were presented in part at Singapore Society of Nephrology Annual Scientific Meeting 2012 by Dr. Weng Kin Wong.

References

[1] National Kidney Foundation, "K/DOQI clinical practice guidelines for chronic kidney disease: evaluation, classification, and stratification," *American Journal of Kidney Diseases*, vol. 39, no. 2, supplement 1, pp. S1–S266, 2002.

[2] G. L. Myers, W. G. Miller, J. Coresh et al., "Recommendations for improving serum creatinine measurement: a report from the Laboratory Working Group of the National Kidney Disease Education Program," *Clinical Chemistry*, vol. 52, no. 1, pp. 5–18, 2006.

[3] R. A. Rodby, R. D. Rohde, Z. Sharon, M. A. Pohl, R. P. Bain, and E. J. Lewis, "The urine protein to creatinine ratio as a predictor of 24-hour urine protein excretion in type 1 diabetic patients with nephropathy," *American Journal of Kidney Diseases*, vol. 26, no. 6, pp. 904–909, 1995.

[4] P. Ruggenenti, F. Gaspari, A. Perna, and G. Remuzzi, "Cross sectional longitudinal study of spot morning urine protein: creatinine ratio, 24 hour urine protein excretion rate, glomerular filtration rate, and end stage renal failure in chronic renal disease in patients without diabetes," *British Medical Journal*, vol. 316, no. 7130, pp. 504–509, 1998.

[5] A. S. Levey, J. Coresh, T. Greene et al., "Expressing the modification of diet in renal disease study equation for estimating glomerular filtration rate with standardized serum creatinine values," *Clinical Chemistry*, vol. 53, no. 4, pp. 766–772, 2007.

[6] W. G. Miller, D. E. Bruns, G. L. Hortin et al., "Current issues in measurement and reporting of urinary albumin excretion," *Clinical Chemistry*, vol. 55, no. 1, pp. 24–38, 2009.

[7] P. Deurenberg and M. Deurenberg-Yap, "Validation of skinfold thickness and hand-held impedance measurements for estimation of body fat percentage among Singaporean Chinese, Malay and Indian subjects," *Asia Pacific Journal of Clinical Nutrition*, vol. 11, no. 1, pp. 1–7, 2002.

[8] A. S. Levey, P. E. de Jong, J. Coresh et al., "The definition, classification, and prognosis of chronic kidney disease: a KDIGO Controversies Conference report," *Kidney International*, vol. 80, no. 1, pp. 17–28, 2011.

[9] "Kidney disease: improving global outcomes (KDIGO) CKD work group: KDIGO 2012 clinical practice guideline for the evaluation and management of chronic kidney disease," *Kidney International Supplements*, vol. 3, pp. 1–150, 2013.

[10] B. W. Teo, H. Xu, D. Wang et al., "GFR estimating equations in a multiethnic asian population," *American Journal of Kidney Diseases*, vol. 58, no. 1, pp. 56–63, 2011.

[11] D. W. Johnson, G. R. D. Jones, T. H. Mathew et al., "Chronic kidney disease and measurement of albuminuria or proteinuria: a position statement," *The Medical Journal of Australia*, vol. 197, no. 4, pp. 224–225, 2012.

[12] A. S. Levey, K.-U. Eckardt, Y. Tsukamoto et al., "Definition and classification of chronic kidney disease: a position statement from kidney disease: improving global outcomes (KDIGO)," *Kidney International*, vol. 67, no. 6, pp. 2089–2100, 2005.

[13] A. S. Levey, L. A. Stevens, C. H. Schmid et al., "A new equation to estimate glomerular filtration rate," *Annals of Internal Medicine*, vol. 150, no. 9, pp. 604–612, 2009.

[14] H. Akaike, "A new look at the statistical model identification," *IEEE Transactions on Automatic Control*, vol. 19, no. 6, pp. 716–723, 1974.

[15] G. Schwarz, "Estimating the dimension of a model," *The Annals of Statistics*, vol. 6, no. 2, pp. 461–464, 1978.

[16] S. Methven, M. S. MacGregor, J. P. Traynor, M. Hair, D. S. J. O'Reilly, and C. J. Deighan, "Comparison of urinary albumin and urinary total protein as predictors of patient outcomes in CKD," *American Journal of Kidney Diseases*, vol. 57, no. 1, pp. 21–28, 2011.

[17] J. Fotheringham, M. J. Campbell, D. G. Fogarty, M. El Nahas, and T. Ellam, "Estimated albumin excretion rate versus urine albumin-creatinine ratio for the estimation of measured albumin excretion rate: derivation and validation of an estimated albumin excretion rate equation," *American Journal of Kidney Diseases*, vol. 63, no. 3, pp. 405–414, 2014.

[18] L. A. Inker, "Albuminuria: time to focus on accuracy," *American Journal of Kidney Diseases*, vol. 63, no. 3, pp. 378–381, 2014.

7

Childhood Nephrotic Syndrome Management and Outcome

Chia-shi Wang,[1,2] **Jia Yan,**[2] **Robert Palmer,**[2] **James Bost,**[2]
Mattie Feasel Wolf,[1] **and Larry A. Greenbaum**[1,2]

[1]*Emory University School of Medicine, 2015 Uppergate Drive NE, Atlanta, GA 30322, USA*
[2]*Children's Healthcare of Atlanta, 1677 Tullie Circle, Atlanta, GA 30329, USA*

Correspondence should be addressed to Chia-shi Wang; chia-shi.wang@emory.edu

Academic Editor: Jochen Reiser

There is a paucity of information on outpatient management and risk factors for hospitalization and complications in childhood nephrotic syndrome (NS). We described the management, patient adherence, and inpatient and outpatient usage of 87 pediatric NS patients diagnosed between 2006 and 2012 in the Atlanta Metropolitan Statistical Area. Multivariable analyses were performed to examine the associations between patient characteristics and disease outcome. We found that 51% of the patients were treated with two or more immunosuppressants. Approximately half of the patients were noted to be nonadherent to medications and urine protein monitoring. The majority (71%) of patients were hospitalized at least once, with a median rate of 0.5 hospitalizations per patient year. Mean hospital length of stay was 4.0 (3.8) days. Fourteen percent of patients experienced at least one serious disease complication. Black race, frequently relapsing/steroid-dependent and steroid-resistant disease, and the first year following diagnosis were associated with higher hospitalization rates. The presence of comorbidities was associated with longer hospital length of stay and increased risk of serious disease complications. Our results highlight the high morbidity and burden of NS and point to particular patient subgroups that may be at increased risk for poor outcome.

1. Introduction

Idiopathic nephrotic syndrome (NS) is one of the most common chronic kidney diseases in children, with a prevalence of approximately 16 cases per 100,000 [1]. It is characterized by heavy proteinuria, hypoalbuminemia, edema, and hyperlipidemia. During active disease, the loss of proteins critical for various biologic functions can result in complications such as infections, thromboembolic disease, and acute kidney injury [1–4]. The current mainstay of treatment is high-dose oral corticosteroids. However, 80 to 90% percent of patients will experience disease relapse, with half relapsing frequently or becoming dependent on corticosteroids to maintain remission. In addition, approximately 7.4–19.6% of children have corticosteroids-resistant disease with poor renal prognosis [5–7]. Repeated and prolonged use of corticosteroids can have adverse effects on metabolism, growth, and behavior [8]. Second-line immunosuppressive agents, such as calcineurin inhibitors, cytotoxic agents, mycophenolate mofetil, and rituximab, are given to those intolerant or resistant to corticosteroids. These agents can cause additional side effects and have expected response rates of only 20–50% [9].

Research has underscored the morbidity and burden of childhood NS. Focal segmental glomerulosclerosis (FSGS), one of the most common histologic variants of NS, is the second-most common cause of end-stage renal disease (ESRD) in the North American Pediatric Renal Transplant Cooperative Study [10]. A cross-sectional analysis of the Kids' Inpatient Database from the Healthcare Cost and Utilization Project (HCUP-KID) revealed that NS resulted in an estimated 48,700 inpatient days and charges totaling $259 million nationally in the years 2006 and 2009. Furthermore, 16% of the discharges had at least one severe complication, including thromboembolism, septicemia, peritonitis, pneumonia, or diabetes [11].

There is a great need to examine the influences on disease outcome in childhood NS. Management of childhood NS involves intense outpatient follow-up and family participation for disease monitoring and treatment. Despite the complexity, few reports exist that describe management patterns. Survey studies have noted significant differences in provider preference for second-line immunosuppressants, glucocorticoid regimens, and when renal biopsies are performed [12, 13]. There are no reports on outpatient clinic visit usage or patient adherence to urine monitoring and medications. There are limited studies on risk factors for increased inpatient usage among pediatric NS patients. Gipson et al. identified patient age 15 years or older, black race, higher socioeconomic status, acute renal failure, thromboembolic disease, hypertension, and infections to be associated with higher inpatient charges [11]. No information is available on predicators for hospitalizations.

We thus performed a retrospective study to assess the relationships between patient characteristics and disease outcome. A thorough review of inpatient and outpatient charts for NS patients was conducted at Children's Healthcare of Atlanta (CHOA), the sole provider of pediatric nephrology care in the Atlanta Metropolitan Statistical Area (MSA). We were able to capture every inpatient and outpatient nephrology encounter and provide descriptions of outpatient management and inpatient usage, which had not previously been reported in pediatric NS. Our goals were to provide an in-depth look at outpatient disease management and to determine risk factors for inpatient utilization and disease complications.

2. Materials and Methods

2.1. Setting. A retrospective chart review was performed on pediatric NS patients diagnosed and managed by the Division of Pediatric Nephrology at Emory University. Outpatient and inpatient charts for up to 3 years from the time of diagnosis were reviewed. The Division of Pediatric Nephrology at Emory University includes all the pediatric nephrologists practicing in the Atlanta MSA and provides all of the nephrology care at the three campuses of CHOA, the only pediatric hospitals within the Atlanta MSA. We were thus able to capture all renal outpatient encounters and all inpatient encounters. The study was approved by the CHOA institutional review board.

2.2. Study Population. We screened patients followed by the Division of Pediatric Nephrology at Emory University for the diagnosis of NS by using *International Classifications of Diseases, Ninth Revision, Clinical Modification* (ICD-9 CM) diagnostic codes 581.3, 581.9, and 582.1. A single pediatric nephrologist (Chia-shi Wang, MD) reviewed each patient's demographic, clinical, laboratory, and histologic information for inclusion and exclusion. We included patients who were >1 and <18 years of age at the onset of NS, met the clinical diagnosis of idiopathic NS (edema, nephrotic range proteinuria, and hypoalbuminemia), resided in the Atlanta MSA at time of diagnosis and during the entire period of

follow-up, and were diagnosed between 1/1/2006 and 1/1/2012. Patients who had been hospitalized outside of CHOA during the follow-up period were excluded. Other exclusion criteria included renal biopsy findings other than minimal change disease (MCD), FSGS, or a variant (mesangial proliferation, IgM deposits, C1q deposits); ESRD; renal transplantation; or secondary causes of nephrotic syndrome (e.g., systemic lupus erythematosus).

2.3. Measurements. Clinical, demographic, and outpatient care adherence characteristics were collected from outpatient records. Variables of interest included sex, age at time of diagnosis, race, ethnicity, insurance type at time of diagnosis, renal histopathology (if biopsy performed), presence of comorbid disease at time of diagnosis (epilepsy, congenital heart disease, inflammatory bowel disease, chronic lung disease, asthma/airway reactive disease, prematurity, or other), NS disease status by corticosteroid response, and use of second-line immunosuppressive agents (e.g., mycophenolate, tacrolimus). NS disease status is classified based on the definitions in Kidney Disease, Improving Global Outcomes [8]. Patients are classified as having steroid-resistant NS (SRNS) if they fail to achieve remission after eight weeks of corticosteroid therapy. Among patients who achieve remission within eight weeks of starting corticosteroid therapy, the disease is classified as frequently relapsing NS (FRNS) if there are two or more relapses within six months of initial response or four or more relapses in any 12-month period; steroid-dependent NS (SDNS) if there are two consecutive relapses during corticosteroid taper, or within 14 days of ceasing therapy; otherwise, the disease is classified as steroid-sensitive, infrequently relapsing NS (SSNS). The classification is made based on the clinical response to corticosteroids in the first three years following diagnosis.

All outpatient nephrology clinic visits pertaining to the treatment and monitoring of NS were reviewed, including both routinely scheduled and acute visits. The numbers of completed and missed clinic appointments were recorded. Percent "no-show" was the number of missed appointments divided by the total number of clinic appointments. A patient was considered as nonadherent with prescribed clinic visits if they had >20% "no-show" during the follow-up period. Assessment of adherence to home urine protein monitoring and medications were based on the documentation of treating physicians who subjectively noted good or poor adherence.

Inpatient records for up to three years from time of diagnosis were reviewed. Each hospitalization was reviewed for its relationship to NS. Only hospitalizations indicated for the management of NS complications or treatment side-effects were included. The number of hospitalizations, length of stay (LOS), intensive care unit (ICU) status, and serious complications were recorded. A serious complication was defined as one of the following: bacterial peritonitis (with or without culture confirmation), septicemia, shock, blood clot(s) (radiologically confirmed), acute kidney injury requiring dialysis, or seizures from hyponatremia or hypertension. Edema, asymptomatic electrolyte abnormalities, and asymptomatic hypertension were not considered serious complications. Disease complications were recorded for each patient if they were the reasons for hospitalization or if they occurred during hospitalization.

2.4. Statistical Analysis. Demographic and clinical characteristics were described by number of patients and percentages. The number of occurrences and percentage of patients were computed for hospitalizations and serious disease complications. Mean and standard deviation or median and interquartile range, where appropriate, were computed for number of outpatient clinic visits, number of clinic appointment "no-shows," hospitalizations, and length of stay (LOS).

Associations of clinical and demographic factors with the number of hospitalizations per year were assessed with Poisson regression. We applied generalized estimating equations to the Poisson distribution to account for within-patient correlation. Independent variables were considered for the model based on clinical relevance and include age, sex, race and ethnicity, insurance status, disease status, comorbidities, and year since diagnosis. Renal histopathology was not included in the model as a large number of patients did not undergo biopsy. Adherence and use of second-line immunosuppressants variables were not included in the model due to difficulty delineating the causal pathway, that is, whether adherence/medications influences the risk of hospitalizations or whether hospitalizations influence the likelihood of adherence to therapy/medications prescribed. Parameter estimates from the model were exponentiated to produce rate ratios.

Associations of clinical and demographic factors with the development of severe disease complications in patients over the duration of follow-up were assessed with logistic regression. Independent variables included in the model were determined a priori based on clinical significance and included age, sex, race and ethnicity, insurance, disease status, and comorbidities. Model fit was assessed by the Hosmer-Lemeshow test.

Linearity of the continuous outcome variable LOS in days per hospitalization was assessed graphically and by skewness and kurtosis measures. Logarithmic transformation of LOS was carried out due to high skewness. Associations between the clinical and demographic factors with LOS were assessed with linear regression. Parameter estimates were then back-transformed to the linear scale to produce mean proportional change in LOS.

Significance level for tests of association was set at 0.05. Statistical analysis was performed using the SAS system, version 9.4 (SAS Institute, Cary, NC).

3. Results

3.1. Patient Characteristics. A total of 87 patients contributed data. All had complete inpatient and outpatient records for 1 year following diagnosis. Eight-two patients (94%) had complete records for 2 years, and 80 patients (92%) had complete records for 3 years. Reasons for lacking year 2 and year 3 records were discharge from clinic (2 out of 87, 2%) and lost to follow-up (5 out of 87, 6%). Clinical and demographic characteristics are shown in Table 1. The majority of patients had steroid sensitive disease (81.6%), with

55% dependent on corticosteroids and relapsing frequently. Eighteen percent of the patients had SRNS. The proportion of patients in each disease category was comparable to prior findings [9, 14]. Patient with SRNS tended to be older and had a more equal male to female ratio compared to those with SSNS and FRNS/SDNS. The majority of SRNS patients were also black, in contrast to patients with SSNS and FRNS/SDNS. The demographic breakdown of our patients was also similar to prior reports [1]. A greater proportion of SRNS patients underwent renal biopsy.

3.2. Outpatient Management. The management and adherence patterns of patients by NS classification are shown in Table 2. Patients had an overall mean (SD) of 3.7 (2.0) clinic visits per year, with a mean of 5.0 (2.0) visits in the first year, 3.0 (1.6) visits in the second year, and 2.8 (1.6) visits in the third year. On average, patients with SSNS had the least number of prescribed clinic visits (2.59, 1.1), followed by patients with FRNS/SDNS (4.33, 1.7). On average, patients with SRNS had the most number of prescribed clinic visits (4.71, 1.7). All patients were initially treated with corticosteroids for a minimum of 6 weeks on presentation. Forty-four patients (51%) were subsequently treated with at least one additional immunosuppressive agent. These 44 patients had either FRNS/SDNS or SRNS disease. The choice of agents differed between FRNS/SDNS and SRNS patients. The preferred agent for patients with FRNS/SDNS was mycophenolate mofetil, selected first in 21 of the 29 (72%) patients who received agents in addition to corticosteroids. In contrast, the preferred agent for patients with SRNS was cyclosporine, selected first in seven out of 12 (58%) patient who received agents in addition to corticosteroids.

Thirty-two out of 71 patients (45%) who were prescribed urine dipsticks for home monitoring were subjectively noted by their treating physicians to be nonadherent with urine monitoring. Thirty-seven out of 87 (43%) patients were noted to be poorly adherent to prescribed NS medications. Twenty-eight out of 87 (32%) of patients had >20% "no-shows" to clinic appointments. Mean percentage of "no-shows" was 14% (22), with a mean of 11% (16) in the first year, 15% (24) in the second year, and 19% (25) in the third year.

3.3. Inpatient Care Utilization. A total of 184 hospitalizations were recorded for the 87 patients. Median hospitalization rate was 0.5 hospitalization per patient year (interquartile range = 0.0 to 1.0). Sixty-two patients (71%) had at least one hospitalization, and 13 patients (15%) had 5 or more hospitalizations in the first 3 years following diagnosis. The mean (SD) LOS per hospitalization was 4.0 (3.8) days.

3.4. Complications. Four out of 184 hospitalizations (2%) resulted in an ICU stay. Reasons for the ICU stays were respiratory distress due to pleural effusion in a child with FRNS/SDNS, respiratory distress due to bacterial pneumonia in a child with FRNS/SDNS, hyponatremia in a child with FRNS/SDNS, and seizures from hypertension in a child with SRNS. Twelve of the 87 (14%) patients experienced serious complications in the first 3 years of disease: two patients with SSNS, seven patients with FRNS/SDNS, and 3 patients

TABLE 1: Characteristics of patients with childhood nephrotic syndrome diagnosed between 2006 and 2012 in the Atlanta MSA.

Characteristic	SSNS ($n = 23$)	FRNS/SDNS ($n = 48$)	SRNS ($n = 16$)	Total ($n = 87$)
Sex				
Male	17 (74)	32 (67)	9 (56)	58 (67)
Female	6 (26)	16 (33)	7 (44)	29 (33)
Age at diagnosis				
1–5 years	17 (74)	27 (56)	3 (19)	47 (54)
6–12 years	6 (26)	15 (31)	5 (31)	26 (30)
13–18 years	0 (0)	6 (13)	8 (50)	14 (16)
Race and ethnicity				
White, non-Hispanic	6 (26)	15 (31)	2 (13)	23 (26)
Black	7 (30)	19 (40)	13 (81)	39 (45)
White, Hispanic	4 (17)	9 (19)	1 (6)	14 (16)
Other	6 (26)	5 (10)	0 (0)	11 (13)
Insurance				
Private	11 (48)	22 (46)	6 (38)	39 (45)
Medicaid	11 (48)	23 (48)	8 (50)	42 (48)
None	1 (4)	3 (6)	2 (13)	6 (7)
Histopathology				
No biopsy	22 (96)	27 (56)	2 (13)	51 (59)
MCD	0 (0)	17 (35)	5 (31)	22 (25)
FSGS	1 (4)	1 (2)	6 (38)	8 (9)
Other	0 (0)	3 (6)	3 (19)	6 (8)
Comorbidity				
None	19 (83)	40 (83)	11 (69)	70 (80)
Asthma	3 (13)	7 (15)	1 (6)	11 (13)
Epilepsy	1 (4)	0 (0)	2 (13)	3 (3)
Inflammatory bowel disease	0 (0)	1 (2)	1 (6)	2 (2)
Prematurity	0 (0)	2 (4)	0 (0)	2 (2)
Other	1 (4)	1 (2)	1 (6)	3 (3)

Data are presented as the number of patients with the percentage in parenthesis.
FRNS, frequently relapsing nephrotic syndrome; MCD, minimal change disease; FSGS, focal segmental glomerulosclerosis; SDNS, steroid-dependent nephrotic syndrome; SRNS, steroid-resistant nephrotic syndrome; SSNS, steroid-sensitive and infrequently relapsing nephrotic syndrome.

with SRNS. Eight patients (9%) experienced bacterial peritonitis, 4 patients (4.6%) experienced septicemia or shock, 2 (2%) experienced blood clots, 1 patient (1%) required renal replacement therapy for acute kidney injury, and 1 patient (1%) developed seizures from hypertension.

3.5. Predictors for NS Morbidity. Our multivariable analysis showed that FRNS/SDNS and SRNS were associated with >4-times higher rates of hospitalization (rate ratio (RR) = 4.43, 95% confidence interval (CI) = 2.74 to 7.15; and RR = 4.14, CI = 1.64 to 10.44; resp.), relative to SSNS. Black race was also significantly associated with increased hospitalization rates (RR = 1.84, CI = 1.04 to 3.25), compared to white race. The hospitalization rates were lower in the second and third year of disease, compared to the first year (RR = 0.35, CI = 0.25 to 0.51; and RR = 0.26, CI = 0.16 to 0.41; resp.). Age at diagnosis, sex, insurance status, and presence of comorbidities were

not significantly associated with the hospitalization rate in this analysis. The results of the analysis are presented in Table 3.

Multivariable analysis of LOS results is presented in Table 4. The presence of comorbidities and severe disease complications were associated with higher LOS (mean increase of 42% (CI = 5% to 93%) and 43% (CI = 6% to 92%), resp.). On average, hospital LOS for black patients was 28% shorter than for white patients (CI = 0.52 to 1.00). Age at diagnosis, sex, insurance status, and disease status were not significantly associated with LOS in this analysis.

Only the presence of comorbidities was found to be associated with the risk of serious complications (OR = 5.36, CI = 1.26 to 22.87). Age at diagnosis, sex, race and ethnicity, insurance status, and disease status were not found to be significantly associated with serious complications. The results of the regression analysis are presented in Table 5.

TABLE 2: Outpatient management and adherence patterns by nephrotic syndrome classification.

Management	SSNS ($n = 23$)	FRNS/SDNS ($n = 48$)	SRNS ($n = 16$)	Total ($n = 87$)
Mean clinic visits per year (SD)	2.59 (1.1)	4.33 (1.7)	4.71 (1.7)	3.7 (2.0)
Immunosuppressive treatment				
Corticosteroids only	23 (100)	19 (40)	4 (25)	46 (53)
Mycophenolate mofetil	0 (0)	24 (50)	6 (38)	30 (34)
Cyclophosphamide	0 (0)	7 (15)	2 (13)	9 (10)
Tacrolimus	0 (0)	7 (15)	3 (19)	10 (11)
Cyclosporine	0 (0)	2 (4)	8 (50)	10 (11)
>1 agents in addition to corticosteroids	0 (0)	10 (21)	4 (25)	14 (16)
Medication adherence				
Adherent	18 (78)	24 (50)	8 (50)	50 (57)
Nonadherent	5 (22)	24 (50)	8 (50)	37 (43)
Clinic follow-up adherence				
Adherent	15 (65)	35 (73)	9 (56)	60 (70)
Nonadherent	8 (35)	13 (27)	7 (44)	28 (32)
				Total ($n = 71$)
Urine monitoring				
Adherent	15 (65)	24 (50)	N/A	39 (55)
Nonadherent	8 (35)	24 (50)	N/A	32 (45)

Data are presented as the number of patients with the percentage in parenthesis or mean and standard deviation in parenthesis.
FRNS, frequently relapsing nephrotic syndrome; MCD, minimal change disease; FSGS, focal segmental glomerulosclerosis; SD, standard deviation; SDNS, steroid-dependent nephrotic syndrome; SRNS, steroid-resistant nephrotic syndrome; SSNS, steroid-sensitive and infrequently relapsing nephrotic syndrome.

4. Discussion

Our findings support previous published reports that childhood NS is a disease of high morbidity and results in significant healthcare burden. The median hospitalization rate of our cohort was high at 0.50 hospitalization per patient year, and the majority of patients were hospitalized at least once (71%). On average, hospitalizations lasted approximately 4 days. Serious complications occurred in 14% of the patients in the first 3 years of follow-up. These results suggest that each NS patient has the potential to contribute significant burden to the healthcare system.

Outpatient management of our patient cohort was also resource-intensive. Clinic visits averaged 3.7 per year in the first 3 years of diagnosis. More than half of the patients were treated with second-line immunosuppressants in addition to corticosteroids, carrying additional monitoring needs. Significantly, providers noted nonadherence to urine monitoring and medications in nearly half of the patients. Furthermore, the rates of "no-shows" to appointments were high at an average of 14%. This is a serious concern as nonadherence is a major cause of treatment failure in pediatric chronic diseases [15].

We hypothesized that disease classification based on steroid response and frequency of relapse would be a predictor of increased hospitalizations and complications, as it is an important determinant of disease prognosis [1]. This was substantiated in our analysis on hospitalizations. FRNS/SDNS and SRNS were associated with increased hospitalization rates compared to children with SSNS. Patients were hospitalized more frequently in the first year of diagnosis. Black race was also found to be associated with increased hospitalization rates despite controlling for disease status and clinical and demographic factors. This may mean that there are other social, economic, or provider/patient factors not captured by our analysis. Disease classification was not associated with increased risk of serious complications as we had hypothesized. It may be possible that our sample size and the number of serious complications were too small to detect a significant difference. Similar to analyses of the HCUP-KID data [11, 16], serious NS complications were associated with longer hospitalizations. In our analysis, black patients had shorter hospitalizations compared to white patients after controlling for disease status, complications, and other clinical and demographic factors. This again suggests the need to explore determinants of health and disease management that result in racial differences. The presence of any comorbid condition, not surprisingly, was significantly associated with increased LOS and development of serious complications. Our analyses suggest that patients with FRNS/SDNS or SRNS with other comorbid conditions may be a particularly vulnerable group.

Our study provided a detailed description of inpatient and outpatient care usage in children with NS. The strengths of our single center analysis include the ability to accurately define a cohort of incident patients with idiopathic NS and capture all instances of disease complications without relying on ICD-9 CM diagnostic codes. We were able to report

TABLE 3: Association between patient characteristics and hospitalization rate.

Variables	Adjusted RR (95% CI)	P value
Age		
1–5 years	1.00 (referent)	
6–12 years	1.10 (0.63 to 1.91)	0.74
13–18 years	1.11 (0.52 to 2.36)	0.79
Sex		
Male	1.00 (referent)	
Female	0.82 (0.55 to 1.23)	0.34
Race and ethnicity		
White, non-Hispanic	1.00 (referent)	
Black	1.84 (1.04 to 3.25)	0.04*
White, Hispanic	1.41 (0.65 to 3.07)	0.38
Other	1.11 (0.56 to 2.21)	0.76
Insurance		
None	1.0 (referent)	
Medicaid	1.15 (0.59 to 2.23)	0.67
Private	0.74 (0.36 to 1.57)	0.45
Disease status		
SSNS	1.00 (referent)	
FRNS/SDNS	4.43 (2.74 to 7.15)	<0.001*
SRNS	4.14 (1.64 to 10.44)	0.003*
Comorbidity		
No	1.00 (referent)	
Yes	1.33 (0.75 to 2.37)	0.33
Year since diagnosis		
1	1.00 (referent)	
2	0.35 (0.24 to 0.51)	<0.001*
3	0.26 (0.16 to 0.41)	<0.001*

CI, confidence interval; FRNS, frequently relapsing nephrotic syndrome; RR, rate ratio; SDNS, steroid-dependent nephrotic syndrome; SRNS, steroid-resistant nephrotic syndrome; SSNS, steroid-sensitive and infrequently relapsing nephrotic syndrome.
*$P < 0.05$.

TABLE 4: Association between patient characteristics and length of stay among hospitalized patients.

Variables	Adjusted β estimate[a] (95% CI)	P value
Age		
1–5 years	1.00 (referent)	
6–12 years	1.21 (0.89 to 1.65)	0.21
13–18 years	1.24 (0.88 to 1.75)	0.21
Sex		
Male	1.00 (referent)	
Female	1.11 (0.86 to 1.43)	0.41
Race and ethnicity		
White, non-Hispanic	1.00 (referent)	
Black	0.72 (0.52 to 1.00)	0.05*
White, Hispanic	0.76 (0.51 to 1.14)	0.18
Other	0.61 (0.37 to 1.01)	0.06
Insurance		
None	1.00 (referent)	
Medicaid	0.83 (0.53 to 1.30)	0.41
Commercial	0.74 (0.46 to 1.19)	0.21
Disease status		
SSNS	1.00 (referent)	
FRNS/SDNS	0.81 (0.59 to 1.12)	0.20
SRNS	0.87 (0.58 to 1.29)	0.47
Comorbidity		
No	1.00 (referent)	
Yes	1.42 (1.05 to 1.93)	0.03*
Complications		
No	1.00 (referent)	
Yes	1.43 (1.06 to 1.92)	0.02*

CI, confidence interval; FRNS, frequently relapsing nephrotic syndrome; SDNS, steroid-dependent nephrotic syndrome; SRNS, steroid-resistant nephrotic syndrome; SSNS, steroid-sensitive and infrequently relapsing nephrotic syndrome.
[a]After exponentiation to give proportional change in mean length of stay (days) compared to the referent.
*$P < 0.05$.

for the first time hospitalization rates, outpatient clinic visit rates, frequency of various immunosuppressant usage, and adherence in children with NS. We were also able to study the influence of NS disease classification on outcomes.

As a single center report, our findings on inpatient and outpatient usage may have limited generalizability. Due to the restrictive inclusion and exclusion criteria with respect to patient address, our sample size is small. This may have affected the validity of our multivariable analyses and reduced our ability to detect significant associations. In addition, as a retrospective study, we were unable to obtain objective measures for medication and urine monitoring adherence or delineate the causal pathway between adherence and NS disease outcome, a variable we suspect to be crucial in chronic disease outcome. Lastly, the duration of follow-up for our cohort is relatively short. Thus, we did not assess rates of important complications such as end-stage renal disease.

5. Conclusions

In conclusion, our study examined NS disease management and inpatient and outpatient usage and described the associations between clinical and demographic characteristics and disease outcome. Our results suggest that patients with FRNS/SDNS and SRNS with other comorbidities are a vulnerable group. Multicenter, prospective studies would enhance our understanding of how outpatient management and adherence patterns of NS patients influence outcome.

TABLE 5: Association between patient characteristics and serious complications.

Variables	Adjusted OR (95% CI)	P value
Age		
1–5 years	1.00 (referent)	
6–12 years	0.64 (0.11 to 3.75)	0.62
13–18 years	1.42 (0.19 to 10.65)	0.74
Sex		
Male	1.00 (referent)	
Female	0.83 (0.18 to 3.86)	0.81
Race and ethnicity		
White, non-Hispanic	1.00 (referent)	
Black	1.90 (0.30 to 12.19)	0.50
White, Hispanic	0.97 (0.06 to 14.89)	0.98
Other	1.36 (0.09 to 21.12)	0.83
Insurance		
None	1.00 (referent)	
Medicaid	0.31 (0.03 to 2.99)	0.31
Commercial	0.29 (0.03 to 3.01)	0.30
Disease status		
SSNS	1.00 (referent)	
FRNS/SDNS	1.81 (0.30 to 10.87)	0.52
SRNS	1.17 (0.10 to 13.89)	0.90
Comorbidity		
No	1.00 (referent)	
Yes	5.36 (1.26 to 22.87)	0.02[*]

CI, confidence interval; FRNS, frequently relapsing nephrotic syndrome; SDNS, steroid-dependent nephrotic syndrome; SRNS, steroid-resistant nephrotic syndrome; SSNS, steroid-sensitive and infrequently relapsing nephrotic syndrome.
[*]$P < 0.05$.

Disclosure

The content is solely the responsibility of the authors and does not necessary represent the official views of the National Institutes of Health.

Acknowledgments

Chia-shi Wang is supported by the National Center for Advancing Translational Sciences of the National Institutes of Health under Award no. UL1TR000454.

References

[1] A. A. Eddy and J. M. Symons, "Nephrotic syndrome in childhood," *Lancet*, vol. 362, no. 9384, pp. 629–639, 2003.

[2] M. N. Rheault, L. Zhang, D. T. Selewski et al., "AKI in children hospitalized with nephrotic syndrome," *Clinical Journal of the American Society of Nephrology*, vol. 10, no. 12, pp. 2110–2118, 2015.

[3] B. A. Kerlin, R. Ayoob, and W. E. Smoyer, "Epidemiology and pathophysiology of nephrotic syndrome-associated thromboembolic disease," *Clinical Journal of the American Society of Nephrology*, vol. 7, no. 3, pp. 513–520, 2012.

[4] C.-C. Wei, I.-W. Yu, H.-W. Lin, and A. C. Tsai, "Occurrence of infection among children with nephrotic syndrome during hospitalizations," *Nephrology*, vol. 17, no. 8, pp. 681–688, 2012.

[5] Symposium on Pediatric Nephrology, "Primary nephrotic syndrome in children: clinical significance of histopathologic variants of minimal change and of diffuse mesangial hypercellularity," *Kidney International*, vol. 20, no. 6, pp. 765–771, 1981.

[6] P. A. McKinney, R. G. Feltbower, J. T. Brocklebank, and M. M. Fitzpatrick, "Time trends and ethnic patterns of childhood nephrotic syndrome in Yorkshire, UK," *Pediatric Nephrology*, vol. 16, no. 12, pp. 1040–1044, 2001.

[7] W. Wong, "Idiopathic nephrotic syndrome in New Zealand children, demographic, clinical features, initial management and outcome after twelve-month follow-up: Results of A Three-year National Surveillance Study," *Journal of Paediatrics and Child Health*, vol. 43, no. 5, pp. 337–341, 2007.

[8] R. M. Lombel, D. S. Gipson, and E. M. Hodson, "Treatment of steroid-sensitive nephrotic syndrome: new guidelines from KDIGO," *Pediatric Nephrology*, vol. 28, no. 3, pp. 415–426, 2013.

[9] R. M. Lombel, E. M. Hodson, and D. S. Gipson, "Treatment of steroid-resistant nephrotic syndrome in children: new guidelines from KDIGO," *Pediatric Nephrology*, vol. 28, no. 3, pp. 409–414, 2013.

[10] M. B. Leonard, L. A. Donaldson, M. Ho, and D. F. Geary, "A prospective cohort study of incident maintenance dialysis in children: An NAPRTC Study," *Kidney International*, vol. 63, no. 2, pp. 744–755, 2003.

[11] D. S. Gipson, K. L. Messer, C. L. Tran et al., "Inpatient health care utilization in the united states among children, adolescents, and young adults with nephrotic syndrome," *American Journal of Kidney Diseases*, vol. 61, no. 6, pp. 910–917, 2013.

[12] N. MacHardy, P. V. Miles, S. F. Massengill et al., "Management patterns of childhood-onset nephrotic syndrome," *Pediatric Nephrology*, vol. 24, no. 11, pp. 2193–2201, 2009.

[13] S. Samuel, S. Scott, C. Morgan et al., "The canadian childhood nephrotic syndrome (CHILDNEPH) project: overview of design and methods," *Canadian Journal of Kidney Health and Disease*, vol. 1, 2014.

[14] R. M. Lombel, D. S. Gipson, E. M. Hodson, and Kidney Disease: Improving Global Outcomes, "Treatment of steroid-sensitive nephrotic syndrome: new guidelines from KDIGO," *Pediatric Nephrology*, vol. 28, no. 3, pp. 415–426, 2013.

[15] M. Santer, N. Ring, L. Yardley, A. W. A. Geraghty, and S. Wyke, "Treatment non-adherence in pediatric long-term medical conditions: systematic review and synthesis of qualitative studies of caregivers' views," *BMC Pediatrics*, vol. 14, article 63, 2014.

[16] R. M. Ayoob, D. S. Hains, and W. E. Smoyer, "Trends in hospitalization characteristics for pediatric nephrotic syndrome in the USA," *Clinical Nephrology*, vol. 78, no. 2, pp. 106–111, 2012.

8

Results in Assisted Peritoneal Dialysis: A Ten-Year Experience

Sara Querido,[1] **Patrícia Quadros Branco,**[2] **Elisabete Costa,**[2] **Sara Pereira,**[2] **Maria Augusta Gaspar,**[2] **and José Diogo Barata**[2]

[1]*Department of Nephrology Centro Hospitalar do Médio Tejo, Avenida Xanana Gusmão, Apartado 45, 2350-754 Torres Novas, Portugal*
[2]*Department of Nephrology, Centro Hospitalar de Lisboa Ocidental, Carnaxide, Portugal*

Correspondence should be addressed to Sara Querido; saraqueridoconde@gmail.com

Academic Editor: Hermann G. Haller

Background/Aims. Peritoneal dialysis is a successful renal replacement therapy (RRT) for old and dependent patients. We evaluated the clinical outcomes of an assisted peritoneal dialysis (aPD) program developed in a Portuguese center. *Methods*. Retrospective study based on 200 adult incident patients admitted during ten years to a PD program. We included all 17 patients who were under aPD and analysed various parameters, including complications with the technique, hospitalizations, and patient and technique survival. *Results*. The global peritonitis rate was lower in helped than in nonhelped patients: 0.4 versus 0.59 episodes/patient/year. The global hospitalization rate was higher in helped than in nonhelped patients: 0.67 versus 0.45 episodes/patient/year (p = NS). Technique survival in helped patients versus nonhelped patients was 92.3%, 92.3%, 83.1%, and 72.7% versus 91.9%, 81.7%, and 72.1%, and 68.3%, at 1, 2, 3, and 4 years, respectively (p = NS), and patient survival in helped patients versus nonhelped patients was 93.3%, 93.3%, 93.3%, and 74.7% versus 95.9% 93.7%, 89%, and 82% at 1, 2, 3, and 4 years, respectively (p = NS). *Conclusions*. aPD offers an opportune, reliable, and effective home care alternative for patients with no other RRT options.

1. Introduction

In the last two decades, most developed countries have seen a continuous growth in the number of patients with end-stage renal disease (ESRD) commencing renal replacement therapy (RRT). It is possible to identify the main factors which influence this growth: aging of the population due to a greater life expectancy; increase in the incidence of chronic kidney disease related to age; better care of patients with chronic diseases; patients with physical limitations who survive now for longer periods of time; and developments in industry and biotechnology [1, 2]. In Portugal in 2014, almost 60% of patients starting dialysis were over the age of 65 years and only 8,73% of all incident patients started PD. Despite this increase in the number of elderly and dependent patients who need RRT [3], a decline in the utilization of peritoneal dialysis (PD) has occurred in a number of countries since the mid-1990s [4]. This decline is particularly acute for the elderly population [5]. Nevertheless, elderly and dependent patients benefit, specially, from PD as it would avoid travelling to dialysis centers, reduce hemodynamic instability

[6], diminish the risk of central venous catheter-associated bacteremia [5], improve blood pressure control [5, 7], and diminish the bacterial translocation and myocardial stunning [8]. Such a population cohort is susceptible to several physical barriers (decreased strength to lift PD bags, decreased manual dexterity, and decreased vision, mobility, and hearing) and cognitive barriers (language, noncompliance, dementia, and psychiatric conditions). Thus, providing home care assistance to support those patients on PD may help increasing the number of individuals that can be safely treated at home [9] as well as reducing hazards related to personal limitations. Assistance to PD patients involves the identification and training of an individual (other than the patient) to perform dialysis-related tasks, such as connecting the patient to the cycler, setting up the cycler, disconnecting the patient from the cycler, or performing continuous ambulatory peritoneal dialysis (CAPD) exchanges. Since 1997 [10], following the publication of the first successful French experience (when home care nurses treated elderly patients with assisted CAPD) assisted PD (aPD) became a valuable alternative to

provide successful RRT for old and dependent patients. Over the past decade, 11,557 patients started PD in France, out of which 44.6% have been on aPD [11]. The nurses who assist at home in France are paid directly by patients, who are partially reimbursed by the French healthcare insurance. Elderly patients are also successfully treated with PD in Hong Kong, where PD is the first treatment option. In March 2007, 80% of patients (median age: 62.3 years) were on PD [12]. Presently aPD is a dialysis modality in evolution all over Western Europe, Canada, South America, and Asia [11–16].

Although aPD is a valuable and successful renal replacement therapy for old and dependent patients we have to consider and face the lack of social support for patients in our country. The aim of this study was to evaluate the results of the aPD program, offered as first option or last resort to elderly or physically incapable end-stage renal disease patients, considering the clinical outcomes of this technique in a single Portuguese center.

2. Material and Methods

This is a retrospective study performed at a single PD Unity in Portugal (PD Unity of Hospital de Santa Cruz, Carnaxide, Portugal), based on the study of 200 adult incident patients admitted during 10 years (2004–2014) to the PD program. We included and studied a total of 17 patients with physical or cognitive debilities who were under aPD. Assisted-care patients were defined as patients who are unable to perform peritoneal fluid exchange at the beginning of PD or who lack the ability to perform their own treatment and have, therefore, to rely on nonprofessional care, including family members or domestic workers. We analyzed demographic, clinical, and laboratory parameters, complications with the technique, hospitalizations, and patient and technique survival through research in clinical processes. The degree of dependence was analyzed through the application of the Davies Score [17] and Karnofsky Index. Normally distributed variables were expressed as mean ± standard deviation and nonnormally distributed variables were expressed as frequency and percentage. Unadjusted analysis was performed by the Kaplan-Meier method to analyse technique survival between self-care and aPD patients. Technique failure classified the dropout from aPD to Hemodialysis due to peritoneal membrane failure or peritonitis. The technique survival was defined in patients who remained on aPD during the observation period and kidney receptors allograft and patients who died during the aPD program due to any reason other than peritonitis or peritoneal membrane failure.

All statistical tests were performed using the Statistical Package for the Social Sciences (SPSS) 14.0 software (SPSS, Inc., Chicago, IL, USA). Categorical variables were described as numbers or percentage of relative frequencies and quantitative variables as mean ± standard deviation (SD) for continuous normally distributed variables. Cox regression was used to compare survival rates.

Differences between clinical data were assessed by Student's t-test for paired samples for normal variables and paired Wilcoxon test for continuous data with nonnormal distribution. A p value of < 0.05 was considered to be statistically significant.

3. Results

We followed a cohort of 17 consecutive incident patients who were engaged in aPD from January 2004 to October 2014. Median age was 58 ± 20 years; 9 patients were men, 12 patients had hypertension, and 6 had diabetes. Fourteen patients had only one helper, like a close relative; 2 patients were treated by multiple family members; and one patient received treatment from 2 home assistance employees. One patient was on PD due to vascular access failure; 5 patients chose PD; and for 11 patients PD was a family's choice. Five patients had physical and cognitive limitations ab initium. The mean age of the ones who had physical limitations was 35.2 years; patients with cognitive limitations had a mean age of 65 years; 7 patients were treated with automated assisted peritoneal dialysis (APD) and 10 patients with CAPD. The Davies Score was greater than 2 in 52.9%; Karnofsky Index was less than 70 in 64.7%. The patients were under PD for 36.98 ± 31.43 months; 4 of them had an acute onset of the technique; kt/V weekly was 2.22 ± 0.60 and nPCR was 0.88 ± 0.30 g/Kg/day. Peritoneal equilibration test (PET) was performed in 14 patients: 8 were low-average and 6 were high-average transporters. The residual renal function was 3.02 ± 3.85 mL/min/1.73 m^2 and 3 patients were anuric. Demographic and PD related parameters in patients under autonomous PD and aPD are compared in Table 1.

Half of the patients have never had a peritonitis episode; 2 patients had a tunnel infection; and 9 patients had one or more episodes of exit-site infection. Six patients needed more than 1 Tenckhoff catheter; 4 patients died during PD technique; 3 patients started haemodialysis (1 due to PD membrane failure and 2 due to peritonitis); and 1 patient received a kidney allograft. The global peritonitis rate was lower in helped than in nonhelped patients: 0.4 versus 0.59 episodes/patient/year. The global hospitalization rate was higher in helped than in nonhelped patients: 0.67 versus 0.45 episodes/patient/year (p = NS). Technique survival in helped patients versus nonhelped patients was 92,3%, 92.3%, 83,1%, and 72.7% versus 91,9%, 81,7%, 72,1%, and 68,3%, at 1, 2, 3, and 4 years, respectively (p = NS) (Figure 1) and patient survival in helped patients versus nonhelped patients was 93,3%, 93,3%, 93,3%, and 74,7% versus 95,9% 93,7%, 89%, and 82% at 1, 2, 3, and 4 years, respectively (p = NS) (Figure 2). Two patients remained on aPD for more than 7 years.

4. Discussion

The outcome of PD is usually assessed by patient survival, technique survival, and peritonitis incidence [18]. PD shows no difference in patient survival, technique survival, and peritonitis rate [19], between elderly and younger patients. Nonetheless, the outcome of assisted-care and self-care in elderly PD patients is not consistent. The RDPLF report showed that patients under assisted-care, either by family

TABLE 1: Demographic and PD related parameters in patients under autonomous PD and aPD.

	Autonomous PD ($n = 183$)		Assisted PD ($n = 17$)	
Age (years)	55,7 ± 15,2		58 ± 20	
Male ($n/\%$)	122 (66,67)		9 (52,94)	
Hypertension ($n/\%$)	172 (93,99)		12 (70,59)	
Diabetes ($n/\%$)	58 (31,69)		6 (35,29)	
APD ($n/\%$)	64 (34,97)		7 (41,18)	
CAPD ($n/\%$)	119 (65,03)		10 (58,82)	
Time under PD (months)	29,7 ± 22,7		36,98 ± 31,43	
Technique survival (months/%)	12 m	91,9	12 m	92,3
	24 m	81,7	24 m	92,3
	36 m	72,1	36 m	83,1
	48 m	68,3	48 m	72,7
Patient survival (months/%)	12 m	95,9	12 m	93,3
	24 m	93,7	24 m	93,3
	36 m	89	36 m	93,3
	48 m	82	48 m	74,7
Weekly kt/V	2,4 ± 0,70		2,22 ± 0,60	
nPCR (g/Kg/day)	0,93		0,88 ± 0,30	
PET	$N = 175$	D/P < 0,5 = 2%	$N = 14$	D/P 0,5–0,64 = 8
		D/P 0,5–0,64 = 35%		
		D/P 0,65–0,81 = 62%		D/P 0,65–0,81 = 6
		D/P > 0,81 = 1%		
Residual renal function (mL/min/1,73 m^2)	$N = 155$	7,14 ± 11	$N = 14$	3,02 ± 3,85

APD: automated peritoneal dialysis; CAPD: continuous ambulatory peritoneal dialysis; PET: peritoneal equilibration test.

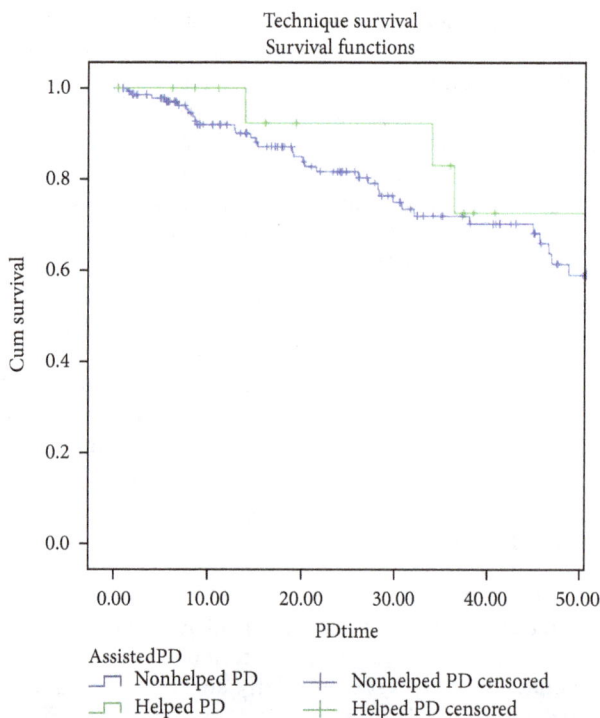

FIGURE 1: Technique survival in helped and nonhelped patients.

members or by nurses, had a poorer survival rate than self-care patients [9]. On the other hand, in a Hong Kong research, no significant differences were found in self-care elderly and nonelderly patients in terms of survival and technique survival. Our study showed that assisted-care PD patients had a poorer outcome in terms of patient survival (12th, 24th, and 48th months) and hospitalization rate but a better performance in terms of peritonitis incidence and technique survival. Lobbedez et al. [11] studied 36 aPD patients and observed a relatively high peritonitis rate, with 50% presenting at least 1 episode per year. Issad et al. showed that peritonitis and exit-site infection rates were not significantly different between aPD and self-care PD patients [10]. Verger et al. revealed that the probability of being peritonitis-free at 2 years was higher for patients assisted by a family member than for those assisted by a private nurse [14]. In our study, the global peritonitis rate was lower in helped than in nonhelped patients (0,4 versus 0,59 episodes/patient/year). As in Verger et al. study, this fact could be explained by the high dedication level of family members.

According to Lobbedez et al. [11] a higher percentage of aPD patients (79%) were hospitalized during the first follow-up year, with peritonitis being the most frequent cause of hospitalization. Our results are similar to the literature with a global hospitalization rate higher in helped than in nonhelped

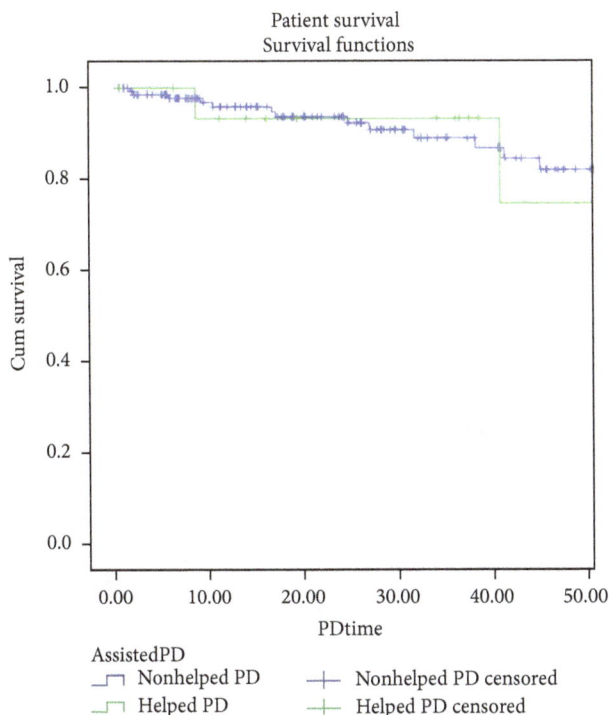

FIGURE 2: Patient survival in helped and nonhelped patients.

patients [0.67 versus 0.45 episodes/patient/year (p = NS)]. This fact could be explained by the high comorbidity index in the aPD patients.

There are not many studies concerning technique survival on assistance method [9, 18]. Those studies showed no association between technique survival and assistance method. We found that technique survival was better in aPD patients. It is difficult to interpret the facts due to the small number of patients in aPD program, but, globally, aPD did not show any disadvantage in terms of technique survival. Lobbedez et al. [11] reported 83% 1-year survival of aPD patients at their center. Povlsen et al. [16] showed that the 1-year and 2-year survival rates of functionally dependent elderly patients on aPD were 58% and 48%, respectively. In our study, the survival rate was 93,3% in the first 3 years under technique, with 2 patients remained on aPD for more than 7 years. The patient who died earlier was a dependent patient with a severe heart disease. Nevertheless, in our series, the survival rate in aPD patients is probably overestimated, considering that these patients had a median age of 58 years, much younger when compared with aPD patients from other series [10, 15].

In UK, aPD is in its infancy. There is no extra funding for providing assistance, so developing a service depends on local enthusiasm. The model of care being developed is based on aPD with one visit per day from a paid carer and the patient or family carrying out the connection and disconnection to/from machine. The community nursing service is not adequately staffed or funded to take on this extra role [20].

5. Conclusions

Our results compare favourably with international reports. In this clinical observation study, aPD offered an opportune, reliable, and effective home care alternative for patients with no other renal replacement therapy options. Due do the lack of support from social institutions the helpers were close relatives in almost every case. It is necessary to adopt measures and institutional support to care for these patients, not forgetting that some of them are young people with a considerable life expectancy, despite cognitive or motor deficits. Nevertheless, larger, longer, and better studies on aPD are warranted. Till now, studies have showed that assistance gives dependent patients an opportunity to have a home-based dialysis modality, increasing the number of patients who can choose an appropriate treatment despite their physical, cognitive, and social conditions.

References

[1] National Institute of Diabetes and Digestive and Kidney Diseases, "United States renal data system 2007 annual data report: atlas of chronic kidney disease & end-stage renal disease in the United States," *American Journal of Kidney Diseases*, vol. 51, supplement 1, pp. S82–S98, 2008.

[2] K. J. Jagger, P. C. W. van Dijk, F. W. Dekker, B. Stengel, K. Simpson, and J. D. Briggs, "The epidemic of aging in renal replacement therapy: an update on elderly patients and their outcomes," *Clinical Nephrology*, vol. 60, no. 5, pp. 352–360, 2003.

[3] E. A. Brown and L. Johansson, "Dialysis options for end-stage renal disease in older people," *Nephron: Clinical Practice*, vol. 119, supplement 1, pp. c10–c13, 2011.

[4] P. Dalal, H. Sangha, and K. Chaudhary, "In peritoneal dialysis, is there sufficient evidence to make 'PD first' therapy?" *International Journal of Nephrology*, vol. 2011, Article ID 239515, 5 pages, 2011.

[5] P. G. Blake, "Peritoneal dialysis—a 'kinder, gentler' treatment for the elderly?" *Peritoneal Dialysis International*, vol. 28, no. 5, pp. 435–436, 2008.

[6] E. A. Brown, L. Johansson, K. Farrington et al., "Broadening Options for Long-term Dialysis in the Elderly (BOLDE): differences in quality of life on peritoneal dialysis compared to haemodialysis for older patients," *Nephrology Dialysis Transplantation*, vol. 25, no. 11, pp. 3755–3763, 2010.

[7] N. Dimkovic, V. Aggarwal, S. Khan, M. Chu, J. Bargman, and D. G. Oreopoulos, "Assisted peritoneal dialysis: what is it and who does it involve?" *Advances in Peritoneal Dialysis*, vol. 25, pp. 165–170, 2009.

[8] N. M. Selby and C. W. McIntyre, "Peritoneal dialysis is not associated with myocardial stunning," *Peritoneal Dialysis International*, vol. 31, no. 1, pp. 27–33, 2011.

[9] C. Castrale, D. Evans, C. Verger et al., "Peritoneal dialysis in elderly patients: report from the French peritoneal dialysis registry (RDPLF)," *Nephrology Dialysis Transplantation*, vol. 25, no. 1, pp. 255–262, 2010.

[10] B. Issad, D. Benevent, M. Allouache et al., "213 Elderly uremic patients over 75 years of age treated with long-term peritoneal dialysis: a French multicenter study," *Peritoneal Dialysis International*, vol. 16, supplement 1, pp. S414–S418, 1996.

[11] T. Lobbedez, R. Moldovan, M. Lecame, B. H. de Ligny, W. El Haggan, and J.-P. Ryckelynck, "Assisted peritoneal dialysis. Experience in a French renal department," *Peritoneal Dialysis International*, vol. 26, no. 6, pp. 671–676, 2006.

[12] P. K.-T. Li and C.-C. Szeto, "Success of the peritoneal dialysis programme in Hong Kong," *Nephrology Dialysis Transplantation*, vol. 23, no. 5, pp. 1475–1478, 2008.

[13] P.-Y. Durand and C. Verger, "The state of peritoneal dialysis in France," *Peritoneal Dialysis International*, vol. 26, no. 6, pp. 654–657, 2006.

[14] C. Verger, M. Duman, P.-Y. Durand, G. Veniez, E. Fabre, and J.-P. Ryckelynck, "Influence of autonomy and type of home assistance on the prevention of peritonitis in assisted automated peritoneal dialysis patients. An analysis of data from the French Language Peritoneal Dialysis Registry," *Nephrology Dialysis Transplantation*, vol. 22, no. 4, pp. 1218–1223, 2007.

[15] D. Paulsen, J. Kronborg, and K. Solbakken, "Organization of peritoneal dialysis in Oppland County, Norway," *Peritoneal Dialysis International*, vol. 26, supplement 2, p. S124, 2006.

[16] J. V. Povlsen, K. Lomholt, and P. Ivarsen, "Assisted APD (aAPD) for the elderly patient dependent on a carer," *Peritoneal Dialysis International*, vol. 26, supplement 2, p. S110, 2006.

[17] S. J. Davies, L. Russell, J. Bryan, L. Phillips, and G. I. Russell, "Comorbidity, urea kinetics, and appetite in continuous ambulatory peritoneal dialysis patients: their interrelationship and prediction of survival," *American Journal of Kidney Diseases*, vol. 26, no. 2, pp. 353–361, 1995.

[18] X. Yang, W. Fang, J. Kothari et al., "Clinical outcomes of elderly patients undergoing chronic peritoneal dialysis: experiences from one center and a review of the literature," *International Urology and Nephrology*, vol. 39, no. 4, pp. 1295–1302, 2007.

[19] P. K.-T. Li, M. C. Law, K. M. Chow et al., "Good patient and technique survival in elderly patients on continuous ambulatory peritoneal dialysis," *Peritoneal Dialysis International*, vol. 27, supplement 2, pp. S196–S201, 2007.

[20] E. A. Brown, "How to address barriers to peritoneal dialysis in the elderly," *Peritoneal Dialysis International*, vol. 31, supplement 2, pp. S83–S85, 2011.

9

Psychosocial Factors in End-Stage Kidney Disease Patients at a Tertiary Hospital in Australia

Charan Bale,[1,2] **Alexandra Douglas,**[1] **Dev Jegatheesan,**[1] **Linh Pham,**[1] **Sonny Huynh,**[1] **Atul Mulay,**[2] **and Dwarakanathan Ranganathan**[1]

[1]*Royal Brisbane and Women's Hospital, Herston, Brisbane, QLD, Australia*
[2]*Dr. D. Y. Patil Medical College, Pune, India*

Correspondence should be addressed to Dwarakanathan Ranganathan; dwarakanathan.ranganathan@health.qld.gov.au

Academic Editor: Anil K. Agarwal

Aim. This study seeks to review the psychosocial factors affecting patients with end-stage kidney disease (ESKD) from a tertiary hospital in Australia. *Methods.* We audited patients with ESKD, referred to social work services from January 2012 to December 2014. All patients underwent psychosocial assessments by one, full-time renal social worker. Patient demographics, cumulative social issues, and subsequent interventions were recorded directly into a database. *Results.* Of the 244 patients referred, the majority were >60 years (58.6%), male (60.7%), born in Australia (62.3%), on haemodialysis (51.6%), and reliant on government financial assistance (88%). Adjustment issues (41%), financial concerns (38.5%), domestic assistance (35.2%), and treatment nonadherence (21.3%) were the predominant reasons for social work consultation. Younger age, referral prior to start of dialysis, and unemployment were significant independent predictors of increased risk of adjustment issues ($p = 0.004$, <0.001, and =0.018, resp.). Independent risk factors for treatment nonadherence included age and financial and employment status ($p = 0.041$, 0.052, and 0.008, resp.). *Conclusion.* Psychosocial and demographic factors were associated with treatment nonadherence and adjustment difficulties. Additional social work support and counselling, in addition to financial assistance from government and nongovernment agencies, may help to improve adjustment to the diagnosis and treatment plans as patients approach ESKD.

1. Introduction

Patients with end-stage kidney disease (ESKD) are exposed to multiple physical and psychological stressors as a result of their illness [1]. Treatment of ESKD in the form of dialysis imposes considerable stress, including potential changes in family relations, social interactions, and occupational demands [1]. The "biopsychosocial" impact of ESKD has been proposed to account for its poorer quality of life (QoL) compared to patients with other chronic diseases [1, 2]. Furthermore, survey data has shown significant correlation between poorer QoL and higher morbidity and mortality in ESKD [3].

As opposed to the mostly invariant biological risk factors, modifiable psychosocial factors may provide avenues for successful intervention and improved clinical outcomes in this population [4].

The renal social worker is the patients' advocate, serving as a bridge in communicating individual's needs to the medical and allied health team [5]. The social worker's expertise encompasses instrumental, informational, and emotional support [6]. Naik et al. commented that "a multidisciplinary team approach is critical to the overall care and QoL of patients with ESKD. Social workers play a central role in the care of these patients, which may be further enhanced by engaging them in the measurement and monitoring of QoL" [7].

There is a paucity of data pertaining to the psychosocial factors affecting patients with ESKD in Australia. This study seeks to identify these issues using the renal social work database of a tertiary hospital. We identify various reasons for initial referral, subsequent consultations, and interventions performed by the renal social worker over a three-year period. We then compare differences across patient demographics and modalities of ESKD management. Ultimately, the study would further explore the significance of social work involvement in the care of patients with ESKD and lead to future improvements in service delivery.

2. Methods

We conducted a single centre retrospective audit of the patients with ESKD (chronic kidney disease stage-V (CKD-V)) who were referred to one, full-time renal social worker from January 2012 to December 2014 at Royal Brisbane & Women's Hospital, Queensland, Australia. Ethics approval was obtained from the Human Research and Ethics committee.

Referrals for social work input were made either by healthcare staff (medical and allied health) or directly by patients and/or family members. The reason for referral varied and many individuals were referred for multiple reasons over the study period. All patients underwent an initial psychosocial assessment by the social worker, typically a 60-minute consultation where issues at index were identified. Subsequent referrals and clinical encounters were recorded directly into a database as they arose. Each issue was analysed separately in the case where an individual patient had many issues identified over the study period.

Social work interventions included instrumental, informational, and emotional supports. Instrumental support included patient advocacy; assistance with paper work/forms; referrals to relevant government agencies (e.g., Department of Housing, welfare services); and allied health services (e.g., psychologist, dietician, and occupational therapist). Informational support included provision of helpful resources across various domains (e.g., predialysis education, treatment adherence, aged care services, management of finances, and employment prospects). Emotional support was provided through counselling sessions and organising family meetings (e.g., for those with adjustment issues, caregiver stress, and palliative care discussions). All clinical reviews, documentation, and data collation were performed by the same social worker over the study period. Deidentified data was transposed into a spreadsheet, including patient demographics, social history, ESKD management modality, summary of social worker encounters, and the respective interventions carried out.

This study only included participants with ESKD defined by estimated glomerular filtration rate (eGFR) < 15 mL/min/1.73 m^2 or those with a functioning renal transplant (CKD-Vt). Patients were subclassified into predialysis, maintenance haemodialysis (HD), peritoneal dialysis (PD), renal transplant, or palliative.

Adherence is defined as "the extent to which a patient complies with the prescribed treatment under limited supervision" [8]. Limited supervision involves monitoring a patient in the community, for example, review at an outpatient appointment or during outpatient dialysis. Adherence also can be defined "as the extent to which a person's behaviour (taking medication, following a diet, and/or executing lifestyle changes) corresponds with agreed recommendations from a healthcare provider" [9]. Adjustment is described in relation to how the patient adapts to the multitude of stressors posed by the routine and restrictions of treatment [10].

Referrals for treatment nonadherence and adjustment were made at the discretion of the treating team, typically when this had serious consequences on the patient's health outcome, for example, hospitalisation due to nonadherence or difficulty coping with life changes associated with ESKD.

Domestic assistance is a service aimed at helping people to remain independent in their home, by helping with the essential light house work tasks necessary to maintain hygiene and safety standards in the home [11].

2.1. Statistical Analysis. Baseline variables are described as proportions or mean (SD) as appropriate. We used cross tabs with chi-square test to assess association of demographic variables with socioeconomic issues that were identified. We used univariate and multivariate logistic regression to determine predictors of adjustment issues and nonadherence. Age, gender, country of origin, financial status, employment status, reimbursement plan, referral before or after starting renal replacement therapy (RRT), and marital status of the patients were considered for inclusion in multivariate model. Since financial status and employment status were highly correlated, separate multivariate models were constructed for each of them to avoid colinearity. A p value < 0.05 was considered as statistically significant and odds ratios with 95% confidence interval were calculated.

3. Results

The study included 244 patients (148 men) with mean age 62.4 (16.9) years. The majority of them were Australian by birth (152). The majority (61.6%) of referrals to social worker were made after dialysis commencement or transplantation. Baseline characteristics of the patients are shown in Table 1. Table 2 shows issues identified after evaluation of the patients by the social worker.

Need for transportation assistance was most prevalent for those patients on HD (46/126 [36.5%]), followed by PD (15/60 [25%]) and transplant patients (7/32 [21.8%]), a significant difference between modality of RRT (p = 0.015) and a more commonly identified issue in patients referred prior to starting RRT (p = 0.004). Child protection was needed significantly more often if the country of birth was other than Australia (5/92 [5.4%] versus 1/152 [0.66%]; p = 0.03). The breakdown of social work interventions is listed in Figure 1.

Adjustment issues problems were the commonest problem identified in 41% of patients. Patients referred prior to starting RRT were more likely to have adjustment problems than those referred after commencement of RRT (72.3% versus 21.3%; p < 0.001, univariate analysis). In multivariate logistic regression, age, referral prior to commencement of RRT, and financial and employment status independently predicted the odds of having adjustment issues (Tables 3(a) and 3(b)). Separate models were created for financial status and employment status to avoid colinearity since the two were highly correlated. Increasing age was associated with a significantly decreased risk of having adjustment issues. Compared to aged pension, patients with financial stability (salary or savings) were significantly less likely to have adjustment issues. Compared to employed patients, unemployed patients

TABLE 1: Baseline characteristics of patients of CKD stage 5.

Characteristics	N	Mean (SD) or n (%)
Gender		
Male	244	148 (60.7%)
Age		62.4 (16.9)
Country of birth		
Australian		152 (62.3%)
Marital status		
Married		93 (38.1%)
Single		55 (22.5%)
Divorced		39 (16%)
Widowed		36 (14.8%)
Partner/Defacto		21 (8.6%)
Financial		
Aged pension		114 (46.3%)
Disability pension		86 (35%)
New-start allowance		12 (4.9%)
Parenting payment		2 (0.8%)
Salary		16 (6.5%)
Savings		13 (5.3%)
Youth allowance		1 (0.4%)
Employment status		
Employed		34%
Retired		77%
Unemployed		130%
Student		3%
Insurance		
Public		213 (87.3%)
Modality of treatment		
Transplant		32 (13.1%)
Haemodialysis		126 (51.6%)
Peritoneal dialysis		60 (24.6%)
None/conservative		26 (10.7%)
Time of referral		
Before RRT		94 (38.4%)

TABLE 2: Social issues present in patients with CKD stage 5.

Issue	n (%)
Adjustment	100 (41)
Finance	94 (38.5)
Domestic assistance	86 (35.2)
Transport	70 (28.7)
Caregiver stress	62 (25.4)
Nonadherence	52 (21.3)
Housing	45 (18.4)
Bereavement	41 (16.8)
Palliative care/advanced care planning	38 (15.4)
Mental health	36 (14.8)
Aged care	31 (12.7)
Employment	24 (9.8)
Child protection	6 (2.5)
Domestic violence	5 (2.0)

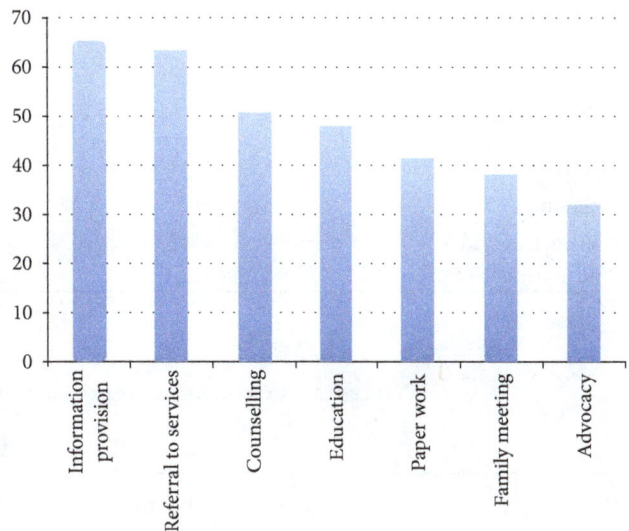

FIGURE 1: Breakdown of social work support services as a percentage. All patients received initial psychosocial assessment (not included in graphic).

were significantly more likely to have adjustment issues (odds ratio 3.34, 95% confidence interval 1.22–9.13, and $p = 0.018$).

Issues related to adherence to treatment were also common and were seen in 21.3% patients. Age and financial/employment status were significant independent predictors of nonadherence in multivariate logistic regression model (Tables 4(a) and 4(b)). Increasing age was associated with a significantly lower risk of nonadherence. Compared to aged pension, disability pension was associated with a significantly greater risk of nonadherence (odds ratio 3.11, 95% confidence interval 1.10 to 8.84, and $p = 0.033$). Compared to employed patients, unemployed patients were significantly more likely to have treatment nonadherence (odds ratio 4.19, 95% confidence interval, 1.46 to 12.01, and $p = 0.008$).

4. Discussion

This study sought to assess the psychosocial challenges faced by patients with ESKD in an Australian population. Among the patients referred to social work, the majority were >60 years of age, male, born in Australia, on HD, unemployed, and reliant on government assistance. The most common social work consults related to patients with difficulties with adjustment, treatment nonadherence, management of finances, and domestic assistance. We found that age, timing of referral (before versus after starting RRT), financial status, and employment status were independent predictors of adjustment issues. Age, financial status, and employment status also were independent predictors of treatment nonadherence.

As defined by Beder, adjustment to dialysis is described in relation to how the patient adapts to the multitude of stressors posed by the routine and restrictions of treatment. Social work intervention aims to stabilise the individual with a view towards maintenance of functionality and return to work after initiation of treatment. Early intervention, especially in

TABLE 3: Multivariate logistic regression for independent predictors of adjustment issues.

(a)

Variables	Odds ratio	95% confidence interval		p value
		Lower	Upper	
Age	0.949	0.916	0.984	0.004
Pre-RRT issues	18.216	8.398	39.514	<0.001
Financial status				0.019
0: aged pension	Ref			Ref
1: disability pension	0.922	0.343	2.476	0.872
2: new-start allowance	0.555	0.086	3.569	0.535
3: parenting payment	0.181	0.002	19.751	0.475
4: salary	0.066	0.011	0.390	0.003
5: savings	0.100	0.16	0.647	0.016
6: youth allowance	5.147	0.000		1.000

(b)

Variables	Odds ratio	95% confidence interval		p value
		Lower	Upper	
Age	0.960	0.933	0.988	0.005
Pre-RRT Issues	14.499	7.139	29.444	<0.001
Employment status				0.048
0: employed	Ref			Ref
1: retired	1.837	0.551	6.120	0.322
2: unemployed	3.344	1.225	9.128	0.018
3: student	0.444	0.018	10.746	0.618

TABLE 4: Multivariate logistic regression showing independent predictors of nonadherence.

(a)

Variables	Odds ratio	95% confidence interval		p value
		Lower	Upper	
Age	0.968	0.938	0.999	0.041
Financial status				0.052
0: aged pension	Ref			Ref
1: disability pension	3.112	1.096	8.839	0.033
2: new-start allowance	0.588	0.072	4.790	0.619
3: parenting payment	4.109	0.000	—	0.999
4: salary	0.996	0.190	5.206	0.996
5: savings	0.766	0.113	5.187	0.785
6: youth allowance	0.000	0.000	—	1.000

(b)

Variables	Odds ratio	95% confidence interval		p value
		Lower	Upper	
Age	0.953	0.930	0.977	<0.001
Employment status				0.008
0: employed	Ref			Ref
1: retired	1.256	0.289	5.461	0.761
2: unemployed	4.191	1.462	12.012	0.008
3: student	0.000	0.000	—	0.999

"at-risk" patient groups, has been shown to significantly decrease the degree of psychosocial maladjustment in new-start dialysis patients [10]. Our current study suggests that patients dependent on government assistance are most at risk of maladjustment in the Australian setting. These patients may therefore also be most likely to benefit from social work intervention. The KHA-CARI guidelines on CKD management suggest the involvement of the social worker in early stages of CKD [12]. Of note the majority (>60%) of patients in this study were referred after commencement of dialysis, whereas a substantial number of patients with adjustment issue were referred prior to RRT. Maladjustment has been associated with loss of employment, which is not uncommon among dialysis patients [10, 13]. Earlier referral to social worker may therefore provide an opportunity to more effectively address adjustment concerns. Importantly, earlier referral may see more new-start dialysis patients maintaining or returning to employment. Treatment nonadherence in ESKD has been widely researched and remains a challenge for the care of these patients globally. Studies in dialysis patients have shown the association between decreased adherence and increased rates of depression, hospitalisation, morbidity, and overall mortality [14–17]. Rates of nonadherence, risk factors, clinical implications, and appropriate interventions have been variably described in the literature, largely owing to the heterogeneity of trials [18]. Treatment nonadherence was identified in 21.3% of patients in this study. We found that younger age, patients on disability pension, and unemployed patients were at a significantly higher independent risk of treatment nonadherence. This suggests that interventions directed at reducing disability and unemployment could improve treatment adherence.

Psychosocial interventions have proven to improve outcomes in randomised trials. Cukor et al. showed that cognitive behavioural therapy improved depressive symptoms, QoL, and treatment compliance in HD patients [18]. A systematic review by Chan et al. showed the association between psychosocial variables and QoL in dialysis patients concluding that targeted interventions to treat psychosocial factors may improve quality of life, morbidity, and ultimately mortality in this population [19]. This has implications for the findings of this study. Firstly the psychosocial factors identified in this population may represent surrogate markers of patient QoL; correlation of the findings with validated QoL scores would be of interest. Secondly, QoL scores may be an appropriate way to assess the outcome of social work interventions over time.

Limitations of our study were that data were collected retrospectively from a single tertiary centre social work database. The findings may therefore underrepresent the true extent and nature of psychosocial issues faced by ESKD patients. Efficacy of social work interventions was not measured, another limitation of our study. Also the number of encounters per patient was not tracked over the study's duration. This could have identified specific risk factors and/or groups that required more intensive social work follow-up.

In conclusion, this study observed the demographics of ESKD patients referred to social work at a tertiary hospital and found the major issues to be related to adjustment,

financial difficulty, and domestic assistance. Risk factors for treatment nonadherence included age, disability pension, and unemployment. Adjustment issues were common and were more likely to be present in patients with younger age and referred before start of RRT. Patients with financial stability were less likely to have adjustment issues compared to patients on aged pension. Age was the common significant variable in adjustment and adherence to treatment. This highlights the need for further financial assistance/support from government and nongovernment agencies. Furthermore, we propose the need for earlier and more comprehensive social work support as patients approach ESKD which may lead to improvements in QoL, morbidity, and mortality.

References

[1] A. Untas, J. Thumma, N. Rascle et al., "The associations of social support and other psychosocial factors with mortality and quality of life in the dialysis outcomes and practice patterns study," *Clinical Journal of the American Society of Nephrology*, vol. 6, no. 1, pp. 142–152, 2011.

[2] C. Loos, S. Briançon, L. Frimat, B. Hanesse, and M. Kessler, "Effect of end-stage renal disease on the quality of life of older patients," *Journal of the American Geriatrics Society*, vol. 51, no. 2, pp. 229–233, 2003.

[3] E. G. Lowrie, R. B. Curtin, N. LePain, and D. Schatell, "Medical outcomes study short form-36: a consistent and powerful predictor of morbidity and mortality in dialysis patients," *American Journal of Kidney Diseases*, vol. 41, no. 6, pp. 1286–1292, 2003.

[4] S. S. Patel, R. A. Peterson, and P. L. Kimmel, "The impact of social support on end-stage renal disease," *Seminars in Dialysis*, vol. 18, no. 2, pp. 98–102, 2005.

[5] N. Avery, "Understanding the role of the renal social worker," American Association of Kidney Patients, https://www.aakp .org/education/resourcelibrary/dialysis-resources/item/understanding-the-role-of-a-renal-social-worker.html.

[6] D. Cukor, S. D. Cohen, R. A. Peterson, and P. L. Kimmen, "Psychosocial aspects of chronic disease: ESRD as a paradigmatic illness," *Journal of the American Society of Nephrology*, vol. 18, no. 12, pp. 3042–3055, 2007.

[7] N. Naik, R. Hess, and M. Unruh, "Measurement of health-related quality of life in the care of patients with ESRD: isn't this the metric that matters?" *Seminars in Dialysis*, vol. 25, no. 4, pp. 439–444, 2012.

[8] Farlex [internet]. Medical Dictionary for the Health Professions and Nursing© Farlex, 2012, http://medical-dictionary.thefree-dictionary.com/adherence.

[9] http://www.who.int/chp/knowledge/publications/adherence_Section1.pdf.

[10] J. Beder, "Evaluation research on the effectiveness of social work intervention on dialysis patients," *Social Work in Health Care*, vol. 30, no. 1, pp. 15–30, 2000.

[11] https://www.adhc.nsw.gov.au/__data/assets/file/0018/228006/Home_Care_Domestic_Assistance_Fact_Sheet_May2012.pdf.

[12] D. W. Johnson, E. Atai, M. Chan et al., "KHA-CARI guideline: early chronic kidney disease: detection, prevention and management," *Nephrology*, vol. 18, no. 5, pp. 340–350, 2013.

[13] A. R. Campbell, "Family caregivers: caring for aging end-stage renal disease partners," *Advances in Renal Replacement Therapy*, vol. 5, no. 2, pp. 98–108, 1998.

[14] J. E. Leggat Jr., "Adherence with dialysis: a focus on mortality risk," *Seminars in Dialysis*, vol. 18, no. 2, pp. 137–141, 2005.

[15] P. L. Kimmel, R. A. Peterson, K. L. Weihs et al., "Psychosocial factors, behavioral compliance and survival in urban hemodialysis patients," *Kidney International*, vol. 54, no. 1, pp. 245–254, 1998.

[16] S. Clark, K. Farrington, and J. Chilcot, "Nonadherence in dialysis patients: prevalence, measurement, outcome, and psychological determinants," *Seminars in Dialysis*, vol. 27, no. 1, pp. 42–49, 2014.

[17] R. Saran, J. L. Bragg-Gresham, H. C. Rayner et al., "Nonadherence in hemodialysis: associations with mortality, hospitalization, and practice patterns in the DOPPS," *Kidney International*, vol. 64, no. 1, pp. 254–262, 2003.

[18] D. Cukor, N. Ver Halen, D. R. Asher et al., "Psychosocial intervention improves depression, quality of life, and fluid adherence in hemodialysis," *Journal of the American Society of Nephrology*, vol. 25, no. 1, pp. 196–206, 2014.

[19] R. Chan, R. Brooks, Z. Steel et al., "The psychosocial correlates of quality of life in the dialysis population: a systematic review and meta-regression analysis," *Quality of Life Research*, vol. 21, no. 4, pp. 563–580, 2012.

10

Classification of Five Uremic Solutes according to Their Effects on Renal Tubular Cells

Takeo Edamatsu, Ayako Fujieda, Atsuko Ezawa, and Yoshiharu Itoh

Pharmaceutical Division, Kureha Corporation, 3-26-2 Hyakunin-cho, Shinjuku-ku, Tokyo 169-8503, Japan

Correspondence should be addressed to Takeo Edamatsu; edamatsu@kureha.co.jp

Academic Editor: Jochen Reiser

Background/Aims. Uremic solutes, which are known to be retained in patients with chronic kidney disease, are considered to have deleterious effects on disease progression. Among these uremic solutes, indoxyl sulfate (IS) has been extensively studied, while other solutes have been studied less to state. We conducted a comparative study to examine the similarities and differences between IS, *p*-cresyl sulfate (PCS), phenyl sulfate (PhS), hippuric acid (HA), and indoleacetic acid (IAA). *Methods.* We used LLC-PK1 cells to evaluate the effects of these solutes on viable cell number, cell cycle progression, and cell death. *Results.* All the solutes reduced viable cell number after 48-hour incubation. N-Acetyl-L-cysteine inhibited this effect induced by all solutes except HA. At the concentration that reduced the cell number to almost 50% of vehicle control, IAA induced apoptosis but not cell cycle delay, whereas other solutes induced delay in cell cycle progression with marginal impact on apoptosis. Phosphorylation of p53 and Chk1 and expression of ATF4 and CHOP genes were detected in IS-, PCS-, and PhS-treated cells, but not in IAA-treated cells. *Conclusions.* Taken together, the adverse effects of PCS and PhS on renal tubular cells are similar to those of IS, while those of HA and IAA differ.

1. Introduction

Uremic solutes are a large number of compounds that are retained in chronic kidney disease (CKD), especially in end-stage renal disease, resulting in elevated serum concentrations compared to normal condition [1]. These solutes are excreted in urine in healthy persons but are accumulated as CKD progresses [2, 3]. Over a hundred uremic solutes have been reported to date, and these solutes are classified into three groups according to the size and protein binding properties [4–6]. Protein-bound solutes have attracted much attention in the last decade, because they are less efficiently removed by dialysis [7] and are possibly associated with CKD-related complications [8].

Indoxyl sulfate (IS) is a representative protein-bound solute and its deleterious effects have been studied in various cell types including renal tubular cells [9], mesangial cells [10], vascular endothelial cells [11], vascular smooth muscle cells [12], osteoclasts [13], osteoblasts [14], erythrocytes [15], and monocytes [16]. Moreover, several studies demonstrate the adverse effects of IS on the kidney [17, 18] and vascular systems [19, 20] of animal models. In humans, several

reports indicate the association of IS with impairment of renal function and development of cardiovascular disease in CKD patients [21–23]. Although these studies imply a causal relationship between IS and progression of CKD and/or CKD-related complications, it is necessary to clarify whether other uremic solutes have similar effects.

Our previous study demonstrated that the serum levels of several solutes are elevated in CKD rats [24]. Most of these solutes are also found to be increased in hemodialysis patients [25]. Among these solutes, we focused on five solutes which were IS, *p*-cresyl sulfate, phenyl sulfate, hippuric acid, and indoleacetic acid. The selection criteria for these solutes were both their high serum concentration in hemodialysis patients and their effect on viable cell number of porcine renal tubular cells (unpublished observation).

Renal tubular cells are the cell component of renal tubules, and tubular injury is thought to be one of the key events causing progression of CKD [26]. Thus we evaluated the effects of the five uremic solutes on viable cell number of renal tubular cells and investigated the underlying mechanisms.

2. Materials and Methods

2.1. Cell Culture. LLC-PK1, a porcine renal tubular epithelial cell line, was obtained from American Type Culture Collection (ATCC, Manassas, VA, USA). LLC-PK1 cells were maintained in Medium 199 (Mediatech, Manassas, VA, USA) supplemented with 10% FBS (BioWest, Nuaillé, France).

2.2. Reagents. Indoxyl sulfate was purchased from Biosynth (Staad, Switzerland). *p*-Cresyl sulfate and phenyl sulfate were synthesized at Eiweiss (Shizuoka, Japan). Hippuric acid and indoleacetic acid were purchased from Tokyo chemical industry (Tokyo, Japan). N-Acetyl-L-cysteine was purchased from Sigma (St. Louis, MO, USA).

2.3. Viable Cell Count. Effects of uremic solutes on viable cell number were determined using the Cell Counting Kit-8 (Dojindo, Wako, Tokyo, Japan), a water-soluble version of the methyl thiazolyl tetrazolium assay, according to the manufacturer's instructions. LLC-PK1 cells were suspended in Medium 199 supplemented with 2% FBS and dispensed into tubes. Each uremic solute was added to the cell suspension and cell density was adjusted to 1.6×10^4 cells/mL. One milliliter/well of the cell suspension was seeded in a 24-well plate and incubated for 48 hours. After incubation, the medium was changed to a medium containing the Cell Counting Kit-8 reagent. The cells were incubated for another 30 min and the optical density at 450 nm (OD450) was measured using a microplate reader (iMark Microplate Reader, Bio-Rad, Hercules, CA, USA). The OD450 of medium containing Cell Counting Kit-8 reagent without cells was measured and was subtracted from the OD450 of each sample.

2.4. Cell Cycle Analysis. Effects of uremic solutes on growth rate were evaluated after adjusting the cell cycle at G1/S or G2/M boundary. Double thymidine block was used for synchronization at G1/S boundary. Cells were incubated overnight in serum-free medium containing 2.5 mmol/L of thymidine, changed to medium supplemented with 10% FBS, and incubated for 7 hours and then in thymidine-containing medium again overnight. For G2/M synchronization, cells were incubated overnight in serum-free medium containing 1.0 μmol/L of nocodazole. After synchronization, the cells were treated with uremic solutes as described above for 4 or 6 hours. Then, the cells were fixed in ethanol and stained with propidium iodide (Propidium Iodide/RNase Staining Solution, Cell Signaling Technology, Danvers, MA, USA). The stained cells were detected by flow cytometer (FACS Calibur, Becton Dickinson, Franklin Lakes, NJ, USA) and the data were analyzed using the Flowjo software (Tomy Digital Biology, Tokyo, Japan).

2.5. Apoptosis. Cells were treated with uremic solutes as described above for 48 hours. After treatment, culture medium that might contain nonadherent cells and adherent cells was harvested. The cells were stained with FITC-conjugated annexin V and propidium (TACS Annexin V-FITC Apoptosis Detection Kit, Trevigen, Gaithersburg, MD, USA). The stained cells were detected by flow cytometer (FACS Calibur) and the data were analyzed using the Flowjo software.

2.6. Western Blotting. Cells were treated with uremic solutes as described above for 5 hours. After treatment, the cells were lysed with RIPA Lysis Buffer (Santa Cruz Biotechnology, Santa Cruz, CA, USA). Antibodies against phosphorylated p53 (at Ser15) and Chk1 (at Ser345) were used (both are supposed to be active forms and were purchased from Cell Signaling Technology). Chemiluminescent signals generated using the ECL Select Western Blotting Detection System (GE Healthcare, Buckinghamshire, UK) were detected by Light-Capture II Cooled CCD Camera Systems (ATTO, Tokyo, Japan). Antibody against β-actin was used as loading control (Biolegend, San Diego, CA, USA).

2.7. Real-Time PCR. Cells were treated with uremic solutes as described above for 5 or 24 hours. After treatment, the cells were lysed in ISOGEN (Nippon Gene, Tokyo, Japan). Total RNA was isolated according to the manufacturer's instructions, and optical density at 260 nm was measured using a spectrophotometer (Gene Spec V, Hitachi High-Tech Manufacturing & Service Corporation, Ibaraki, Japan). The RNA (300 ng) was reverse-transcribed using the PrimeScript RT Reagent Kit (Takarabio, Shiga, Japan) in a 10 μL reaction volume. Using 0.6 μL of complementary DNA, SYBR Premix Ex Taq II Tli RNaseH Plus (Takarabio), and 10 pmol of each of the primer sets for various target genes (Table 1), real-time PCR was performed in a 25 μL reaction volume and analyzed using the Thermal Cycler Dice Real Time System (TP800, Takarabio) at the following thermal cycling conditions: denaturation at 95°C for 30 sec, followed by 40 cycles of 95°C denaturation for 5 sec and 60°C annealing/extension for 30 sec.

2.8. Statistical Analysis. Statistical analysis was performed by Student's *t*-test, and $P < 0.01$ was considered as significant.

3. Results

3.1. Effects on Cell Viability. All five uremic solutes decreased viable cell number dose-dependently upon incubating with LLC-PK1 cells for 48 hours (Figure 1). To compare the mechanisms of action of the five solutes, the concentration of each solute that reduces the cell number by almost 50% was used in subsequent experiments. For IAA, two or three different concentrations were always used, because the reduction rates differed in different experiments. In some experiments, two concentrations of IS were used for the same reason. Viable cell numbers were evaluated in each experiment for confirmation purpose. The results of viable cell numbers for various experimental conditions are shown in Supplementary Figures available online at http://dx.doi.org/10.1155/2014/512178.

TABLE 1: Primers for real-time PCR.

Target	Regulation	Forward	Reverse
p21	p53-regulated	5′-catgtggacctgttgctgtc-3′	5′-cctcttggagaagatcagcc-3′
ATF4	ER stress responsive	5′-ggtcagtgcctcagacaaca-3′	5′-tctggcatggtttccaggtc-3′
CHOP	ER stress responsive	5′-cttcaccactcttgaccctg-3′	5′-gagctctgactggaatcagg-3′
Cdc20	p53-regulated	5′-aatgtcctggcaactggagg-3′	5′-tgagctccttgtagtgggga-3′
Skp2	p53-regulated	5′-acctccacccagatgtgact-3′	5′-gtgctgtacacgaaaagggc-3′
Puma	p53-regulated	5′-gatctcaacgcgctgtacga-3′	5′-caggcacctaattaggctcc-3′
GAPDH	house-keeping gene	5′-ccatcaccatcttccaggag-3′	5′-gagatgatgaccctcttggc-3′

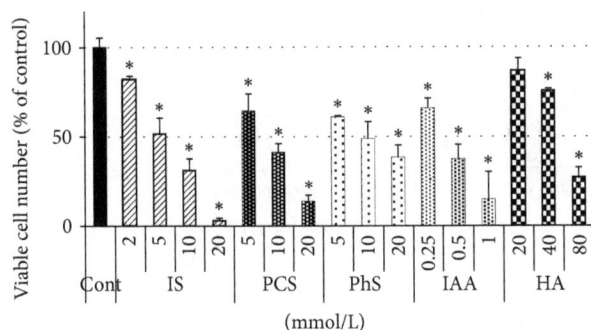

FIGURE 1: Effects of five uremic solutes on viable cell number. Porcine renal tubular cells were treated with each uremic solute for 48 hours. Viable cell number was evaluated using Cell Counting Kit-8. Optical density at 450 nm was measured and the values were calculated as percent of control. Data are shown as mean ± S.D ($n = 4$). Asterisks indicate significant reduction of viable cell population compared to control ($P < 0.01$). Cont, control; IS, indoxyl sulfate; PCS, p-cresyl sulfate; PhS, phenyl sulfate; HA, hippuric acid.

3.2. *Effects on Cell Cycle Progression.* The decrease in viable cell number is supposed to be due to either reduction in growth rate or induction of cell death. To investigate these two possibilities, the effects of uremic solutes on growth rate and apoptosis were evaluated.

First, to determine the effects on growth rate, cells were synchronized at G1/S boundary, and the synchronized cells were released to grow with or without uremic solutes. In this experimental setting, the cell cytometry histogram shifts from left to right in a time-dependent manner, according to the increase in DNA content (Figure 2(a)). Therefore, delayed growth will appear as a lag of the histogram on the left hand side of the corresponding control. Under these experimental conditions, IS, p-cresyl sulfate (PCS), and phenyl sulfate (PhS) delayed growth rate (Figure 2(b)), whereas hippuric acid (HA) and IAA (Figure 2(c)) had no impact on growth rate. In this experiment, 0.25 and 0.5 mmol/L of IAA decreased viable cell number by 26 and 84%, respectively (Supplementary Figure 1).

Next, cells were synchronized at G2/M boundary, and then the cells were released to grow with or without uremic solutes. In this experimental setting, the histogram of untreated control cells at 0 hours shows a predominant cell population on the right (cells in G2 phase, Figure 3(a)) with negligible amount on the left (cells in G1 phase). As mitosis progresses, cells in G2 phase decrease and cells in G1 phase increase. Data are shown as percent of cells in G1 and G2 phases. IS, PCS, PhS, and HA retarded both the decrease of cells in G2 phase and the increase of cells in G1 phase (Figure 3(b)). In sharp contrast to these four solutes, IAA had no effect on the rate of G2 to G1 transition (Figure 3(c)). In this experiment, 0.25, 0.5, and 1 mmol/L of IAA decreased viable cell number by 12, 42, and 79%, respectively (Supplementary Figure 2).

3.3. *Effects on Cell Death.* Because IAA had no effects on growth rate as described above, the effect on cell death was examined. Annexin V-FITC and propidium iodide were used to detect dying and dead cells, respectively. As a result, only IAA induced significant increase of dying cells (Figure 4), while marginal increases of dying cells were observed in PCS or HA-treated groups ($P = 0.044$ and 0.021, resp.). IAA also induced marginal increase of dead cells ($P = 0.013$).

3.4. *Inhibition of Cell Viability Reduction by Antioxidant.* Previous studies have reported that IS induces reactive oxygen species (ROS) and that ROS could be involved in IS-induced inhibition of cell proliferation in several cell types [27, 28]. Therefore, we examined the effect of N-acetyl-L-cysteine, an antioxidant, on reduction of viable cell number induced by each solute. Incubation with N-acetyl-L-cysteine partially inhibited reduction of viable cell number in IS, PCS, or PhS groups and completely inhibited the reduction in IAA group (Figure 5). Meanwhile, N-acetyl-L-cysteine did not inhibit the effect of HA.

3.5. *Phosphorylation of p53 and Chk1.* IS has been reported to inhibit cellular proliferation in a p53-dependent manner in HK-2, a human proximal tubular cell line [29]. Therefore, we examined phosphorylation of p53. We also examined phosphorylation of Chk1 that is also involved in DNA damage response like p53. The results showed that IS and PCS induced p53 phosphorylation (Figure 6), while IS, PCS, and PhS induced Chk1 phosphorylation. IAA and HA had no effect on phosphorylation of these proteins. In this experiment, 0.25 and 0.5 mmol/L of IAA decreased viable cell number by 30 and 55%, respectively, and 5 and 10 mmol/L of IS decreased viable cell number by 42 and 76%, respectively (Supplementary Figure 4).

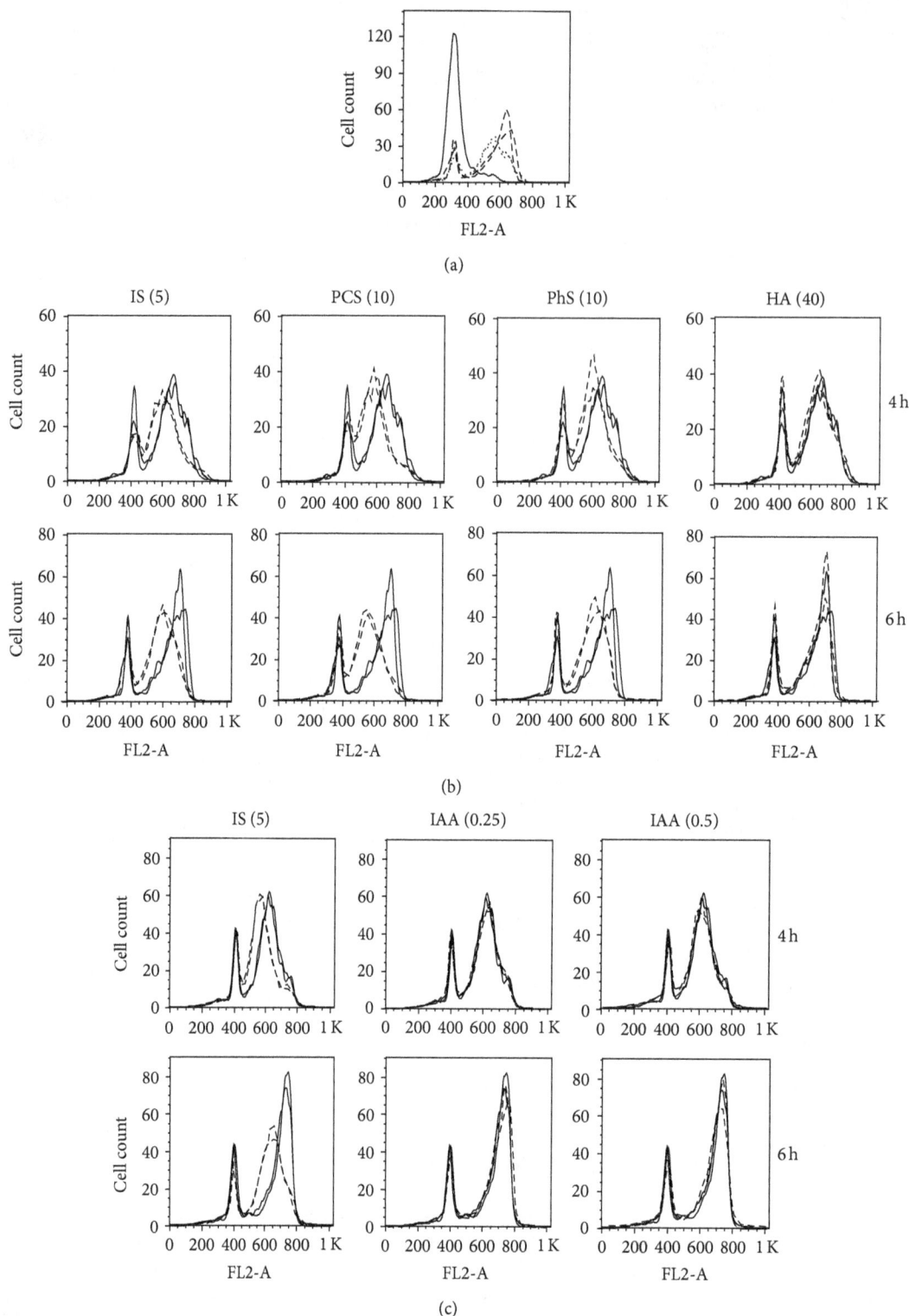

FIGURE 2: Effects of uremic solutes on cell cycle progression after porcine renal tubular cells were synchronized at G1/S boundary. (a) Time-dependent shift of histograms of untreated control cells. Each line indicates time after release from synchronization. Solid line: 0 hours, dotted line: 4 hours, and dashed line: 6 hours. Duplicate data for each time point are shown except for 0 hours. (b) and (c) Histograms of uremic solute-treated cells and corresponding control cells at indicated time points. After synchronization, cells were released to grow with (dashed line) or without (solid line) uremic solute for indicated periods. Cont, control; IS, indoxyl sulfate; PCS, p-cresyl sulfate; PhS, phenyl sulfate; HA, hippuric acid; IAA, indoleacetic acid. Concentrations of solutes (mmol/L) are shown in parentheses. Duplicate data are shown. Data are representative of two independent experiments.

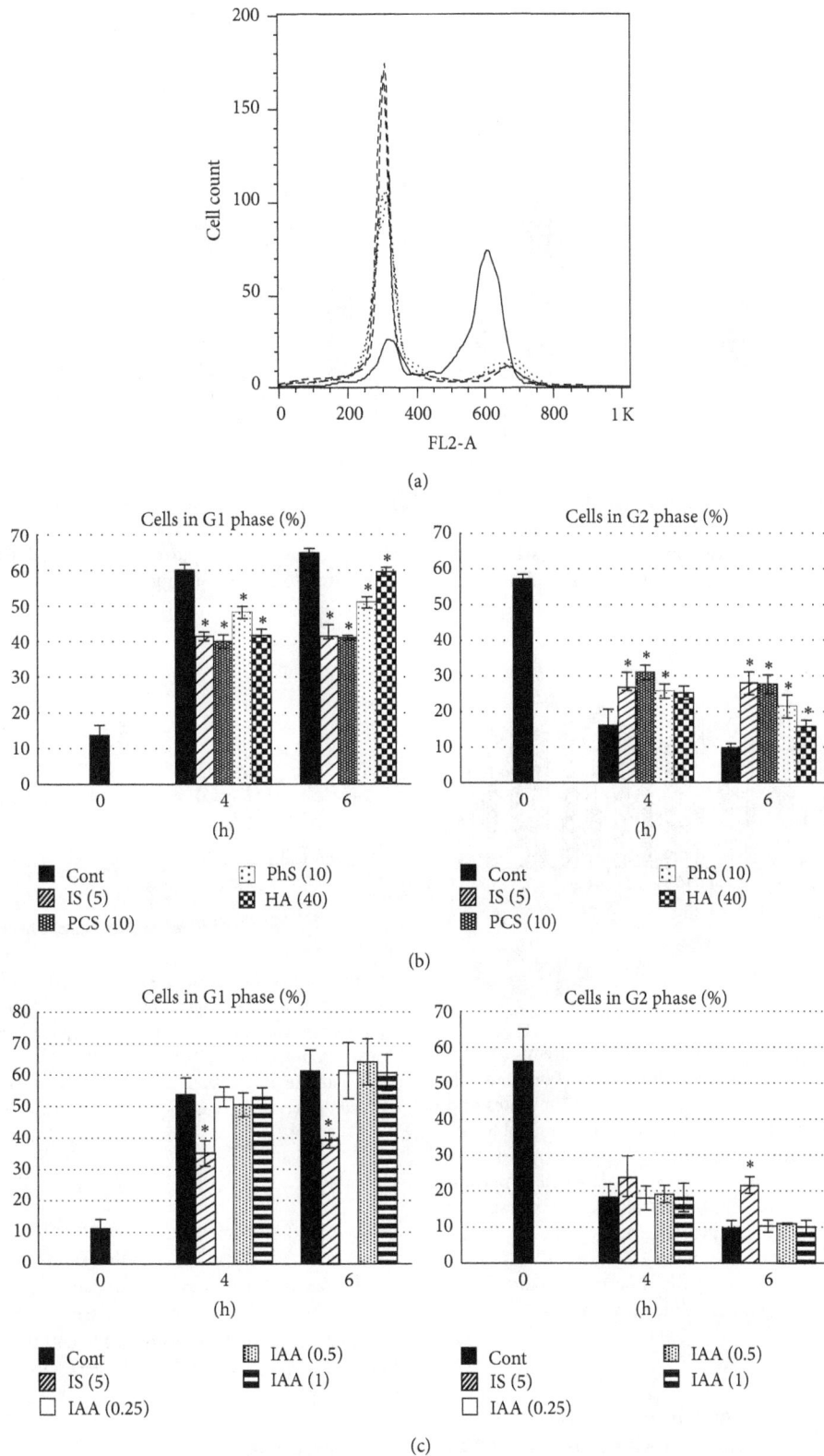

FIGURE 3: Effects of uremic solutes on cell cycle progression after porcine renal tubular cells were synchronized at G2/M boundary. (a) Time-dependent shift of histograms of untreated control cells. Each line indicates time after release from synchronization. Solid line: 0 hours, dotted line: 4 hours, and dashed line: 6 hours. Duplicate data for each time point are shown except for 0 hours. (b) and (c) Percent of cells in G1 or G2 phase. After synchronization, cells were released to grow with or without uremic solutes for indicated periods. Percent of cells in each phase was analyzed and calculated. Cont, control; IS, indoxyl sulfate; PCS, p-cresyl sulfate; PhS, phenyl sulfate; HA, hippuric acid; IAA, indoleacetic acid. Data are shown as mean ± S.D. (n = 4). Asterisks indicate significant difference compared to corresponding control ($P < 0.01$). Concentrations of solutes (mmol/L) are shown in parentheses.

Annexin V-FITC positive cells (%)   Annexin V-FITC/PI positive cells (%)

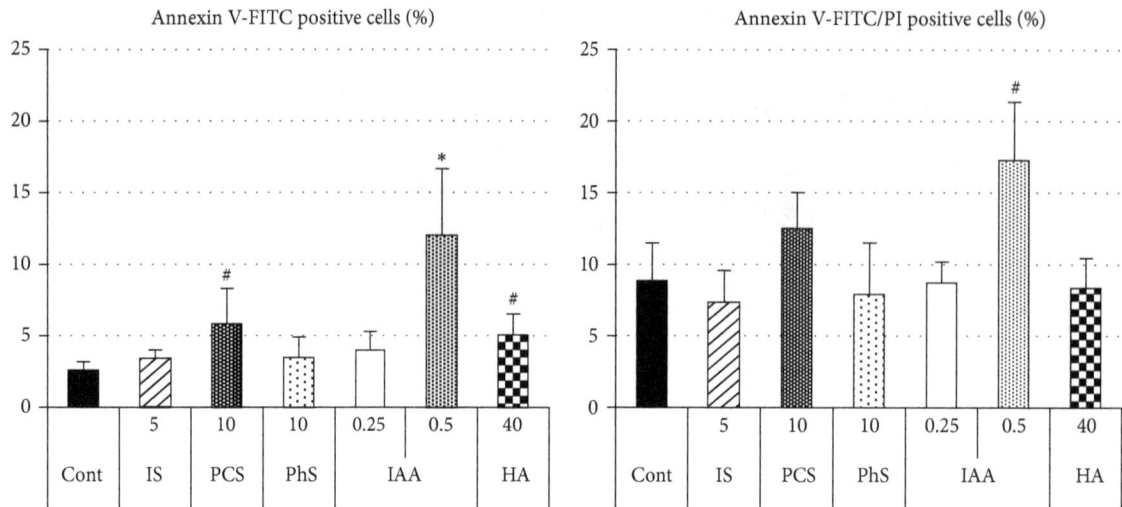

FIGURE 4: Effects of uremic solutes on cell death. After 48-hour incubation with each uremic solute, porcine renal tubular cells were stained with annexin V-FITC and propidium iodide (PI). Percent of annexin V-positive cells and annexin V/PI-positive cells was analyzed and calculated. Cont, control; IS, indoxyl sulfate; PCS, p-cresyl sulfate; PhS, phenyl sulfate; HA, hippuric acid; IAA, indoleacetic acid. Data are shown as mean ± S.D. (n = 4). Asterisk indicates significant difference compared to corresponding control ($P < 0.01$). Sharp marks (#) indicate $P < 0.05$.

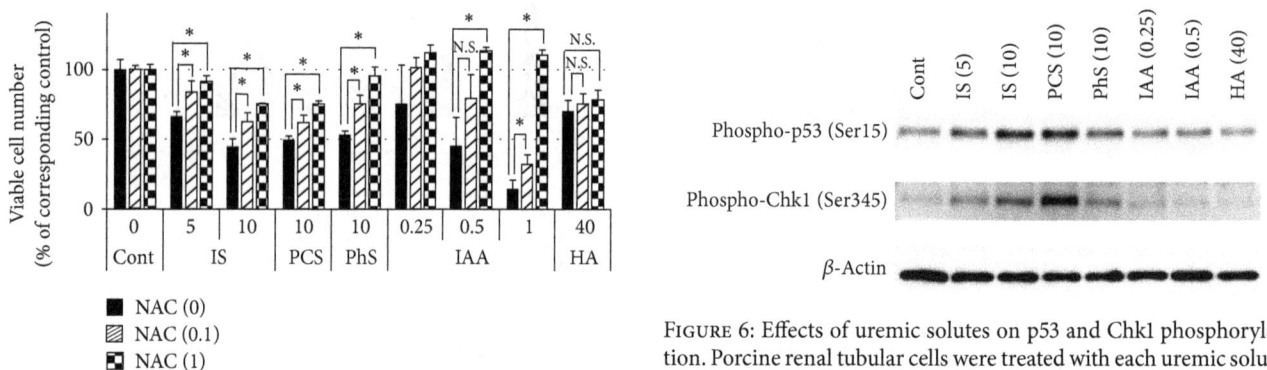

FIGURE 5: Effect of N-acetyl-L-cysteine (NAC) on uremic solute-induced decrease in viable cell number. Porcine renal tubular cells were treated with NAC (0, 0.1 or 1 mmol/L) for 20 minutes and further treated with each uremic solute for 48 hours. Viable cell number was evaluated using Cell Counting Kit-8. Optical density at 450 nm was measured and the values were calculated as percent of the corresponding control. Cont, control; IS, indoxyl sulfate; PCS, p-cresyl sulfate; PhS, phenyl sulfate; HA, hippuric acid; IAA, indoleacetic acid. Data are shown as mean ± S.D. (n = 4). Asterisks indicate significant difference each pairs described in this figure ($P < 0.01$). N.S. means nonsignificant difference.

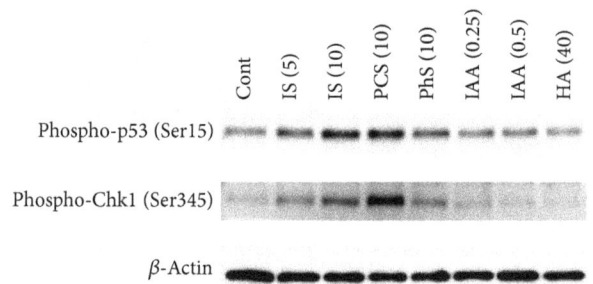

FIGURE 6: Effects of uremic solutes on p53 and Chk1 phosphorylation. Porcine renal tubular cells were treated with each uremic solute for 5 hours. Cell lysates were obtained and subjected to Western blotting. Cont, control; IS, indoxyl sulfate; PCS, p-cresyl sulfate; PhS, phenyl sulfate; HA, hippuric acid; IAA, indoleacetic acid. Images are representative of two independent experiments.

3.6. Expression of Genes Involved in Growth Delay or Cell Death. To further explore molecules which are involved in uremic solute-induced cell cycle delay and/or cell death, we examined the expression of genes known to play important roles in these processes (Figure 7). IS and PCS significantly induced p21 mRNA expression at 24 hours after treatment. IS (10 mmol/L), PCS, and HA significantly induced Puma (p53 upregulated modulator of apoptosis) mRNA expression at 5 hours after treatment. PCS and PhS suppressed Cdc20 and Skp2 mRNA expression at 24 hours after treatment. IS, PCS, PhS, and HA induced ATF4 and CHOP mRNA. On the other hand, IAA did not affect the expression of all these genes at all concentrations tested. In this experiment, 0.25, 0.5, and 1 mmol/L of IAA decreased viable cell number by 16, 49, and 72%, respectively (Supplementary Figure 5).

4. Discussion

To the best of our knowledge, this is the first study that systematically compared the effects of five uremic solutes on porcine renal tubular cells. Our results are schematized in Figure 8. The five solutes evaluated in this study were categorized into three groups by the difference in mechanism of reducing viable cell number upon 48-hour treatment.

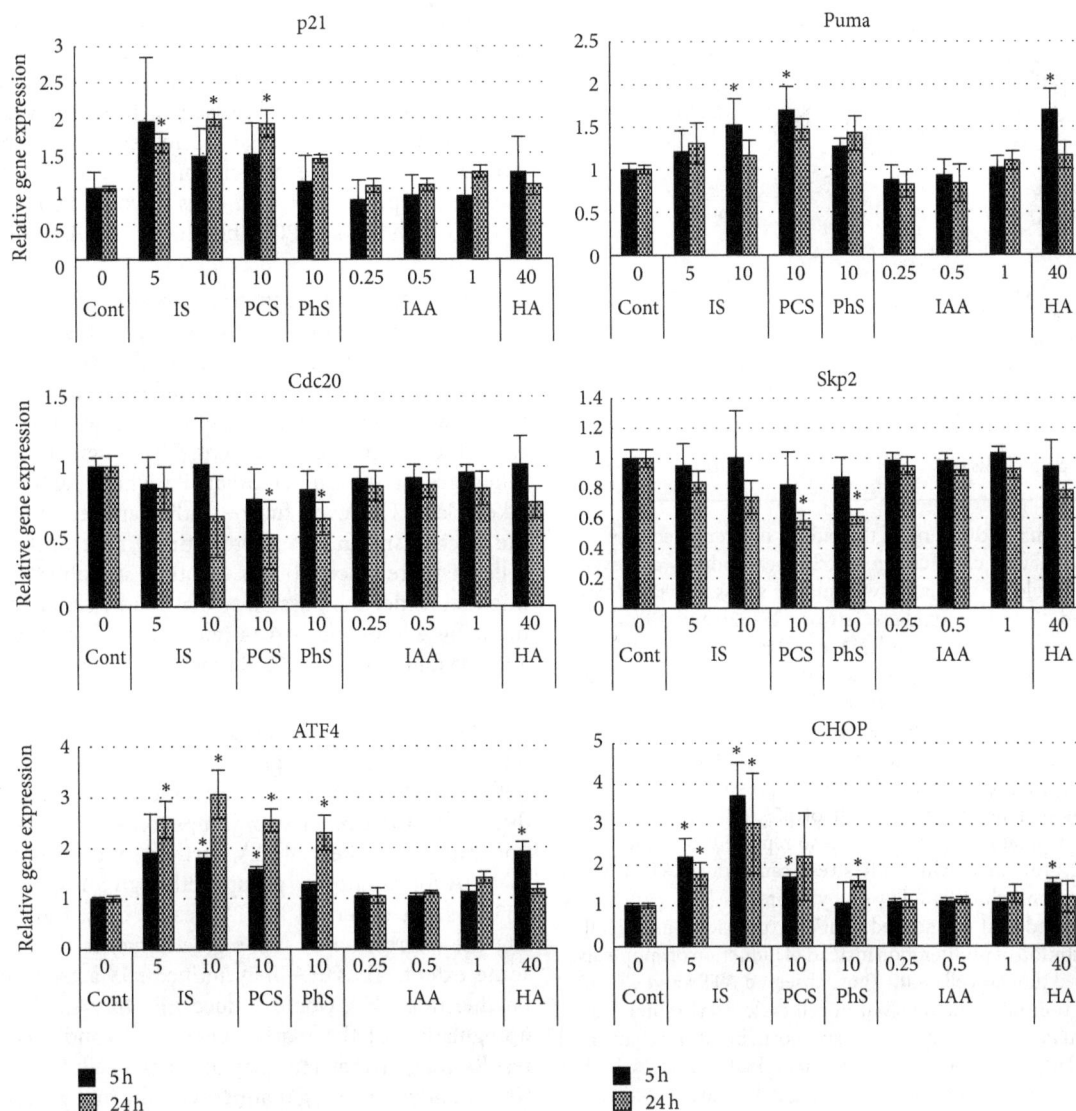

FIGURE 7: Effects of uremic solutes on gene expression. Porcine renal tubular cells were treated with each uremic solute for 5 and 24 hours. Total RNA was extracted and subjected to real-time PCR. Gene expression level relative to GAPDH expression was calculated by $\Delta\Delta$Ct method. Data are expressed as relative values to the corresponding control. Cont, control; IS, indoxyl sulfate; PCS, p-cresyl sulfate; PhS, phenyl sulfate; HA, hippuric acid; IAA, indoleacetic acid. Data are shown as mean ± S.D. ($n = 6$). Asterisks indicate more than 1.5-fold increase or decrease with statistical significance compared to corresponding control ($P < 0.01$).

The first group is composed of IS, PCS, and PhS. This group of solutes induces delay in cell cycle progression rather than cell death to reduce the viable cell number. Oxidative stress is presumably involved in these processes, because viable cell number was partly recovered by incubation with N-acetyl-L-cysteine. Moreover IS is reported to induce oxidative stress in several cell types including renal tubular cells [27–32]. This oxidative stress would induce DNA damage, which is followed by activation of Chk1 and p53 [33]. Subsequent modulation or regulation of their downstream targets would eventually delay cell cycle progression [31, 32, 34–38]. Meanwhile, upregulation of ATF4 and CHOP, known as a hallmark of one of the three pathways of endoplasmic reticulum stress (ER stress) response, was also observed. ER stress response is an adaptive response in

nature, but prolonged ER stress overwhelms the adaptive response and eventually results in apoptosis through CHOP upregulation [39]. Thus, upregulation of these genes could induce apoptosis, but only marginal increase of dying cells was observed with this group of solutes. A possible reason is that the incubation time was too short to observe apoptosis. On the other hand, it is reported that CHOP induction by IS inhibits cellular proliferation in human proximal tubular cells [40]. Therefore upregulation of ATF4 and CHOP might also contribute to delay in cell cycle progression in addition to activation of the p53 pathway.

IS has been reported to inhibit proliferation of human proximal tubular cells through inducing oxidative stress, p53 activation, and ER stress [29, 32, 40]. The present study confirms these phenomena in porcine tubular cells

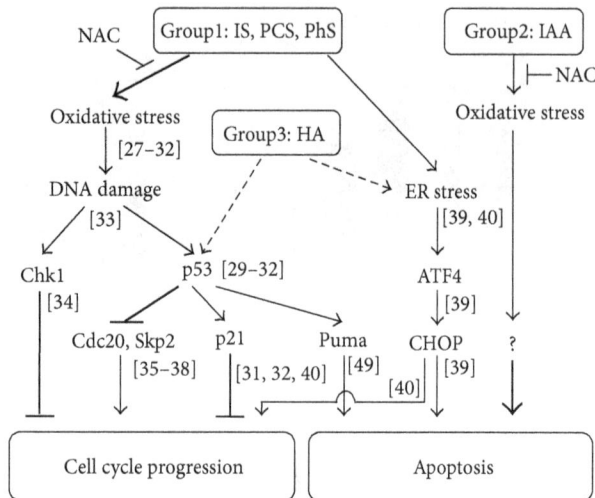

FIGURE 8: Schematic diagram of the effects of uremic solutes on porcine renal tubular cells. *Group 1* exclusively induces cell cycle delay, which would be mediated by oxidative stress and ER stress. IS is reported to induce oxidative stress [27–32] and ER stress [40]. Oxidative stress can cause DNA damage, which is followed by Chk1 and p53 activation [33]. Activated Chk1 can arrest cell cycle progression [34]. Activation of p53 by IS is also reported [29–32]. Activated p53 can repress transcription of Cdc20 [38] and Skp2 [36, 37]. Because both Cdc20 and Skp2 have important roles in cell cycle progression [35], their repression might delay cell cycle. Another downstream target of p53, p21, which is also an important regulator of cell cycle, is also reported to be induced by IS [31, 32, 40]. Meanwhile, ER stress can induce ATF4 and CHOP expression, which is followed by apoptosis [39]. However, it is also reported that IS induced CHOP expression and CHOP mediates inhibition of proliferation instead of induction of apoptosis in human renal tubular cells [40]. Thus, observed ATF4 and CHOP mRNA induction might be involved in cell cycle delay rather than apoptosis. *Group 2* exclusively induces apoptosis, but its mechanism of action is largely unknown. *Group 3* marginally induces both cell cycle delay and apoptosis, which might be partly mediated by p53 and ER stress. More detailed explanation is in Section 4. Cont, control; IS, indoxyl sulfate; PCS, *p*-cresyl sulfate; PhS, phenyl sulfate; HA, hippuric acid; IAA, indoleacetic acid; NAC, N-acetyl-L-cysteine. Number in brackets corresponds to the number of reference literature.

and additionally reveals that PCS and PhS induce growth retardation in a similar manner as IS. Administration of PCS to CKD rat model has been shown to cause further renal tubular damage by mechanisms similar to that of IS [41]. Moreover another report reveals that IS and PCS induce similar inflammatory gene expressions in renal tubular cells [42]. Thus, IS, PCS, and PhS might aggravate renal function via p53 activation and ER stress in an additive manner. Activation of p53 and resultant cellular senescence have been proposed to increase sensitivity to insult and decrease repair ability in the renal system, further impairing renal function [43]. ER stress is also known to be involved in the progression of kidney disease [44]. Future studies are necessary to clarify the involvement of these solutes in the induction of cellular senescence and/or ER stress in clinical settings.

IS also induces cellular senescence via p53 activation in other cell types such as endothelial cells [30] and vascular smooth muscle cells [31], which implies involvement of IS in the progression of cardiovascular disease (CVD) in CKD patients, as has been suggested in several epidemiological studies [22, 23]. The association of PCS with CVD has also been reported [45–47]. Thus it would be interesting to evaluate the effects of PCS and PhS in vascular cells.

The second group comprises only IAA, but other solutes not tested in this study may also belong to this group. In sharp contrast to IS, IAA induces cell death rather than delay of cell cycle progression to reduce viable cell number. Although the effects of both IAA and IS seemed to be mediated by ROS, the results were different. This might be due to the difference of subcellular organelle where ROS production takes place. However, future studies are required to clarify the mechanisms in detail. Interestingly, senescent endothelial cells are more susceptible to apoptotic stimuli [48]. Thus one might consider the possibility that IS (a cellular senescence-inducing solute) and IAA (a cell death-inducing solute) may affect viability of certain cell types in a cooperative manner.

The third group comprises HA, but again other solutes may also belong to this group. HA marginally induces delay both in cell cycle progression and in cell death, which differs from the other two groups. N-Acetyl-L-cysteine did not inhibit the effect of HA, further supporting the notion that HA forms another group. Although phosphorylation of p53 was not observed in HA-treated cells, HA did modulate the expression of p53-regulated genes (Puma) [49] to some extent. Thus HA may induce p53 activation slightly. Furthermore, HA would induce ER stress, as indicated by upregulation of the marker gene ATF4 and CHOP. These results suggest that HA may affect the cellular system in a somewhat overlapping manner with the first group.

This study has some limitations. First, the concentrations of the uremic solute tested in this experiment were much higher than the serum concentrations in CKD patients [2, 5, 25]. In clinical settings, multiple uremic solutes exist and may affect biological systems in an additive or synergistic manner. However, only a single solute was tested in each experiment. Thus, high concentrations were necessary to obtain measurable effects on cellular function and to evaluate the mechanisms of each solute.

In conclusion, this study suggests that uremic solutes can be categorized into groups depending on their mechanisms of action on cells. We speculate that solutes within a group exert their effects in an additive manner while solutes in different groups act in a cooperative manner. Future studies are necessary to verify these possibilities.

References

[1] R. Vanholder, R. de Smet, G. Glorieux et al., "Review on uremic toxins: classification, concentration, and interindividual

variability," *Kidney International*, vol. 63, no. 5, pp. 1934–1943, 2003.

[2] J. Boelaert, F. Lynen, G. Glorieux et al., "A novel UPLC-MS-MS method for simultaneous determination of seven uremic retention toxins with cardiovascular relevance in chronic kidney disease patients," *Analytical and Bioanalytical Chemistry*, vol. 405, no. 6, pp. 1937–1947, 2013.

[3] C.-J. Lin, H.-H. Chen, C.-F. Pan et al., "p-Cresylsulfate and indoxyl sulfate level at different stages of chronic kidney disease," *Journal of Clinical Laboratory Analysis*, vol. 25, no. 3, pp. 191–197, 2011.

[4] N. Neirynck, R. Vanholder, E. Schepers, S. Eloot, A. Pletinck, and G. Glorieux, "An update on uremic toxins," *International Urology and Nephrology*, vol. 45, no. 1, pp. 139–150, 2013.

[5] F. Duranton, G. Cohen, R. De Smet et al., "Normal and pathologic concentrations of uremic toxins," *Journal of the American Society of Nephrology*, vol. 23, no. 7, pp. 1258–1270, 2012.

[6] R. Vanholder, S. van Laecke, and G. Glorieux, "The middle-molecule hypothesis 30 years after: lost and rediscovered in the universe of uremic toxicity?" *Journal of Nephrology*, vol. 21, no. 2, pp. 146–160, 2008.

[7] R. Vanholder, R. De Smet, and N. Lameire, "Protein-bound uremic solutes: the forgotten toxins," *Kidney International*, vol. 59, pp. S266–S270, 2001.

[8] S. Liabeuf, T. B. Drüeke, and Z. A. Massy, "Protein-bound uremic toxins: new insight from clinical studies," *Toxins*, vol. 3, no. 7, pp. 911–919, 2011.

[9] M. Motojima, A. Hosokawa, H. Yamato, T. Muraki, and T. Yoshioka, "Uremic toxins of organic anions up-regulate PAI-1 expression by induction of NF-κB and free radical in proximal tubular cells," *Kidney International*, vol. 63, no. 5, pp. 1671–1680, 2003.

[10] A. K. Gelasco and J. R. Raymond, "Indoxyl sulfate induces complex redox alterations in mesangial cells," *The American Journal of Physiology—Renal Physiology*, vol. 290, no. 6, pp. F1551–F1558, 2006.

[11] L. Dou, E. Bertrand, C. Cerini et al., "The uremic solutes p-cresol and indoxyl sulfate inhibit endothelial proliferation and wound repair," *Kidney International*, vol. 65, no. 2, pp. 442–451, 2004.

[12] G. Muteliefu, A. Enomoto, P. Jiang, M. Takahashi, and T. Niwa, "Indoxyl sulphate induces oxidative stress and the expression of osteoblast-specific proteins in vascular smooth muscle cells," *Nephrology Dialysis Transplantation*, vol. 24, no. 7, pp. 2051–2058, 2009.

[13] A. Mozar, L. Louvet, C. Godin et al., "Indoxyl sulphate inhibits osteoclast differentiation and function," *Nephrology Dialysis Transplantation*, vol. 27, no. 6, pp. 2176–2181, 2012.

[14] T. Nii-Kono, Y. Iwasaki, M. Uchida et al., "Indoxyl sulfate induces skeletal resistance to parathyroid hormone in cultured osteoblastic cells," *Kidney International*, vol. 71, no. 8, pp. 738–743, 2007.

[15] M. S. E. Ahmed, M. Abed, J. Voelkl, and F. Lang, "Triggering of suicidal erythrocyte death by uremic toxin indoxyl sulfate," *BMC Nephrology*, vol. 14, no. 1, article 244, 2013.

[16] S. Ito, Y. Higuchi, Y. Yagi et al., "Reduction of indoxyl sulfate by AST-120 attenuates monocyte inflammation related to chronic kidney disease," *Journal of Leukocyte Biology*, vol. 93, no. 6, pp. 837–845, 2013.

[17] T. Miyazaki, M. Ise, M. Hirata et al., "Indoxyl sulfate stimulates renal synthesis of transforming growth factor-β1 and progression of renal failure," *Kidney International*, vol. 51, no. 63, pp. S211–S214, 1997.

[18] T. Miyazaki, M. Ise, H. Seo, and T. Niwa, "Indoxyl sulfate increases the gene expressions of TGF-β1, TIMP-1 and pro-α1(I) collagen in uremic rat kidneys," *Kidney International, Supplement*, vol. 51, no. 62, pp. S15–S22, 1997.

[19] A. Adijiang, S. Goto, S. Uramoto, F. Nishijima, and T. Niwa, "Indoxyl sulphate promotes aortic calcification with expression of osteoblast-specific proteins in hypertensive rats," *Nephrology Dialysis Transplantation*, vol. 23, no. 6, pp. 1892–1901, 2008.

[20] S. Ito, M. Osaka, Y. Higuchi, F. Nishijima, H. Ishii, and M. Yoshida, "Indoxyl sulfate induces leukocyte-endothelial interactions through up-regulation of E-selectin," *The Journal of Biological Chemistry*, vol. 285, no. 50, pp. 38869–38875, 2010.

[21] I.-W. Wu, K.-H. Hsu, C.-C. Lee et al., "P-cresyl sulphate and indoxyl sulphate predict progression of chronic kidney disease," *Nephrology Dialysis Transplantation*, vol. 26, no. 3, pp. 938–947, 2011.

[22] C.-J. Lin, H.-L. Liu, C.-F. Pan et al., "Indoxyl sulfate predicts cardiovascular disease and renal function deterioration in advanced chronic kidney disease," *Archives of Medical Research*, vol. 43, no. 6, pp. 451–456, 2012.

[23] F. C. Barreto, D. V. Barreto, S. Liabeuf et al., "Serum indoxyl sulfate is associated with vascular disease and mortality in chronic kidney disease patients," *Clinical Journal of the American Society of Nephrology*, vol. 4, no. 10, pp. 1551–1558, 2009.

[24] K. Kikuchi, Y. Itoh, R. Tateoka, A. Ezawa, K. Murakami, and T. Niwa, "Metabolomic analysis of uremic toxins by liquid chromatography/electrospray ionization-tandem mass spectrometry," *Journal of Chromatography B: Analytical Technologies in the Biomedical and Life Sciences*, vol. 878, no. 20, pp. 1662–1668, 2010.

[25] Y. Itoh, A. Ezawa, K. Kikuchi, Y. Tsuruta, and T. Niwa, "Protein-bound uremic toxins in hemodialysis patients measured by liquid chromatography/tandem mass spectrometry and their effects on endothelial ROS production," *Analytical and Bioanalytical Chemistry*, vol. 403, no. 7, pp. 1841–1850, 2012.

[26] K. S. Hodgkins and H. W. Schnaper, "Tubulointerstitial injury and the progression of chronic kidney disease," *Pediatric Nephrology*, vol. 27, no. 6, pp. 901–909, 2012.

[27] Z. Tumur and T. Niwa, "Indoxyl sulfate inhibits nitric oxide production and cell viability by inducing oxidative stress in vascular endothelial cells," *The American Journal of Nephrology*, vol. 29, no. 6, pp. 551–557, 2009.

[28] V.-C. Wu, G.-H. Young, P.-H. Huang et al., "In acute kidney injury, indoxyl sulfate impairs human endothelial progenitor cells: modulation by statin," *Angiogenesis*, vol. 16, no. 3, pp. 609–624, 2013.

[29] H. Shimizu, D. Bolati, A. Adijiang et al., "Senescence and dysfunction of proximal tubular cells are associated with activated p53 expression by indoxyl sulfate," *American Journal of Physiology: Cell Physiology*, vol. 299, no. 5, pp. C1110–C1117, 2010.

[30] Y. Adelibieke, H. Shimizu, G. Muteliefu, D. Bolati, and T. Niwa, "Indoxyl sulfate induces endothelial cell senescence by increasing reactive oxygen species production and p53 activity," *Journal of Renal Nutrition*, vol. 22, no. 1, pp. 86–89, 2012.

[31] G. Muteliefu, H. Shimizu, A. Enomoto, F. Nishijima, M. Takahashi, and T. Niwa, "Indoxyl sulfate promotes vascular smooth muscle cell senescence with upregulation of p53, p21,

and prelamin A through oxidative stress," *American Journal of Physiology—Cell Physiology*, vol. 303, no. 2, pp. C126–C134, 2012.

[32] H. Shimizu, D. Bolati, A. Adijiang et al., "NF-κb plays an important role in indoxyl sulfate-induced cellular senescence, fibrotic gene expression, and inhibition of proliferation in proximal tubular cells," *American Journal of Physiology: Cell Physiology*, vol. 301, no. 5, pp. C1201–C1212, 2011.

[33] H. Niida and M. Nakanishi, "DNA damage checkpoints in mammals," *Mutagenesis*, vol. 21, no. 1, pp. 3–9, 2006.

[34] C. S. Sørensen and R. G. Syljuåsen, "Safeguarding genome integrity: the checkpoint kinases ATR, CHK1 and WEE1 restrain CDK activity during normal DNA replication," *Nucleic Acids Research*, vol. 40, no. 2, pp. 477–486, 2012.

[35] P. Fasanaro, M. C. Capogrossi, and F. Martelli, "Regulation of the endothelial cell cycle by the ubiquitin-proteasome system," *Cardiovascular Research*, vol. 85, no. 2, pp. 272–280, 2010.

[36] T. Zuo, R. Liu, H. Zhang et al., "FOXP3 is a novel transcriptional repressor for the breast cancer oncogene SKP2," *Journal of Clinical Investigation*, vol. 117, no. 12, pp. 3765–3773, 2007.

[37] D.-J. Jung, D.-H. Jin, S.-W. Hong et al., "Foxp3 expression in p53-dependent DNA damage responses," *The Journal of Biological Chemistry*, vol. 285, no. 11, pp. 7995–8002, 2010.

[38] T. Banerjee, S. Nath, and S. Roychoudhury, "DNA damage induced p53 downregulates Cdc20 by direct binding to its promoter causing chromatin remodeling," *Nucleic Acids Research*, vol. 37, no. 8, pp. 2688–2698, 2009.

[39] R. Sano and J. C. Reed, "ER stress-induced cell death mechanisms," *Biochimica et Biophysica Acta—Molecular Cell Research*, vol. 1833, no. 12, pp. 3460–3470, 2013.

[40] T. Kawakami, R. Inagi, T. Wada, T. Tanaka, T. Fujita, and M. Nangaku, "Indoxyl sulfate inhibits proliferation of human proximal tubular cells via endoplasmic reticulum stress," *American Journal of Physiology—Renal Physiology*, vol. 299, no. 3, pp. F568–F576, 2010.

[41] H. Watanabe, Y. Miyamoto, D. Honda et al., "*p*-Cresyl sulfate causes renal tubular cell damage by inducing oxidative stress by activation of NADPH oxidase," *Kidney International*, vol. 83, no. 4, pp. 582–592, 2013.

[42] C.-Y. Sun, H.-H. Hsu, and M.-S. Wu, "*P*-Cresol sulfate and indoxyl sulfate induce similar cellular inflammatory gene expressions in cultured proximal renal tubular cells," *Nephrology Dialysis Transplantation*, vol. 28, no. 1, pp. 70–78, 2013.

[43] H. Yang and A. B. Fogo, "Cell senescence in the aging kidney," *Journal of the American Society of Nephrology*, vol. 21, no. 9, pp. 1436–1439, 2010.

[44] R. Inagi, "Endoplasmic reticulum stress as a progression factor for kidney injury," *Current Opinion in Pharmacology*, vol. 10, no. 2, pp. 156–165, 2010.

[45] B. K. I. Meijers, K. Claes, B. Bammens et al., "*p*-Cresol and cardiovascular risk in mild-to-moderate kidney disease," *Clinical Journal of the American Society of Nephrology*, vol. 5, no. 7, pp. 1182–1189, 2010.

[46] I.-W. Wu, K.-H. Hsu, H.-J. Hsu et al., "Serum free p-cresyl sulfate levels predict cardiovascular and all-cause mortality in elderly hemodialysis patients—a prospective cohort study," *Nephrology Dialysis Transplantation*, vol. 27, no. 3, pp. 1169–1175, 2012.

[47] C.-J. Lin, C.-K. Chuang, T. Jayakumar et al., "Serum *p*-cresyl sulfate predicts cardiovascular disease and mortality in elderly hemodialysis patients," *Archives of Medical Science*, vol. 9, no. 4, pp. 662–668, 2013.

[48] J. Hoffmann, J. Haendeler, A. Aicher et al., "Aging enhances the sensitivity of endothelial cells toward apoptotic stimuli: important role of nitric oxide," *Circulation Research*, vol. 89, no. 8, pp. 709–715, 2001.

[49] K. Nakano and K. H. Vousden, "PUMA, a novel proapoptotic gene, is induced by p53," *Molecular Cell*, vol. 7, no. 3, pp. 683–694, 2001.

11

Anti-VEGF Cancer Therapy in Nephrology Practice

Hassan Izzedine[1,2]

[1] Department of Nephrology, Pitie-Salpetriere Hospital, 75013 Paris, France
[2] Department of Nephrology, Monceau Park International Clinic, 75017 Paris, France

Correspondence should be addressed to Hassan Izzedine; hassan.izzedine@psl.aphp.fr

Academic Editor: Danuta Zwolinska

Expanded clinical experience with the antivascular endothelial growth factor (VEGF) agents has come with increasing recognition of their renal adverse effects. Although renal histology is rarely sought in antiangiogenic-treated cancer patients, kidney damage related to anti-VEGF is now established. Its manifestations include hypertension, proteinuria, and mainly glomerular thrombotic microangiopathy. Then, in nephrology practice, should we continue to perform kidney biopsy, and what should be done with the anti-VEGF agents in case of renal toxicity?

1. Introduction

Angiogenesis is a vital physiologic process needed for growth and development [1, 2]. In the renal glomeruli, podocytes express vascular endothelial growth factor (VEGF), whereas VEGF receptor tyrosine kinases are expressed by both podocytes and glomerular endothelial cells [3]. The biological functions of VEGF are mediated by its binding to one of the VEGF receptor tyrosine kinases, which include VEGFR-1 (Flt-1), VEGFR-2 (KDR/Flk-1), and VEGFR-3 (Flt-4). A major regulator of angiogenesis is VEGF and its cognate receptor VEGFR2. Antiangiogenesis agents are among the most commonly used anticancer agents in oncology practice today. Therapeutic approaches target the VEGF ligand (bevacizumab (anti-VEGF monoclonal antibody), aflibercept (VEGF Trap)) or the tyrosine kinase receptor [sunitinib, sorafenib, and pazopanib] TKI interfere with the activity of VEGFR and other growth factors, among them PDGF receptors (PDGFRs), stem cell factor receptor (c-kit), FMS-like tyrosine kinase-3 (Flt-3), and b-raf and Bcl-Abl. They are, thus, commonly named as multitargeted TKI. Table 1 summarized several selected FDA approved targeted antiangiogenic agents.

2. Renal Adverse Effects

The filtration barrier of the renal glomeruli is formed by endothelial cells (ECs), podocytes, and basement membrane components. VEGF, which is expressed by podocytes both during development and in the adult, activates VEGFR-2 on glomerular capillary endothelial cells. Interaction of VEGF produced by podocytes with VEGFR2 on glomerular ECs is critical to the normal function and repair of the system. Clinically, renal adverse effects following anti-VEGF therapies may present as hypertension, asymptomatic proteinuria, and, rarely, nephrotic syndrome or acute renal failure. The underlying pathological changes are not always clear. In the few cases where renal biopsies were performed, pathological findings have included proliferative glomerulopathies, thrombotic microangiopathy [4], and, rarely, interstitial nephritis [5]. In preclinical murine models, heterozygous deletion of *VEGF* in podocytes led to loss of EC fenestration, loss of podocytes, mesangiolysis, and proteinuria [6, 7] suggesting that VEGF have a critical protective role in the pathogenesis of microangiopathic process [8].

2.1. Hypertension. Hypertension is one of the best-documented and most frequently observed AE of VEGF/VEGFr inhibitors [9–16]. It is a VEGF inhibitor class dependent, dose-dependent, and additive adverse event [11]. Hypertension can occur any time after the initiation of treatment and may be involved after prolonged treatment. This side effect usually can be managed with oral antihypertensive agents, and anti-VEGF treatment can be continued without reduction in dose. The effect of anti-VEGF agents on blood pressure

TABLE 1: Selected FDA approved targeted anticancer drugs.

Generic (trade) names	Target gene or receptor	Indication
IV antiangiogenic drugs		
Bevacizumab (Avastin)	VEGF-A	Metastatic colorectal cancer (mCRC) (with chemotherapy) Metastatic NSCLC (with chemotherapy) Metastatic breast cancer (with chemotherapy) Recurrent glioblastoma (monotherapy) Metastatic renal cell carcinoma (RCC) (with IFN-a)
VEGF Trap (Aflibercept)	VEGF A, PlGF	mCRC (second-line)
Temsirolimus (Toricel)	mTOR	Advanced RCC
Oral antiangiogenic drugs		
Dasatinib (Syrcell)	BCR-ABL	Philadelphia chromosome-positive (Ph+) CML
Imatinib (Gleevec)	BCR-ABL	Ph+ CML; gastrointestinal stromal tumor (GIST)
Nilotinib (Tasigna)	BCR-ABL	Ph+ CML
Bosutinib (Bosulif)	BCR-ABL, Src	Ph+ CML
Ponatinib (Iclusig)	BCR-ABL	ALL and CML
Vemurafenib (Zelboraf)	BRAFV600E	Melanoma
Vismodegib (Erivedge)	SMO	Basal cell carcinoma
Ruxolitinib (Jakafi)	JAK1/2	Myelofibrosis
Gefinitib (Iressa)	EGFR	NSCLC
Erlotinib (Tarceva)	EGFR	NSCLC and pancreatic cancer
Crizotinib (Xalkori)	EML4-ALK	NSCLC
Abiraterone (Zytiga)	CYP17A1	Prostate cancer
Enzalutamide (Xtandi)	AR	Prostate cancer
Regorafenib (Stivarga)	VEGFR2, PDGFR, FGFRs, Tie2, RAF-1, BRAF, BRAFV600E, Abl	Metastatic colorectal cancer (refractory disease)
Lenalidomide (Revlimid)	Anti-tumor, immunomodulatory	Multiple myeloma
Lapatinib (Tykreb)	EGFR, HER2/neu	Breast cancer
Sunitinib (Sutent)	VEGFRs, PDGFR, VEGF, cKIT, RET, CSF-1R, flt3	GIST; advanced RCC; Unresectable locally advanced or metastatic pancreatic neuroendocrine tumours
Sorafenib (Nexavar)	VEGFR, PDGFR, C-Raf, B-Raf, MAP Kinase, cKIT	Advanced RCC Unresectable hepatocellular carcinoma
Pazopanib (Votrient)	VEGF, c-kit, PDGFR	RCC; advanced soft tissue sarcoma chemotherapy treated
Vandetanib	VEGFRs, EGFRs and RET	Unresectable locally advanced or metastatic medullary thyroid cancer
Everolimus (Afinitor)	mTOR	Advanced HER2-negative Breast Cancer, Progressive Neuroendocrine Tumours of Pancreatic Origin (PNET), Subependymal Giant Cell Astrocytoma (SEGA), Advanced RCC; soft tissue sarcoma; renal angiomyolipoma

VEGFR, vascular endothelial growth factor receptor; NSCLC, non-small cell lung cancer; BCR-ABL, fusion of abelson (Abl) tyrosine kinase gen at chromosome 9 and break point cluster (Bcr) gene at chromosome 22; CML, chronic myeloid leukemia; EGFR, epidermal growth factor receptor; EML4-ALK, rearrangement of echinoderm microtubule-associated protein-like 4-anaplastic lymphoma kinase; HER2/neu, one of four membrane proteins in EGFR family; PDGFG, platelet-derived growth factor receptor RET: proto-oncogene, encodes receptor kinase for the neurotrophic factor family; CSF-1R, colony stimulating factor; flt3, encodes receptor tyrosine kinase that regulates hematopoiesis; MAP kinase, family of serine threonine proteins responsible for regulating cellular activities, such as apoptosis; c-kit, tyrosine kinase stem cell factor receptor; SMO, smoothened, e transmembrane protein involved in Hodgebog signal transduction; mTOR, mammalian target of rapamycin inhibitor; BRAF, gene encoding for B-Raf, member of raf kinase family.

is dose-dependent and the extent of hypertension might reflect the extent of target inhibition. In a phase 2 study in patients with renal-cell carcinoma (RCC) treated with either placebo, 3 mg/kg bevacizumab, or 10 mg/kg bevacizumab, the rate of hypertension was significantly higher in the high-dose group (36%) compared with the low dose group (3%) [17]. With small-molecule VEGFr TKis, the increment rise in blood pressure was also proportional to dose [18]. More-specific and potent VEGFr TKIs, such as cediranib and axi-tinib, are associated with a higher rate of hypertension compared to sunitinib or sorafenib at the MTD [19]. Because blood pressure is a known on-target effect for anti-VEGF

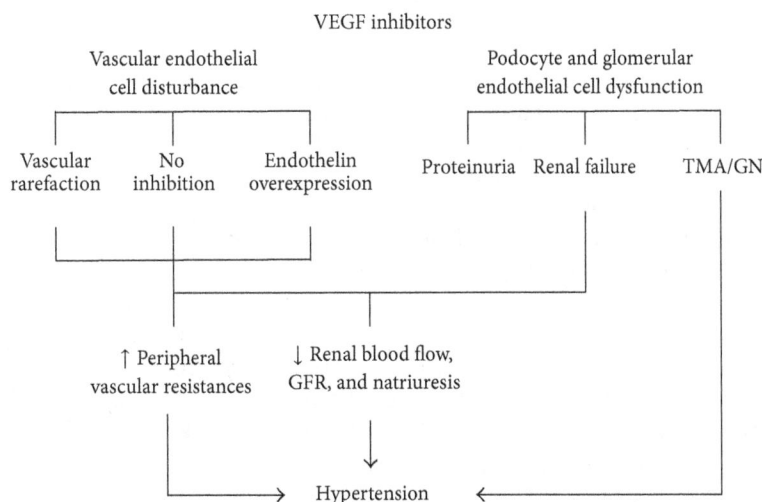

FIGURE 1: Potential mechanisms of hypertension related to anti-VEGF agents.

agents, blood pressure is a potential pharmacodynamic marker for anti-VEGF therapy. In a retrospective analysis of sunitinib in 40 patients with cytokine-refractory RCC, only hypertension, particularly grade 3, was associated with a higher treatment response rate [20]. A similar finding was demonstrated in a prospective study of 43 patients with metastatic RCC treated with bevacizumab. In that study, a significantly longer median time to progression was observed for patients with hypertension than for patients with BP <150/100 mmHg (8.1 versus 4.2; $P = .036$) [21]. Ravaud and Sire [22] evaluated hypertension and efficacy in 93 patients receiving either sunitinib, sorafenib, or bevacizumab as first-, second-, or third-line therapy. Among the eligible patients with grade ≥2 hypertension, 88% had a clinical benefit (defined as an objective response or stable disease) and 53% benefited for ≥6 months, versus 55% and 35%, respectively. More recently, the predictive power of hypertension was evaluated in a retrospective analysis of the phase III CALGB 90206 study, which demonstrated that patients on bevacizumab plus interferon who developed grade ≥2 hypertension had significantly greater progression-free survival and overall survival times than patients who did not develop hypertension [23]. For this reason, there have been several reports correlating treatment related blood pressure changes with clinical outcome [20, 21, 24–26]. However, one analysis used patient-specific data including individual blood pressure values from eight phase III controlled trials with bevacizumab conducted by Genentech or Roche [27] found that treatment-related hypertension did not predict benefit from bevacizumab. Prospective trials are needed to clarify this issue.

VEGFr2 signaling generates nitric oxide and prostaglandin, which induces EC-dependent vasodilatation in arterioles and venules [28, 29] the component of vasculature that has most impact on blood pressure. Hence, blockage of VEGF would lead to vasoconstriction [29–31]. Vascular rarefaction has also been hypothesized as a mechanism of hypertension induced by anti-VEGF therapy [32]. Hypertension may

also reflect a renal parenchymal disorder (i.e., acute renal injury, glomerulopathy, and thrombotic microangiopathy) (Figure 1).

Furthermore, many factors, including preexisting hypertension, cancer type, VEGF polymorphism, chemotherapy and its side effects, other medications, and activity and diet may play a role. Patients with preexisting hypertension are generally more likely to develop further elevation in blood pressure when receiving anti-VEGF therapy. The risk of hypertension related to anti-VEGF therapy is also higher in patients with metastatic RCC compared to other indications as reported in sorafenib (17% and 5% of RCC [33] and hepatocellular carcinoma [34] treated patients the same dose of sorafenib, resp.) and sunitinib [35, 36] phase 3 trials. Certain VEGF polymorphisms might be associated with a lower risk of grade 3 or 4 hypertension in bevacizumab-treated breast cancer patients [37] and under sunitinib therapy [38].

Hypertension is a known risk for more severe complications, such as reversible posterior leukoencephalopathy syndrome. RPLS is attributed to hypertensive encephalopathy and endothelial dysfunction leading to breakdown of the blood-brain barrier, focal cerebral oedema, or vasospasm. RPLS is a serious but reversible condition characterised by onset of headache, altered mental function, seizures, visual impairment or blindness, and occipital-parietal subcortical cerebral oedema evident by computed tomography and magnetic resonance imaging. RPLS has been reported in patients on bevacizumab [39], sunitinib, or sorafenib [40].

In patients with cancer, the primary goal of hypertension management is to maintain an acceptable blood pressure level to allow safe delivery of antiangiogenesis therapy. In order to prevent life-threatening complications, while minimizing delay and/or dose attenuation of anticancer therapy, close monitoring of blood pressure and timely initiation or titration of hypertension medications are critical. The Joint National Committee on Prevention, Detection, Evaluation, and Treatment of High Blood Pressure (JNC7) stipulate that target blood pressure control should be <140/90 mmHg in the general population and <120/80 mmHg in patients with diabetes or renal dysfunction [41]. Although this ideal blood pressure target does not need be reached to allow continuation of antiangiogenesis therapies, given the effectiveness of hypertensive medication, this goal should be achievable in most patients. Hypertension can be controlled with standard oral hypertensive medications in most cases where therapeutic doses of these anti-VEGF agents are used. In patients who develop hypertensive crisis, permanent discontinuation of anti-VEGF therapy is recommended.

2.2. Proteinuria. As for hypertension, proteinuria is a VEGF inhibitor class dependent, dose-dependent, and additive adverse event [11]. Proteinuria was found in 23% of 1132 patients in clinical trials of bevacizumab in various types of cancer and was more common in patients receiving bevacizumab plus chemotherapy than in patients on chemotherapy alone [12, 13]. Significant increase in urine protein (grade 3, >3.5 g protein per 24 h urine) is less common, occurring in 3% of patients in most clinical trials [42–45] and in up to 7-8% of patients with RCC [17, 46]. In rare cases, patients with asymptomatic proteinuria can progress to nephrotic syndrome (<0.5% of patients) [47]. In a follow-up review of more than 12,000 patients, Zhu et al. identified the incidence of high-grade proteinuria (grade 3 or worse) at 2.2% with a relative risk (RR) of 4.79 (95% CI: 2.71–8.46). The RR of developing nephrotic syndrome with chemotherapy containing bevacizumab (when compared with chemotherapy without bevacizumab) was 7.78 [48]. Proteinuria is typically asymptomatic and decreases after treatment ends. Proteinuria is rarely reported in clinical trials with sunitinib or sorafenib, although how closely patients were monitored for this adverse effect is unclear. With axitinib, a potent and specific VEGFr TKi, 32% of patients (17 of 52) with RCC developed grade 2 or higher proteinuria (as measured by a dipstick) and a few patients had proteinuria >1 g per 24 h urine [49]. The common occurrence of proteinuria after inhibition of VEGF signalling reflects the importance of VEGF in normal renal function [6, 7]. Targeted heterozygous deletion of VEGF in podocytes results in renal pathology manifested by loss of endothelial fenestrations in glomerular capillaries, proliferation of glomerular endothelial cells (endotheliosis), loss of podocytes, and proteinuria in mice [6, 7]. Pharmacological inhibition of VEGF signalling in mice also reduces endothelial fenestrations in glomerular capillaries [50]. Inhibition of VEGF-dependent interactions between podocytes and glomerular endothelial cells disrupts the filtration barrier, which in turn leads to dose-dependent proteinuria [6, 50]. Patients treated with anti-VEGF agent should be monitored for proteinuria, by either dipstick or calculation of the urine protein/creatinine ratio on spot urine samples. Anti-VEGF agents should be interrupted if 24 h urine protein exceeds 2.0 or 3.5 g, and these agents should be permanently discontinued upon development of nephrotic syndrome. Serious impairment of renal function is rare. Indeed, in clinical practice, oncologists and nephrologists usually manage proteinuria related to anti VEGF treatment only when at nephrotic range or when associated with renal insufficiency. However, we found that proteinuria induced by anti VEGF therapy, even if weak and without associated renal insufficiency, may reflect a renal TMA in 35% of cases [51]. Hence, proteinuria, even if weak and without associated renal insufficiency, may reflect a serious histological renal disease.

2.3. Renal Thrombotic Microangiopathy. Thrombotic microangiopathy (TMA) has been described in biopsy samples from case reports of patients treated with bevacizumab [8, 52, 53], VEGF-Trap [54], and sunitinib [55–57]. TMA associated with VEGF/VEGFr inhibitors was mostly localized to the kidney, and systemic manifestations (e.g., thrombocytopenia or schistocytosis) were present only in half of these patients [58]. Available data indicate that systemically evident TMA is very rare with anti-VEGF therapies. However, the use of more than one anti-VEGF agent in combination might enhance the risk. In a phase 1 dose escalation trial of concurrent bevacizumab (10 mg/kg every 2 weeks) and escalating doses of sunitinib (25 mg, 37.5 mg, or 50 mg daily for 4 out of 6 weeks) in patients with RCC, 5 of the 12 patients at the highest dose level developed systemic TMA, or microangiopathic haemolytic anemia; clinical presentations in these cases included thrombocytopenia, schistocytes, hypertension, and varying degrees of proteinuria [11, 59].

3. In Nephrology Clinical Practice

3.1. Comparing the Anti-VEGF Agents: Are There (Renal) Toxicity Differences? Anti-VEGF treatments in general have been relatively well tolerated when compared with traditional chemotherapy. This may relate to the tumor specificity of VEGF expression and/or the redundancy of angiogenesis in the host. Common toxicities thought to be related to on-target effects include fatigue, hypertension [60–62], proteinuria, delayed wound healing, and chemical hypothyroidism (often without clinical symptoms) [63–66]. Several rare side effects have also been reported in multiple trials and include bleeding and/or thrombosis (which can be severe or fatal), intestinal and nasal septal perforation [67], effects on growth plates [68], and posterior reversible encephalopathy syndrome (PRES), also known as reversible posterior leukoencephalopathy syndrome (RPLS) [69].

The differences in binding and complex formation between VEGF ligand targeting agents bevacizumab and aflibercept could have important implications in terms of the AE profile, for example, in terms of renal damage and proteinuria resulting from the deposition of VEGF-A-bevacizumab complexes in the kidney [70, 71]. Indeed, unlike bevacizumab VEGF, aflibercept formed stable complexes in the circulation that remained bound to VEGF-A. In addition, although aflibercept formed inert 1 : 1 complexes with VEGF-A, bevacizumab formed heterogeneous multimeric immune complexes that were rapidly cleared from the circulation [71]. Many of TKI agents have unwanted "off-target" AEs associated with their inhibition of non-VEGFR kinases compared with VEGF ligand targeting agents [72, 73]. These off-target AEs included fatigue, diarrhea, nausea, anorexia, and hand-foot reaction [73, 74]. In the past 7 years, we have managed

78 patients who developed biopsy-proven kidney disease under anti VEGF therapy. Those patients were referred for proteinuria, hypertension, and/or renal insufficiency after the initiation of anti VEGF therapy. Of those patients, 65.4% (51 pts) experienced renal thrombotic microangiopathy (TMA) and twenty-seven patients (34.6%) had variable glomerulopathies mainly minimal change disease and/or focal segmental glomerulosclerosis (MCN/FSGS) sometimes in collapsing variant [58]. We found that MCN/FSGS-like lesions developed mainly under TKIs, whereas TMA complicated anti-VEGF ligand [58]. Immunomorphological and molecular studies suggest that RelA and c-mip define two separate glomerular damages associated with anti-angiogenic drugs, based on two distinct pathophysiological mechanisms. Indeed, we show that MCN/FSGS lesions are associated with high abundance of c-mip. In contrast, in TMA resulting from anti-VEGF therapy, c-mip is not detected, while RelA is produced at high levels by podocytes and glomerular endothelial cells [58].

3.2. Kidney Biopsy: Why Is It Done? Proteinuria after inhibition of VEGF signalling will frequently and promptly disappear upon stopping the responsible agent and achieving blood pressure control, and rarely acute renal failure can develop. Furthermore, bleeding is one of the most severe and potentially life-threatening toxicities of antiangiogenic drugs, particularly bevacizumab which retains the highest frequency. Hence, renal biopsy is rarely performed in patients with proteinuria or renal insufficiency under VEGF targeted therapies with the result of an unassessable true rate of glomerulopathy or renal-localized TMA. Therefore, should we reserve the renal biopsy only for research? In my personal view, we must continue to make kidney biopsy in clinical practice for the following reasons: (a) half and 100% of TMA under anti-VEGF are exclusive renal-localized clinically and histologically, respectively [58], (b) proteinuria induced by anti-VEGF therapy, even if weakly and without associated renal insufficiency, may reflect a serious histological renal disease (35% of our 78 TMA patients had proteinuria less than 1 gram per 24 h) [51], and (c) proteinuria may be related to a paraneoplastic membranous nephropathy (2 unpublished personal cases) requiring instead a therapeutic strengthening rather than stopping the anti-VEGF. Moreover, to minimize the hemorrhagic risk, the biopsy should be performed by an interventional nephrologist and/or by transjugular way.

3.3. Once Kidney Disease Related to Anti-VEGF Is Diagnosed, Do We Continue, Discontinue, or Change the Treatment? In clinical practice, the decision to continue, discontinue, or change a treatment is a daily problem. "When to stop" may be interpreted in 2 ways: either the temporary suspension of anti-VEGF agents without any loss of benefit or a final decision to stop. In many cases, this decision depends strongly on the interpretation of the outcome change from baseline. When the change in outcome indicates effectiveness, contin-

uing the treatment is a logical decision. Similarly, discontinuing the treatment is appropriate when it has not been effective. Often, the problem is whether we stop or not an effective treatment due to its renal side effects.

I think we should distinguish two groups of patients: those with glomerular disease type MCN/FSGS for which antihypertensive and antiproteinuric treatments can stabilize kidney disease and those with renal TMA. There are only few published data on renal outcome in this setting. In one case of sunitinib induced renal TMA, blood pressure and renal function remained stable and proteinuria became undetectable under irbesartan over 3 months while sunitinib was continued [55]. Another patient who developed TMA under bevacizumab had favourable response after stopping bevacizumab (normalising blood pressure, disappearance of haemolysis, and return of renal function to previous baseline level). Sunitinib, introduced 2 months later, was stopped after 3 weeks of treatment as a result of the recurrence of a severe TMA. Once again, the response of this second episode was favourable in the days after stoppage of sunitinib, although ten courses of plasma exchange were initially needed [52]. In my own experience, four patients required maintains of an anti-VEGF treatment despite renal TMA. One patient who experienced TMA under VEGF Trap was switched to bevacizumab displaying an absence of proteinuria and stable renal function two years later without TMA recurrence. Two patients with TMA related to bevacizumab continued this therapy in association with antihypertensive drugs for 8 months despite persistent proteinuria and the occurrence of systemic manifestations (such as hemolysis, thrombocytopenia, and schistocytosis) but renal function remained stable. For the last patient, the reintroduction of bevacizumab resulted in a more severe recurrence of TMA (hematological and renal signs). It, therefore, seems more reasonable to stop the culprit drug in case of TMA. In case the offender treatment is the only active one, a temporary halt is still necessary time to obtain an optimal blockade of the renin angiotensin aldosterone system before its reintroduction at half dose if possible and to adjust the dosage according to efficacy and clinical tolerance. Treatment reintroduction or continuation must meet two requirements: a rigorous and necessary monitoring of renal and hematological parameters and discontinuation of treatment in case of recurrence of TMA. Careful risk-benefit assessment for individual patients is important and should take into account risk factors related to the host and the tumour.

In conclusion, anti-VEGF agents may induce hypertension proteinuria and TMA related to endothelial cell dysfunction and regression of fenestrated capillaries. At the current time, approaches to toxicity management and treatment modifications are largely empirical. Therapeutic or observational studies are needed to identify baseline risk factors and early signs of serious AEs and collect data on safety if antiangiogenesis agents be resumed after recovery from AEs.

References

[1] H. F. Dvorak, "Angiogenesis: update 2005," *Journal of Thrombosis and Haemostasis*, vol. 3, no. 8, pp. 1835–1842, 2005.

[2] S. V. Bhadada, B. R. Goyal, and M. M. Patel, "Angiogenic targets for potential disorders," *Fundamental and Clinical Pharmacology*, vol. 25, no. 1, pp. 29–47, 2011.

[3] J. Müller-Deile, K. Worthmann, M. Saleem, I. Tossidou, H. Haller, and M. Schiffer, "The balance of autocrine VEGF-A and VEGF-C determines podocyte survival," *American Journal of Physiology-Renal Physiology*, vol. 297, no. 6, pp. F1656–F1667, 2009.

[4] H. Izzedine, C. Massard, J. P. Spano, F. Goldwasser, D. Khayat, and J. C. Soria, "VEGF signalling inhibition-induced proteinuria: mechanisms, significance and management," *European Journal of Cancer*, vol. 46, no. 2, pp. 439–448, 2010.

[5] R. K. Barakat, N. Singh, R. Lal, R. R. Verani, K. W. Finkel, and J. R. Foringer, "Interstitial nephritis secondary to bevacizumab treatment in metastatic leiomyosarcoma," *Annals of Pharmacotherapy*, vol. 41, no. 4, pp. 707–710, 2007.

[6] V. Eremina, M. Sood, J. Haigh et al., "Glomerular-specific alterations of VEGF-A expression lead to distinct congenital and acquired renal diseases," *The Journal of Clinical Investigation*, vol. 111, no. 5, pp. 707–716, 2003.

[7] B. F. Schrijvers, A. Flyvbjerg, and A. S. de Vriese, "The role of vascular endothelial growth factor (VEGF) in renal pathophysiology," *Kidney International*, vol. 65, no. 6, pp. 2003–2017, 2004.

[8] V. Eremina, J. A. Jefferson, J. Kowalewska et al., "VEGF inhibition and renal thrombotic microangiopathy," *The New England Journal of Medicine*, vol. 358, no. 11, pp. 1129–1136, 2008.

[9] D. C. Sane, L. Anton, and K. B. Brosnihan, "Angiogenic growth factors and hypertension," *Angiogenesis*, vol. 7, no. 3, pp. 193–201, 2004.

[10] W. J. van Heeckeren, J. Ortiz, M. M. Cooney, and S. C. Remick, "Hypertension, proteinuria, and antagonism of vascular endothelial growth factor signaling: clinical toxicity, therapeutic target, or novel biomarker?" *Journal of Clinical Oncology*, vol. 25, no. 21, pp. 2993–2995, 2007.

[11] J. C. Soria, C. Massard, and H. Izzedine, "From theoretical synergy to clinical supra-additive toxicity," *Journal of Clinical Oncology*, vol. 27, no. 9, pp. 1359–1361, 2009.

[12] H. Hurwitz and S. Saini, "Bevacizumab in the treatment of metastatic colorectal cancer: safety profile and management of adverse events," *Seminars in Oncology*, vol. 33, no. 10, pp. S26–S34, 2006.

[13] F. F. Kabbinavar, J. Schulz, M. McCleod et al., "Addition of bevacizumab to bolus fluorouracil and leucovorin in first-line metastatic colorectal cancer: Results of a randomized phase II trial," *Journal of Clinical Oncology*, vol. 23, no. 16, pp. 3697–3705, 2005.

[14] R. J. Motzer, B. I. Rini, R. M. Bukowski et al., "Sunitinib in patients with metastatic renal cell carcinoma," *Journal of the American Medical Association*, vol. 295, no. 21, pp. 2516–2524, 2006.

[15] G. D. Demetri, A. T. van Oosterom, M. Blackstein et al., "Phase 3, multicenter, randomized, double-blind, placebo-controlled trial of SU11248 in patients following failure of imatinib for metastatic GIST," *Journal of Clinical Oncology*, vol. 34, p. 308s, 2005, (Abstract 4000).

[16] R. C. Kane, A. T. Farrell, H. Saber et al., "Sorafenib for the treatment of advanced renal cell carcinoma," *Clinical Cancer Research*, vol. 12, no. 24, pp. 7271–7278, 2006.

[17] J. C. Yang, L. Haworth, R. M. Sherry et al., "A randomized trial of bevacizumab, an anti-vascular endothelial growth factor antibody, for metastatic renal cancer," *The New England Journal of Medicine*, vol. 349, no. 5, pp. 427–434, 2003.

[18] M. L. Maitland et al., "Blood pressure (BP) as a biomarker for sorafenib, an inhibitor of the vascular endothelial growth factor (VEGF) signalling pathway [abstract]," *ASCO Meeting Abstracts*, vol. 24, p. 2035, 2035.

[19] J. Drevs, P. Siegert, M. Medinger et al., "Phase I clinical study of AZD2171, an oral vascular endothelial growth factor signaling inhibitor, in patients with advanced solid tumors," *Journal of Clinical Oncology*, vol. 25, no. 21, pp. 3045–3054, 2007.

[20] O. Rixe, B. Billemont, and H. Izzedine, "Hypertension as a predictive factor of Sunitinib activity," *Annals of Oncology*, vol. 18, no. 6, p. 1117, 2007.

[21] P. Bono, H. Elfving, T. Utriainen et al., "Hypertension and clinical benefit of bevacizumab in the treatment of advanced renal cell carcinoma," *Annals of Oncology*, vol. 20, no. 2, pp. 393–394, 2009.

[22] A. Ravaud and M. Sire, "Arterial hypertension and clinical benefit of sunitinib, sorafenib and bevacizumab in first and second-line treatment of metastatic renal cell cancer," *Annals of Oncology*, vol. 20, no. 5, pp. 966–967, 2009.

[23] B. I. Rini, S. Halabi, J. E. Rosenberg et al., "Phase III trial of bevacizumab plus interferon alfa versus interferon alfa monotherapy in patients with metastatic renal cell carcinoma: final results of CALGB 90206," *Journal of Clinical Oncology*, vol. 28, no. 13, pp. 2137–2143, 2010.

[24] G. Friberg, K. Kasza, E. E. Vokes, and H. L. Kindler, "Early hypertension (HTN) as a potential pharmacodynamic (PD) marker for survival in pancreatic cancer (PC) patients (pts) treated with bevacizumab (B) and gemcitabine (G)," *Journal of Clinical Oncology*, vol. 23, p. 16S, 2005.

[25] S. N. Holden, S. G. Eckhardt, R. Basser et al., "Clinical evaluation of ZD6474, an orally active inhibitor of VEGF and EGF receptor signaling, in patients with solid, malignant tumors," *Annals of Oncology*, vol. 16, no. 8, pp. 1391–1397, 2005.

[26] B. I. Rini, J. H. Schiller, J. P. Fruehauf et al., "Association of diastolic blood pressure (dBP) 90 mmHg with overall survival (OS) in patients treated with axitinib (AG- 013736)," *Journal of Clinical Oncology*, vol. 26, no. 20, abstract 3543, 2008.

[27] H. Hurwitz, P. S. Douglas, J. P. Middleton et al., "Analysis of early hypertension (HTN) and clinical outcome with bevacizumab (BV)," *Journal of Clinical Oncology*, vol. 28, no. 15s, 2010.

[28] J. D. Hood, C. J. Meininger, M. Ziche, and H. J. Granger, "VEGF upregulates ecNOS message, protein, and NO production in human endothelial cells," *American Journal of Physiology: Heart and Circulatory Physiology*, vol. 274, no. 3, pp. H1054–H1058, 1998.

[29] J. R. Horowitz, A. Rivard, R. van der Zee et al., "Vascular endothelial growth factor/vascular permeability factor produces nitric oxide-dependent hypotension: Evidence for a maintenance role in quiescent adult endothelium," *Arteriosclerosis, Thrombosis, and Vascular Biology*, vol. 17, no. 11, pp. 2793–2800, 1997.

[30] C. S. Facemire, A. B. Nixon, R. Griffiths, H. Hurwitz, and T. M. Coffman, "Vascular endothelial growth factor receptor 2 controls blood pressure by regulating nitric oxide synthase expression," *Hypertension*, vol. 54, no. 3, pp. 652–658, 2009.

[31] A. Nixon, J. Allen, E. Miller et al., "Clinical evaluation of nitric oxide responses to anti-VEGF therapy with bevacizumab," *Journal of Clinical Oncology*, vol. 25, no. 18S, 2007.

[32] N. Steeghs, M. Hovens, and A. Rabelink, "VEGFr2 blockade in patients with solid tumors: mechanisms of hypertension and effects on vascular function," *Journal of Clinical Oncology*, vol. 24, abstract 3037, no. 130s, 2006.

[33] B. Escudier, T. Eisen, W. M. Stadler et al., "Sorafenib in advanced clear-cell renal-cell carcinoma," *The New England Journal of Medicine*, vol. 356, no. 2, pp. 125–134, 2007.

[34] J. M. Llovet, S. Ricci, V. Mazzaferro et al., "Sorafenib in advanced hepatocellular carcinoma," *New England Journal of Medicine*, vol. 359, no. 4, pp. 378–390, 2008.

[35] G. D. Demetri, A. T. van Oosterom, C. R. Garrett et al., "Efficacy and safety of sunitinib in patients with advanced gastrointestinal stromal tumour after failure of imatinib: a randomised controlled trial," *The Lancet*, vol. 368, no. 9544, pp. 1329–1338, 2006.

[36] R. J. Motzer, T. E. Hutson, P. Tomczak et al., "Sunitinib versus interferon alfa in metastatic renal-cell carcinoma," *The New England Journal of Medicine*, vol. 356, no. 2, pp. 115–124, 2007.

[37] B. P. Schneider, M. Wang, M. Radovich et al., "Association of vascular endothelial growth factor and vascular endothelial growth factor receptor-2 genetic polymorphisms with outcome in a trial of paclitaxel compared with paclitaxel plus bevacizumab in advanced breast cancer: ECOG 2100," *Journal of Clinical Oncology*, vol. 26, no. 28, pp. 4672–4678, 2008.

[38] K. Eechoute, A. A. M. van der Veldt, S. Oosting et al., "Polymorphisms in endothelial nitric oxide synthase (eNOS) and vascular endothelial growth factor (VEGF) predict sunitinib-induced hypertension," *Clinical Pharmacology and Therapeutics*, vol. 92, no. 4, pp. 503–510, 2012.

[39] J. A. Allen, A. Adlakha, and P. R. Bergethon, "Reversible posterior leukoencephalopathy syndrome after bevacizumab/FOLFIRI regimen for metastatic colon cancer," *Archives of Neurology*, vol. 63, no. 10, pp. 1475–1478, 2006.

[40] R. Govindarajan, J. Adusumilli, D. L. Baxter, A. El-Khoueiry, and S. I. Harik, "Reversible posterior leukoencephalopathy syndrome induced by RAF kinase inhibitor BAY 43-9006," *Journal of Clinical Oncology*, vol. 24, no. 28, article e48, 2006.

[41] A. V. Chobanian, G. L. Bakris, H. R. Black et al., "National Heart, Lung, and Blood Institute Joint National Committee on Prevention, Detection, Evaluation, and Treatment of High Blood Pressure; National High Blood Pressure Education Program Coordinating Committee. The Seventh Report of the Joint National Committee on Prevention, Detection, Evaluation, and Treatment of High Blood Pressure: the JNC 7 report," *Journal of the American Medical Association*, vol. 289, pp. 2560–2572, 2003.

[42] H. Hurwitz, L. Fehrenbacher, W. Novotny et al., "Bevacizumab plus irinotecan, fluorouracil, and leucovorin for metastatic colorectal cancer," *The New England Journal of Medicine*, vol. 350, no. 23, pp. 2335–2342, 2004.

[43] K. Miller, M. Wang, J. Gralow et al., "Paclitaxel plus bevacizumab versus paclitaxel alone for metastatic breast cancer," *The New England Journal of Medicine*, vol. 357, no. 26, pp. 2666–2676, 2007.

[44] B. J. Giantonio, P. J. Catalano, N. J. Meropol et al., "Bevacizumab in combination with oxaliplatin, fluorouracil, and leucovorin (FOLFOX4) for previously treated metastatic colorectal cancer: results from the Eastern Cooperative Oncology Group Study E3200," *Journal of Clinical Oncology*, vol. 25, no. 12, pp. 1539–1544, 2007.

[45] A. Sandler, R. Gray, M. C. Perry et al., "Paclitaxel-carboplatin alone or with bevacizumab for non-small-cell lung cancer," *The New England Journal of Medicine*, vol. 355, no. 24, pp. 2542–2550, 2006.

[46] B. Escudier, A. Pluzanska, P. Koralewski et al., "Bevacizumab plus interferon alfa-2a for treatment of metastatic renal cell carcinoma: a randomised, double-blind phase III trial," *The Lancet*, vol. 370, no. 9605, pp. 2103–2111, 2007.

[47] Avastin, (bevacizumab) package insert, Genentech Inc., 2008.

[48] X. Zhu, S. Wu, W. L. Dahut, and C. R. Parikh, "Risks of proteinuria and hypertension with bevacizumab, an antibody against vascular endothelial growth factor: systematic review and meta-analysis," *The American Journal of Kidney Diseases*, vol. 49, no. 2, pp. 186–193, 2007.

[49] O. Rixe, R. M. Bukowski, M. D. Michaelson et al., "Axitinib treatment in patients with cytokine-refractory metastatic renal-cell cancer: a phase II study," *The Lancet Oncology*, vol. 8, no. 11, pp. 975–984, 2007.

[50] T. Kamba, B. Y. Y. Tam, H. Hashizume et al., "VEGF-dependent plasticity of fenestrated capillaries in the normal adult microvasculature," *The American Journal of Physiology: Heart and Circulatory Physiology*, vol. 290, no. 2, pp. H560–H576, 2006.

[51] H. Izzedine, J. C. Soria, and B. Escudier, "Proteinuria and VEGF-targeted therapies: an underestimated toxicity?" *Journal of Nephrology*, vol. 26, no. 5, pp. 807–810, 2013.

[52] C. Frangié, C. Lefaucheur, J. Medioni, C. Jacquot, G. S. Hill, and D. Nochy, "Renal thrombotic microangiopathy caused by anti-VEGF-antibody treatment for metastatic renal-cell carcinoma," *The Lancet Oncology*, vol. 8, no. 2, pp. 177–178, 2007.

[53] D. Roncone, A. Satoskar, T. Nadasdy, J. P. Monk, and B. H. Rovin, "Proteinuria in a patient receiving anti-VEGF therapy for metastatic renal cell carcinoma," *Nature Clinical Practice Nephrology*, vol. 3, no. 5, pp. 287–293, 2007.

[54] H. Izzedine, I. Brocheriou, G. Deray, and O. Rixe, "Thrombotic microangiopathy and anti-VEGF agents," *Nephrology Dialysis Transplantation*, vol. 22, no. 5, pp. 1481–1482, 2007.

[55] G. Bollée, N. Patey, G. Cazajous et al., "Thrombotic microangiopathy secondary to VEGF pathway inhibition by sunitinib," *Nephrology Dialysis Transplantation*, vol. 24, no. 2, pp. 682–685, 2009.

[56] E. Kapiteijn, A. Brand, J. Kroep, and H. Gelderblom, "Sunitinib induced hypertension, thrombotic microangiopathy and reversible posterior leukencephalopathy syndrome," *Annals of Oncology*, vol. 18, no. 10, pp. 1745–1747, 2007.

[57] S. A. Levey, R. S. Bajwa, M. M. Picken, J. I. Clark, K. Barton, and D. J. Leehey, "Thrombotic microangiopathy associated with sunitinib, a VEGF inhibitor, in a patient with factor V Leiden mutation," *NDT Plus*, vol. 1, no. 3, pp. 154–156, 2008.

[58] H. Izzedine, M. Mangier, V. Ory et al., "Expression patterns of RelA and c-mip are associated with different glomerular diseases following anti-VEGF therapy," *Kidney International*, vol. 85, no. 2, pp. 457–470, 2014.

[59] D. R. Feldman, M. S. Baum, M. S. Ginsberg et al., "Phase I trial of bevacizumab plus escalated doses of sunitinib in patients with metastatic renal cell carcinoma," *Journal of Clinical Oncology*, vol. 27, no. 9, pp. 1432–1439, 2009.

[60] H. Izzedine, O. Rixe, B. Billemont, A. Baumelou, and G. Deray, "Angiogenesis inhibitor therapies: focus on kidney toxicity and hypertension," *American Journal of Kidney Diseases*, vol. 50, no. 2, pp. 203–218, 2007.

[61] H. Izzedine, S. Ederhy, F. Goldwasser et al., "Management of hypertension in angiogenesis inhibitor-treated patients," *Annals of Oncology*, vol. 20, no. 5, pp. 807–815, 2009.

[62] A. Pande, J. Lombardo, E. Spangenthal, and M. Javle, "Hypertension secondary to anti-angiogenic therapy: experience with bevacizumab," *Anticancer Research*, vol. 27, no. 5, pp. 3465–3470, 2007.

[63] M. L. Veronese, A. Mosenkis, K. T. Flaherty et al., "Mechanisms of hypertension associated with BAY 43-9006," *Journal of Clinical Oncology*, vol. 24, no. 9, pp. 1363–1369, 2006.

[64] S. Boehm, C. Rothermundt, D. Hess, and M. Joerger, "Antiangiogenic drugs in oncology: a focus on drug safety and the elderly—a mini-review," *Gerontology*, vol. 56, no. 3, pp. 303–309, 2010.

[65] S. Geiger-Gritsch, B. Stollenwerk, R. Miksad, B. Guba, C. Wild, and U. Siebert, "Safety of bevacizumab in patients with advanced cancer: a meta-analysis of randomized controlled trials," *Oncologist*, vol. 15, no. 11, pp. 1179–1191, 2010.

[66] E. S. Robinson, U. A. Matulonis, P. Ivy et al., "Rapid development of hypertension and proteinuria with cediranib, an oral vascular endothelial growth factor receptor inhibitor," *Clinical Journal of the American Society of Nephrology*, vol. 5, no. 3, pp. 477–483, 2010.

[67] S. Hapani, D. Chu, and S. Wu, "Risk of gastrointestinal perforation in patients with cancer treated with bevacizumab: a meta-analysis," *The Lancet Oncology*, vol. 10, no. 6, pp. 559–568, 2009.

[68] A. P. Hall, F. Russell Westwood, and P. F. Wadsworth, "Review of the effects of anti-angiogenic compounds on the epiphyseal growth plate," *Toxicologic Pathology*, vol. 34, no. 2, pp. 131–147, 2006.

[69] O. Artunay, E. Yuzbasioglu, R. Rasier, A. Sengul, and H. Bahcecioglu, "Posterior reversible encephalopathy syndrome after intravitreal bevacizumab injection in patient with choroidal neovascular membrane secondary to age-related maculopathy," *Journal of Ocular Pharmacology and Therapeutics*, vol. 26, no. 3, pp. 301–303, 2010.

[70] Q. S. Chu, "Aflibercept (AVE0005): an alternative strategy for inhibiting tumour angiogenesis by vascular endothelial growth factors," *Expert Opinion on Biological Therapy*, vol. 9, no. 2, pp. 263–271, 2009.

[71] J. S. Rudge, J. Holash, D. Hylton et al., "VEGF Trap complex formation measures production rates of VEGF, providing a biomarker for predicting efficacious angiogenic blockade," *Proceedings of the National Academy of Sciences of the United States of America*, vol. 104, no. 47, pp. 18363–18370, 2007.

[72] P. Bhargava and M. O. Robinson, "Development of second-generation VEGFR tyrosine kinase inhibitors: Current status," *Current Oncology Reports*, vol. 13, no. 2, pp. 103–111, 2011.

[73] S. P. Ivy, J. Y. Wick, and B. M. Kaufman, "An overview of small-molecule inhibitors of VEGFR signaling," *Nature Reviews Clinical Oncology*, vol. 6, no. 10, pp. 569–579, 2009.

[74] Y. Wu, Z. Zhong, J. Huber et al., "Anti-vascular endothelial growth factor receptor-1 antagonist antibody as a therapeutic agent for cancer," *Clinical Cancer Research*, vol. 12, no. 21, pp. 6573–6584, 2006.

12

Impact of Pediatric Chronic Dialysis on Long-Term Patient Outcome

Daniella Levy Erez,[1,2] **Irit Krause,**[1,2] **Amit Dagan,**[1,2] **Roxana Cleper,**[1,2] **Yafa Falush,**[1] **and Miriam Davidovits**[1,2]

[1]*Institute of Nephrology, Schneider Children's Medical Center of Israel, 49202 Petah Tikva, Israel*
[2]*Sackler Faculty of Medicine, Tel Aviv University, 6997801 Tel Aviv, Israel*

Correspondence should be addressed to Daniella Levy Erez; levy.erez.daniella@gmail.com

Academic Editor: David B. Kershaw

Objective. Owing to a shortage of kidney donors in Israel, children with end-stage renal disease (ESRD) may stay on maintenance dialysis for a considerable time, placing them at a significant risk. The aim of this study was to understand the causes of mortality. *Study Design.* Clinical data were collected retrospectively from the files of children on chronic dialysis (>3 months) during the years 1995–2013 at a single pediatric medical center. *Results.* 110 patients were enrolled in the study. Mean age was 10.7 ± 5.27 yrs. (range: 1 month–24 yrs). Forty-five children (42%) had dysplastic kidneys and 19 (17.5%) had focal segmental glomerulosclerosis. Twenty-five (22.7%) received peritoneal dialysis, 59 (53.6%) hemodialysis, and 6 (23.6%) both modalities sequentially. Median dialysis duration was 1.46 years (range: 0.25–17.54 years). Mean follow-up was 13.5 ± 5.84 yrs. Seventy-nine patients (71.8%) underwent successful transplantation, 10 (11.2%) had graft failure, and 8 (7.3%) continued dialysis without transplantation. Twelve patients (10.9%) died: 8 of dialysis-associated complications and 4 of their primary illness. The 5-year survival rate was 84%: 90% for patients older than 5 years and 61% for younger patients. *Conclusions.* Chronic dialysis is a suitable temporary option for children awaiting renal transplantation. Although overall long-term survival rate is high, very young children are at high risk for life-threatening dialysis-associated complications.

1. Introduction

End-stage renal disease (ESRD) is a major cause of morbidity and mortality in children. In the pediatric population, ESRD is mainly due to congenital anomalies of the kidney and urinary tract (CAKUT) and glomerular diseases [1–3]. The prevalence of ESRD in children in the United States is 8.3 per 100,000 [4] and 1.5/100,000 in Israel [5]. Kidney transplantation provides the best long-term results and optimum quality of life [6–10]. Because of the shortage of kidney sources in Israel, more than 75% of children waiting for a renal transplant are on dialysis for more than 2 years due to the shortage of available kidneys [5] placing them at high risk of dialysis-associated complication. Data on the long-term outcome of this patient group are scarce.

In children, peritoneal dialysis (PD) is preferred over hemodialysis (HD) in terms of quality of life, growth, and preservation of residual renal function [7]. Hemodialysis poses greater risks of access failure, vascular thrombosis, and obliteration of the great veins, which can be compromised for life [2, 6, 11]. In addition, multisystem involvement in ESRD in this population can lead to growth retardation [12, 13], cardiovascular complications [14, 15], and hematological complications [16–18].

The life span of children with ESRD is significantly lower than that of the age- and gender-matched general population. In studies of children on dialysis from Australia and New Zealand, survival rates were 85.7% at 3 years, 79% at 10 years, and 66% at 20 years [19]. Lower survival rates were found in children less than 12 months; 3-year survival for this age group was 68% in the North American Pediatric Renal Transplant Cooperative Study (NAPRTCS) annual report [20]. Similar results were reported in other studies from Netherlands [21, 22], with little change in more recent studies

[3] despite significant progress made in renal replacement therapy. The most important risk factors for poor treatment outcome were younger age at onset of dialysis and type of nonrenal comorbidities [1, 3, 19, 20]. The leading causes of death in children on dialysis are cardiovascular disease and infections [6, 19, 21].

The aim of the present study was to evaluate the long-term outcome of a large cohort of pediatric patients on chronic dialysis in a single tertiary medical center. Attention was focused on mortality rate and causes of death.

2. Materials and Methods

The study cohort included all patients with ESRD maintained on dialysis for at least 3 months in the Dialysis Unit of Schneider Children's Medical Center of Israel from January 1995 through December 2013. The following data were retrospectively recorded from the medical files of each patient: *clinical parameters* such as cause of ESRD, age at diagnosis, associated diseases, age at initiation of dialysis, type of dialysis (PD, HD, and both), duration of dialysis, dialysis complications; *laboratory parameters* such as complete blood cell count and blood chemistry (iron status was evaluated by recommended parameters); *parameters related to treatment of chronic kidney disease* such as weight and height standard deviation scores (SDS) at dialysis onset and study end, use of recombinant growth hormone (rGH) therapy, blood pressure percentiles and SDS by gender, age and height percentile, presence of left ventricular hypertrophy (LVH) measured by echocardiography (mass index > 51 gr/m$^{2.7}$), use and number of antihypertensive drugs, administration of recombinant erythropoietin (rEPO), and need for blood transfusions throughout treatment.

2.1. Definitions

2.1.1. Exit Site/Tunnel Infection.
Exit site/tunnel infection was diagnosed by the presence of purulent drainage with negative peritoneal fluid culture [23]. *Peritonitis* was diagnosed by the presence of at least 2 of the following criteria: cloudy effluent and/or abdominal pain or fever; effluent leukocyte count of >100 cells/mm^3 with >50% neutrophils; bacterial growth in the peritoneal culture [24].

2.1.2. Anemia.
Anemia was diagnosed when hemoglobin level was less than 11 g/dL [18] or when there was a need for blood transfusions.

2.1.3. Hypertension.
Hypertension was diagnosed by either blood pressure values over the 95th percentile for age and heights at 3 visits or a need for antihypertensive therapy. Data were presented by SDS scores.

2.2. Outcome Measures

2.2.1. Primary Outcome.
Primary outcome was as follows: death or survival at the end of the study period, survival with successful kidney transplant, or continuing dialysis at the end of the study period.

TABLE 1: Causes of ESRD leading to need for dialysis.

Major causes of ESRD	Number (%)
CAKUT	45 (40.9%)
Nephronophthisis	6 (5.45%)
FSGS	19 (17.27%)
Congenital nephrotic syndrome	4 (3.63%)
Metabolic diseases	5 (4.54%)
Alport	2 (1.81%)
Denys-Drash syndrome	3 (2.72%)
Glomerulonephritis	12 (10.9%)
Hypoxic injury	1 (0.9%)
Familial HUS	2 (1.81%)
Secondary HUS	2 (1.81%)
PCKD	2 (1.81%)
Other/unknown	7 (6.36%)

2.2.2. Secondary Outcome.
Secondary outcome was as follows: dialysis complications (number of infections, number of access failures, and need for exchange), changes in growth, recorded in z scores, cardiovascular disease defined as z scores of hypertension, and LVH and anemia (percent of the population and hemoglobin level.)

Outcome was analyzed overall and by dialysis modality (PD versus HD), age at onset of dialysis (>5 years versus <5 years), and year of initiation of dialysis (1995–2003 versus 2004–2013).

2.3. Statistical Analysis.
Data were analyzed using BMDP statistical software [25]. Analysis of variance (ANOVA) was used to compare continuous variables (biological parameters) between groups, with Bonferroni's corrections for multiple comparisons and Pearson's chi-square test for discrete variables (such as complications). Mann-Whitney nonparametric U test was used to analyze parameters such as number of blood pressure drugs. Comparing changes over time, we used ANOVA with repeated measures or Wilcoxon test, as appropriate. Survival curves were formulated according to the Kaplan-Meier method. Patient survival was calculated per 100 patient dialysis years. A p value of ≤0.05 was considered significant.

The study was approved by the Ethics Committee of Rabin Medical Center.

3. Results

3.1. Background Characteristics.
One hundred and ten children met the study criteria, 63 boys (57.3%) and 47 girls (42.7%) of mean age 10.67 ± 5.27 years (range: 1 month–24 yrs.) at onset of dialysis. Twenty-three patients were <5 years and 87 > 5 years; Seventy-four patients (67%) were adolescents (age: over 12 years). Eighty-two patients (74%) were of Jewish and 28 (26%) were of Arab origin. Maintenance dialysis duration was as follows: median 1.46 years (range: 0.25–17.54 years) and mean 2.48 ± 3.02 years. Mean duration of follow-up was 13.5 years ± 5.84. The major causes of ESRD are shown in Table 1.

TABLE 2: Study parameters related to dialysis modality.

Parameters	HD exclusively ($n = 59$, 53.6%)	PD exclusively ($n = 25$, 22.7%)	Both modalities* ($n = 26$, 23.6%)	p value
Age at dialysis onset (yr.), mean ± SD	12.41 ± 4.58[†]	7.58 ± 5.36[†]	9.68 ± 5.21	<0.001
Duration of dialysis (yr.), mean ± SD	1.41 ± 0.79	1.32 ± 0.47	1.41 ± 0.76	0.87
Number of patients by period of treatment, n (%)				
1995–2003	33 (55.9%)	9 (15.3%)	17 (28.8%)	0.09[‡]
2004–2013	26 (51.0%)	16 (31.4%)	9 (17.6%)	
Hb level, g/dL, mean ± SD				
At dialysis onset	9.18 ± 1.62	9.22 ± 1.61	8.8 ± 1.96	0.6
At study end	10.88 ± 1.41	10.55 ± 1.75	10.32 ± 1.46	0.3
Growth SDS, mean ± SD				
At dialysis onset				
Height SDS	−1.25 ± 0.94	−1.01 ± 1.50	−1.4 ± 0.83	0.52
Weight SDS	−0.64 ± 0.70	−0.31 ± 1.20	−0.55 ± 0.64	0.25
At study end				
Height SDS	−1.47 ± 1.22	−1.46 ± 1.44	−2.3 ± 0.8[†]	0.009
Weight SDS	−0.81 ± 0.62	−0.37 ± 0.79	−1.22 ± 0.46	<0.001

*PD and HD sequentially. [†]$p < 0.001$. [‡]The number of patients treated by PD increased significantly in the later period.

Table 2 shows clinical parameters of the patients analyzed according to dialysis modality. Significance was found only in patient mean age ($p < 0.001$). The later period (2004–2013) was characterized by a twofold increase in the proportion of patients treated with PD (15% versus 31% of all dialyzed patients).

3.2. Dialysis Access. For PD, a two-cuffed peritoneal catheter was inserted by a specialized pediatric surgeon in the operating room. Prophylaxis with Cefamezine was administered in all patients during the later period of the study (2004–2013). All the caregivers were instructed for appropriate performance of the procedure emphasizing aseptic techniques and were managed by automated PD. For HD, an arteriovenous graft or fistula was used in 44 patients (all of whom weighed > 20 kg, 52%) [23] and a central venous perm-cuffed catheter (Permacath [26]) in 41 (48%). Noncuffed central catheters were only used when there was an acute indication for dialysis and used as a bridge until a permanent access could be secured. Overall, 5 vascular access exchanges per 1000 patient-years were needed; in 35 patients (59% of patients on HD exclusively) there was no need for a change of access throughout the treatment course. The main reason for catheter removal was infection.

3.3. Dialysis Complications

3.3.1. Exit Site. Exit site infection rate was 5.9 episodes per 1000 patient-years.

3.3.2. Hemodialysis. At least one episode of exit site infection occurred in 22 patients on HD both exclusively and sequentially (25%). Bacteremia was documented at least once in 19 patients on HD (22%). The average bacteremia rate was 4.4 episodes per 1000 patient-years.

3.3.3. Peritoneal Dialysis. 16 patients developed exit site infection (31%). The average peritonitis rate was 20 episodes per 1000 patient-years. Tunnel infections were 2.2 episodes per 1000 patient-years. No bacteremia episodes were noted in patients on PD.

The rate of total catheter-related infections was significantly higher for PD than for HD ($p < 0.001$). The earlier treatment period was characterized by a significantly higher rate of exit site infections (68.8% versus 28%, $p < 0.001$) and of bacteremia (19.1% versus 40.8%, $p < 0.02$). The peritonitis rate in the patients on PD was also higher in the earlier period, but the difference did not reach statistical significance (68% versus 81%, $p = 0.35$).

3.4. Anemia. Anemia was documented in 101 patients (92%) before onset of dialysis. Mean hemoglobin level was 9.11 ± 1.69 gr/dL at onset of dialysis and 10.66 ± 1.52 gr/dL ($p < 0.001$) at study end. The rate of rEPO administration was 85.3% at onset of dialysis, increasing to 97.8% at study end ($p = 0.01$).

Findings by dialysis modality are shown in Table 2. Blood transfusion was necessary in 21 patients (19.8%) during the first 3 months on dialysis and in 5 patients (4.5%) during the last 3 months on dialysis.

3.5. Growth and Nutrition. Mean weight SDS was −0.56 ± 0.84 at dialysis onset and −0.84 ± 0.69 at study end ($p = 0.01$). Respective values for height were −1.22 ± 1.11 and −1.62 ± 1.26; this difference was not statistically significant ($p = 0.13$). Growth parameters analyzed by dialysis modality are shown in Table 2. Patients were placed on an age- and weight-adjusted diet under careful follow-up by a renal dietitian. A gastrostomy tube was inserted in 13 cases (14%). Forty-seven patients (43%) were treated with rGH.

3.6. Hypertension. Seventy-seven patients (70%) were hypertensive (systolic, diastolic, or both) at onset of dialysis. Mean systolic blood pressure SDS decreased from 3.35 ± 2.19 at onset of dialysis to 2.14 ± 2.83 at study end ($p < 0.001$). Respective values for diastolic blood pressure SDS were 2.51 ± 1.72 and 1.36 ± 2.22 ($p < 0.001$). The number of medications needed to control hypertension ranged from 1 to 4 (median 1) at onset of dialysis and decreased to 0 to 5 (median 0) at study end. Seventy patients (63%) needed treatment at dialysis onset compared to 46 (42%) at study end ($p < 0.001$).

LVH was found in 50 patients (46%) at onset of dialysis and 37 (34%) at study end ($p = 0.01$). During treatment, LVH developed in 11 patients (10.5%) who had not had LVH at dialysis onset.

3.7. Outcome. Eighty-nine patients (90.3%) received a kidney graft during the study period, of whom 79 (88.8%) had a functioning graft at study end and 10 (11.2%) lost graft function and returned to dialysis. Causes for loss of graft included 5 patients with noncompliance; 1 with FSGS recurrence; 2 with acute rejection; 1 with graft renal artery thrombosis; 1 with chronic antibody mediated rejection. Eighty-six patients had one renal transplant and 2 patients had 2 transplants. Sixty-four grafts originated from deceased donors, 15 were from living-related donors, and 9 were from living nonrelated donors. Another 8 patients (7.3%) continued dialysis; this group age was on average 11 ± 6.4 years at onset of dialysis and were on maintenance dialysis for an average of 2.85 ± 3.9 years (range: 0.25–6.64). One child with CAKUT ceased dialysis with stable kidney function.

12 patients died during the study period, with a mortality rate of 10.9%. Causes of death are detailed in Table 3. Two patients who died suffered from Schimke immunoosseous dysplasia complicated by moyamoya phenomenon. Their death was attributed to cerebrovascular accidents. Three patients who died from hyperkalemia were on Kayexalate and a low potassium diet.

On Kaplan-Meier analysis, the 5-year overall survival rate on dialysis was 84%: 90% in children > 5 years and 61% in children < 5 years at dialysis onset (Figure 1). Patients treated with PD exclusively had survival rates of 100% at 1 year and 78% at 5 years; the rate for HD exclusively was 93% at both time points and for combined modalities 95% and 68%. There was no statistically significant difference in overall survival among the groups ($p = 0.56$).

Mortality rates analyzed by patient-years on dialysis were 4.3 deaths per 100 patient-years for the whole cohort, 2.39 deaths per 100 patient-years for patients > 5 years at onset of dialysis, and 11.6 deaths per 100 patient-years for patients < 5 years at onset of dialysis. The mortality rate for PD exclusively was 9 per 100 patient-years, for HD exclusively was 7.26 per 100 patient-years, and for combined treatment was 3.93 per 100 patient-years. By treatment period, 5-year survival rates were 73% in patients treated in 1995–2003 and

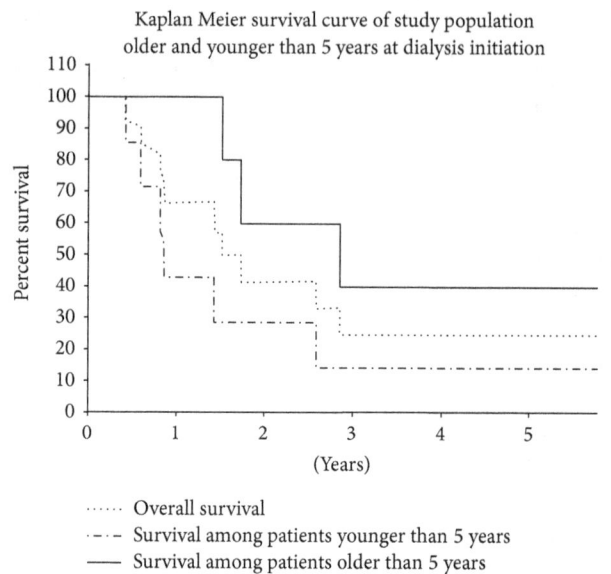

FIGURE 1: Kaplan Meier survival curve of study population and Kaplan Meier survival curves of children beginning dialysis at age > 5 years or <5 years.

90% in patients treated in 2004–2013; the difference was not statistically significant ($p = 0.81$).

4. Discussion

To the best of our knowledge, this is one of the largest single-center longitudinal outcome series of paediatric ESRD managed with long-term maintenance dialysis in the medical literature. Previous studies described smaller cohorts of 34 [27] and 98 children [8] with shorter follow-up times of 9 and 14 years, respectively. Males were slightly overrepresented in our study (57.3% versus 42.7% for females), in agreement with findings that ESRD is more common in males [6, 21, 22, 24, 25]. Also expected was the younger age of patients who started with PD compared to patients who started with HD (7.58 versus 12.41 years) given the considerable technical difficulties with dialysis in younger children [2, 11].

Maintenance dialysis duration in our study, median 1.46 years, range 0.25–17.54 years, and mean 2.48 ± 3.02 years, was similar to that in centers in Europe and USA [6, 8, 28] despite the limited graft sources in a small country such as Israel. The limited amount of potential donors in Israel can be explained by various religious beliefs causing individuals not to donate organs.

Our dialysis unit can provide both HD and PD. PD is known to have several advantages over HD in children, including better preservation of native renal function, lack of long-term compromise of the main venous vascular tree, and freedom from frequent hospital visits with significantly less interference with everyday life activities and quality of life. Nevertheless, only 35% of our patients were started on PD compared to 80% in other series [8]; this can be explained by the reasonable travel distances to the pediatric dialysis unit from most parts of our country; therefore patients who

TABLE 3: Characteristics of patients on maintenance dialysis who died during the study period (12/110).

Pt. number	Age at dialysis initiation (years)	Sex	Cause of ESRD	Duration of dialysis (years)	Modality of dialysis	Access	Age at death (years)	Cause of death
1	1.58	M	Familial HUS	0.86	HD	P	2.42	Cardiac arrest due to hyperkalemia
2	3.69	M	CAKUT	2.35	Combined	P + T	6.04	Sepsis
3	1.98	M	HUS s/p BMT	0.42	Combined	P + T	2.41	Sepsis
4	2	F	Bilateral Nephrectomy due to Wilms tumor	0.59	Combined	P + T	2.59	Cardiac arrest due to hyperkalemia
5	3.54	F	Familial HUS	9.57	HD	AVF	13.11	Access failure
6	14.51	F	Systemic Lupus Erythematosus	6.23	HD	AVF	20.74	Mesenteric event
7	7.96	M	FSGS	1.52	Combined	P + T	9.48	Access failure
8	7.8	M	FSGS-Schimke syndrome	2.86	PD	T	10.66	CVA
9	9.08	M	FSGS-Schimke syndrome	1.73	PD	T	10.81	CVA
10	3.2	M	Congenital nephrotic syndrome	0.81	HD	P	4.01	Cardiac arrest due to hyperkalemia
11	9.55	F	Nephrotoxic kidney injury	5.91	HD	AV	15.46	Metastatic Neuroblastoma
12	4.62	M	CAKUT	1.43	Combined	P + T	6.05	Sepsis

AVF: arterial venous fistula; BMT: bone marrow transplantation; CAKUT: congenital anomalies of the kidney and urinary tract; CVA: cerebrovascular accident due to moyamoya phenomenon; ESRD: end-stage renal disease, FSGS: focal segmental glomerulosclerosis; HD: hemodialysis, HUS: hemolytic uremic syndrome; P: permacath; PD: peritoneal dialysis; s/p: status post; T: tenckhoff peritoneal catheter.

cannot be managed with PD at home are easily switched to HD when it is in their best interest. Furthermore, 67% of our cohort were adolescents, many of whom may have declined PD because of its major impact on body image.

Primary graft/arteriovenous fistulas are considered the best permanent vascular access for HD with lowest risks of secondary failure and complications [26]; they were used in 52% of our patients, a significantly higher rate than reported in the literature (36% and 21.3%) [22, 28]. The rate of infections was low in our study compared to NAPRTCS [20]: 2 episodes per 100 patient-years versus 8.1 per 100 patient-years. Low rates of secondary failure and infection rates have been associated with high surgical skills and expertise and use of standardized PD education programs, administration of prophylactic antibiotics prior to insertion of PD catheters, and aseptic techniques.

Anemia may be caused by a multitude of factors and poses a challenging problem in patients on chronic dialysis similar to other studies. Ninety-two percent of our patients were anemic at onset of dialysis, with a mean hemoglobin level of 9.11 ± 1.69 gr%. By the end of the study, this value increased significantly to 10.66 ± 1.52 gr% ($p < 0.001$), concomitant with a decrease in the need for blood transfusions (from 19.8% of patients to 4.5%; $p < 0.001$). A similar positive trend was found in the annual NAPRTCS report with a hematocrit range of 29.9% to 32% at onset of dialysis, which improved after 6 months to 32.3%–33% as found in [20]. It is possible that the more intensive rEPO treatment given during dialysis compared to the predialysis period was responsible for this finding. In addition, we suspect that compliance was better for intravenous than subcutaneous rEPO administration.

Cardiovascular disease is a major cause of death in adolescents and young adults [15]. In their nationwide Dutch study partly focused on cardiovascular disease, Groothoff et al. [15] reported LVH rates of 47% and 39% in male and female adolescents, respectively, and in an analysis of a large European registry, Fadrowski et al. [16] found that uncontrolled hypertension was present in 45.5% of patients on HD and 35.5% on PD; rates of antihypertensive drug use in these groups were 69.7% and 68.2% male/female, respectively, and in 51.9% of all patients. In our study, 70% of children presented with hypertension at onset of dialysis. By study end, there was a significant improvement in blood pressure SDS, with a decrease in the LVH rate from 46% to 34% ($p = 0.01$). Improvement in LVH over time on dialysis can be explained by good fluid volume control and close monitoring of cardiovascular parameters and better patient compliance and adherence to treatment.

Growth retardation is a complication of chronic kidney disease and has a significant influence on both final adult height and quality of life [7, 13]. In the NAPRTCS reports, growth rate improved significantly, from −2.8 to −1.9 ($p = 0.078$), in patients treated with rGH (9.4% of patients on PD and 8.7% of patients on HD) but worsened in the remainder [8, 20]. We did not observe a significant improvement in growth in the present study, perhaps our patients were not as growth retarded initially as in the NAPRTCS data which may explain their relative lack of response to GH. Also some of our patients may have already reached their adult height.

According to the NAPRTCS reports [20, 22] survival in paediatric patients on dialysis, calculated by deaths per 100 patient-years, varied from 13.6 at age 1 year, to 8.2 at age 1-2 years, 6.1 at age 2–5 years, and 2.8 at age > 6 years. Overall survival rates were 95% at 1 year and 85.7% at 3 years [20, 22]. In the long-term study from Australia and New Zealand by McDonald and Craig [19], 10-year and 20-year survival rates of children on dialysis were 79% and 66%, respectively. The United States Renal Data System (USRDS) study by Mitsnefes et al. [3] reported an overall mortality of 9.88 per 100 patient-years in patients younger than 5 years and 3.86 per 100 patient-years in patients older than 5 years. Shroff et al. [8] in a single-Center 14-year study reported 17 deaths in 98 patients, for an overall survival rate of 83%. In our present 18-year study, of 110 young patients on maintenance dialysis, 12 died. Eight deaths (7.2%) were related to dialysis complications. The 5-year overall survival rate was 84%: 61% in patients younger than 5 years and 90% in patients older than 5 years at onset of dialysis. Calculating survival in patient-years of dialysis yielded a better outcome than in the study of Mitsnefes et al. [3]: 4.3 deaths for the whole cohort, 11.6 in the younger group, and 2.39 in the older group. Only 2 patients who died were exclusively on PD and those 2 died due to complications of their primary illness. It was not found statistically significant, probably because of a small number of deaths.

The limitation of the present study is its retrospective design, a small sample size which for a single center is relatively large but not compared with multicenter studies, and a specific population which may defer from other centers/groups.

In conclusion, despite the relatively long period on maintenance dialysis, pediatric patients with ESRD in our center have a similar outcome in terms of survival and dialysis complications to that reported in other industrialized countries. We suggest that efforts be made to broaden the use of arteriovenous fistulas and minimize the use of central cuffed catheters in order to avoid infections and thrombosis. Implementation of standardized PD education programs, prophylactic antibiotics prior to insertion of PD catheters, and strict adherence to aseptic techniques may reduce the rate of PD -associated infections.

The findings may have important implications for decreasing the risks of dialysis-associated complications especially for very young ESRD patients, thereby lowering hospitalization and improving survival.

References

[1] D. Miklovicova, M. Cornelissen, K. Cransberg, J. W. Groothoff, L. Dedik, and C. H. Schroder, "Etiology and epidemiology of end-stage renal disease in Dutch children 1987–2001," *Pediatric Nephrology*, vol. 20, no. 8, pp. 1136–1142, 2005.

[2] R. Shroff, E. Wright, S. Ledermann, C. Hutchinson, and L. Rees, "Chronic hemodialysis in infants and children under 2 years of age," *Pediatric Nephrology*, vol. 18, no. 4, pp. 378–383, 2003.

[3] M. M. Mitsnefes, B. L. Laskin, M. Dahhou, X. Zhang, and B. J. Foster, "Mortality risk among children initially treated with dialysis for end-stage kidney disease, 1990–2010," *The Journal of the American Medical Association*, vol. 309, no. 18, pp. 1921–1929, 2013.

[4] United States Renal Data System, http://www.usrds.org.

[5] Israel National Dialysis Registry Follow-up 1989–2001, http://www.old.health.gov.il/download/docs/units/comp/dia/1.pdf.

[6] E. Verrina, A. Edefonti, B. Gianoglio et al., "A multicenter experience on patient and technique survival in children on chronic dialysis," *Pediatric Nephrology*, vol. 19, no. 1, pp. 82–90, 2004.

[7] B. A. Warady, A. M. Neu, and F. Schaefer, "Optimal care of the infant, child, and adolescent on dialysis: 2014 update," *American Journal of Kidney Diseases*, vol. 64, no. 1, pp. 128–142, 2014.

[8] R. Shroff, L. Rees, R. Trompeter, C. Hutchinson, and S. Ledermann, "Long-term outcome of chronic dialysis in children," *Pediatric Nephrology*, vol. 21, no. 2, pp. 257–264, 2006.

[9] L. Rees, R. Shroff, C. Hutchinson, O. N. Fernando, and R. S. Trompeter, "Long-term outcome of paediatric renal transplantation: follow-up of 300 children from 1973 to 2000," *Nephron—Clinical Practice*, vol. 105, no. 2, pp. c68–c76, 2007.

[10] J. A. Kari, J. Romagnoli, P. Duffy, O. N. Fernando, L. Rees, and R. S. Trompeter, "Renal transplantation in children under 5 years of age," *Pediatric Nephrology*, vol. 13, no. 9, pp. 730–736, 1999.

[11] Y. Kovalski, R. Cleper, I. Krause, and M. Davidovits, "Hemodialysis in children weighing less than 15 kg: a single-center experience," *Pediatric Nephrology*, vol. 22, no. 12, pp. 2105–2110, 2007.

[12] L. Rees, M. Azocar, D. Borzych et al., "Growth in very young children undergoing chronic peritoneal dialysis," *Journal of the American Society of Nephrology*, vol. 22, no. 12, pp. 2303–2312, 2011.

[13] R. N. Fine, "Etiology and treatment of growth retardation in children with chronic kidney disease and end-stage renal disease: a historical perspective," *Pediatric Nephrology*, vol. 25, no. 4, pp. 725–732, 2010.

[14] A. M. Kramer, K. J. van Stralen, K. J. Jager et al., "Demographics of blood pressure and hypertension in children on renal replacement therapy in Europe," *Kidney International*, vol. 80, no. 10, pp. 1092–1098, 2011.

[15] J. W. Groothoff, M. R. Lilien, N. C. J. van de Kar, E. D. Wolff, and J. C. Davin, "Cardiovascular disease as a late complication of end-stage renal disease in children," *Pediatric Nephrology*, vol. 20, no. 3, pp. 374–379, 2005.

[16] J. J. Fadrowski, S. L. Furth, and B. A. Fivush, "Anemia in pediatric dialysis patients in end-stage renal disease network 5," *Pediatric Nephrology*, vol. 19, no. 9, pp. 1029–1034, 2004.

[17] D. Borzych-Duzalka, Y. Bilginer, I. S. Ha et al., "Management of anemia in children receiving chronic peritoneal dialysis," *Journal of the American Society of Nephrology*, vol. 24, no. 4, pp. 665–676, 2013.

[18] "KDOQI Clinical Practice Guideline and Clinical Practice Recommendations for anemia in chronic kidney disease: 2007 update of hemoglobin target," *American Journal of Kidney Diseases*, vol. 50, no. 3, pp. 471–530, 2007.

[19] S. P. McDonald and J. C. Craig, "Long-term survival of children with end-stage renal disease," *The New England Journal of Medicine*, vol. 350, no. 26, pp. 2654–2662, 2004.

[20] A. M. Neu, P. L. Ho, R. A. McDonald, and B. A. Warady, "Chronic dialysis in children and adolescents. The 2001 NAPRTCS Annual Report," *Pediatric Nephrology*, vol. 17, no. 8, pp. 656–663, 2002.

[21] J. W. Groothoff, M. P. Gruppen, M. Offringa et al., "Mortality and causes of death of end-stage renal disease in children: a Dutch cohort study," *Kidney International*, vol. 61, no. 2, pp. 621–629, 2002.

[22] M. B. Leonard, L. A. Donaldson, M. Ho, and D. F. Geary, "A prospective cohort study of incident maintenance dialysis in children: An NAPRTC Study," *Kidney International*, vol. 63, no. 2, pp. 744–755, 2003.

[23] D. Shemesh, O. Olsha, D. Berelowitz, and C. Zigelman, "An integrated vascular management programme," *EDTNA-ERCA Journal*, vol. 30, no. 4, pp. 201–207, 2004.

[24] D.-J. Leehey, C.-C. Szeto, and P. K.-T. Li, "Peritonitis and exit site infection," in *Handbook of Dialysis*, J. T. Daugirdas, P. G. Blake, and T. S. Ing, Eds., pp. 417–439, Wolterrs Kluwer Lippincott, Williams & Wilkins, Philadelphia, Pa, USA, 4th edition, 2007.

[25] W. J. Dixon, Ed., *BMDP Statistical Software*, University of California Press, Los Angeles, Los Angeles, Calif, USA, 1993.

[26] W. N. Hayes, A. R. Watson, N. Callaghan, E. Wright, and C. J. Stefanidis, "Vascular access: choice and complications in European paediatric haemodialysis units," *Pediatric Nephrology*, vol. 27, no. 6, pp. 999–1004, 2012.

[27] S. Feinstein, C. Rinat, R. Becker-Cohen, E. Ben-Shalom, S. B. Schwartz, and Y. Frishberg, "The outcome of chronic dialysis in infants and toddlers—advantages and drawbacks of haemodialysis," *Nephrology Dialysis Transplantation*, vol. 23, no. 4, pp. 1336–1345, 2008.

[28] North American Pediatric Renal Transplant Cooperative study (NAPRTCS) 2011 Annual Report, https://web.emmes.com/study/ped/annlrept/annualrept2011.pdf.

13

Hydration Status is Associated with Aortic Stiffness, but Not with Peripheral Arterial Stiffness, in Chronically Hemodialysed Patients

Daniel Bia,[1] **Cintia Galli,**[2,3] **Rodolfo Valtuille,**[4] **Yanina Zócalo,**[1] **Sandra A. Wray,**[5] **Ricardo L. Armentano,**[3,5] **and Edmundo I. Cabrera Fischer**[2,3,5]

[1]*Physiology Department, School of Medicine, CUiiDARTE, Republic University, 11800 Montevideo, Uruguay*
[2]*National Council of Technical and Scientific Research (CONICET), C1033AAJ Buenos Aires, Argentina*
[3]*Technological National University, C1179AAQ Buenos Aires, Argentina*
[4]*Fresenius FME Burzaco, B1852FZD Buenos Aires, Argentina*
[5]*Favaloro University, Solis, C1093AAS Buenos Aires, Argentina*

Correspondence should be addressed to Daniel Bia; dbia@fmed.edu.uy

Academic Editor: Alessandro Amore

Background. Adequate fluid management could be essential to minimize high arterial stiffness observed in chronically hemodialyzed patients (CHP). *Aim.* To determine the association between body fluid status and central and peripheral arterial stiffness levels. *Methods.* Arterial stiffness was assessed in 65 CHP by measuring the pulse wave velocity (PWV) in a central arterial pathway (carotid-femoral) and in a peripheral pathway (carotid-brachial). A blood pressure-independent regional arterial stiffness index was calculated using PWV. Volume status was assessed by whole-body multiple-frequency bioimpedance. Patients were first observed as an entire group and then divided into three different fluid status-related groups: normal, overhydration, and dehydration groups. *Results.* Only carotid-femoral stiffness was positively associated ($P < 0.05$) with the hydration status evaluated through extracellular/intracellular fluid, extracellular/Total Body Fluid, and absolute and relative overhydration. *Conclusion.* Volume status and overload are associated with central, but not peripheral, arterial stiffness levels with independence of the blood pressure level, in CHP.

1. Introduction

The increased mortality observed in chronic kidney disease compelled analyzing the role of the traditional risk factors and those derived from recent studies that are particularly relevant in chronically hemodialyzed patients (CHP). Consequently, left ventricular hypertrophy, malnutrition, and hydration status (i.e., overhydration, OH) in end stage renal disease have become "novel risk factors" [1–4]. Volume overload is considered a predictor of outcome in CHP [5], in which systemic hypertension is also well documented; however OH is not always accompanied by volume-dependent high blood pressure (BP). Previous reports demonstrated that hypertension is not always fluid-dependent in CHP [6]. Consequently, at present, a Normal Hydration State is

a very important target to be taken into account during renal replacement therapy.

At least in theory, an adequate fluid management could be essential to minimize the high arterial stiffness observed in CHP. Even so, it is not still clear how volume overload affects the arterial system and the nature of the association with other novel risk factors [7]. Recently, Hur et al. have reported that fluid evaluation with bioimpedance spectroscopy (BIS) determines an improvement in the management of CHP and decreases in arterial stiffness [8]. However, the mentioned authors were incapable of determining if the origin of the arterial stiffness improvement was due to volume overload [8]. In other words, whether volume overload determines a BP dependent or independent arterial stiffness increase and whether these potential effects are similar in central (i.e., elastic) and peripheral (i.e., muscular) arteries remain to be analyzed.

From a different point of view, cardiovascular disease is a well-known leading cause of the increased mortality observed in CHP and is associated with aortic stiffening [9, 10]. More than a decade ago, Blacher et al. demonstrated that the measurement of arterial pulse wave velocity (PWV; "gold standard" parameter to measure regional arterial stiffness) has prognostic power to predict mortality in end stage renal disease [9]. However, the physiopathological mechanisms that determine the increased risk have not been properly elucidated.

At present, the hydration status of the human body can be assessed by multifrequency bioimpedance [11]. Furthermore, using BIS and applying a 2-compartment (2-C) model of body composition (BC; fat-free mass and fat mass), a significant association between volume overload (evaluated as extracellular [ECF] to intracellular water [ICF] ratio) and aortic stiffness was reported [7, 12]. Nevertheless, at least four aspects of this association should be noted: (a) Is the volume overload-arterial stiffness relationship the same in elastic and muscular arteries? (b) Does the mentioned association persist when the hydration status is quantified using another model, such as the three compartment (3-C) model? (c) Does this hydration status-arterial stiffness association persist if vascular stiffness is obtained with independence of the BP levels of the patient? (d) Is the association similar when a comparison between right and left arterial territories of the human body is performed?

In this context, the aim of this study was to determine the hydration status using a 3-C model and the central (i.e., elastic artery) and peripheral (i.e., muscular artery) arterial stiffness levels in CHP, in order to evaluate the potential BP dependent and/or independent association between body fluid status (OH, OH/ECF, ECF/ICF, and ECF/Total Body Fluid (TBF)) and central (carotid-femoral pathway) and peripheral (carotid-brachial) arterial stiffness levels.

2. Methods

This research was carried out in a single health care institution (Fresenius Medical Care FME Burzaco, Buenos Aires, Argentina). From an initial cohort of ambulatory CHP ($n = 104$), sixty-five patients were enrolled in this cross-sectional research. The inclusion criteria were as follows: (1) patients are on hemodialysis for more than 3 months, (2) the vascular access is placed in the upper limb, and (3) patients have had no acute cardiovascular events in the last 3 months. The exclusion criteria were as follows: (1) patients abusing alcohol, (2) patients with lower or upper extremity amputation, (3) patients with symptomatic carotid artery stenosis, (4) patients with uncontrolled diabetes mellitus, (5) patients unwilling to participate in the investigation, (6) patients with cardiac arrhythmias, and (7) patients with metallic implants (stents, pacemakers, etc.). Our Institutional Review Board and Ethics Committee approved this study. All patients gave their written consent to participate in the study.

2.1. Measurements. Before their midweek hemodialysis session, patients were subjected to the measurement of PWV and of other physical parameters, such as arterial BP, body weight, standing height, and waist and hip perimeter. The hydration status was determined through a bioimpedance study. Blood was drawn from each patient and routine chemical analyses were performed to quantify haematocrit, haemoglobin, serum creatinine, calcium, phosphate, serum albumin, parathyroid hormone (PTH), urea, total cholesterol, HDL and LDL cholesterol, and triglyceride.

In all patients, brachial BP was measured in the contralateral upper limb to which the functioning vascular access was confectioned. The patients were allowed to rest in supine position during 15 minutes before the BP measurement. Pressure was determined using a digital automatic BP monitor (Omron model HEM 781 INT). Heart rate, waist circumference, and hip perimeter were also measured, and the body mass index (BMI) was calculated by dividing weight by height squared.

The study of body fluids was done using a bioimpedance monitor (Fresenius Medical Care, (BCM) Body Composition Monitor OP-ES, software version: 3.2.x edition: 8/03.12). The BCM is a BIS device that measures 50 different frequencies that range from 5 to 1000 kHz, analyzing the whole-body bioimpedance. The BCM discriminates fluid of the intra- and extracellular water content of lean tissue mass (LTM), adipose tissue mass (ATM), and excess fluid (OH). LTM, ATM, and OH are obtained from measurements of body weight, height, and whole-body ICF and ECF determined by BIS. The body composition model determines whether changes in ICF and ECF reflect an increase or a loss of ATM or LTM. This is the only device that identifies OH as a third compartment on the basis of a unique body composition model. OH represents the excess fluid (fluid overload) stored almost exclusively in the extracellular volume of a patient and is therefore part of the ECF, whereas the water of LTM and ATM consists of differing proportions of ECF and ICF, in addition to solid components. Applying the 3-C model, the following parameters were recorded in each patient: Lean Tissue Index (LTI (kg/m^2)); Fat Tissue Index (FTI (kg/m^2)); Total Body Fluid (TBF (L)); ECF (L); ICF (L); and OH (L). Three volume ratios were quantified: ECF/ICF, ECF/TBF, and OH/ECF. Over and subhydration were defined when the OH/ECF ratio was >15% or <0%, respectively [4, 6].

Measurements of PWV were performed on the right and left carotid-femoral and carotid-brachial pathways, using a previously validated instrument (Arteriometer V100, OxyTech, Buenos Aires, Argentina), according to the technique previously and widely described [13–15]. In order to evaluate the aortic and upper limb regional arterial stiffness by means of PWV, the carotid and femoral (or brachial) pulse waves were recorded using mechanotransducers, simultaneously placed on the skin over the carotid and femoral (or brachial) arteries, with the subjects in supine position. Once adequate pulse waveforms were recorded, the time delay between the waveforms (pulse transit time) was measured. To this end, the well-known algorithm to detect the pulse waveform "foot," called the maximal systolic upstroke algorithm, was used [15]. The distance between the carotid and the femoral (or brachial) sites was used together with the pulse transit time to calculate PWV. The reported value of PWV for each subject was the average of at least 8 consecutive beats automatically calculated. Before calculating PWV, brachial pressure and heart rate were recorded.

PWV is essentially dependent on BP. Studies have shown a significant association between PWV and systolic BP in CHP. To overcome this disadvantage, a BP-normalized stiffness index (β) was recently developed and proposed as a new parameter for evaluating regional arterial stiffness, independently of BP level [16]. The equation to quantify β is derived from the Bramwell-Hill equation and the stiffness parameter β may be less influenced by BP than PWV, and its measurement has been shown to be reproducible. We quantify β as $\beta = \mathrm{Ln}(SBP/DBP) \cdot (2 \cdot \rho \cdot PWV^2/PP)$, where Ln is the natural logarithm and SBP, PP, and DBP are the systolic, pulse, and diastolic BP, respectively [16].

2.2. Statistical Analysis. Continuous variables are expressed as mean value ± standard deviation. ANOVA (Bonferroni test) and χ^2 analysis were used to analyze differences among the normal hydration state (NHS) group, the overhydration (OH) group, and the subhydration (SH) group. Pearson's correlation was run to determine the relationship between PWV (or β) and volume status parameters (ECF/ICF, ECF/TBF, OH, andOH/ECF). All analyses were completed with SPSS software, version 20.0 (SPSS, Chicago, IL, USA). A P value of <0.05 was regarded as statistically significant.

3. Results

Data collection was successful for all patients included in this study. In all patients, arterial BP and the hydration status were routinely monitored allowing, when necessary, the fluid correction during the renal replacement therapy session and/or the use of pharmacological resources.

Table 1 shows the anthropometric, hemodynamic, and blood characteristics for the entire analyzed population and the three hydric state-related groups. There were no differences in age among groups and in BP levels between the normal and OH group.

Table 2 shows the body water parameters quantified for the entire population and the three hydric state-related groups. Note that the net levels of ECF, ICF, and TBF were not different among groups, but the relative distribution of the water in the extracellular and intracellular components was different, determining differences in ECF/ICF, ECF/TBF, OH, and OH/TBF.

Table 3 shows the arterial stiffness levels for the entire group and the three hydric state-related groups. The OH group showed higher carotid-femoral (but not carotid-brachial) arterial stiffness level than the normal hydric state group ($P < 0.05$). Additionally, note that differences in carotid-femoral arterial stiffness between OH and dehydration groups disappeared when a BP-independent stiffness index (β) was calculated. Additionally, there were no differences in carotid-brachial arterial stiffness among groups, with independence of the employed parameter (PWV or β).

The carotid-femoral PWV was positively correlated ($P < 0.05$) with the extracellular-to-intracellular fluid volume ratio (ECF/ICF), as seen in Figure 1(a). Our analysis shows the same results, for carotid-femoral PWV obtained both for the left and right body side. Furthermore, the mentioned association has shown to be independent of the BP level as it is when calculating β (Figure 1(b)). However, these results could not be confirmed when the right and left aorto-axilo-humeral pathway was considered and evaluated using PWV and β (Figures 1(c) and 1(d)).

The ECF/TBF was found to be associated with the PWV value in the carotid-femoral pathway, but not in the aorto-axilo-humeral pathway. As seen in Figure 2(a), a positive correlation ($P < 0.05$) was found in both the left and the right PWV carotid-femoral pathways. Moreover, the β-ECF/TBF relationship ($P < 0.05$) shows that the mentioned changes are independent of the BP level (Figure 2(b)). Nevertheless, the right and left carotid-brachial pathway β level were not correlated with the ECF/TBF ratio (Figures 2(c) and 2(d)).

Overhydration (OH) measured in absolute units (liters) showed a low (but significant) correlation ($P < 0.05$) with the right and left carotid-femoral PWV (Figure 3(a)). This positive relationship was not confirmed when β value was used, not in the right carotid-femoral pathway, or in the left one. Additionally, the right and left carotid-humeral PWV did not show correlation with OH. Finally, when OH was quantified in relative terms (%), the right and left arterial stiffness OH/ECF relationship, analyzed in the carotid-femoral and carotid-brachial pathway, showed similar results that those obtained using absolute values (see Figure 4).

4. Discussion

In this work, the relationship between the hydration status and arterial stiffness is analyzed using, for the first time, a modern device that measures 50 different frequencies (from 5 to 1000 kHz), in order to characterize the whole-body bioimpedance. This technology allows using a 3-C model that ensures a reliable quantification of the body fluid compartment. According to the aim of this research, we characterized the arterial stiffness (1) of elastic and muscular arteries and (2) in both the right and left arterial territories of the patients. These approaches allow us to conclude the following:

(1) Fluid overload, quantified in terms of absolute values (OH) and of relative estimations (OH/ECF) through BCM, showed a significant BP dependent association with aortic stiffness, but not with peripheral arterial stiffness evaluated in the carotid-brachial pathway.

(2) Extracellular fluid relative increases (ECF/ICF and ECF/TBF) were significantly associated with aortic stiffness and with independence of the BP levels. This relationship was not observed when peripheral arterial stiffness was considered. This is an important, original finding [7, 12], which proves that the association of aortic stiffness and hydration status should not be extrapolated to other arterial territories, such as the upper limbs.

TABLE 1: Anthropometric, hemodynamic, and blood characteristics for the entire population and the hydric state-related groups.

	Entire group MV ± SD	Normal Hydration State (NHS) MV ± SD	Overhydration (OH) MV ± SD	Subhydration (SH) MV ± SD	P value NHS versus OH	NHS versus SH	OH versus SH
n	65	40	12	13			
Gender (female, %)	30.8%	32.5%	25.0%	30.8%			
Time of hemodialysis (month)	65.35 ± 60.54	71.65 ± 59.07	67.75 ± 73.18	43.77 ± 51.50	0.850	0.134	0.350
Age (years)	58.34 ± 15.93	55.98 ± 17.54	64.75 ± 12.48	59.69 ± 12.25	0.114	0.482	0.317
Height (m)	1.63 ± 0.10	1.63 ± 0.10	1.66 ± 0.09	1.62 ± 0.10	0.446	0.643	0.303
Body weight (kg)	71.76 ± 13.98	72.11 ± 11.74	63.75 ± 10.31	78.07 ± 19.75	0.031	0.189	0.035
BMI (kg/m^2)	26.93 ± 4.69	27.12 ± 3.91	23.28 ± 3.81	29.71 ± 5.72	0.004	0.071	0.003
Systolic blood pressure (mmHg)	127.97 ± 26.49	133.25 ± 24.89	132.92 ± 25.11	107.15 ± 23.76	0.968	0.002	0.015
Mean blood pressure (mmHg)	92.61 ± 16.40	94.92 ± 14.66	98.19 ± 14.27	80.33 ± 18.39	0.497	0.005	0.013
Diastolic blood pressure (mmHg)	74.92 ± 13.63	75.75 ± 11.98	80.83 ± 12.16	66.92 ± 16.78	0.205	0.042	0.027
Heart rate (beats/min)	87.69 ± 15.04	86.63 ± 14.83	88.42 ± 16.42	90.31 ± 15.23	0.722	0.443	0.768
Hemoglobin (g/dL)	10.54 ± 1.77	10.49 ± 1.70	10.94 ± 2.01	10.34 ± 1.83	0.445	0.782	0.440
Hematocrit (%)	33.69 ± 5.38	33.59 ± 5.40	34.61 ± 5.91	33.16 ± 5.13	0.575	0.805	0.519
Serum albumin (g/dL)	3.99 ± 0.34	4.07 ± 0.30	3.74 ± 0.39	3.97 ± 0.29	0.004	0.332	0.104
Calcium (mg/dL)	8.63 ± 0.44	8.61 ± 0.49	8.63 ± 0.28	8.72 ± 0.42	0.849	0.468	0.575
Phosphates (mg/dL)	4.63 ± 0.86	4.66 ± 0.86	4.41 ± 0.95	4.72 ± 0.83	0.387	0.822	0.387
Parathyroid hormone (pg/mL)	357.60 ± 280.32	425.04 ± 313.01	303.27 ± 192.62	205.45 ± 159.58	0.210	0.019	0.179
Serum urea (mg/dL)	147.88 ± 39.00	147.03 ± 42.43	141.92 ± 38.23	156.00 ± 28.46	0.710	0.481	0.304
Total cholesterol (mg/dL)	175.49 ± 40.20	178.90 ± 39.50	154.75 ± 36.55	184.15 ± 42.10	0.065	0.683	0.076
HDL cholesterol (mg/dL)	40.12 ± 13.07	38.10 ± 12.36	46.33 ± 17.44	40.62 ± 9.17	0.073	0.503	0.310
LDL cholesterol (mg/dL)	101.45 ± 34.87	98.25 ± 35.13	97.33 ± 31.48	115.11 ± 36.19	0.936	0.142	0.205
Total triglycerides (mg/dL)	177.23 ± 98.81	195.96 ± 105.95	128.50 ± 83.96	164.58 ± 73.54	0.049	0.327	0.264

MV: mean value, SD: standard deviation, BMI: body mass index, PWV: pulse wave velocity, and β: arterial stiffness index. A $P < 0.05$ was considered statistically significate.

TABLE 2: Hydric status for the entire population and the hydric state-related groups.

	Entire group	Normal Hydration State (NHS)	Overhydration (OH)	Subhydration (SH)	P value		
	MV ± SD	MV ± SD	MV ± SD	MV ± SD	NHS versus OH	NHS versus SH	OH versus SH
ECF (L)	16.67 ± 3.03	16.75 ± 3.00	17.63 ± 2.40	15.52 ± 3.47	**0.361**	**0.219**	**0.093**
ICF (L)	17.53 ± 4.24	17.81 ± 4.55	16.21 ± 2.82	17.88 ± 4.36	**0.257**	**0.962**	**0.272**
TBF (L)	34.19 ± 6.88	34.55 ± 7.26	33.86 ± 4.88	33.38 ± 7.66	**0.760**	**0.623**	**0.857**
ECF/EIF	0.97 ± 0.14	0.97 ± 0.14	1.10 ± 0.12	0.88 ± 0.09	**0.003**	**0.029**	**0.000**
ECF/TBF	0.49 ± 0.04	0.49 ± 0.04	0.52 ± 0.03	0.47 ± 0.02	**0.005**	**0.033**	**0.000**
OH (L)	1.42 ± 1.55	1.42 ± 0.70	3.68 ± 1.13	−0.66 ± 0.48	**0.000**	**0.000**	**0.000**
OH/TBF (%)	8.04 ± 8.60	8.32 ± 3.41	20.63 ± 4.49	−4.45 ± 3.30	**0.000**	**0.000**	**0.000**

MV: mean value, SD: standard deviation, and ECF and ICF: extracellular and intracellular fluid volume, respectively. TBF: Total Body Fluid volume. OH: overhydration. A $P < 0.05$ was considered statistically significate.

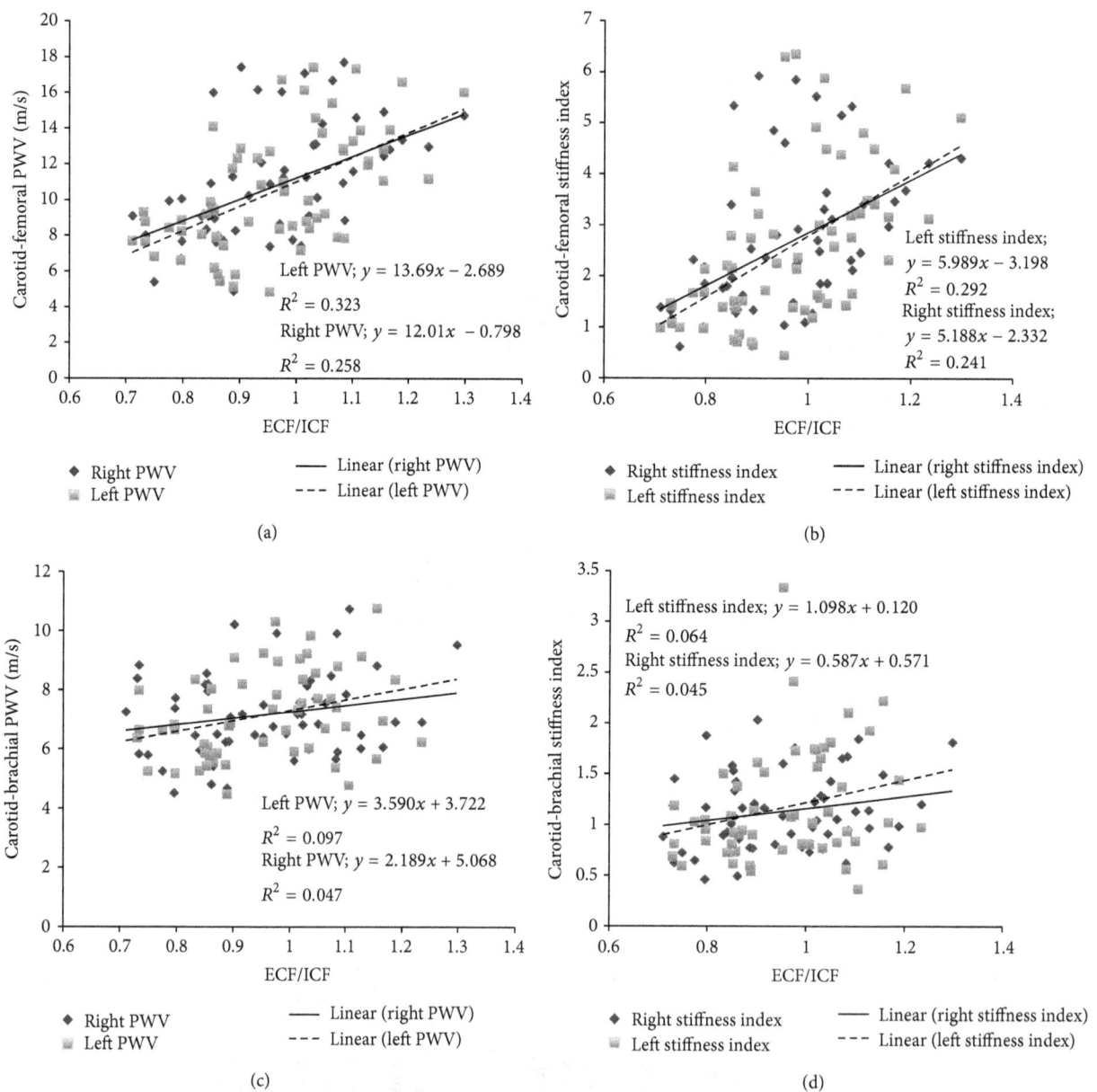

(a)

(b)

(c)

(d)

FIGURE 1: Pulse wave velocity (PWV) and hydration status evaluated through extracellular/intracellular fluid ratio (ECF/ICF) measured using a multi-impedancimetric technique. The carotid-femoral PWV-ECF/ICF relationship shows a significant relationship ($P < 0.05$), as does the stiffness index (β)-ECF/ICF relationship ($P < 0.05$).

TABLE 3: Arterial stiffness levels for the entire population and the hydric state-related groups.

	Entire group MV ± SD	Normal Hydration State (NHS) MV ± SD	Overhydration (OH) MV ± SD	Subhydration (SH) MV ± SD	P value NHS versus OH	NHS versus SH	OH versus SH
Carotid-femoral (aortic) stiffness							
Right carotid-femoral PWV (m/s)	10.74 ± 3.25	10.40 ± 3.44	12.84 ± 2.27	9.78 ± 2.69	0.032	0.586	0.009
Left carotid-femoral PWV (m/s)	10.48 ± 3.30	10.08 ± 3.37	12.57 ± 3.38	9.84 ± 2.33	0.036	0.821	0.034
Right carotid-femoral β	2.65 ± 1.45	2.44 ± 1.52	3.45 ± 1.03	2.54 ± 1.41	0.046	0.847	0.100
Left carotid-femoral β	2.56 ± 1.52	2.31 ± 1.47	3.41 ± 1.52	2.60 ± 1.49	0.036	0.553	0.214
Carotid-brachial stiffness							
Right carotid-brachial PWV (m/s)	7.17 ± 1.38	7.11 ± 1.33	7.65 ± 1.84	7.00 ± 1.20	0.321	0.796	0.341
Left carotid-brachial PWV (m/s)	7.15 ± 1.47	7.19 ± 1.34	7.83 ± 1.97	6.58 ± 1.36	0.273	0.179	0.109
Right carotid-brachial β	1.15 ± 0.40	1.08 ± 0.37	1.24 ± 0.43	1.30 ± 0.47	0.283	0.105	0.758
Left carotid-brachial β	1.17 ± 0.55	1.14 ± 0.46	1.32 ± 0.66	1.17 ± 0.74	0.362	0.879	0.646

MV: mean value, SD: standard deviation, PWV: pulse wave velocity, β: regional arterial stiffness index. A $P < 0.05$ was considered statistical significative.

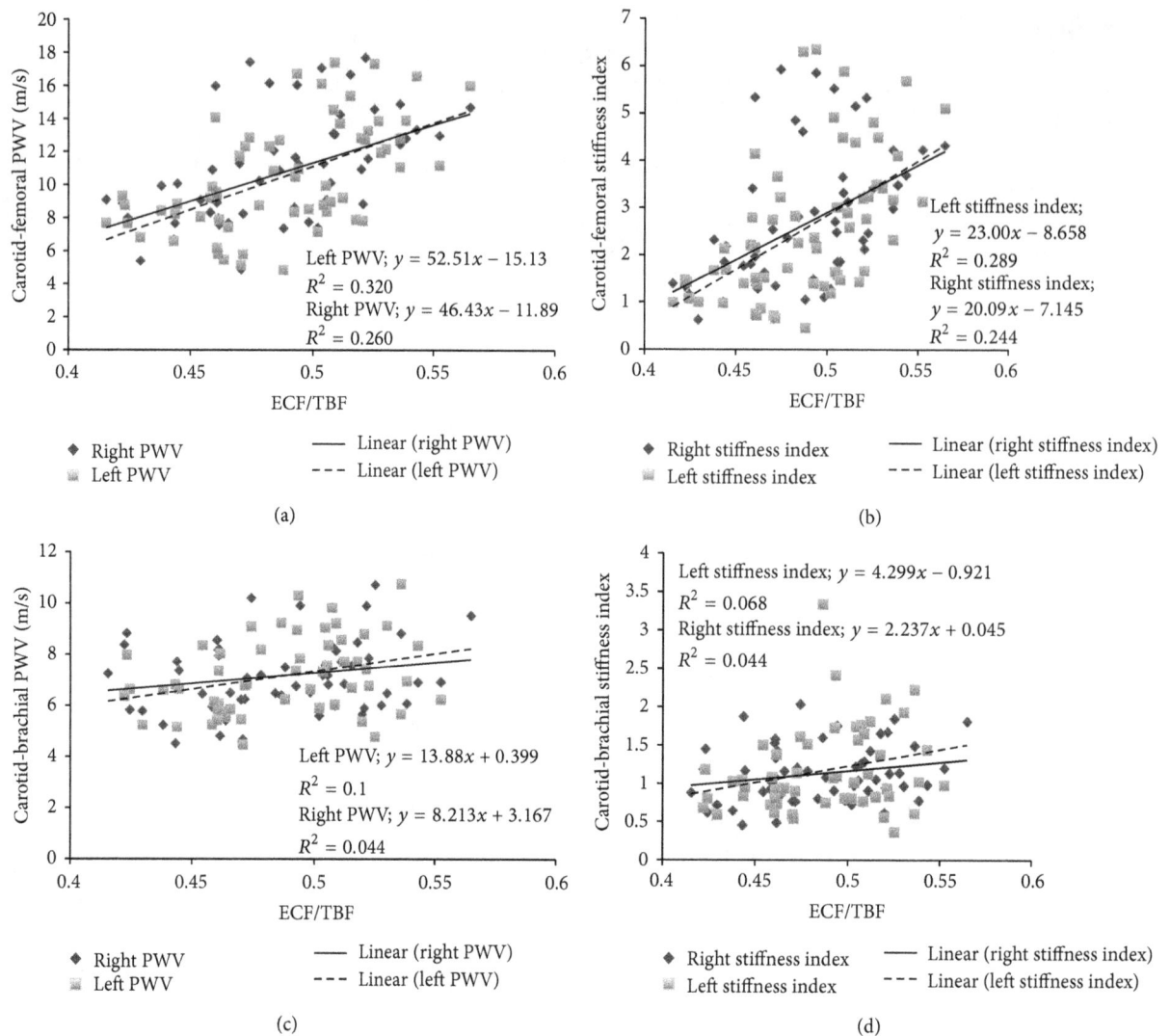

FIGURE 2: Pulse wave velocity (PWV) and hydration status evaluated through extracellular/Total Body Fluid ratio (ECF/TBF) measured using multi-impedancimetric technique. The carotid-femoral PWV-ECF/TBF relationship shows a significant relationship ($P < 0.05$), as the stiffness index (β)-ECF/TBF relationship ($P < 0.05$).

(3) Fluid overload patients showed significant higher levels of arterial stiffness, evaluated through carotid-femoral PWV, with respect to those that exhibit normal or low hydration status. This difference was not observed when arterial stiffness was analyzed in terms of the β index, indicating that the observed differences were BP dependent (Table 3). On the contrary, the analysis in terms of peripheral arterial stiffness showed nonsignificant differences between overhydrated and normally hydrated patients, with independence of blood pressure levels.

(4) Dehydratated patients showed nonsignificant differences in terms of arterial stiffness with respect to hemodialyzed patients with normal hydration status, both in terms of aortic and in terms of peripheral stiffness (Table 3).

Our results showed that ECF/ICF and ECF/TBF ratios are associated with carotid-femoral PWV, with independence of BP, but not with carotid-brachial PWV (Figure 1). These findings are partially coincident with those previously reported by Lin et al. [12] and Zheng et al. [7]. In the mentioned reports, the carotid-femoral PWV was correlated with ECF/ICF [12] and ECF/TBF [7], respectively. However, the authors omitted mentioning if such association persists when arterial stiffness is analyzed with independence of arterial BP. Moreover, Lin et al. and Zheng et al. results could not be confirmed when the aorto-axilo-humeral pathway was considered and evaluated using carotid-brachial PWV. Therefore, our results indicate (for the first time) that the increase in the ECF/ICF or ECF/TBF ratio did not provoke a similar change in the arterial stiffness of different arterial pathways. In other words, to affirm that ECF/ICF or ECF/TBF ratio is associated with the arterial stiffness increase in large arteries, as previously

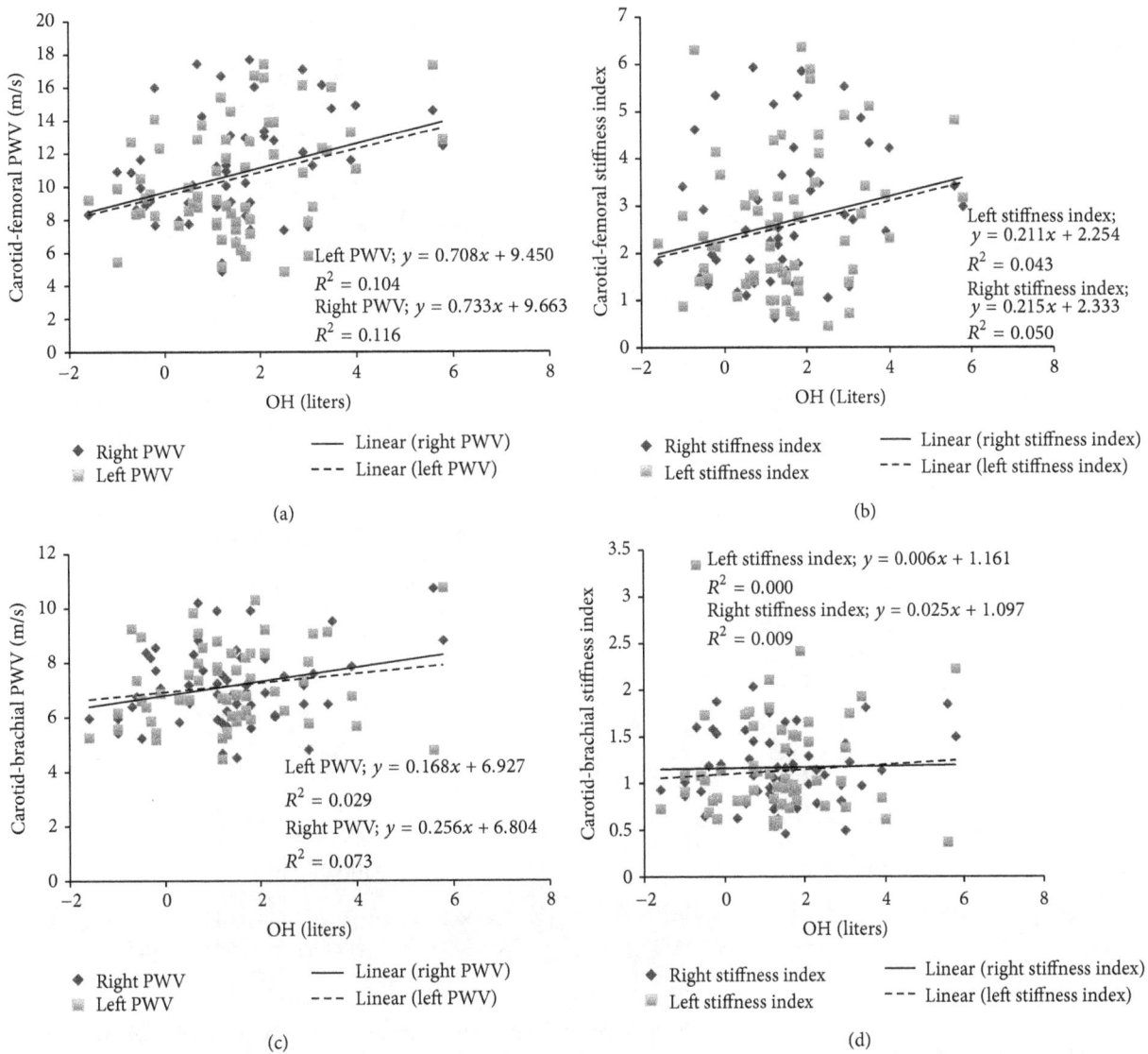

FIGURE 3: Pulse wave velocity (PWV) and hydration status evaluated through extracellular/overhydration ratio (OH) measured in absolute values using the multi-impedancimetric technique. The carotid-femoral PWV-OH relationship shows a significant relationship ($P < 0.05$), as does the stiffness index (β)-OH relationship ($P < 0.05$).

mentioned [12], is an incorrect generalization. The research reported by Lin et al. and Zheng et al. was carried out using a similar bioimpedance technique but not the same one. Consequently, the effect of overhydration on arterial stiffness only could be correctly evaluated analyzing the aortic stiffness (carotid-femoral PWV), but not peripheral stiffness. This result has practical importance for noninvasive vascular laboratories evaluation.

In theory, an ECF overload could be the origin of high levels of BP that increase arterial stiffness due to acute vascular passive overdistension (enlargement). This pressure dependent increase of arterial stiffness is determined by the collagen fiber recruitment in response to vascular diameter increases [15]. However, our results showed that the association between ECF/ICF and arterial stiffness is independent of the arterial BP levels. This important finding was evident

when arterial stiffness was analyzed using indexes of vascular function that are independent of arterial BP.

It is important to mention that the above-described results include compartment fluid evaluations in absolute (OH) and relative (OH/ECF) indexes, obtained through a widely employed 3-C model. The significant correlation between PWV and indexes associated specifically with overload (OH and OH/ECF) has not been reported previously. Furthermore, we found that arterial stiffness/overhydration status significant relationship should be restricted to the carotid-femoral pathway and not muscular or transitional arteries.

To quantify OH/TBF and mainly OH is important to reach a more integrative evaluation of the hydric status of the patient. These parameters can be obtained from the model published by Chamney et al. in 2007 [17], which stated OH

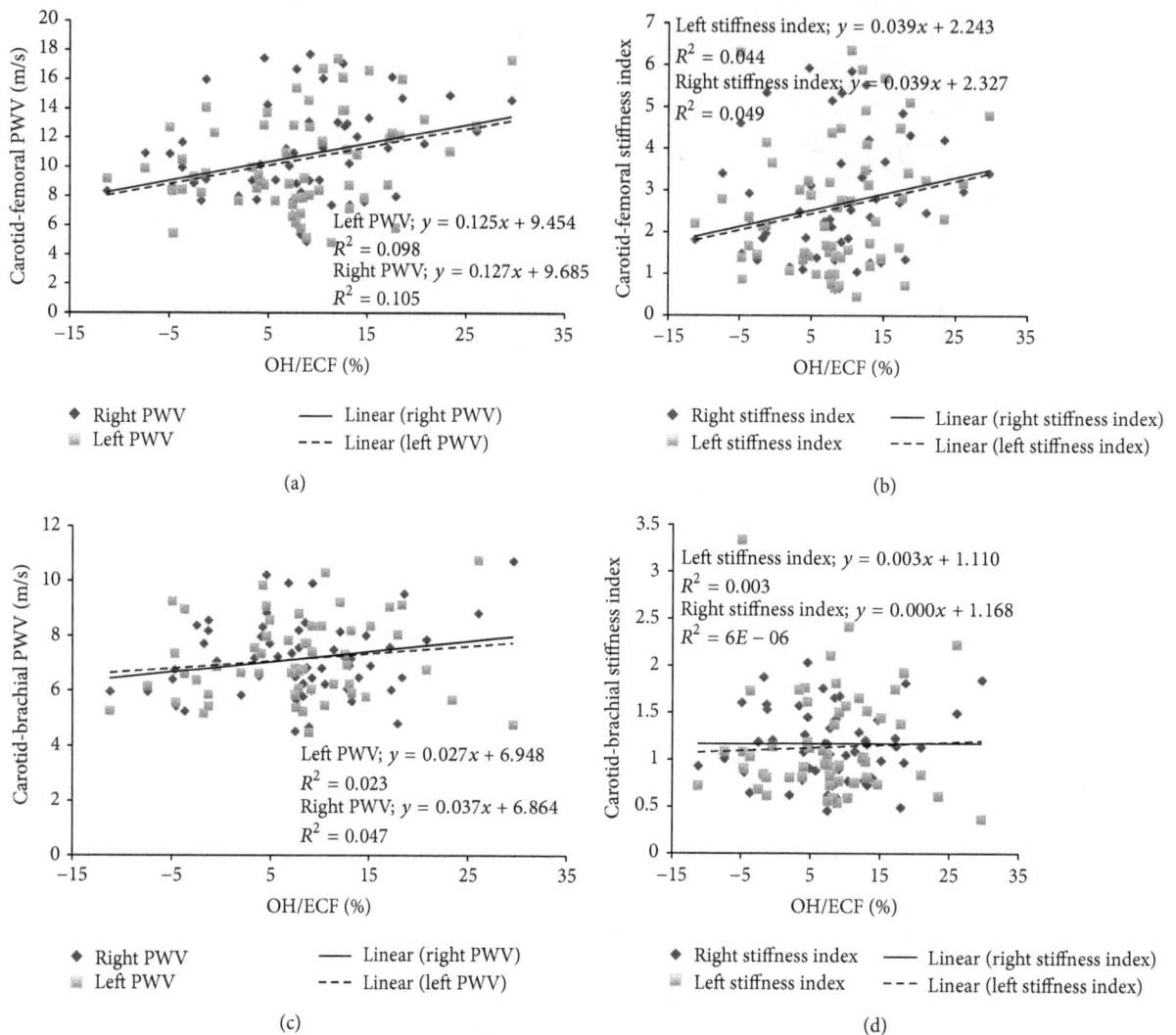

FIGURE 4: Pulse wave velocity (PWV) and hydration status evaluated through overhydration/Extracellular fluid ratio (OH/ECF) measured in relative values using multi-impedancimetric technique. The carotid-femoral PWV-OH/ECF relationship shows a significant relationship ($P < 0.05$), as does the stiffness index (β)-OH/ECF relationship ($P < 0.005$).

("MExF") as a function of ECF, ICF, and weight. A few years ago a novel prediction model was validated, in which body composition and fluid overload (OH) are estimated using a 3-C model. The model uses a correction factor for BMI which was introduced into the body composition monitor (BCM). The 3-C model includes three compartments calculated from ECF and TBF estimations: OH, LTM, and ATM. To this end, constant hydration ratios of the normohydrated LTM and ATM are assumed [17] and the model determines whether changes in ICF and ECF reflect increase or loss of ATM or LTM. OH represents the excess fluid (fluid overload) stored almost exclusively in the extracellular volume of a patient and is therefore part of the ECF, whereas the water of LTM and ATM consists of differing proportion of extracellular and intracellular water in addition to solid components. Healthy individuals are considered to be "normally hydrated" and therefore have virtually no OH. These individuals may be characterized in terms of ATM and LTM only. As the extra-cellular hydration of LTM and ATM is known, the expected "normal" volume of ECF of these tissues can be calculated. The difference between "normal" ECF and measured ECF is the excess fluid, OH. A negative OH means that the patient is under- or dehydrated. Both in healthy subjects and in chronic kidney disease patients, the distribution of LTM and ATM will lead to significant differences in the ECF/ICF ratio. Therefore ECF/ICF alone does not provide enough information about the hydration status. Therefore, in order to quantify the absolute and/or relative overhydration, other parameters than ECF/ICF are needed.

4.1. Methodological Aspects and Limitations. The β index used to evaluate the arterial stiffness provided information of the vascular wall state with independence of the BP level. This is not a minor issue since significant improvements of arterial wall stiffness without changes in BP levels have been reported [7].

Aortic PWV was evaluated in all cases using right and left carotid-femoral pathways in order to provide a complete screening of the elastic arteries involved in this vascular territory. According to a recent publication there were some differences between the right and the left carotid-femoral pathways [18]. As shown in the four figures that summarize this research, the above-mentioned differences seem to have minimal relevance in the analyzed population.

A limitation of this study is the lack of data about arterial stiffness before the beginning of renal function replacement therapy. However, as shown, significant association between arterial stiffness and the hydration status could be found.

Finally, as recently commented by Covic et al. [19], despite the extensive use of the modern bioimpedance technique as the bedside technology, there are some potential limitations. Among them, extreme or morbid obesity (BMI ≥ 40) is a significant limitation of the use of bioimpedance [19]. It is important to point out that SH patients included in our study showed lower values of BMI ($29.71 \pm 5.72 \, kg/m^2$) and no values of BMI ≥ 40 were observed, with $38,22 \, kg/m^2$ as the highest observed value.

4.2. Clinical Relevance. Elastin is the main constituent of the aortic wall, determining a high level of vascular distensibility. On the other hand, peripheral muscular arteries have lower compliance levels than the aorta. In physiological states, there is an arterial stiffness gradient between the aorta and the peripheral muscular arteries. The mentioned gradient of arterial stiffness determines the existence of reflection sites that dampen the transmission of travelling pressure waves from the aorta to the microcirculation. Additionally, peripheral arterial waves in the diastolic period arrive to the aortic root increasing coronary blood flow. In physiological condition, the aging process determines an aortic stiffness increase that is higher than that observed in muscular peripheral arteries. Consequently, the above-mentioned gradient between elastic and muscular arteries decreases. The reversal of the aortic-peripheral arteries stiffness gradient has been proposed as an index of vascular damage [20, 21]. Recently, Fortier et al. [22] showed that the measurement of the aortic (a central elastic artery) and brachial arteries stiffness (a peripheral muscular artery) and the quantification of the "stiffness gradient" (i.e., aortic-brachial arterial stiffness mismatch) could be useful in adult hemodialyzed patients and has been proposed as a new index and as a prognostic marker. The mentioned authors evaluate arterial stiffness mismatch through the PWV ratio, which is the aortic PWV divided by the upper-arm PWV [22]. The PWV ratio was strongly and independently associated with increased mortality in patients on dialysis [22]. This is why when hemodialyzed patients are evaluated, the inclusion of arterial territories different from the carotid-femoral pathway is important. In theory, if we included the mentioned PWV ratio index, our results would show that overhydration (measured as OH and OH/ECF) or an increased ECF/ICF ratio could be associated with an increased PWV ratio. According to

our results, overhydration could lead to the attenuation (or even reversion) of the expected arterial stiffness gradient, promoting end-organ damage. In other words, our work suggests a potential mechanism by which overhydration is associated with aortic stiffness in a different way than that evidenced when peripheral arterial stiffness is analyzed with respect to the hydration status. This is not a minor issue, since coronary blood flow could be modified determining changes in the circulatory system dynamics.

Another clinical connotation derived from our results is suggested if we consider that normalization of fluid overload could not be accompanied by changes in arterial stiffness in the peripheral vessels. Unfortunately, previous studies that have evaluated the association between arterial stiffness and hydration status only evaluated elastic arteries (i.e., carotid artery, aorta), without considering that they cannot respond like the muscular arteries [7, 12]. The different response to renal replacement therapy, in terms of arterial stiffness of both arterial evaluated territories, could be explained by the quantitative variation of the amount of arterial wall constituents observed in brachial and aortic arteries. Previous research has pointed out that changes induced by age on arterial elasticity are not uniform and depend on the vascular territory [23].

Finally, as mentioned, considering that in a 2-C model variations in hydration state may have a strong effect on the prediction of fat-free mass, a recent novel prediction model was validated, in which body composition and net and relative OH are estimated using a 3-C model [17]. As mentioned above, our results show that aortic stiffness is associated with indexes of fluid overload, with independence of arterial BP levels.

5. Conclusion

In hemodialysis patients, volume status and overload, expressed as extracellular/intracellular fluid ratio (ECF/ICF), extracellular/Total Body Fluid ratio (ECF/TBF), or overhydration (OH), are associated with central (aortic), but not peripheral (axilo-brachial) arterial stiffness values, independently of BP. Guiding the patients towards this target of normohydration leads to improved aortic but not peripheral arteries function.

Acknowledgments

The authors gratefully acknowledge the Agencia Nacional de Investigación e Innovación (ANII), and Espacio Interdisciplinario (EI) and Comisión Sectorial de Investigación Científica (CSIC-Udelar) of the Republic University, Uruguay. This work was supported by the René Favaloro University Foundation and funds of "PICT 2008 OC AR 0340" (Argentina) and Agencia Nacional de

Investigación e Innovación and funds of PRSCT-008-020 and FCE-2007-635 (Uruguay).

References

[1] G. M. London, B. Pannier, A. P. Guerin et al., "Alterations of left ventricular hypertrophy in and survival of patients receiving hemodialysis: follow-up of an interventional study," *Journal of the American Society of Nephrology*, vol. 12, no. 12, pp. 2759–2767, 2001.

[2] G. M. London, S. J. Marchais, A. P. Guérin, P. Boutouyrie, F. Métivier, and M.-C. de Vernejoul, "Association of bone activity, calcium load, aortic stiffness, and calcifications in ESRD," *Journal of the American Society of Nephrology*, vol. 19, no. 9, pp. 1827–1835, 2008.

[3] L. Segall, N.-G. Mardare, S. Ungureanu et al., "Nutritional status evaluation and survival in haemodialysis patients in one centre from Romania," *Nephrology Dialysis Transplantation*, vol. 24, no. 8, pp. 2536–2540, 2009.

[4] V. Wizemann, P. Wabel, P. Chamney et al., "The mortality risk of overhydration in haemodialysis patients," *Nephrology Dialysis Transplantation*, vol. 24, no. 5, pp. 1574–1579, 2009.

[5] S.-C. Hung, K.-L. Kuo, C.-H. Peng et al., "Volume overload correlates with cardiovascular risk factors in patients with chronic kidney disease," *Kidney International*, vol. 85, no. 3, pp. 703–709, 2014.

[6] P. Wabel, U. Moissl, P. Chamney et al., "Towards improved cardiovascular management: the necessity of combining blood pressure and fluid overload," *Nephrology Dialysis Transplantation*, vol. 23, no. 9, pp. 2965–2971, 2008.

[7] D. Zheng, L.-T. Cheng, Z. Zhuang, Y. Gu, L.-J. Tang, and T. Wang, "Correlation between pulse wave velocity and fluid distribution in hemodialysis patients," *Blood Purification*, vol. 27, no. 3, pp. 248–252, 2009.

[8] E. Hur, M. Usta, H. Toz et al., "Effect of fluid management guided by bioimpedance spectroscopy on cardiovascular parameters in hemodialysis patients: a randomized controlled trial," *American Journal of Kidney Diseases*, vol. 61, no. 6, pp. 957–965, 2013.

[9] J. Blacher, M. E. Safar, A. P. Guerin, B. Pannier, S. J. Marchais, and G. M. London, "Aortic pulse wave velocity index and mortality in end-stage renal disease," *Kidney International*, vol. 63, no. 5, pp. 1852–1860, 2003.

[10] B. Pannier, A. P. Guérin, S. J. Marchais, M. E. Safar, and G. M. London, "Stiffness of capacitive and conduit arteries: prognostic significance for end-stage renal disease patients," *Hypertension*, vol. 45, no. 4, pp. 592–596, 2005.

[11] J. T. Daugirdas, "Bioimpedance technology and optimal fluid management," *The American Journal of Kidney Diseases*, vol. 61, no. 6, pp. 861–864, 2013.

[12] Y.-P. Lin, W.-C. Yu, T.-L. Hsu, P. Y.-A. Ding, W.-C. Yang, and C.-H. Chen, "The extracellular fluid-to-intracellular fluid volume ratio is associated with large-artery structure and function in hemodialysis patients," *American Journal of Kidney Diseases*, vol. 42, no. 5, pp. 990–999, 2003.

[13] E. I. C. Fischer, D. Bia, R. Valtuille, S. Craf, C. Galli, and R. L. Armentano, "Vascular access localization determines regional changes in arterial stiffness," *Journal of Vascular Access*, vol. 10, no. 3, pp. 192–198, 2009.

[14] D. Bia, E. I. Cabrera-Fischer, Y. Zócalo et al., "Vascular accesses for haemodialysis in the upper arm cause greater reduction in the carotid-brachial stiffness than those in the forearm: study of gender differences," *International Journal of Nephrology*, vol. 2012, Article ID 598512, 10 pages, 2012.

[15] S. Laurent, J. Cockcroft, L. van Bortel et al., "Expert consensus document on arterial stiffness: methodological issues and clinical applications," *European Heart Journal*, vol. 27, no. 21, pp. 2588–2605, 2006.

[16] K. Shirai, N. Hiruta, M. Song et al., "Cardio-ankle vascular index (CAVI) as a novel indicator of arterial stiffness: theory, evidence and perspectives," *Journal of Atherosclerosis and Thrombosis*, vol. 18, no. 11, pp. 924–938, 2011.

[17] P. W. Chamney, P. Wabel, U. M. Moissl et al., "A whole-body model to distinguish excess fluid from the hydration of major body tissues," *The American Journal of Clinical Nutrition*, vol. 85, no. 1, pp. 80–89, 2007.

[18] M. Dzeko, C. D. Peters, K. D. Kjaergaard, J. D. Jensen, and B. Jespersen, "Aortic pulse wave velocity results depend on which carotid artery is used for the measurements," *Journal of Hypertension*, vol. 31, no. 1, pp. 117–122, 2013.

[19] A. Covic, L. Voroneanu, and D. Goldsmith, "Routine bioimpedance-derived volume assessment for all hypertensives: a new paradigm," *American Journal of Nephrology*, vol. 40, no. 5, pp. 434–440, 2014.

[20] G. F. Mitchell, H. Parise, E. J. Benjamin et al., "Changes in arterial stiffness and wave reflection with advancing age in healthy men and women: the Framingham Heart Study," *Hypertension*, vol. 43, no. 6, pp. 1239–1245, 2004.

[21] M. Briet, P. Boutouyrie, S. Laurent, and G. M. London, "Arterial stiffness and pulse pressure in CKD and ESRD," *Kidney International*, vol. 82, no. 4, pp. 388–400, 2012.

[22] C. Fortier, F. Mac-Way, S. Desmeules et al., "Aortic-brachial stiffness mismatch and mortality in dialysis population," *Hypertension*, vol. 65, no. 2, pp. 378–384, 2015.

[23] J. J. Van der Heijden-Spek, J. A. Staessen, R. H. Fagard, A. P. Hoeks, H. A. Struijker Boudier, and L. M. Van Bortel, "Effect of age on brachial artery wall properties differs from the aorta and is gender dependent: a population study," *Hypertension*, vol. 35, no. 2, pp. 637–642, 2000.

14

Effect of Pentoxifylline on Microalbuminuria in Diabetic Patients

Shahrzad Shahidi,[1] **Marziyeh Hoseinbalam,**[2] **Bijan Iraj,**[2] **and Mojtaba Akbari**[3]

[1]*Isfahan Kidney Disease Research Center, Isfahan University of Medical Sciences, Isfahan, Iran*
[2]*Isfahan Endocrine and Metabolism Research Center, Isfahan University of Medical Sciences, Isfahan, Iran*
[3]*Department of Epidemiology, School of Health and Nutrition, Shiraz University of Medical Sciences, Shiraz, Iran*

Correspondence should be addressed to Marziyeh Hoseinbalam; drhoseinbalam@yahoo.com

Academic Editor: Jochen Reiser

Background. Pentoxifylline is a nonspecific phosphodiesterase inhibitor with anti-inflammatory properties. Human studies have proved its antiproteinuric effect in patients with glomerular diseases, but this study was designed to assess the effects of add-on pentoxifylline to available treatment on reduction of microalbuminuria in diabetic patients without glomerular diseases. *Methods.* In a double-blind placebo-controlled, randomized study we evaluated the influence of pentoxifylline on microalbuminuria in type 2 diabetic patients. 40 diabetic patients with estimated glomerular filtration rate (eGFR) of more than $60 \, \text{mL/min/1.73} \, \text{m}^2$ in eight weeks and microalbuminuria were randomized to two groups which will receive pentoxifylline 1200 mg/day or placebo added to regular medications for 6 months. albuminuria; eGFR was evaluated at three- and six-month follow-up period. *Results.* Baseline characteristics were similar between the two groups. At six months, the mean estimated GFR and albuminuria were not different between two groups at 3- and 6-month follow-up. Trend of albumin to creatinine ratio, systolic and diastolic blood pressure, and eGFR in both groups were decreased, but no significant differences were noted between two groups (P value > 0.05). *Conclusion.* Pentoxifylline has not a significant additive antimicroalbuminuric effect compared with placebo in patients with type 2 diabetes with early stage of kidney disease; however, further clinical investigations are necessary to be done.

1. Introduction

Diabetes is among the most common and major diseases in the world and recently in most countries the number of patients with diabetes has strikingly increased. Diabetic nephropathy is enlisted as one of the chronic microvascular complications of diabetes which is associated with considerable morbidity and mortality [1, 2] and is a main cause for approximately 50% of all end stage renal disease, and this results in increasing renal replacement therapy and healthcare costs [3, 4]. Though many pathophysiologic processes are involved in the pathogenesis of diabetic nephropathy, the fundamental mechanisms of it are not fully established [5]. Diabetic nephropathy is characterized by proteinuria, hypertension, and advanced renal insufficiency. More than 350 million people will be afflicted by diabetes by 2030 [6]; and about 20 to 30 percent of these diabetic patients, either type 1 or type 2, will be suffering from diabetic nephropathy, which has a greater incidence as the disease becomes more chronic [7].

Recently, the focus has moved to much earlier stages in renal disease as established by the presence of microalbuminuria [8, 9] and this is an early sign of diabetic nephropathy and premature cardiovascular disease [9, 10]. Biannual control of microalbuminuria in patients with diabetes is recommended in American and European guidelines [11, 12]. Microalbuminuria indicates a possibility of ongoing renal involvement due to diabetic nephropathy which ultimately results in end stage renal disease [13]. In type 2 diabetes, microalbuminuria or overt proteinuria may be present by the time of diagnosis and the latter is often accompanied by hypertension in these patients; however conditions such as congestive heart failure, hypertension, and infections can also lead to microalbuminuria in diabetic patients [2, 14]. It is reported that approximately a total of 3.7 percent of type 2 diabetic patients go toward advanced renal complications, and the risk for major renal involvements in patients with microalbuminuria is two times greater than normoalbuminuric patients [15]. This reinforces the necessity of early detection and treatment of microalbuminuria.

One effective treatment is the use of angiotensin converting enzyme inhibitor (ACEI) which delivers its effect in delaying the development of diabetic nephropathy through inhibition of renin-angiotensin system; however these treatments are being shown to be not only time consuming, but also not preventive enough. Studies have shown that beside metabolic and hemodynamic changes, inflammatory phenomena are also involved in progression of diabetic nephropathy, implying that the anti-inflammatory drugs could be beneficial [16–18].

Pentoxifylline is a nonselective phosphodiesterase inhibitor that is used in peripheral vascular diseases. There have been several theories for its mechanism of action, including anti-cell proliferation, and being anti-inflammatory and anti-fibrotic [19–22]. Clinically, pentoxifylline has been shown to be beneficial in nephropathies by reducing proteinuria and TNF-α level; however its overall advantage for nephropathies is still a matter of debate [23–25]. Few studies have shown that coapplication of pentoxifylline with ACEI drugs in diabetic patients or its use together with immunosuppressant drugs in nephrotic syndrome of lupus patients resulted in a reduction of proteinuria [26, 27]. It is yet not clear whether or not pentoxifylline is effective on reduction of proteinuria. So, the present study was designed to assess the effects of pentoxifylline on microalbuminuria in diabetic patients.

2. Materials and Methods

The present study was a randomized, parallel-group, double blind study which was conducted between Sep. 2012 and Sep. 2013, on 50 adult patients with diabetic nephropathy in our city endocrine and metabolism research center outpatient clinic. The ethics committee of our University of Medical Sciences approved the study. Eligibility was defining as age older than 18 years in both genders, with an estimated glomerular filtration rate (GFR) higher than 60 mL/min/1.73 m^2 in the last six months. GFR was estimated using the 4-variable Modification of Diet in Renal Disease (MDRD). Also, patients were screened only if blood pressure (BP) was less than 140/90 mm Hg by using beta blockers, ACEI or ARB, without pressure alterations, under interventions, on a diet with protein intake levels less than 0.8 gr/kg/d, and glycosylated hemoglobin (HbA1c) less than 8%. Patients were eligible for enrollment if spot urine albumin-creatinine ratio was less than 300 mg/g in 3 consecutive measurements during a 3-month screening period.

Patients were excluded if they had myocardial infarction, had undergone coronary artery bypass grafting or percutaneous transluminal coronary angioplasty, or had a stroke or a retinal hemorrhage within the prior 6 months. Additional exclusion criteria included abnormal liver function test results, congestive heart failure (New York Heart Association class III or IV), obstructive uropathy, active malignancy, and being not able to discontinue immunosuppressive or nonsteroidal anti-inflammatory drugs, as well as pregnant women or those who do breast feeding, or any changes in patient's medications during the examination on any basis including high blood pressure and patient's disinclination for enrollment or intolerance to pentoxifylline.

After obtaining written informed consent from studied patients, all participating patients underwent primary examinations by a physician. Age, sex, weight, height, systolic and diastolic blood pressure, GFR (based on the MDRD formula), and urinary albumin/creatinine ratio in a morning spot urine sample were measured and calculated. Then, using randommaker software "Random Allocation" eligible patients were randomly divided into two 20-member groups. Case group includes patients who received 400 mg pentoxifylline pills (manufactured by Amin Pharmaceutical, three times a day) besides the patients' regular medications, and control group includes patients who received placebo similar to pentoxifylline pills besides the patients' regular medications. During the study patients' blood pressure was monitored and controlled via their routine monthly examinations by their physicians; no changes were made in neither the type nor the dosage of their hypertensive drugs. Also, three and six months later, the participants' albumin/creatinine ratio in spot urine sample, systolic and diastolic blood pressure, and GFR were measured.

All statistical analyses were done using SPSS software for Windows, version 20. Descriptive data are reported as mean ± SD, or number (percent) as appropriate. Independent Samples Test and Chi-square test and ANOVA were used for comparing all studied variables between groups as appropriate. The level of significance is considered to be less than 0.05.

3. Results

Of 98 reviewed patients, 48 patients did not enter to the study (39 patients were not eligible and nine patients refused informed consent). Fifty patients were eligible and randomly assigned into two treatment groups. Patients were followed up for 6 months. During the follow-up, 10 patients (5 patients in control and 5 patients in case groups) in both groups were excluded due to gastrointestinal problems and, finally, 40 patients in both groups completed the study and were analyzed (Figure 1).

The mean age of the studied patients was 53.2 ± 10.2 years; 25 patients (62.5%) were female and 15 patients (37.5%) were male. Table 1 shows baseline characteristics of studied patients. No significant differences were noted between case and control groups for mean of age and sex combination, weight, GFR, duration of being diabetic, BMI, and HbA1C (P value > 0.05).

Table 2 shows the comparison of patients' ratio of albumin to creatinine between study groups, systolic and diastolic blood pressure, and GFR at studied time points. As shown the ratio of albumin to creatinine was similar between two groups and no significant difference was noted between cases and controls (P value > 0.05). Patients' systolic and diastolic blood pressure and GFR at studied time points, in both

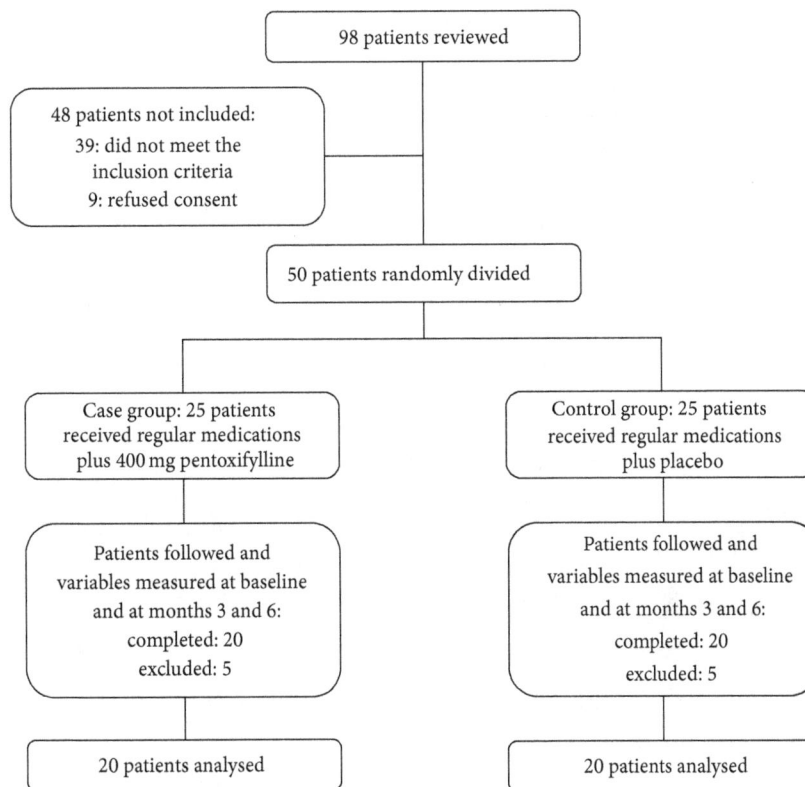

FIGURE 1: Patients who entered to the study, divided into the study groups and analyzed.

TABLE 1: Baseline characteristics in 40 studies patients by groups.

	Case group ($n = 20$)	Control group ($n = 20$)	P value
Age (year)	50.3 ± 9	55.6 ± 10.7	0.1^*
Sex			
Male	9 (40.9)	6 (33.3)	$0.8^\dagger$
Female	13 (59.1)	12 (66.7)	
Weight (kg)	79.60 ± 2.40	78.45 ± 1.68	0.86^*
Body mass index	30.51 ± 7.13	30.75 ± 4.22	0.90^*
GFR (mL/min/1.73 m^2)	73.93 ± 1.05	71.54 ± 9.29	0.45^*
HbA1C (%)	7.76 ± 1.62	7.4 ± 1.6	0.55^*
Duration of being diabetic	5.95 ± 5.58	5.54 ± 5.87	0.82^*

Data expressed as mean ± SD or number (percent). GFR: glomerular filtration rate; HbA1C: glycosylated hemoglobin.
Case group included 20 patients who received regular medications plus 400 mg pentoxifylline. Control group included 20 patients who received regular medications plus placebo.
P values calculated by *Independent Samples Test, †Chi-square test.

case and control groups, were not statistically significantly different (P value > 0.05). Also trend of ratio of albumin to creatinine, systolic and diastolic blood pressure, and GFR between groups during six-month follow-up were analyzed by ANOVA and results are reported in Figure 2. As shown trend of ratio of albumin to creatinine, systolic and diastolic blood pressure, and GFR in both groups were similar and no significant differences were noted between groups (P values > 0.05).

Drugs used by patients before and during study period were reported in all patients (Table 3) including eight patients in pentoxifylline group and 11 patients in control group for ARBs (P value = 0.12), three of patients in pentoxifylline group and two patients in control group for ACEI (P value = 0.81), two patients in pentoxifylline groups and one in control group for β-blocker (P value = 0.67), and two patients in both pentoxifylline and control groups for Ca-blocker (P value = 0.83). Also, four patients in both pentoxifylline and control groups reported use of diuretic (P value = 0.68), and 17 in pentoxifylline group and 14 patients in control group reported use of statin (P value = 0.97).

TABLE 2: Parameters of patients during the study.

	Baseline	Time points Month 3	Month 6
Albumin/creatinine ratio			
Case	60.69 ± 22.04	56.98 ± 25.28	59.37 ± 28.24
Control	63.87 ± 23.26	64.51 ± 31.27	64.63 ± 27.86
P value	0.77	0.41	0.58
Systolic blood pressure			
Case	115.68 ± 11.16	117.73 ± 9.72	114.32 ± 11.37
Control	115.28 ± 9.15	115.28 ± 11.17	112.50 ± 11.15
P value	0.90	0.46	0.61
Diastolic blood pressure			
Case	75.45 ± 8.15	76.50 ± 5.72	75 ± 5.34
Control	77.29 ± 8.26	77.22 ± 6.69	77.50 ± 8.44
P value	0.50	0.88	0.26
Glomerular filtration rate			
Case	73.93 ± 1.05	—	73.05 ± 11.80
Control	71.54 ± 9.29	—	80.22 ± 11.97
P value	0.45	—	0.06

Data expressed as mean ± SD.
Case group included patients who received regular medications plus 400 mg pentoxifylline. Control group included patients who received regular medications plus placebo.
P values calculated by Independent Samples Test.

TABLE 3: Baseline characteristics in 40 studies patients by groups.

	Case group (n = 20)	Control group (n = 20)	P value
ARB	8 (40)	11 (55)	0.12
ACEI	3 (15)	2 (10)	0.81
Beta-blocker	2 (10)	1 (5)	0.67
Ca blocker	2 (10)	2 (10)	0.83
Diuretics	4 (20)	4 (20)	0.99
Statins	17 (85)	14 (70)	0.97

Data expressed as number (percent). ARB: angiotensin receptor blocker; ACEI: angiotensin converting enzyme inhibitor.
Case group included 20 patients who received regular medications plus 400 mg pentoxifylline. Control group included 20 patients who received regular medications plus placebo.
P values calculated by Chi-square test.

4. Discussion

Microalbuminuria is one of the first clinical symptoms of diabetic nephropathy that may progress to macroalbuminuria and the progressive loss of glomerular filtration rate and finally the end stage renal disease [2]. Early recognition and treatment of microalbuminuria can prevent irreversible complications such as kidney problems [10]. Antihypertensive treatments, renoprotective treatments such as angiotensin converting enzyme inhibitors or angiotensin II receptor blockers, antihyperlipidemia medications, and protein intake restriction are treatments that have been used to control diabetic nephropathy [11, 16, 17, 28, 29]. Due to report of some side effects, in all of the diabetic patients these treatments cannot always be used with the proper dosage of the medications and different medications have been assessed in these patients. The present study was undertaken to answer the question whether add-on pentoxifylline to available treatment in diabetic patients would improve microalbuminuria, and we found that the add-on pentoxifylline to available treatment does not decrease microalbuminuria during six-month treatment in these patients compared with placebo. Also differences in the mean of albumin/creatinine ratio of random urine sample and urine creatinine level before and after treatment between groups were not statistically significant. Totally our results showed that add-on pentoxifylline to available treatment does not provide additive antimicroalbuminuric effects in patients with early stage of diabetic nephropathy (stages 1 to 3).

Pentoxifylline is one of a number of anti-inflammatory drugs that have been used for clinical trials in diabetic patients with nephropathy. Effect of pentoxifylline on albuminuria among these has been evaluated in several studies with different findings. Some studies have clearly shown significant decrease in albuminuria in the pentoxifylline group compared with placebo or routine treatment. In a prospective and randomized study, Navarro et al. showed an additional effect on the reduction of urinary albumin excretion of treatment with pentoxifylline in a group of patients with type 2 diabetes and diabetic nephropathy and residual albuminuria despite long-term therapy with angiotensin II receptor blockers at the recommended dosage [27]. Rodríguez-Morán et al. [30] have also compared the efficacy of pentoxifylline and captopril on the reduction of albuminuria in 130 normotensive diabetic patients with normal renal function and concluded that pentoxifylline is an effective alternative

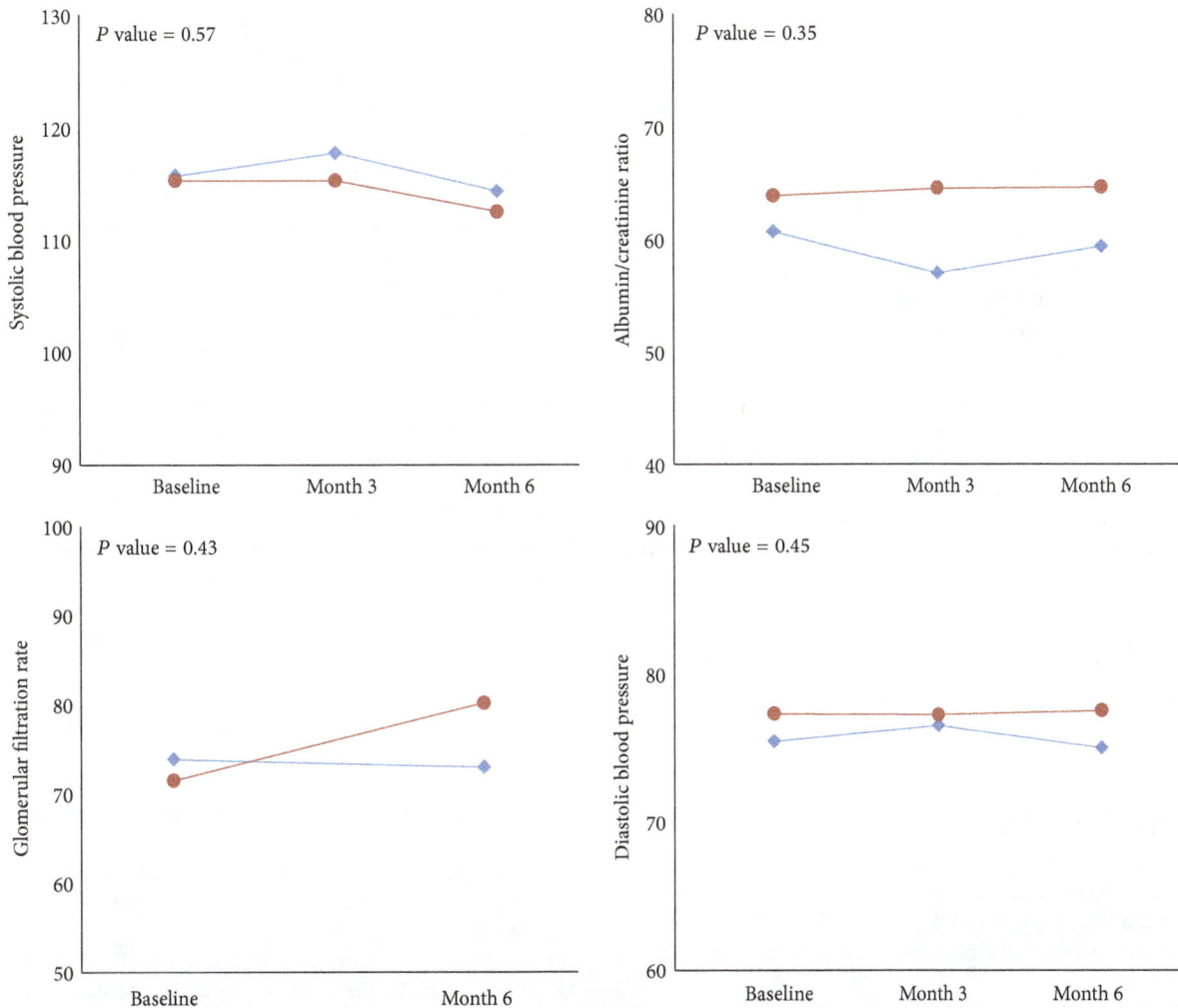

FIGURE 2: Comparison of trend of studied variables in time points between case and control groups. Case group included 20 patients who received regular medications plus 400 mg pentoxifylline. Control group included 20 patients who received regular medications plus placebo. Statistical analyses were done using ANOVA and no significant differences were noted between groups for trend of albumin/creatinine ratio, systolic and diastolic blood pressure, and glomerular filtration rate at time points (P values > 0.05).

agent to ACE inhibitors in reducing albuminuria. In the study of Solerte et al., 21 diabetic patients received pentoxifylline and results showed a significant reduction of albuminuria and arterial blood pressure in these patients compared to other groups with treatment with antihypertensive drugs [31]. Another study by Harmankaya et al. was done on 25 hypertensive type 2 diabetic patients with persistent microalbuminuria and normal renal function under treatment with combining pentoxifylline with an angiotensin converting enzyme inhibitor, lisinopril, on urinary albumin excretion compared with those obtained in a control group of 25 type 2 diabetic patients treated with lisinopril only and reporting a significant reduction in urinary albumin excretion in pentoxifylline group [32]. All the results in these studies concluded that pentoxifylline is an effective alternative agent for reducing albuminuria. Results of the present study were different from these findings and reported no significant reduction in albuminuria in studied patients after add-on pentoxifylline to available treatment compared to placebo.

The reason for differences between these studies could be justified by the different medications; whereas in some studies patients were treated only with pentoxifylline, in some other studies some other different medications were included. Other possible reasons of differences between findings are differences in doses of pentoxifylline, time of patients' follow-up, or lack of placebo group.

Currently, to treat peripheral vascular and bronchoconstrictive diseases pentoxifylline is used. Various conditions such as antiphospholipid syndrome, alcoholic hepatitis, and wound healing have a role in the determination of pentoxifylline effects [33, 34]. But in patients with diabetic nephropathy the effects of pentoxifylline are unclear and this might be because of the heterogeneous clinical nature of diabetic nephropathy [35, 36]. It is reported that urinary albumin excretion is the most powerful marker for subsequent renal events in patient with type 2 diabetes and nephropathy and that the degree of albuminuria reduction is linearly related to the subsequent renal protection [37]; thus any further reduction of albuminuria in patients with diabetes is of great importance. Unfortunately, data on this aspect are scarce and additive antimicroalbuminuric effect of pentoxifylline is an interesting question which is sustained over time. Therefore, the reduction of the residual albuminuria by additional approaches needs to be considered.

After excluding 10 patients during follow-up period small sample size is the possible main limitation of the present study. So, future studies with large sample size are suggested to evaluate the effects of body pentoxifylline in patients with diabetic nephropathy.

In conclusion, the results of our study show that, in patients who have type 2 diabetes and are under long-term treatment, pentoxifylline does not have a significant additive antimicroalbuminuric effect compared with placebo; however, further clinical investigation is necessary to determine this effect.

Ethical Approval

This work complies with all relevant ethical and privacy requirements.

Authors' Contribution

All authors have read and approved the paper and hereby confirm that this paper has not been published elsewhere and has not been submitted simultaneously to another journal.

References

[1] G. Danaei, M. M. Finucane, Y. Lu et al., "National, regional, and global trends in fasting plasma glucose and diabetes prevalence since 1980: systematic analysis of health examination surveys and epidemiological studies with 370 country-years and 2.7 million participants," *The Lancet*, vol. 378, no. 9785, pp. 31–40, 2011.

[2] M. A. Ahmed, G. Kishore, H. A. Khader, and M. N. Kasturirangan, "Risk factors and management of diabetic nephropathy," *Saudi Journal of Kidney Diseases and Transplantation*, vol. 24, no. 6, pp. 1242–1247, 2013.

[3] M. C. Korrapati, L. H. Howell, B. E. Shaner, J. K. Megyesi, L. J. Siskind, and R. G. Schnellmann, "Suramin: a potential therapy for diabetic nephropathy," *PLoS ONE*, vol. 8, no. 9, Article ID e73655, 2013.

[4] M. E. Molitch, R. A. DeFronzo, M. J. Franz et al., "Nephropathy in diabetes," *Diabetes Care*, vol. 27, no. 1, pp. 79–83, 2004.

[5] J. D. Kopple and U. Feroze, "The effect of obesity on chronic kidney disease," *Journal of Renal Nutrition*, vol. 21, no. 1, pp. 66–71, 2011.

[6] World Health Organization, *The Diabetes Program*, WHO, Geneva, Switzerland, 2004.

[7] G. Remuzzi, A. Schieppati, and P. Ruggenenti, "Nephropathy in patients with type 2 diabetes," *The New England Journal of Medicine*, vol. 346, no. 15, pp. 1145–1151, 2002.

[8] S. Agewall, J. Wikstrand, S. Ljungman, and B. Fagerberg, "Usefulness of microalbuminuria in predicting cardiovascular mortality in treated hypertensive men with and without diabetes mellitus," *The American Journal of Cardiology*, vol. 80, no. 2, pp. 164–169, 1997.

[9] C. E. Mogensen and P. L. Poulsen, "Microalbuminuria, glycemic control, and blood pressure predicting outcome in diabetes type 1 and type 2," *Kidney International, Supplement*, vol. 66, no. 92, pp. S40–S41, 2004.

[10] D. de Zeeuw, H.-H. Parving, and R. H. Henning, "Microalbuminuria as an early marker for cardiovascular disease," *Journal of the American Society of Nephrology*, vol. 17, no. 8, pp. 2100–2105, 2006.

[11] G. Mancia, G. de Backer, A. Dominiczak et al., "Guidelines for the management of arterial hypertension: The Task Force for the Management of Arterial Hypertension of the European Society of Hypertension and of the European Society of Cardiology," *Journal of Hypertension*, vol. 25, pp. 1105–1187, 2007.

[12] American Diabetes Association, "Standards of medical care in diabetes—2009," *Diabetes Care*, vol. 32, no. 1, pp. 13–61, 2008.

[13] E. Ritz, "Albuminuria and vascular damage—the vicious twins," *The New England Journal of Medicine*, vol. 348, no. 23, pp. 2349–2352, 2003.

[14] S. F. Dinneen and H. C. Gerstein, "The association of microalbuminuria and mortality in non-insulin-dependent diabetes mellitus: a systematic overview of the literature," *Archives of Internal Medicine*, vol. 157, no. 13, pp. 1413–1418, 1997.

[15] A. I. Adler, R. J. Stevens, S. E. Manley, R. W. Bilous, C. A. Cull, and R. R. Holman, "Development and progression of nephropathy in type 2 diabetes: the United Kingdom Prospective Diabetes Study (UKPDS 64)," *Kidney International*, vol. 63, no. 1, pp. 225–232, 2003.

[16] E. J. Lewis, L. G. Hunsicker, R. P. Bain, and R. D. Rohde, "The effect of angiotensin-converting-enzyme inhibition on diabetic nephropathy. The Collaborative Study Group," *The New England Journal of Medicine*, vol. 329, no. 20, pp. 1456–1462, 1993.

[17] E. J. Lewis, L. G. Hunsicker, W. R. Clarke et al., "Renoprotective effect of the angiotensin-receptor antagonist irbesartan in patients with nephropathy due to type 2 diabetes," *The New England Journal of Medicine*, vol. 345, no. 12, pp. 851–860, 2001.

[18] B. M. Brenner, M. E. Cooper, D. de Zeeuw et al., "Effects of losartan on renal and cardiovascular outcomes in patients with type 2 diabetes and nephropathy," *The New England Journal of Medicine*, vol. 345, no. 12, pp. 861–869, 2001.

[19] S.-L. Lin, Y.-M. Chen, C.-T. Chien, W.-C. Chiang, C.-C. Tsai, and T.-J. Tsai, "Pentoxifylline attenuated the renal disease progression in rats with remnant kidney," *Journal of the American Society of Nephrology*, vol. 13, no. 12, pp. 2916–2929, 2002.

[20] S.-L. Lin, R.-H. Chen, Y.-M. Chen, W.-C. Chiang, T.-J. Tsai, and B.-S. Hsieh, "Pentoxifylline inhibits platelet-derived growth factor-stimulated cyclin D1 expression in mesangial cells by blocking Akt membrane translocation," *Molecular Pharmacology*, vol. 64, no. 4, pp. 811–822, 2003.

[21] Y.-M. Chen, Y.-Y. Ng, S.-L. Lin, W.-C. Chiang, H. Y. Lan, and T.-J. Tsai, "Pentoxifylline suppresses renal tumour necrosis factor-α and ameliorates experimental crescentic glomerulonephritis in rats," *Nephrology Dialysis Transplantation*, vol. 19, no. 5, pp. 1106–1115, 2004.

[22] T.-J. Tsai, R.-H. Lin, C.-C. Chang et al., "Vasodilator agents modulate sat glomerular mesangial cell growth and collagen synthesis," *Nephron*, vol. 70, no. 1, pp. 91–99, 1995.

[23] J. F. Navarro, C. Mora, A. Rivero et al., "Urinary protein excretion and serum tumor necrosis factor in diabetic patients with advanced renal failure: effects of pentoxifylline administration," *American Journal of Kidney Diseases*, vol. 33, no. 3, pp. 458–463, 1999.

[24] Y.-M. Chen, S.-L. Lin, W.-C. Chiang, K.-D. Wu, and T.-J. Tsai, "Pentoxifylline ameliorates proteinuria through suppression of renal monocyte chemoattractant protein-1 in patients with proteinuric primary glomerular diseases," *Kidney International*, vol. 69, no. 8, pp. 1410–1415, 2006.

[25] D. Ducloux, C. Bresson-Vautrin, and J.-M. Chalopin, "Use of pentoxifylline in membranous nephropathy," *The Lancet*, vol. 357, no. 9269, pp. 1672–1673, 2001.

[26] G. Galindo-Rodríguez, R. Bustamante, G. Esquivel-Nava et al., "Pentoxifylline in the treatment of refractory nephrotic syndrome secondary to lupus nephritis," *Journal of Rheumatology*, vol. 30, no. 11, pp. 2382–2384, 2003.

[27] J. F. Navarro, C. Mora, M. Muros, and J. García, "Additive antiproteinuric effect of pentoxifylline in patients with type 2 diabetes under angiotensin II receptor blockade: a short-term, randomized, controlled trial," *Journal of the American Society of Nephrology*, vol. 16, no. 7, pp. 2119–2126, 2005.

[28] P. Jacobsen, S. Andersen, K. Rossing, B. R. Jensen, and H.-H. Parving, "Dual blockade of the renin-angiotensin system versus maximal recommended dose of ACE inhibition in diabetic nephropathy," *Kidney International*, vol. 63, no. 5, pp. 1874–1880, 2003.

[29] R. Cetinkaya, A. R. Odabas, and Y. Selcuk, "Anti-proteinuric effects of combination therapy with enalapril and losartan in patients with nephropathy due to type 2 diabetes," *International Journal of Clinical Practice*, vol. 58, no. 5, pp. 432–435, 2004.

[30] M. Rodríguez-Morán, G. González-González, M. V. Bermúdez-Barba et al., "Effects of pentoxifylline on the urinary protein excretion profile of type 2 diabetic patients with microproteinuria—a double-blind, placebo-controlled randomized trial," *Clinical Nephrology*, vol. 66, no. 1, pp. 3–10, 2006.

[31] S. B. Solerte, M. Fioravanti, A. L. Patti et al., "Increased plasma apolipoprotein B levels and blood hyperviscosity in non-insulin-dependent diabetic patients: role in the occurrence of arterial hypertension," *Acta Diabetologica Latina*, vol. 24, no. 4, pp. 341–349, 1987.

[32] Ö. Harmankaya, S. Seber, and M. Yilmaz, "Combination of pentoxifylline with angiotensin converting enzyme inhibitors produces an additional reduction in microalbuminuria in hypertensive type 2 diabetic patients," *Renal Failure*, vol. 25, no. 3, pp. 465–470, 2003.

[33] M. Boolell, M. J. Allen, S. A. Ballard et al., "Sildenafil: an orally active type 5 cyclic GMP-specific phosphodiesterase inhibitor for the treatment of penile erectile dysfunction.," *International journal of impotence research*, vol. 8, no. 2, pp. 47–52, 1996.

[34] M. M. Teixeira, R. W. Gristwood, N. Cooper, and P. G. Hellewell, "Phosphodiesterase (PDE)4 inhibitors: anti-inflammatory drugs of the future?" *Trends in Pharmacological Sciences*, vol. 18, no. 5, pp. 164–170, 1997.

[35] H. J. Kramer, Q. D. Nguyen, G. Curhan, and C.-Y. Hsu, "Renal insufficiency in the absence of albuminuria and retinopathy among adults with type 2 diabetes mellitus," *The Journal of the American Medical Association*, vol. 289, no. 24, pp. 3273–3277, 2003.

[36] R. Retnakaran, C. A. Cull, K. I. Thorne, A. I. Adler, R. R. Holman, and UKPDS Study Group, "Risk factors for renal dysfunction in type 2 diabetes: U.K. prospective diabetes study 74," *Diabetes*, vol. 55, no. 6, pp. 1832–1839, 2006.

[37] D. De Zeeuw, G. Remuzzi, H.-H. Parving et al., "Proteinuria, a target for renoprotection in patients with type 2 diabetic nephropathy: lessons from RENAAL," *Kidney International*, vol. 65, no. 6, pp. 2309–2320, 2004.

15

NT-proBNP, Cardiometabolic Risk Factors, and Nutritional Status in Hemodialysis Patients

Jacques Ducros,[1,2] **Laurent Larifla,**[3,4] **Henri Merault,**[1,2] **and Lydia Foucan**[1,4]

[1]*Centre de Dialyse AUDRA, Hôpital RICOU, Pointe-à-Pitre, Guadeloupe, France*
[2]*Service de Néphrologie, Centre Hospitalier Universitaire, Guadeloupe, France*
[3]*Service de Cardiologie, Centre Hospitalier Universitaire, Guadeloupe, France*
[4]*Equipe de Recherche Epidémiologie Clinique et Médecine sur le Risque Cardio Métabolique, ECM/LAMIA,*
*   EA 4540, Université des Antilles, Centre Hospitalier Universitaire, Guadeloupe, France*

Correspondence should be addressed to Lydia Foucan; lfoucan29@yahoo.com

Academic Editor: David B. Kershaw

Background. We aimed to evaluate the association between NT-proBNP and malnutrition in HD patients while taking into account the four established categories of parameters for diagnosis of protein energy wasting (PEW). *Methods.* A cross-sectional study was performed in Afro-Caribbean dialysis patients. One component in each of the 4 categories for the wasting syndrome was retained: serum albumin ≤ 38 g/L, BMI ≤ 23 Kg/m^2, serum creatinine ≤ 818 μmol/L, and normalized protein catabolic rate (nPCR) ≤ 0.8 g/kg/day. NT-proBNP was assessed using a chemiluminescence immunoassay. Two multivariate logistic regression models were performed to determine the parameters associated with high NT-proBNP concentrations. *Results.* In 207 HD patients, 16.9% had PEW (at least three components). LVEF lower than 60% was found in 13.8% of patients. NT-proBNP levels ranged from 125 to 33144 pg/mL. In model 1, high levels of NT-proBNP (≥6243 pg/mL) were independently associated with PEW OR 14.2 (3.25–62.4), male gender 2.80 (1.22–6.57), hsCRP > 5 mg/L 3.90 (1.77–8.57), and dialysis vintage > 3 years 3.84 (1.35–10.8). In model 2, LVEF OR was 0.93 (0.88–0.98). NT-proBNP concentrations were significantly higher when the PEW component number was higher. *Conclusion.* In dialysis patients, high NT-proBNP levels must draw attention to cardiac function but also to nutritional status.

1. Introduction

Uremic malnutrition, also called, protein energy wasting (PEW), corresponding to a decrease in energy and body protein, is a common problem in patients with end stage renal disease (ESRD) undergoing hemodialysis (HD) [1–3]. This syndrome found approximately in 20 to 70% of HD patients [1] has been associated with inflammation [4], overhydration [5], and high morbidity and mortality [2, 6]. Previous studies have also reported association between N-terminal pro-brain natriuretic peptide (NT-proBNP) levels and malnutrition assessed using the subjective global assessment and malnutrition-inflammation score [7, 8] and it was suggested that PEW might have a direct effect on the level of NT-proBNP by affecting ventricular remodeling in HD patients [7]. The International Society of Renal Nutrition

and Metabolism (ISRNM) proposed, in 2008, a uniformed nomenclature to define malnutrition in individuals with kidney disease [3] from several parameters among four established categories (biochemical criteria; body mass and composition, muscle mass, and dietary intakes). The severity of malnutrition can then be identified according to the number of malnutrition parameters.

Brain natriuretic peptide (BNP), one member of the natriuretic family, is synthesized by ventricular cardiomyocytes, in response to wall stress, and plays a major role in regulation of blood pressure and extracellular volume [9]. In the circulation, the enzyme-mediated cleavage of proBNP results in BNP, the active peptide, and NT-proBNP, an inactive N-terminal fragment. NT-proBNP is cleared essentially by the kidney, while BNP is cleared by its specific natriuretic peptide receptors and by an endopeptidase, independently of glomerular filtration rate [10–12]. Blood concentration of NT-proBNP has been associated with left ventricular disorders, hypervolemia [13, 14], and identified as a predictive factor of cardiac events and mortality in the HD population [13–15].

Since NT-proBNP level is directly influenced by kidney function, elevated levels of this inactive fragment are often observed in HD patients without clinical evidence of cardiovascular disease [15, 16].

The question of whether NT-proBNP is a marker of malnutrition in HD is still asked. Thus, we tested the hypothesis that NT-proBNP concentrations vary according to the number of malnutrition markers.

2. Objectives

We aimed to evaluate the association between NT-proBNP and malnutrition taking into account the four categories of the ISRMN definition for PEW and to analyze the relationships between NT-proBNP concentrations and the number of malnutrition markers in HD patients.

3. Subjects and Methods

This study was approved by the Institutional Review Board Committee of the dialysis centre which has waived the need for informed consent since the current study reported the results of the annual checkup of HD patients.

3.1. Patient Population. In a cross-sectional study, we included Afro-Caribbean patients who underwent maintenance HD treatment for more than three months and who were checked in December 2015 in the AUDRA centre (one of the dialysis facilities in the island of Guadeloupe, France). For the purpose of the study, patients included had no acute cardiac insufficiency, acute coronary complication, or chronic obstructive pulmonary disease.

Standard dialysis treatment consisted of three weekly sessions using bicarbonate buffer and synthetic high flux membrane. The dialysate electrolytes prescription usually includes sodium (140 mmol/L), potassium (2 mmol/L), bicarbonates (35 mmol/L), and calcium (1.5 mmol/L). Sodium prescription is adapted according to blood pressure and fluid status.

Weekly dialysis time was twelve hours in 83% of patients. The ultrafiltration rate was between 0.8 to 1.5 l per hour. Dialysis dose delivery was estimated from the urea Kt/V (urea clearance over time).

3.2. Data Collection. Demographic and clinical data such as age, gender, dialysis vintage, anthropometric parameters, cardiovascular risk factors, history of cardiovascular events, and use of nutritional supplementation were recorded. Body mass index (BMI) in kg/m^2 was calculated as dry weight divided by height squared. This dry weight is regularly assessed and calculated for each patient on the basis of clinical status and bioimpedance analysis performed at the end of dialysis.

Predialysis and postdialysis systolic blood pressure (SBP) and diastolic blood pressure (DBP) were recorded with automated monitors for every dialysis session. Average SBP and DBP over a 1-month period were calculated.

Dialysis vintage was defined as the duration of time between the first day of HD treatment and December 31, 2015.

3.3. Laboratory Measures. All laboratory values were measured by automated and standardized methods, before the start of dialysis (on the day of the midweek dialysis session). Laboratory data refer to single measures.

Samples were collected for serum albumin, creatinine, and highly sensitive C-reactive protein (hsCRP) measurements. Serum albumin and serum creatinine (SCr) concentrations were determined.

The normalized protein catabolic rate (nPCR) [17] was used to assess the dietary protein intake.

NT-proBNP was assessed using a Siemens (DPC) Immulite 2000 chemiluminescence immunoassay based on N-terminal polyclonal sheep antibody.

3.4. Echocardiography. Standard transthoracic echocardiographic examination was performed by a cardiologist, who was blinded to the clinical data of the study subjects. All echocardiographic measurements were done according to the guidelines of the American Society of Echocardiography [9]. Left ventricular ejection fraction (LVEF) was calculated using the Simpson biplane method from 2 chambers and 4 chambers' apical views. Left ventricular mass (LVM) was calculated using the Devereux formula [18]. Left ventricular mass index (LVMI) was calculated as LVM/body surface area. Left ventricular hypertrophy (LVH) was defined by a LVMI > 134 g/m^2 in men or >110 g/m^2 in women.

3.5. Definition of Clinical Factors and Events

Nutritional Status. One component in each of the 4 categories of the wasting syndrome [3] was retained: serum albumin ≤ 38 g/L, BMI ≤ 23 Kg/m^2, SCr ≤ 818 μmol/L [2], and nPCR ≤ 0.8 g/kg/day.

Slight malnutrition was defined when one criterion for PEW was present, moderate malnutrition when two criteria were present, and severe malnutrition (PEW) in presence of three or four criteria [19].

(i) *Inflammation* was defined as a serum concentration of hsCRP of >5 mg/L.

(ii) *Preexisting* cardiovascular (CV) *complications* included coronary event occurring before December 2015.

(iii) Weight loss was defined as −5% over 3 months [3].

(iv) Interdialytic weight gain (IDWG) was calculated by subtracting the postdialysis weight of previous HD session from the predialysis weight of the index HD session. The average IDWG of six previous sessions was considered.

3.6. Statistical Methods. Data are presented as percentages for categorical variables and as means ± standard deviations (SD) and medians (interquartile ranges, IQR) for continuous variables.

The chi-squared test and ANCOVA with adjustment for age, gender, or Mann–Whitney test were used to test percentage and mean differences between groups according to the presence or absence of high NT-proBNP levels. NT-proBNP values were logarithmically transformed to approach a normal distribution. The Pearson correlation test, adjusted for age and gender, was used to study the relationships between log NT-proBNP and other continuous variables.

The individuals were classified into 5 categories according to the number of criteria for PEW (ISRNM definition) with individuals exhibiting 0, 1, 2, 3, and 4 criteria.

We also used multivariate logistic regressions in the overall study population to determine the parameters associated with high NT-proBNP concentrations. In model 1, age/10 years, gender, predialysis SBP, dialysis vintage > 3 years, IDWG, diabetes, hsCRP > 5 mg/L, and nutritional status were included as covariates. In model 2, LVEF was included, in addition to the aforementioned covariates. The adjusted odds ratios and 95% confidence intervals (OR 95% CI) were provided.

Statistical analyses were performed by using IBM-SPSS statistical software package version 21 (IBM, Armonk, NY, USA). Statistical significance was defined as $P < 0.05$.

4. Results

Overall, 207 stable patients, undergoing HD at the dialysis centre, were included in the current study. The population was 54% male. Mean ± SD age was 64 ± 13 years and the mean dialysis vintage 7.2±0.4 years. The major comorbidities were hypertension (90%), diabetes (41.5%), obesity (26.5%), and past history of coronary artery disease (CAD) (9.7%). Antihypertensive medications were prescribed to 82% of HD patients. All the patients had diuresis lower than 500 mL/day (i.e., no residual renal function).

Thirty-five patients (16.9%) had PEW (at least three parameters). Echocardiography was available for 159 patients for whom median [IQR] LVEF was 68% [63%–70%]. Among them, 13.8% had a LVEF lower than 60% and 3 patients (1.9%) had a LVEF lower than 40%. Characteristics of the patients are presented in Table 1.

NT-proBNP ranged from 125 to 33144 pg/mL with mean and median of 5243 ± 6573 and 2405 [1121–6243] pg/mL, respectively.

Since there was no threshold-consensus for HD patients, for the purpose of the study, participants with NT-proBNP ≥ 6243 pg/mL (75th percentile) were categorized as having high NT-proBNP levels.

Patients with high NT-proBNP levels were more likely to have higher dialysis vintage, higher frequencies of weight loss, low BMI (≤23 Kg/m²), low serum albumin levels (≤38 g/L), low serum creatinine levels (≤818 μmol/L), low nPCR (≤0.8 g/kg/d), lower mean hemoglobin rate, higher frequencies of hsCRP > 5 (mg/L), nutritional supplementation, moderate malnutrition, and PEW. They also had lower frequency of diabetes, lower mean IDWG, and lower mean LVEF (Table 1). No significant difference was noted for age and frequencies of CAD history and of left ventricular hypertrophy.

Patients with PEW had a higher median NT-proBNP values and lower mean IDWG than those without PEW 6243 [1833–18721] versus 2132 [1100–5200] pg/mL, $P = 0.002$, and 1.7 ± 0.9 versus 2.5 ± 1.0 Kg, $P < 0.001$, respectively.

Median NT-proBNP in patients with and without diabetes was 2362 [1090–5245] versus 2453 [1162–7816], respectively, $P = 0.219$, and frequencies of PEW were 13% in patients with diabetes and 20% in those without diabetes, $P = 0.183$.

In 77 diabetic subjects with available glycated hemoglobin (A1CHb), there was no significant difference in mean A1CHb levels between those with ($n = 11$) and without ($n = 66$) high NT-proBNP levels: 7.04 ± 1.37% versus 7.03 ± 1.75%, respectively, $P = 0.771$.

4.1. Correlations of Log NT-proBNP with Clinical and Biological Parameters (Table 2). There were positive correlations between log NT-proBNP and dialysis vintage ($r = 0.18$; $P = 0.008$), predialysis SBP ($r = 0.18$; $P = 0.010$), predialysis DBP ($r = 0.20$; $P = 0.007$), postdialysis SBP ($r = 0.18$; $P = 0.009$), and hsCRP ($r = 0.21$; $P = 0.002$) and negative correlations with BMI ($r = -0.19$; $P = 0.005$), nPCR ($r = -0.15$; $P = 0.028$), and LVEF ($r = -0.24$; $P = 0.002$).

4.2. Logistic Regression for High Values of NT-proBNP (≥6243 pg/mL). In model 1 concerning 207 subjects, the following factors were identified: gender OR 2.80 (1.22–6.57), $P = 0.010$; dialysis vintage OR 3.80 (1.35–10.8), $P = 0.012$; hsCRP > 5 mg/L OR 3.90 (1.77–8.57), $P = 0.001$; and PEW OR 14.2 (3.25–62.4), $P < 0.001$. Having PEW (presence of 3 or 4 criteria) was associated with a 14-fold increase in the odds of having high NT-proBNP levels, Table 3.

In model 2 concerning 159 subjects with available echocardiographic data, independent factors for high values of NT-proBNP included gender OR 3.17 (1.18–8.49), $P = 0.022$; hsCRP > 5 mg/L OR 3.81 (1.45–10.0), $P = 0.007$; PEW OR 11.7 (2.01–64.2), $P = 0.006$; and LVEF OR 0.93 (0.88–0.98), $P = 0.011$.

The odds ratios for having moderate malnutrition (defined as the presence of 1 to 2 criteria) were nearly significant 3.28 (0.98–10.9), $P = 0.052$ in model 1, and 3.73 (1.83–16.7), $P = 0.080$ in model 2.

Of note, age, SBP, IDWG, and diabetes history were not independently associated with high levels of NT-proBNP.

4.3. Distribution of NT-proBNP and IDWG according to the Number of PEW Criteria. The five groups of subjects according to the number of criteria (0, 1, 2, 3, and 4) for PEW according to the ISRNM definition included 41 (19.8%), 67 (32.4%), 64 (30.9%), 21 (10.1%), and 14 (6.8%) subjects, respectively.

NT-proBNP (median [IQR]) concentrations were significantly higher when the number of malnutrition criteria was higher, for 0 criteria: 1858 [1143–2706] pg/mL, 1: 2276 [1092–4070] pg/mL, 2: 2676 [1045–7149] pg/mL, 3: 4025 [701–14340] pg/mL, and 4: 12289 [2507–23451] pg/mL ($P < 0.001$ for comparison of mean log NT-proBNP) (Figure 1).

TABLE 1: Characteristics of hemodialysis patients according to NT-proBNP levels.

		All patients $N = 207$	NT-proBNP (pg/mL) $N = 207$		
			<6243 $n = 155$	≥6243 $n = 52$	P
Age (y)	207	64 ± 13	63 ± 14	65 ± 12	0.382
Dialysis vintage (y)	207	7.2 ± 0.4	6.9 ± 0.8	7.9 ± 0.9	0.342
Dialysis vintage ≥ 3 y (%)	207	73.4	69.0	86.5	**0.013**
Sex (men)	207	54.1	51.0	63.5	0.118
Diabetes (%)	207	41.5	46.5	26.9	**0.013**
Previous CAD (%)	207	9.7	9.0	11.5	0.597
Hypertension (%)	207	89.9	89.7	90.4	0.884
Predialysis SBP (mmHg)	207	146 ± 24	145 ± 24	149 ± 26	0.280
Predialysis DBP (mmHg)	207	81 ± 17	80 ± 14	83 ± 17	0.091
Postdialysis SBP (mmHg)	207	137 ± 26	135 ± 26	143 ± 27	**0.048**
Postdialysis DBP (mmHg)	207	76 ± 16	75 ± 16	77 ± 17	0.453
Hemoglobin (g/dL)	207	11.8 ± 1.5	11.9 ± 1.4	11.3 ± 1.6	**0.008**
Serum sodium (mmol/L)	207	139 ± 3	139 ± 2	138 ± 3	0.184
IDWG (Kg)	207	2.3 ± 1.0	2.4 ± 1.1	2.1 ± 0.8	**0.014**
KT/V	207	1.3 ± 0.2	1.3 ± 0.2	1.4 ± 0.2	0.475
Nutritional supplementation	207	26.6	22.6	38.5	**0.025**
Nutritional parameters					
Body mass index (Kg/m^2)	207	26.1 ± 6.7	26.9 ± 6.9	23.8 ± 5.2	**0.004**
Body mass index ≤ 23 Kg/m^2 (%)	207	35.7	29.0	55.8	**<0.001**
Serum albumin (g/L)	207	38.2 ± 4.5	38.5 ± 4.5	37.3 ± 4.4	0.095
Serum albumin ≤ 38 g/L (%)	207	47.3	43.2	59.6	**0.041**
Serum creatinine (μmol/L)	207	884 ± 278	915 ± 275	793 ± 268	**0.001**
Serum creatinine ≤ 818 μmol/L (%)	207	41.1	34.2	61.5	**0.001**
NPCR (g/kg/D)	207	0.94 ± 0.21	0.96 ± 0.21	0.87 ± 0.21	**0.010**
NPCR ≤ 0.8 g/kg/D (%)	207	27.5	23.9	38.5	**0.042**
Malnutrition (≥1 factor) (%)	207	80.2	76.1	92.3	**0.011**
PEW (≥3 factors) (%)	207	16.9	11.0	34.6	**<0.001**
hsCRP > 5 (mg/L)	207	48.5	40.6	71.2	**<0.001**
Echocardiographic parameters		All patients $N = 159$	NT-proBNP (pg/mL)		
			<6243 $N = 122$	≥6243 $N = 37$	P
LVEF (%)	159	65.1 ± 8.5	66.3 ± 7.3	60.9 ± 10.9	**<0.001**
LVEF < 60 (%)	159	13.8	10.7	24.3	**0.035**
Left ventricular hypertrophy (%)	159	40.3	38.5	45.9	0.420

Data in this table are presented as column percentages or mean ± SD. Significant P values are in bold.

Similar trends were found in both genders for median NT-proBNP and as follows: in men: for 0 criteria: 1883 pg/mL, 1: 1905 pg/mL, 2: 3001 pg/mL, 3: 12482 pg/mL, and 4: 14495 pg/mL and in women: for 0 criteria: 1505 pg/mL, 1: 2723 pg/mL, 2: 2662 pg/mL, 3: 3332 pg/mL, and 4: 6939 pg/mL.

The IDWG (median [IQR]) values decreased significantly with the number of malnutrition criteria: 0: 3 [2–4] Kg, 1: 2.1 [2-3] Kg, 2: 2 [1.5–3] Kg, 3: 2 [1–3] Kg, and 4: 1.25 [1-2] Kg ($P < 0.001$) (Figure 1).

5. Discussion

In the current study, in a cohort of Afro-Caribbean stable adult hemodialysis patients, we evaluated the association of NT-proBNP plasma levels and nutritional status using the ISRNM definition for protein energy wasting [3]. Our HD patients exhibited high levels of NT-proBNP as previously reported in ESRD patients [16, 20, 21]. NT-proBNP was associated with PEW and with left ventricular ejection fraction,

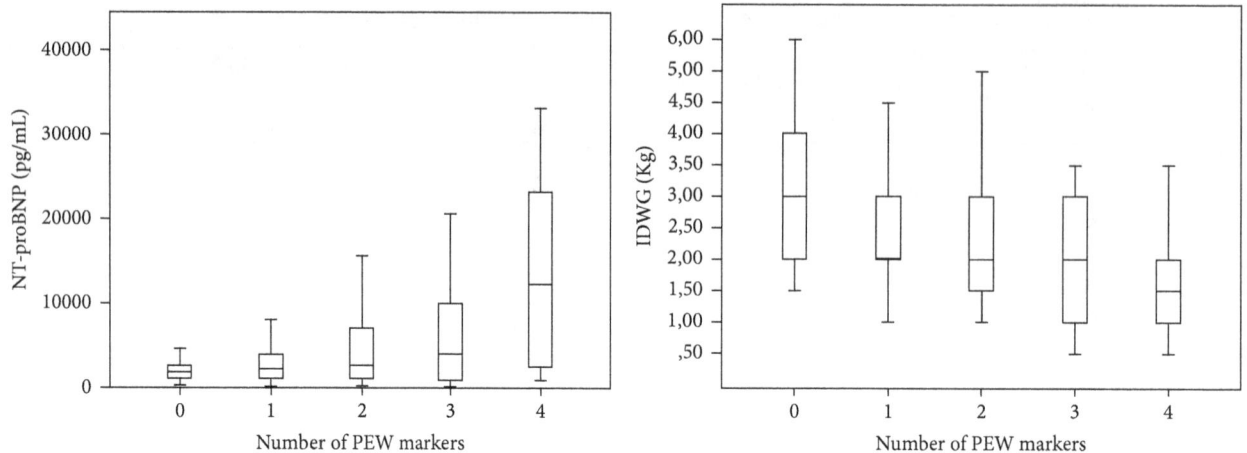

FIGURE 1: Distribution of NT-proBNP levels ($P < 0.001$) and IDWG ($P < 0.001$) according to the number of malnutrition criteria.

TABLE 2: Correlations between log NT-proBNP and clinical, biological, and echocardiographic parameters.

	n	r	P
Age (y)	207	0.03	0.600
Dialysis vintage (y)	207	0.18	**0.008**
Kt/V	207	0.09	0.176
IDWG	207	−0.11	0.121
Predialysis SBP (mmHg)	207	0.18	**0.010**
Predialysis DBP (mmHg)	207	0.20	**0.007**
Postdialysis SBP (mmHg)	207	0.18	**0.009**
Postdialysis DBP (mmHg)	207	0.11	**0.143**
hsCRP (mg/L)	207	0.21	**0.002**
Hemoglobin (g/dL)	207	−0.15	**0.032**
Nutritional parameters			
Body mass index (Kg/m^2)	207	−0.19	**0.005**
Serum albumin (g/L)	207	−0.09	0.197
Serum creatinine (μmol/L)	207	−0.14	0.078
NPCR (g/kg/D)	207	−0.15	**0.028**
Echocardiography			
LVEF (%)	159	−0.24	**0.002**

Correlations adjusted for age and sex.

independently of age, SBP, diabetes, hsCRP, and IDWG. In addition, we have also shown that NT-proBNP was higher and IDWG lower when the number of malnutrition criteria was higher. Our findings highlight the relationship between malnutrition and NT-proBNP concentrations.

5.1. NT-proBNP and Cardiometabolic Risk Factors. In the present study, we considered NT-proBNP values ≥ 6243 pg/mL (75th percentile) as the highest NT-proBNP levels, since there was no threshold-consensus for HD patients. In a recent study in 238 Japanese HD patients, NT-proBNP values ≥

5760 pg/mL (higher tertile) were considered as the higher values [22]. Predialysis median NT-proBNP levels were previously found markedly elevated in HD patients, 4079 pg/ml [1893–15076] [14], compared to median population-based normal values, 20 pg/ml [10–30] [23].

The role of natriuretic peptides in cardiovascular homeostasis is well established. Brain natriuretic peptide is secreted by the heart mainly in response to the stretching of the myocardium induced by volume overload or in response to hypertrophy [24].

In this study, predialysis SBP was not associated with high levels of NT-proBNP in the multivariate logistic regression although high blood pressure is a common cause of increased left ventricular wall stress [25, 26]. The high frequencies of hypertension (90%) in this study population might contribute to these results.

The prevalence of abnormal left ventricular function (LVEF < 60%) was not high in this population (13.8%) and only 1.9% had a LVEF lower than 40%. In addition, no significant difference in frequencies of left ventricular hypertrophy was noted between NT-proBNP groups suggesting that factors other than cardiac status impact on NT-proBNP concentrations.

Insulin resistance has been associated with lower natriuretic peptide levels [27]. In this line, frequency of diabetes was higher in our patients with the lower levels of NT-proBNP (<6243 pg/mL) than in the others (46.5% versus 26.9%; $P = 0.013$). Recently, in patients without chronic kidney disease, prospective studies have shown that low levels of NT-proBNP are a positive predictor of incident type 2 diabetes [28, 29].

Inflammation (hsCRP > 5 mg/L) was associated with high NT-proBNP levels. Some authors described hsCRP as the most powerful cardiac biomarker for predicting all-cause of death when compared with NT-proBNP [16]. Inflammation also induces anorexia, reduces the effective use of dietary protein and energy intake, and augments protein catabolism [30].

TABLE 3: Multivariate logistic regression for high values of NT-proBNP ($\geq$6243 pg/mL).

	Model 1 N = 207		Model 2 N = 159	
	OR (95% CI)	P	OR (95% CI)	P
Age/10 y	1.01 (0.99–1.03)	0.831	1.01 (0.98–1.04)	0.420
Sex (M)	2.80 (1.22–6.57)	**0.015**	3.17 (1.18–8.49)	**0.022**
Predialysis SBP	1.01 (0.99–1.02)	0.175	1.01 (0.99–1.02)	0.310
Dialysis vintage > 3 y (yes/no)	3.80 (1.35–10.8)	**0.012**	2.40 (0.80–7.21)	0.118
IDWG (Kg)	0.68 (0.43–1.08)	0.107	0.57 (0.32–1.01)	0.050
Diabetes (Yes/No)	0.50 (0.22–1.13)	0.099	0.46 (0.18–1.17)	0.110
hsCRP > 5 mg/L (Yes/No)	3.90 (1.77–8.57)	**0.001**	3.81 (1.45–10.0)	**0.007**
Moderate malnutrition/normal nutritional status	3.28 (0.98–10.9)	0.052	3.73 (1.83–16.7)	0.081
Severe malnutrition (PEW)/normal nutritional status	14.2 (3.25–62.4)	**<0.001**	11.7 (2.01–64.2)	**0.006**
Left ventricular ejection fraction %	—	—	0.93 (0.88–0.98)	**0.011**

5.2. NT-proBNP and PEW Components. In a previous study, malnutrition was accompanied by volume overload and was associated with increased NT-proBNP levels, independently of volume status [7].

Our patients with the highest levels of NT-proBNP exhibited higher frequencies of the four parameters used for the identification of PEW (ISRNM definition). Since there is no recognized threshold for low creatinine levels, we kept the creatinine value of our previous study in which patients who had SCr below 818 μmol/L had a hazard ratio of death two times higher than those with SCr above this threshold [2]. The multivariate logistic regression showed that patients with PEW had a 14-fold higher odds of having high values of NT-proBNP compared with those with no criteria, independently of predialysis SBP, dialysis vintage, IDWG, and LVEF.

5.2.1. Role of Body Mass Index. Several arguments are in favor of an important role of BMI and especially adipose tissue in the relationship between malnutrition and NT-proBNP levels. Negative linear relationships between BMI and plasma natriuretic peptide levels have been reported [31, 32]. In patients without renal insufficiency and without history of cardiomyopathy, obese patients have reduced concentrations of BNP and NT-proBNP compared to nonobese patients despite having elevated left ventricular end diastolic pressures [33].

In our study, patients with high levels of NT-proBNP were more likely to have a BMI $\leq$ 23 Kg/m^2 (55.8%) than the others (29%) (Table 1) and also more likely to have had a weight loss that is also a malnutrition criterion according to the ISRMN definition [3]. In obese subjects undergoing weight loss surgery, weight loss was found associated with early increases in NT-proBNP concentrations [34].

Each of the three other malnutrition criteria used in our study (low nPCR values, low albumin, and low creatinine levels) was also associated with high NT-proBNP concentrations.

That could be explained by their own relationships with weight status. In fact, HD patients with greater protein and energy intakes usually have a greater BMI [35] and inversely. Hypoalbuminemia is the result of the combined effects of inflammation and inadequate protein and caloric intake [30] that may lead to low BMI. Creatinine levels are a surrogate of muscle mass in HD patients [36]. Anorexia and low nutrient intake may also lead to lower muscle mass, lower creatinine levels, and possibly lower BMI.

Weight gain and obesity have been associated with increased expression of natriuretic peptide receptors-C, in adipose tissue and increased degradation of natriuretic peptides [37]. NT-proBNP is essentially eliminated by the kidney, thus, in patient with low BMI or reduced adipose tissue, an increased synthesis or secretion of NT-proBNP by myocardial cells has been suggested [38]. Moreover, the existence of a heart-gut-brain axis, involving the ghrelin-appetite-hormone, was also evoked [39]. In this line, intravenous administration of BNP [34] or of human synthetic ghrelin [35] argued for an association between BNP concentrations and appetite regulation. The natriuretic peptides would participate in body weight regulation and energy homeostasis [35]. Thus NT-proBNP concentrations might reflect pathophysiological implication of BNP in these processes.

5.3. NT-proBNP, IDWG, and the Number of PEW Criteria. Interestingly, in our study, NT-proBNP concentrations were higher when the number of malnutrition criteria were higher while IDWG were lower (Figure 1). Interdialytic weight gain has been regarded as a surrogate of volume overload, in ESRD patients on HD but also as an index of good appetite and nutritional status [40, 41]. Our results concerning NT-proBNP concentrations suggest that the heart-gut-brain axis is particularly stimulated when the degree of malnutrition is high.

This study has some limitations including the single measurement of NT-proBNP and other laboratory parameters and also the lack of other anthropometric parameters (such as mid-arm circumference) and other markers of malnutrition. Results of bioelectrical impedance were not available and the hydration status was not taken into account. The cross-sectional design did not let us draw any causality link.

But our study also has several strengths. Data were obtained in a homogenous population of Afro-Caribbean subjects and it is known that measures of serum creatinine and other nutritional markers may vary according to ethnic groups. There was no difference in dialysis quality and age between NT-proBNP groups whereas NT-proBNP concentrations were reported to increase with age. There was also no bias in relation to type of dialysis or dialysis membrane since dialysis modalities were identical for all subjects and performed with synthetic high flux membranes.

6. Conclusion

The results of the present study confirm the association between malnutrition and NT-proBNP concentrations. In addition we demonstrated that NT-proBNP concentrations are higher when the number of malnutrition criteria is higher. Since high NT-proBNP levels and a worse nutritional status are both prognostic factors of survival, in dialysis patients, high NT-proBNP levels must draw attention to cardiac function but also to nutritional status.

Acknowledgments

The authors would like to acknowledge the nurses and the physicians of the AUDRA hemodialysis centre and all individuals who participated in this study.

References

[1] M. Aparicio, N. Cano, P. Chauveau et al., "Nutritional status of haemodialysis patients: a French national cooperative study," *Nephrology Dialysis Transplantation*, vol. 14, no. 7, pp. 1679–1686, 1999.

[2] L. Foucan, H. Merault, F.-L. Velayoudom-Cephise, L. Larifla, C. Alecu, and J. Ducros, "Impact of protein energy wasting status on survival among Afro-Caribbean hemodialysis patients: a 3-year prospective study," *SpringerPlus*, vol. 4, no. 1, article 452, 2015.

[3] D. Fouque, K. Kalantar-Zadeh, J. Kopple et al., "A proposed nomenclature and diagnostic criteria for protein-energy wasting in acute and chronic kidney disease," *Kidney International*, vol. 73, no. 4, pp. 391–398, 2008.

[4] E. Streja, C. P. Kovesdy, M. Z. Molnar et al., "Role of nutritional status and inflammation in higher survival of African American and hispanic hemodialysis patients," *American Journal of Kidney Diseases*, vol. 57, no. 6, pp. 883–893, 2011.

[5] M. Antlanger, M. Hecking, M. Haidinger et al., "Fluid overload in hemodialysis patients: a cross-sectional study to determine its association with cardiac biomarkers and nutritional status," *BMC Nephrology*, vol. 14, no. 1, article 266, 2013.

[6] B. A. Cooper, E. L. Penne, L. H. Bartlett, and C. A. Pollock, "Protein malnutrition and hypoalbuminemia as predictors of vascular events and mortality in ESRD," *American Journal of Kidney Diseases*, vol. 43, no. 1, pp. 61–66, 2004.

[7] Y.-J. Lee, B. G. Song, M. S. Kim et al., "Interaction of malnutrition, N-terminal pro-B-type natriuretic peptide and ventricular remodeling in patients on maintenance hemodialysis," *Clinical Nephrology*, vol. 79, no. 4, pp. 253–260, 2013.

[8] Q. Guo, P. Bárány, A. R. Qureshi et al., "N-terminal pro-brain natriuretic peptide independently predicts protein energy wasting and is associated with all-cause mortality in prevalent HD patients," *American Journal of Nephrology*, vol. 29, no. 6, pp. 516–523, 2009.

[9] E. R. Levin, D. G. Gardner, and W. K. Samson, "Natriuretic peptides," *New England Journal of Medicine*, vol. 339, no. 5, pp. 321–328, 1998.

[10] N. Schlueter, A. De Sterke, D. M. Willmes, J. Spranger, J. Jordan, and A. L. Birkenfeld, "Metabolic actions of natriuretic peptides and therapeutic potential in the metabolic syndrome," *Pharmacology and Therapeutics*, vol. 144, no. 1, pp. 12–27, 2014.

[11] L. R. Potter, "Natriuretic peptide metabolism, clearance and degradation," *FEBS Journal*, vol. 278, no. 11, pp. 1808–1817, 2011.

[12] P. A. McCullough and K. R. Sandberg, "B-type natriuretic peptide and renal disease," *Heart Failure Reviews*, vol. 8, no. 4, pp. 355–358, 2003.

[13] C. Kamano, H. Osawa, K. Hashimoto et al., "N-terminal pro-brain natriuretic peptide as a predictor of heart failure with preserved ejection fraction in hemodialysis patients without fluid overload," *Blood Purification*, vol. 33, no. 1-3, pp. 37–43, 2012.

[14] L. H. Madsen, S. Ladefoged, P. Corell, M. Schou, P. R. Hildebrandt, and D. Atar, "N-terminal pro brain natriuretic peptide predicts mortality in patients with end-stage renal disease in hemodialysis," *Kidney International*, vol. 71, no. 6, pp. 548–554, 2007.

[15] C. Sommerer, J. Beimler, V. Schwenger et al., "Cardiac biomarkers and survival in haemodialysis patients," *European Journal of Clinical Investigation*, vol. 37, no. 5, pp. 350–356, 2007.

[16] F. S. Apple, M. A. M. Murakami, L. A. Pearce, and C. A. Herzog, "Multi-biomarker risk stratification of N-terminal pro-B-type natriuretic peptide, high-sensitivity C-reactive protein, and cardiac troponin T and I in end-stage renal disease for all-cause death," *Clinical Chemistry*, vol. 50, no. 12, pp. 2279–2285, 2004.

[17] J. T. Daugirdas, "The post: pre-dialysis plasma urea nitrogen ratio to estimate K.t/V and NPCR: mathematical modeling," *The International journal of Artificial Organs*, vol. 12, no. 7, pp. 411–419, 1989.

[18] R. B. Devereux, D. R. Alonso, and E. M. Lutas, "Echocardiographic assessment of left ventricular hypertrophy: comparison

to necropsy findings," *The American Journal of Cardiology*, vol. 57, no. 6, pp. 450–458, 1986.

[19] T. A. Ikizler, N. J. Cano, H. Franch et al., "Prevention and treatment of protein energy wasting in chronic kidney disease patients: A consensus statement by the International Society of Renal Nutrition and Metabolism," *Kidney International*, vol. 84, no. 6, pp. 1096–1107, 2013.

[20] W. H. Hörl, "Natriuretic peptides in acute and chronic kidney disease and during renal replacement therapy," *Journal of Investigative Medicine*, vol. 53, no. 7, pp. 366–370, 2005.

[21] P. Jourdain, G. Lefevre, C. Oddoze et al., "NT-proBNP in practice: from chemistry to medicine," *Annales de Biologie Clinique*, vol. 67, no. 3, pp. 255–271, 2009.

[22] M. Ikeda, H. Honda, K. Takahashi, K. Shishido, and T. Shibata, "N-Terminal Pro-B-Type natriuretic peptide as a biomarker for loss of muscle mass in prevalent hemodialysis patients," *PLoS ONE*, vol. 11, no. 11, Article ID e0166804, 2016.

[23] T. A. McDonagh, S. Holmer, I. Raymond, A. Luchner, P. Hildebrant, and H. J. Dargie, "NT-proBNP and the diagnosis of heart failure: a pooled analysis of three European epidemiological studies," *European Journal of Heart Failure*, vol. 6, no. 3, pp. 269–273, 2004.

[24] B. A. Groenning, J. C. Nilsson, L. Sondergaard et al., "Detection of left ventricular enlargement and impaired systolic function with plasma N-terminal pro brain natriuretic peptide concentrations," *American Heart Journal*, vol. 143, no. 5, pp. 923–929, 2002.

[25] A. R. Pries and T. W. Secomb, "Structural adaptation of microvascular networks and development of hypertension," *Microcirculation*, vol. 9, no. 4, pp. 305–314, 2002.

[26] C. Mouly-Bertin, A. Bissery, H. Milon et al., "N-terminal pro-brain natriuretic peptide—a promising biomarker for the diagnosis of left ventricular hypertrophy in hypertensive women," *Archives of Cardiovascular Diseases*, vol. 101, no. 5, pp. 307–315, 2008.

[27] A. M. Khan, S. Cheng, M. Magnusson et al., "Cardiac natriuretic peptides, obesity, and insulin resistance: Evidence from two community-based studies," *Journal of Clinical Endocrinology and Metabolism*, vol. 96, no. 10, pp. 3242–3249, 2011.

[28] M. Lazo, J. H. Young, F. L. Brancati et al., "NH2-terminal pro-brain natriuretic peptide and risk of diabetes," *Diabetes*, vol. 62, no. 9, pp. 3189–3193, 2013.

[29] M. Magnusson, A. Jujic, B. Hedblad et al., "Low plasma level of atrial natriuretic peptide predicts development of diabetes: The prospective Malmö diet and cancer study," *Journal of Clinical Endocrinology and Metabolism*, vol. 97, no. 2, pp. 638–645, 2012.

[30] B. R. Don and G. Kaysen, "Serum albumin: relationship to inflammation and nutrition," *Seminars in Dialysis*, vol. 17, no. 6, pp. 432–437, 2004.

[31] S. Collins, "A heart-adipose tissue connection in the regulation of energy metabolism," *Nature Reviews Endocrinology*, vol. 10, no. 3, pp. 157–163, 2014.

[32] T. J. Wang, M. G. Larson, D. Levy et al., "Impact of obesity on plasma natriuretic peptide levels," *Circulation*, vol. 109, no. 5, pp. 594–600, 2004.

[33] J. A. Taylor, R. H. Christenson, K. Rao, M. Jorge, and S. S. Gottlieb, "B-Type natriuretic peptide and N-terminal pro B-type natriuretic peptide are depressed in obesity despite higher left ventricular end diastolic pressures," *American Heart Journal*, vol. 152, no. 6, pp. 1071–1076, 2006.

[34] A. Chen-Tournoux, A. M. Khan, A. L. Baggish et al., "Effect of weight loss after weight loss surgery on plasma N-terminal pro-B-type natriuretic peptide levels," *American Journal of Cardiology*, vol. 106, no. 10, pp. 1450–1455, 2010.

[35] K. Kalantar-Zadeh, T. A. Ikizler, G. Block, M. M. Avram, and J. D. Kopple, "Malnutrition-inflammation complex syndrome in dialysis patients: causes and consequences," *American Journal of Kidney Diseases*, vol. 42, no. 5, pp. 864–881, 2003.

[36] K. Kalantar-Zadeh, E. Streja, M. Z. Molnar et al., "Mortality prediction by surrogates of body composition: an examination of the obesity paradox in hemodialysis patients using composite ranking score analysis," *American Journal of Epidemiology*, vol. 175, no. 8, pp. 793–803, 2012.

[37] P. Dessi-Fulgheri, R. Sarzani, P. Tamburrini et al., "Plasma atrial natriuretic peptide and natriuretic peptide receptor gene expression in adipose tissue of normotensive and hypertensive obese patients," *Journal of Hypertension*, vol. 15, no. 12, part 2, pp. 1695–1699, 1997.

[38] A. Bayes-Genis, C. DeFilippi, and J. L. Januzzi Jr., "Understanding amino-terminal Pro-B-type natriuretic peptide in obesity," *American Journal of Cardiology*, vol. 101, no. 3, pp. S89–S94, 2008.

[39] G. Vila, G. Grimm, M. Resl et al., "B-type natriuretic peptide modulates ghrelin, hunger, and satiety in healthy men," *Diabetes*, vol. 61, no. 10, pp. 2592–2596, 2012.

[40] J. M. López-Gómez, M. Villaverde, R. Jofre, P. Rodriguez-Benítez, and R. Pérez-García, "Interdialytic weight gain as a marker of blood pressure, nutrition, and survival in hemodialysis patients," *Kidney International*, vol. 67, supplement 93, pp. S63–S68, 2005.

[41] S. Sezer, F. N. Özdemir, Z. Arat, Ö. Perim, M. Turan, and M. Haberal, "The association of interdialytic weight gain with nutritional parameters and mortality risk in hemodialysis patients," *Renal Failure*, vol. 24, no. 1, pp. 37–48, 2002.

16

Prognostic Value of Serum Uric Acid in Patients on the Waiting List before and after Renal Transplantation

Henrique Cotchi Simbo Muela,[1,2] Jose Jayme Galvão De Lima,[1] Luis Henrique W. Gowdak,[1] Flávio J. de Paula,[3] and Luiz Aparecido Bortolotto[1]

[1]*Heart Institute (InCor), Hospital das Clínicas, University of São Paulo Medical School, 05403-000 São Paulo, SP, Brazil*
[2]*Faculty of Medicine, Agostinho Neto University, Luanda, Angola*
[3]*Renal Transplant Unit, Urology, Hospital das Clínicas, University of São Paulo Medical School, 05403-000 São Paulo, SP, Brazil*

Correspondence should be addressed to Jose Jayme Galvão De Lima; jose.lima@incor.usp.br

Academic Editor: Danuta Zwolinska

Background. High serum uric acid (UA) is associated with increased cardiovascular (CV) risk in the general population. The impact of UA on CV events and mortality in CKD is unclear. *Objective.* To assess the relationship between UA and prognosis in hemodialysis (HD) patients before and after renal transplantation (TX). *Methods.* 1020 HD patients assessed for CV risk and followed from the time of inception until CV event, death, or TX (HD) or date of TX, CV event, death, or return to dialysis (TX). *Results.* 821 patients remained on HD while 199 underwent TX. High UA ($\geq$428 mmol/L) was not associated with either composite CV events or mortality in HD patients. In TX patients high UA predicted an increased risk of events ($P = 0.03$, HR 1.6, and 95% CI 1.03–2.54) but not with death. In the Cox proportional model UA was no longer significantly associated with CV events. Instead, a reduced GFR (<50 mL/min) emerged as the independent risk factor for events ($P = 0.02$, HR 1.79, and % CI 1.07–3.21). *Conclusion.* In recipients of TX an increased posttransplant UA is related to higher probability of major CV events but this association probably caused concurrent reduction in GFR.

1. Introduction

An elevated serum uric acid (UA) is consistently associated with increased cardiovascular (CV) risk in the general population, in part because patients with hypertension, metabolic syndrome, and chronic kidney disease (CKD) frequently have elevated uric acid levels [1, 2]. Although hyperuricemia is common in patients with chronic kidney disease, the impact of uric acid on mortality and CV events remains unclear.

There are experimental and epidemiological evidences indicating that uric acid and hyperuricemia may play a role in the pathogenesis of renal and CV diseases [3]. Also, hyperuricemia after kidney transplantation seems to have an adverse effect on renal allograft survival. For instance, patients with hyperuricemia demonstrated a 5-year graft survival rate of 68.8%, compared with 83.3% in patients with normouricemia [4]. However, the Symphony study observed no significant association between uric acid concentration and worsening of renal allograft function in the first 3 years after transplantation [5].

Serum UA has also been associated with coronary artery calcification and carotid intimal thickening [6, 7]. A number of epidemiological studies have found an independent association between hyperuricemia and myocardial infarction, ischemic stroke, CV events, and all-cause and CV mortality [8, 9]. It is well known that all the above-mentioned complications are common in patients with renal disease, including those who underwent renal transplantation.

Based on these evidences, it is plausible to hypothesize an adverse effect of increased UA level on CV outcomes in patients with CKD candidates to renal transplantation. In this study we aimed to assess the relationship between baseline serum uric acid and the risk of cardiovascular events and all-cause mortality in a group of patients on the waiting list for renal transplantation evaluated before and after renal transplantation.

2. Methods

2.1. Participants and Measurements. This was a longitudinal observational study conducted in 1020 hemodialysis (HD) patients, listed to receive their first kidney graft from a deceased donor, assessed for cardiovascular risk at the Hypertension Unit, Heart Institute (InCor), University of São Paulo Medical School, Brazil, and followed from July 1999 to June 2011. Inclusion criteria were age of 18 years or older and having serum uric acid level measurement at the first visit. Patients, who had been included on the waiting list before July 1, 1999, were excluded since before that date serum UA was not measured on inception. For patients who underwent renal transplantation, we excluded those who did not have UA measurement at the first evaluation after renal transplantation.

Patients were being treated by hemodialysis, performed in 4 h sessions, three times per week with a target Kt/V of 1.3. Routine medication for patients on dialysis included aspirin, rennin-angiotensin system inhibitors, statins, and beta-blockers for all individuals independent of risk stratification. Asymptomatic hyperuricemia was not treated. Hemodialysis patients were followed from the time of placement on the waiting list until death, renal transplantation, or occurrence of CV events. Patients who underwent transplantation were followed from the time of engraftment until death, occurrence of CV event, or return to dialysis. Routine immunosuppression consisted of prednisone, mycophenolate, and tacrolimus or cyclosporine. Cardioprotective medication was maintained after transplantation, as stated above. All individuals provided a signed, written informed consent and the study was approved by the institutional ethics committee and conducted according to the Declaration of Helsinki.

2.2. Laboratories Parameters. Serum UA, along with routine laboratory tests, was measured on baseline in patients on the waiting list and at the first laboratory evaluation performed after transplantation. Serum UA was determined using the URCA method (Dimension Clinical Chemistry System, Siemens Healthcare Diagnosis, Newark, USA). The cut-off 428 mmol/L was used according to the reference values of our laboratory so patients were divided into two groups: those with serum acid uric level less than 428 mmol/L and those with that value or higher. For patients on the waiting list, high-sensitivity C-reactive protein levels were also determined. Increased C-reactive protein was defined by serum levels of the enzyme higher than 5 mg/L. Dyslipidemia was defined by either total cholesterol or triglycerides higher 5.18 mmol/L. For patients who underwent renal transplantation, the glomerular filtration rate (GFR) was assessed by the MDRD formula. We used the median of GFR for the whole renal transplant group (50 mL/min/1.73 m^2) measured at the end of the follow-up, as a cut-off to define an adequate graft function. That figure is also justified because it corresponds, roughly, to a normal renal function of an individual with one functional kidney, as occurs after a successful renal transplantation.

2.3. Outcomes. We assessed 2 outcomes: all-cause mortality and major CV events (fatal/nonfatal), defined as sudden death, unstable angina, myocardial infarction, stroke, new-onset heart failure, and acute arterial syndrome requiring intervention. When more than one event occurred, only the first event was considered for analysis. We initially analyzed the impact of increased baseline serum UA on outcomes in patients on dialysis and in patients undergoing renal transplantation. Subanalysis was also performed separately in patients with diabetes or with increased levels of C-reactive protein. For patients who underwent renal transplantation the impact of serum UA on prognosis was also evaluated in patients with reduced (<50 mL/min/1.73 m^2) estimated GFR.

2.4. Statistical Analysis. All statistical analyses were performed using the JMP statistical program (JMP for Windows, version 6.0, SAS Institute, Cary, NC, USA). Continuous variables were presented as mean and standard deviation and the categorical values as percentage. Differences between uric acid groups were tested by χ^2 test for categorical variables and Student's t-test for continuous variables. Survival curves were compared by Kaplan-Meier method and compared by log-rank; Cox regression model was used to assess the variables related to CV events after renal transplantation and $P < 0.05$ was considered statistically significant.

3. Results

3.1. Characteristics of Patients before and after Renal Transplantation. Table 1 shows the main clinical characteristics for patients on dialysis according to serum UA levels. Serum uric acid < 428 was observed in 838 (82%) patients whereas, in 182 (18%), serum UA was increased. For the whole dialysis population, the mean age was 54 ± 11 years and 72% were Caucasians, 59% males, 40% diabetics, 38% with associated CVD (heart failure, previous stroke, myocardial infarction, and coronary or peripheral vascular intervention), and median follow-up was 26 months. Hypertension was the most frequent risk factor affecting more than 80% of our patients. Patients with higher serum UA were younger (52.3 ± 9.9 versus 54.1 ± 11.3 years old, resp., $P < 0.05$) and dyslipidemia was more frequent in patients with elevated uric acid (41.1% versus 34.1%, resp., $P < 0.05$). All other variables were comparable between the two groups.

Table 2 shows the clinical characteristics of 199 patients that underwent renal transplantation. Serum uric acid was increased in 66 patients (33%). The main baseline characteristics for the totality of transplanted subjects were the following: age, 52 ± 11 years, 72% Caucasians, 55% males, 34% diabetics, 26% with associated CVD, and median follow-up, 19 months. There were no significant differences in clinical characteristics of transplanted patients according to their uric acid levels. However, GFR was higher in patients with serum uric acid < 428 mmol/L from the first posttransplant week onward (Table 3).

TABLE 1: Main characteristics of hemodialysis patients on the waiting list for renal transplantation.

	Total (1020)	Uric acid < 428[¥] (838)	Uric acid ≥ 428[¥] (182)
Age (years)	53.7 ± 11.1	54.1 ± 11.3	52.3 ± 9.9*
Sex (males) (%)	58.9	59.3	65.4
Race (Caucasians) (%)	71.5	71.5	71.4
Body mass index (kg/m²)	25.5 ± 4.8	25.2 ± 4.6	27.1 ± 4.6
Diabetes mellitus (%)	39.6	41.7	37.9
Dyslipidemia (%)	35.6	34.1	41.1*
Smoking (%)	24.4	25.0	24.8
Hypertension (%)	80.7	79.1	82.4
Associated CVD (%)	38.1	39.7	34.8
C-reactive protein > 5 mg/L (%)	56.5	56.0	57.9
Uric acid[¥] (mean)	346 ± 104	310 ± 63	511 ± 89

[¥]mmol/L; *$P < 0.05$.

TABLE 2: Characteristics of the patients after renal transplantation.

	Total (199)	Uric acid[¥] < 428 (133)	Uric acid[¥] ≥ 428 (66)
Age, years (mean ± sd)	52.1 ± 10.7	52.1 ± 11.1	51.9 ± 10.1
Sex (males) (%)	55.3	51.9	62.1
Race (Caucasians) (%)	71.8	71.4	72.7
BMI* (kg/m²) (mean ± sd)	24.8 ± 4.5	24.7 ± 4.6	25.1 ± 4.3
Diabetes mellitus (%)	33.7	33.8	33.3
Dyslipidemia (%)	35.3	34.7	36.7
Smoking (%)	17.1	17.3	16.6
Hypertension (%)	82.9	81.2	86.4
Associated CVD (%)	26.1	27.1	24.2
Uric acid[¥] (mean ± sd)	377 ± 126	305 ± 64	521 ± 89

*Body mass index; [¥]mmol/L.

TABLE 3: Mean GFR value on different time intervals after renal transplantation.

	Mean value of GFR (mL/min/1.73 m²)		
	Uric acid[¥] < 428 value (n)	Uric acid[¥] ≥ 428 value (n)	P value
First day	12.09 (124)	9.58 (59)	0.093
7 days	27.15 (123)	17.75 (59)	0.013
30 days	52.7 (125)	38.75 (59)	0.003
>30 days	54.85 (117)	40.72 (57)	0.0003

[¥]mmol/L; GFR: glomerular filtration rate.

Figures 1(a) and 1(b) depict the incidence of major CV events and death by any cause in patients on dialysis with normal and increased baseline serum UA, respectively. In the dialysis group high baseline serum UA was not associated with either major CV events or all-cause mortality. In the subgroups of patients with diabetes or increased C-reactive protein an elevated UA also did not alter the incidence of events or death (data not shown).

For patients who underwent renal transplantation post-transplant baseline UA ≥ 428 mmol/L was associated with increased probability of CV events ($P = 0.03$, HR 1.6, and 95% CI 1.03–2.54) but did not correlate with death (Figures 2(a) and 2(b)). In patients with estimated GFR < 50 mL/min an elevated UA had no significant impact on the incidence of events (log-rank = 0.59, HR = 1.16%, and CI 0.65–1.99) or death (log-rank = 0.61, HR = 0.90%, and CI 0.59–1.34).

Table 4 shows the multivariate analysis (Cox model) that included, as independent variables, increased serum UA, age, reduced GFR, diabetes, hypertension, and associated CV disease. Reduced GFR was the only independent predictor of major adverse CV events after renal transplantation (HR 1.79, % CI 1.07–3.21, and $P = 0.02$). Increased serum AU, age, pretransplantation diabetes, hypertension, and associated CV disease were not predictors of adverse CV events.

4. Discussion

In this study we examined the relationship between serum UA and cardiovascular events and all-cause mortality risk in dialysis patients before and after renal transplantation.

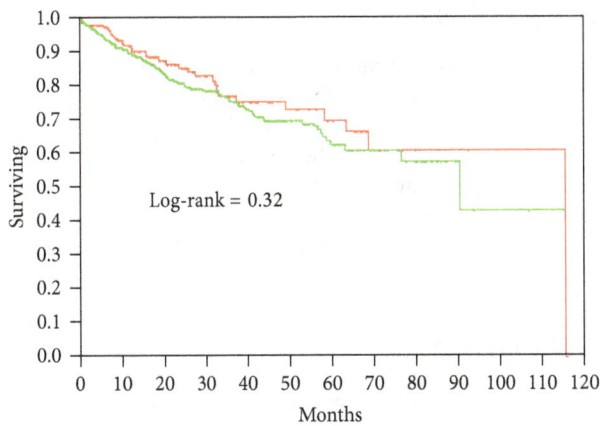

(a) Cardiovascular events

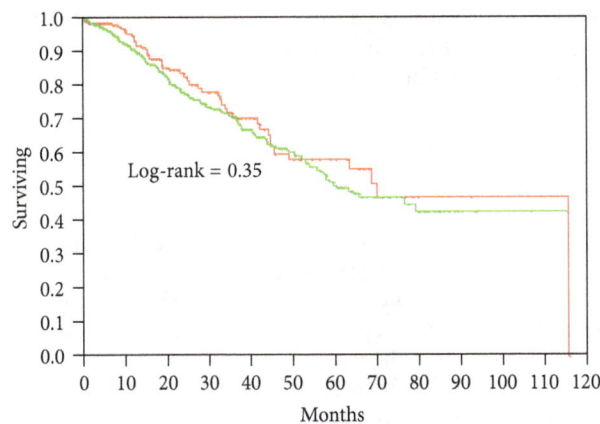

(b) Death by any cause

FIGURE 1: (a) and (b) Cardiovascular events and mortality in patients on the waiting list for renal transplantation according to uric acid level.

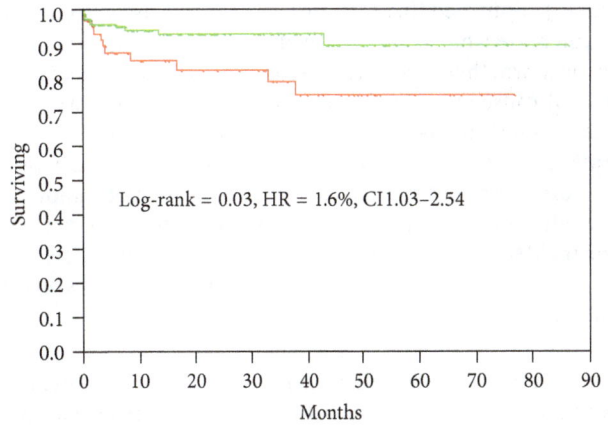

(a) Cardiovascular events

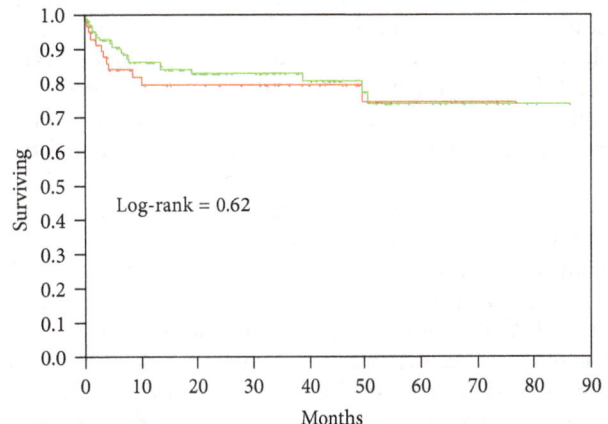

(b) Death by any cause

FIGURE 2: (a) and (b) Cardiovascular events and mortality in renal transplant patients according to uric acid level.

TABLE 4: Results of Cox regression model with cardiovascular events as dependent variable in renal allograft recipients.

Variable	HR	%CI	P
Age at time of transplantation ($\geq$52 yrs)	1.50	0.99–1.11	0.09
Serum uric acid ($\geq$428 mmol/L)	1.41	0.88–2.28	0.15
GFR < 50 mL/min/1.73 m^2	**1.79**	**1.07–3.21**	**0.02**
Diabetes mellitus	0.78	0.48–1.30	0.342
Hypertension	0.80	0.32–0.52	0.54
Cardiovascular disease	0.73	0.45–1.20	0.208

GFR: glomerular filtration rate.

The main finding was that higher UA ($\geq$ 428 mmol/L) was associated with higher risk for cardiovascular events after renal transplantation. However, after adjusting for confounding factors, including GFR, that association was no longer significant. Instead, it was a reduced graft function that predicted future events. On the other hand, an increased UA did not influence the outcome of patients on dialysis or the incidence of death in allograft recipients.

Our data show that elevated serum UA was not predictor of cardiovascular events or death in dialysis patients on the waiting list for transplant. Likewise, analysis in the subgroups of diabetics and in subjects with elevated C-reactive protein showed no significant differences relative to cardiovascular events or mortality in patients with high or normal uric acid levels.

Many but not all observational studies suggest that hyperuricemia is an independent risk factor for cardiovascular mortality and/or all-cause mortality in the general population [10–12]. Culleton et al. [13], using Framingham Heart Study data, reported that an elevated serum uric acid level at baseline was not independently associated with increased risk of cardiovascular mortality. They concluded that the apparent association of serum uric acid to cardiovascular events was probably due to confounding cardiovascular risk factors.

Hyperuricemia is also common in subjects with end-stage renal disease, where it has been reported in up to 50% of subjects [14–16]. Consistent with studies in the general population, 2 studies performed in hemodialysis patients

[15, 16] confirmed that hyperuricemia is also associated with an increased mortality risk in the dialysis population. It is unclear whether uric acid level is a marker for CV disease and all-cause mortality in this patient population or whether the relationship between uric acid level and mortality is independent of traditional CVD risk factors [17]. Perhaps it is more important that there is no definitive information on the effect of correction or prevention of hyperuricemia and the incidence of cardiovascular complications due to the lack of sufficient data from randomized, prospective studies on the subject.

Herein, we found that an elevated UA was associated with an increased incidence of CV events in renal transplant patients. We also observed that the proportion of patients with increased serum UA was higher in patients with reduced estimated GFR, as shown in Table 3. Since a compromised allograft function is an important predictor of CV event and death it is conceivable that the increased risk associated with higher serum UA may be explained by a compromised graft function. Indeed, in the Cox proportional model that included, besides serum UA, age, comorbidities, and GFR, an elevated serum UA was no longer significantly associated with CV events. Instead, a reduced GFR (<50 mL/min) emerged as the sole independent risk factor for major CV events. Also, in patients with reduced GFR an increased serum UA did not correlate with prognosis, contrary with that observed in the totality of patients undergoing renal transplantation. It is of interest that hyperuricemia is a common complication of cyclosporine and tacrolimus-based immunosuppression and that this alteration is attributed to reduced GFR [18, 19].

Therefore, our results favor the concept that the association of serum uric acid to cardiovascular events is probably due to confounding risk factors, especially a reduced GFR, at least in recipients of kidney transplant.

In the present investigation, pretransplant diabetes, hypertension, or concomitant cardiovascular disease was not associated with death or events in renal transplant recipients. This probably reflects the exclusion of patients with more severe comorbidities from the waiting list, leaving only individuals with mild diabetes and less advanced cardiovascular disease to be transplanted.

Why were only renal transplant recipients and not patients on dialysis affected by an increased serum UA? It was not the purpose of this investigation to answer this question. Notwithstanding, it is possible that the very high risk associated with dialysis would have superseded the relatively low impact related to an increased UA. Also, removal of UA by dialysis could have made it impossible to detect associations between increased UA and prognosis. Finally, since renal function appears to be the critical factor explaining the negative effect of UA on prognosis, in patients with no significant renal function, any association between serum UA and events would be impossible to infer.

5. Conclusions

Our data suggest that an increased posttransplant uric acid is related to higher probability of major CV events but suggest that this association probably caused concurrent reduction in GFR. Even so, the data may be useful to identify renal transplant patients at increased risk for cardiovascular events. More investigations are necessary to verify the impact of control in serum UA on prognosis of renal transplant recipients.

6. Limitations

The retrospective nature or our study may have limited the analysis of confounder factors that could influence the elevation of uric acid either before or after renal transplantation. Information regarding the use of diuretics or other drugs that could interfere with UA levels is lacking. Serum UA was measured only on inception.

References

[1] R. J. Johnson, D.-H. Kang, D. Feig et al., "Is there a pathogenetic role for uric acid in hypertension and cardiovascular and renal disease?" *Hypertension*, vol. 41, no. 6, pp. 1183–1190, 2003.

[2] W.-C. Liu, C.-C. Hung, S.-C. Chen et al., "Association of Hyperuricemia with renal outcomes, cardiovascular disease, and mortality," *Clinical Journal of the American Society of Nephrology*, vol. 7, no. 4, pp. 541–548, 2012.

[3] A. Haririan, J. M. Noguiera, K. Zandi-Nejad et al., "The independent association between serum uric acid and graft outcomes after kidney transplantation," *Transplantation*, vol. 89, pp. 573–579, 2010.

[4] U. Gerhardt, M. G. Hüttmann, and H. Hohage, "Influence of hyperglycemia and hyperuricemia on long-term transplant survival in kidney transplant recipients," *Clinical Transplantation*, vol. 13, no. 5, pp. 375–379, 1999.

[5] H.-U. Meier-Kriesche, J. D. Schold, Y. Vanrenterghem, P. F. Halloran, and H. Ekberg, "Uric acid levels have no significant effect on renal function in adult renal transplant recipients: evidence from the Symphony Study," *Clinical Journal of the American Society of Nephrology*, vol. 4, no. 10, pp. 1655–1660, 2009.

[6] F. Viazzi, D. Parodi, G. Leoncini et al., "Serum uric acid and target organ damage in primary hypertension," *Hypertension*, vol. 45, no. 5, pp. 991–996, 2005.

[7] R. D. Santos, K. Nasir, R. Orakzai, R. S. Meneghelo, J. A. M. Carvalho, and R. S. Blumenthal, "Relation of uric acid levels to presence of coronary artery calcium detected by electron beam tomography in men free of symptomatic myocardial ischemia with versus without the metabolic syndrome," *The American Journal of Cardiology*, vol. 99, no. 1, pp. 42–45, 2007.

[8] J. Fang and M. H. Alderman, "Serum uric acid and cardiovascular mortality: the NHANES I Epidemiologic Follow-up Study, 1971–1992," *Journal of the American Medical Association*, vol. 283, no. 18, pp. 2404–2410, 2000.

[9] S. D. Navaneethan and S. Beddhu, "Associations of serum uric acid with cardiovascular events and mortality in moderate chronic kidney disease," *Nephrology Dialysis Transplantation*, vol. 24, no. 4, pp. 1260–1266, 2009.

[10] A. Høieggen, M. H. Alderman, S. E. Kjeldsen et al., "The impact of serum uric acid on cardiovascular outcomes in the LIFE Study," *Kidney International*, vol. 65, no. 3, pp. 1041–1049, 2004.

[11] A. Hozawa, A. R. Folsom, H. Ibrahim, F. J. Nieto, W. D. Rosamond, and E. Shahar, "Serum uric acid and risk of ischemic stroke: the ARIC Study," *Atherosclerosis*, vol. 187, no. 2, pp. 401–407, 2006.

[12] M. Chonchol, M. G. Shlipak, R. Katz et al., "Relationship of uric acid with progression of kidney disease," *The American Journal of Kidney Diseases*, vol. 50, no. 2, pp. 239–247, 2007.

[13] B. F. Culleton, M. G. Larson, W. B. Kannel, and D. Levy, "Serum uric acid and risk for cardiovascular disease and death: the Framingham heart study," *Annals of Internal Medicine*, vol. 131, no. 1, pp. 7–13, 1999.

[14] S. M. K. Lee, A. L. Lee, T. J. Winters et al., "Low serum uric acid level is a risk factor for death in incident hemodialysis patients," *American Journal of Nephrology*, vol. 29, no. 2, pp. 79–85, 2009.

[15] S.-P. Hsu, M.-F. Pai, Y.-S. Peng, C.-K. Chiang, T.-I. Ho, and K.-Y. Hung, "Serum uric acid levels show a 'J-shaped' association with all-cause mortality in haemodialysis patients," *Nephrology Dialysis Transplantation*, vol. 19, no. 2, pp. 457–462, 2004.

[16] M. E. Suliman, R. J. Johnson, E. García-López et al., "J-shaped mortality relationship for uric acid in CKD," *American Journal of Kidney Diseases*, vol. 48, no. 5, pp. 761–771, 2006.

[17] M. Madero, M. J. Sarnak, X. Wang et al., "Uric acid and long-term outcomes in CKD," *The American Journal of Kidney Diseases*, vol. 53, no. 5, pp. 796–803, 2009.

[18] M. Mazzali, "Uric acid and transplantation," *Seminars in Nephrology*, vol. 25, no. 1, pp. 50–55, 2005.

[19] M. Kanbay, A. Akcay, B. Huddam et al., "Influence of cyclosporine and tacrolimus on serum uric acid levels in stable kidney transplant recipients," *Transplantation Proceedings*, vol. 37, no. 7, pp. 3119–3120, 2005.

17

Sleep Parameters in Short Daily versus Conventional Dialysis

Ludimila D'Avila e Silva Allemand,[1] **Otávio Toledo Nóbrega,**[1] **Juliane Pena Lauar,**[2] **Joel Paulo Russomano Veiga,**[1] **and Einstein Francisco Camargos**[1]

[1]*Universidade de Brasília (UnB), Brasília, DF, Brazil*
[2]*Centro Brasiliense de Nefrologia, Brasília, DF, Brazil*

Correspondence should be addressed to Einstein Francisco Camargos; einsteinfc@gmail.com

Academic Editor: Jochen Reiser

Previous studies have observed worse sleep quality in patients undergoing conventional dialysis as compared to daily dialysis. Our aim was to compare the sleep parameters of patients undergoing daily or conventional dialysis using an objective measure (actigraphy). This cross-sectional study was performed in three dialysis centers, including a convenience sample (nonprobability sampling) of 73 patients (36 patients on daily hemodialysis and 37 patients on conventional hemodialysis). The following parameters were evaluated: nocturnal total sleep time (NTST), expressed in minutes; wake time after sleep onset (WASO), expressed in minutes; number of nighttime awakenings; daytime total sleep time (DTST), expressed in minutes; number of daytime naps; and nighttime percentage of sleep (% sleep). The Mini-Mental State Examination and the Beck Depression Inventory were also administered. The mean age was 53.4 ± 17.0 years. After adjustment of confounding factors using multiple linear regression analysis, no difference in actigraphy parameters was detected between the groups: NTST ($p = 0.468$), WASO ($p = 0.88$), % sleep ($p = 0.754$), awakenings ($p = 0.648$), naps ($p = 0.414$), and DTST ($p = 0.805$). Different from previous studies employing qualitative analysis, the present assessment did not observe an influence of hemodialysis modality on objective sleep parameters in chronic renal patients.

1. Introduction

The literature provides evidence that chronic diseases may compromise the quality of sleep. One example is end-stage renal disease (ESRD), in which 80% of affected individuals experience insomnia and other sleep disturbances [1, 2]. Additionally, an independent association has been observed between ESRD and reduced total and REM sleep times, possibly as a result of uremia, fluid overload, or both [3].

The clinical management of ESRD relies on renal replacement therapy through dialysis. Conventional dialysis, the most traditional modality, involves thrice weekly sessions lasting up to 4 hours. Recent studies have shown significant improvement in survival with the use of high-flux membranes, ultrafiltration control, bicarbonate dialysate, and other more efficient water treatments [4]. These advancements have led to the introduction of daily dialysis that has some advantages over conventional dialytic therapy,

including shorter daily treatment times. On the other hand, the study of Locatelli and coworkers showed that only a subset of patients with low serum albumin experience increased survival [5]. Daily hemodialysis is indeed associated with better control of blood pressure, ventricular hypertrophy, depression, cognitive function, and also survival. The mechanisms are probably related to a decreased ultrafiltration rate and better volume control and not the use of high-flux membranes. Daily dialysis is provided five to seven times per week, with sessions lasting 1.5 to 2.5 hours per day. Improvements in clinical parameters in daily dialysis have been cited, such as treatment tolerance, blood pressure control, nutritional status, and adverse events (anemia and hospital admissions, among others), with increase in survival and quality of life as well as patient well-being [6].

Enhancement in sleep quality, which is often poor in individuals on maintenance hemodialysis, has also been suggested in association with daily dialysis, although the findings are inconclusive. A study performed by Jaber et al. [7] with individuals undergoing short daily hemodialysis (6 times a week) has shown significant improvement in the prevalence and severity of restless legs symptoms after 12 months. Sleep disturbances, assessed with a self-administered survey, were also significantly improved. In addition, a recent study comparing polysomnographic parameters of 15 patients on daily hemodialysis versus 15 patients on conventional hemodialysis did not detect significant differences in the prevalence of obstructive sleep apnea between the groups (33.3% for daily dialysis versus 53.3% for conventional dialysis, $p = 0.08$) [8]. Similarly, a study using the Medical Outcomes Study Sleep Problems Index II instrument did not detect statistically significant differences between frequent versus conventional dialysis in sleep quality at 12 months [9].

Thus, the aim of the present study was to compare the sleep profile of patients undergoing daily or conventional dialysis using an objective measure (actigraphy). We hypothesized that sleep parameters, especially total nocturnal sleep time, would be more favorable with daily dialysis.

2. Methods

2.1. Setting. The present cross-sectional study included non-probability sampling of ESRD patients undergoing daily or conventional dialysis in three facilities in Brasília, Brazil. The first facility (*Centro Brasiliense de Nefrologia* (CBN)) is a private clinic providing daily dialysis (1.5 to 2.5 h sessions) exclusively to private insurance patients. The second facility, located in a university hospital (*Centro de Diálise do Hospital Universitário de Brasília* (HUB/UnB)), provides conventional dialysis (3 to 4 h sessions) exclusively to patients from the public health care system (Unified Health System (SUS)). The third facility (*Nephron-Unidade de Diálise*) provides care to both private and public health care patients, with focus on conventional dialysis (sessions lasting 3 to 4 hours). Baseline data were collected from medical records. The study was approved by the Research Ethics Committee at the School of Medicine, Universidade de Brasília (protocol CAAE 31399514.9.0000.5558). All participants included in the final sample signed an informed consent form before the procedures. All procedures performed in studies involving human participants were in accordance with the ethical standards of the institutional and/or national research committee and with the 1964 Declaration of Helsinki and its later amendments or comparable ethical standards.

2.2. Participants. We included community-dwelling patients aged ≥18 years with a confirmed diagnosis of ESRD, receiving hemodialysis treatment for at least 3 months, and living in the same address for the study period. Patients who were not capable of understanding or answering questionnaires were not included, as well as those with movement disorders, upper limb paralysis that could compromise actigraphy, psychiatric disorders or disabling cognitive disorders, history of traumatic brain injury with residual neurological deficit, or any other detectable unstable medical condition that could prevent the patient from completing the research protocol.

All interviews were performed by the principal investigator (Ludimila D'Avila e Silva Allemand) on two different occasions during hemodialysis sessions. Data were collected between October 2014 and April 2016.

2.3. Measurements. A brief questionnaire was administered for collection of demographic clinical data: age (years), sex (m/f), body mass index (BMI; kg/m^2), schooling (years), income, ESRD etiology, duration of dialysis (hemodialysis vintage, in months), and dialysis shift (morning/afternoon/night). The use of hypnotics, antidepressants, or other psychotropic medications was investigated (yes/no), as well as tobacco and alcohol consumption (yes/no). Medical records were reviewed to obtain the most recent data on hemoglobin (g/dL), iron (μg/dL), ferritin (μg/L), phosphorus (mg/dL), calcium (mg/dL), albumin (g/dL), potassium (mmol/L), and pre- and postdialysis urea (mg/dL) levels. The following tests were performed in all patients: the Mini-Mental State Examination (MMSE) (cognitive profile) [10] and the Beck Depression Inventory (BDI-II) [11].

Sleep parameters were assessed using an actigraph (Actiwatch, Respironics, Inc., Mini-Mitter, Bend, OR) and a data analysis software platform (Actiware, version 5.59.0015, 2010). The following parameters were used: (1) wake threshold selection = medium; (2) wake threshold value = 40; and (3) sleep interval detection algorithm = 10 immobile minutes for sleep onset and sleep end.

The actigraph was placed on the arm without arteriovenous fistula for continuous monitoring over nine days. To reduce the possibility of bias, the first and last days were disregarded, and data referring to 7 days and 7 nights were analyzed. Patients kept a sleep diary to document the time at which they went to bed and turned off the lights, as well as any occasions when they had to remove the device. The diary was used for adjustment of actigraphy data if necessary. Participants also used the "event" marker in the actigraph to record the time getting into bed and out of bed. Actigraphy data for each participant were extracted after 9 days. Data were analyzed in a blind fashion, with the evaluator blinded to the type of dialysis.

The following outcomes were evaluated: nocturnal total sleep time (NTST), expressed in minutes; wake time after sleep onset (WASO), that is, the sum of wake times from sleep onset to final awakening, expressed in minutes; number of nighttime awakenings from sleep onset to final awakening (awakenings); daytime total sleep time (DTST), expressed in minutes; number of daytime naps (naps), that is, daytime sleep periods lasting more than 10 minutes; and nighttime percentage of sleep (% sleep) from sleep onset to final awakening.

2.4. Statistical Analysis. Student's *t*-test was used to compare continuous variables with close-to-Gaussian distribution in both treatment groups. The Mann–Whitney test was used for variables with non-Gaussian distribution regardless of treatment modality. Pearson's chi-square test was used to compare proportions between treatments.

The influence of potential confounding factors was tested by multiple linear regression models having sleep parameters

TABLE 1: Demographic and clinical variables of patients undergoing dialysis ($n = 73$).

Variable[*]	Daily hemodialysis $n = 36$	Conventional hemodialysis $n = 37$	p[#]
Age (years)	59.3 ± 18.6	47.6 ± 13.3	0.002
Sex			0.044
Male	24 (66.7)	16 (43.2)	
Female	12 (33.3)	21 (56.8)	
Schooling (years)	2.7 ± 0.5	1.6 ± 0.6	<0.0001
Hemodialysis vintage (months)	50.9 ± 38.5	59.2 ± 50.3	0.650
Treatment shift			0.074
Morning	22 (61.1)	27 (73.0)	
Afternoon	9 (25.0)	10 (27.0)	
Night	5 (13.9)	0 (0.0)	
Use of hypnotics			0.091
Yes	8 (22.2)	3 (8.1)	
No	28 (77.8)	34 (91.9)	
Use of antidepressants			0.0004
Yes	16 (44.4)	3 (8.1)	
No	20 (55.6)	34 (91.9)	
Other psychotropic medications			0.590
Yes	6 (16.7)	8 (21.6)	
No	30 (83.3)	29 (78.4)	
Use of tobacco			0.674
Yes	3 (8.3)	2 (5.4)	
No	33 (91.7)	35 (94.6)	
Use of alcohol			0.188
Yes	8 (22.2)	4 (10.8)	
No	28 (77.8)	33 (89.2)	
Scales			
MMSE	27.9 ± 1.9	27.6 ± 2.2	0.378
BDI-II	10.6 ± 7.0	14.6 ± 6.9	0.013
Body mass index (kg·m^2)	25.1 ± 5.0	25.7 ± 3.8	0.577
Hemoglobin (g/dL)	11.7 ± 1.3	10.9 ± 2.0	0.071
Iron (μg/dL)	62.9 ± 28.7	64.4 ± 26.1	0.742
Ferritin (ng/mL)	331.2 ± 326	379.2 ± 275	0.499
Albumin (g/dL)	4.0 ± 0.6	4.0 ± 0.3	0.563
Predialysis urea level (mg/dL)	107.8 ± 34.9	132.6 ± 34.5	0.003
Postdialysis urea level (mg/dL)	51.1 ± 19.0	35.4 ± 17.7	0.0005
Potassium (mEq/L)	5.0 ± 0.7	5.4 ± 0.9	0.031
Phosphorus (mg/dL)	5.4 ± 1.5	5.5 ± 1.5	0.725
Calcium (mg/dL)	9.1 ± 0.8	9.0 ± 0.7	0.393

[*]Mean ± standard deviation or frequency (%). [#]Student's t-test, Mann–Whitney test, or Pearson's chi-square.

(NTST, WASO, % sleep, awakenings, naps, and DTST) as dependent variables. Potential confounders, sex, age, schooling, income, hemodialysis duration and shift, use of medications, tobacco, and alcohol, and MMSE, BDI-II, and BMI scores, were entered into the model in a stepwise manner. The contribution of each variable to the model was estimated and compared according to specified entry or removal criteria. Independent variables were kept in the model if $p = 0.15$. A $p < 0.05$ was established as limit for significance. Statistical analyses were carried out using SAS 9.4 software (SAS Institute, Cary, USA).

3. Results

Of 80 eligible patients, six refused to participate (4 patients on daily dialysis and 2 patients on conventional dialysis) and one patient died. Thus, the final sample included 73 patients (36 patients on daily hemodialysis and 37 patients on conventional hemodialysis).

The mean age of participants was 53.4 ± 17 years (59.3 years for daily hemodialysis and 47.5 years for conventional hemodialysis, $p = 0.002$); 40 patients were male and 33 were female. Table 1 describes the study population. ESRD

TABLE 2: Actigraphic variables, sleep quality, and daytime sleepiness in patients undergoing two modalities or hemodialysis ($n = 73$).

Variable	Hemodialysis[*]		p value[#]
	Daily ($n = 36$)	Conventional ($n = 37$)	
NTST (min)	348.0 ± 95.2	349.9 ± 63.9	0.468
WASO	76.0 ± 41.1	66.4 ± 33.4	0.188
% sleep	82.5 ± 8.4	84.8 ± 7.1	0.754
Awakenings (number)	26.8 ± 10.2	23.6 ± 8.1	0.648
Naps	43.6 ± 18.1	38.1 ± 15.7	0.414
DTST	188.9 ± 99.7	175.2 ± 93.7	0.805

[*]Mean ± standard deviation or frequency (%). [#]Linear or multiple regression models adjusted for age, dialysis shift, use of hypnotics, use of antidepressants, and BDI-II score. NTST: nocturnal total sleep time; WASO: wake time after sleep onset; DTST: daytime total sleep time.

was caused by hypertensive nephropathy ($n = 24$, 32.8%), diabetic nephropathy ($n = 13$, 17.8%), glomerulonephritis ($n = 8$, 10.9%), polycystic kidney disease ($n = 8$, 10.9%), lupus nephritis ($n = 3$, 4.1%), and other causes ($n = 15$, 20.5%).

There was no statistical difference between the groups in actigraphy parameters. Mean NTST, WASO, % sleep, awakenings, naps, and DTST were similar in the daily dialysis and conventional dialysis groups even after adjustment of confounding factors using multiple regression analysis (Table 2). However, when considering the overall sample ($n = 73$), multiple linear regression analysis showed that dialysis shift (morning, afternoon, or night) significantly influenced specific sleep variables. Patients undergoing hemodialysis in the afternoon or night had an additional 40.3 minutes of NTST as compared to patients undergoing dialysis in the morning (95% CI: 3.56–77.09; $p = 0.032$); and patients undergoing dialysis in the morning had a mean of 69 additional minutes of DTST as compared to patients undergoing hemodialysis in the afternoon or at night (95% CI: 25.59–112.33; $p = 0.002$).

BDI-II scores were negatively associated with WASO. Patients with lower BDI-II scores (higher total scores indicate more severe depressive symptoms) had higher mean WASO (95% CI: −2.25–−0.11; $p = 0.030$). In addition, patients using antidepressants had an additional 34 minutes of WASO and 8 additional awakenings as compared to patients who were not using antidepressants (95% CI: 17.75–49.96; $p < 0.0001$).

4. Discussion

In this sample of 36 patients undergoing daily dialysis and 37 patients undergoing conventional dialysis, no differences were observed between the groups in terms of objective sleep parameters. To the best of our knowledge, there are no available comparative studies employing objective parameters to assess sleep in patients with this profile. To date, studies have employed qualitative, nonparametric measures or overnight polysomnography [8, 9, 12].

Previous studies have demonstrated that actigraphy is sensitive to detecting sleep patterns associated with specific sleep disorders as well as with other medical or neurobehavioral disorders [13]. A high correlation has also been reported between the gold standard polysomnography and actigraphic estimates of total sleep time and sleep efficiency, with 88% accuracy of actigraphy to distinguish sleep from wakefulness [14].

The present study corroborates frequent reports from the literature which describe poor sleep quality in hemodialysis patients, as reflected in our sample by an overall mean NTST of 5.8 hours. A systematic review of the literature has shown high prevalence of sleep disturbances in ESRD patients on conventional dialysis [15]. Bastos et al. have also reported poor sleep quality (Pittsburgh Sleep Quality Index ≥ 6) in 75% of conventional dialysis patients ($n = 100$) [16]. However, few studies have addressed the impact of daily hemodialysis on sleep parameters. Most studies have focused on conventional dialysis, peritoneal dialysis, or nocturnal hemodialysis.

Elias et al. [3] have compared polysomnographic parameters in 15 patients on daily dialysis versus 15 patients on conventional dialysis strictly regarding the presence of obstructive sleep apnea (OSA). The difference in OSA prevalence between the groups reached only borderline significance (33.3% for daily dialysis and 53.3% for conventional dialysis, $p = 0.08$). That study did not compare variables such as sleep efficiency, daytime sleepiness, naps, or total sleep time, providing only evidence of associations between OSA and both low dialysis dose and poor cardiovascular outcomes.

Another study has been recently performed to compare the effect of daily and nocturnal dialysis versus conventional dialysis on self-reported sleep quality [8]. A standardized questionnaire was used (Medical Outcomes Study Sleep Problems Index II) to evaluate sleep disturbances (scored from 0 to 100, with higher value indicating poorer quality of sleep). The authors did not find statistically significant differences between the two dialysis modalities in terms of sleep quality at 12 months.

Sabbatini et al. [17] investigated whether the technical and therapeutic advancements of hemodialysis had any impact on sleep disturbances in 694 patients. A (nonvalidated) questionnaire was used, in addition to clinical data obtained from the medical chart, dialysis data, and lifestyle information. The authors observed that 86% of patients presented some sleep disturbance (nocturnal awakening in 92%, difficulty falling asleep in 67%, and early waking in the morning in 62%); insomnia was detected in 45%. That study also associated the presence of insomnia with longer duration of dialysis (>12 months) in patients undergoing dialysis in the morning and in those with high levels of parathyroid hormone.

Similarly, studies have demonstrated excessive daytime sleepiness in chronic dialysis patients (about 30%) [18, 19]. In our sample, actigraphy also revealed increased daytime sleepiness. DTST was about 3 hours per day in both groups, which could explain why patients take naps during dialysis sessions. Nevertheless, this finding may be overestimated, since actigraphy records body movements and the arm is often at rest during dialysis sessions.

The findings of the present study regarding depressive symptoms deserve special attention. In our sample, patients with fewer depressive symptoms according to the BDI-II had worse nocturnal sleep quality, represented by higher WASO. This disagrees with the report by Trbojevic-Stankovic et al. [20] who observed that individuals with depression undergoing dialysis had significantly worse sleep quality than nondepressed individuals. However, that study analyzed sleep quality (by the Pittsburgh Sleep Quality Index) as a parametric variable, which is not methodologically adequate. The fewer depressive symptoms detected in our daily hemodialysis group [versus conventional hemodialysis group] might be explained by the significantly higher use of antidepressants in this group.

It is possible that sleep disturbances may be related to other aspects beyond the renal/dialytic component. It is likely that the etiology of sleep disorders in these patients has a multifactorial nature [21]. Aspects linked to social and work activities (which are restricted in individuals undergoing dialysis), genetic and psychological factors, and lifestyle habits may interfere with sleep [22, 23]. However, other factors, which have not often been evaluated, may also be related to sleep disorders in these patients, such as anemia, levels of urea and uremic toxins in blood, cardiovascular diseases, arterial hypertension, diabetes, advanced age, time since the onset of dialysis, alcohol and tobacco abuse, and depression. As previously mentioned in the literature, a plausible cause might be the influence of biochemical parameters, such as hemoglobin, urea, and phosphorus levels [23]. In clinical practice, increased levels of phosphorus may be associated with bone pain, pruritus, and, consequently, sleep fragmentation.

Variations in urinary volume during sleep, associated with reduced sodium, calcium, and potassium excretion, may also be associated with sleep disorders, which are frequent in ESRD [24]. In addition, it is known that ESRD is associated with increased inflammation, which, according to some authors, could also influence sleep quality in these individuals [25].

Another important aspect in the evaluation of sleep in chronic renal patients is related to the shift during which the treatment is usually performed. Some studies have demonstrated that morning dialysis is significantly associated with worse sleep quality; it is possible that, beyond behavioral factors that may disturb sleep, such as early waking in the morning, metabolic factors may also affect the circadian rhythm [17, 21, 25]. A better quality of sleep has been observed after nocturnal dialysis [26]. Conversely, the patients in the present study who underwent morning dialysis had less nocturnal sleep and more daytime sleep as compared to those undergoing dialysis in the afternoon or at night. One hypothesis that could explain this finding is that the need to wake up very early for treatment sessions affects total sleep time, with an increase in the number of naps during the day.

Some methodological limitations of the present study must be addressed. First, the older age of patients on daily hemodialysis (59.3 years versus 47.5 years for participants on conventional dialysis) may have counterbalanced the worse biochemical parameters of patients on conventional dialysis, despite the statistical adjustment. Nevertheless, Sabry et al. [27] have identified high prevalence of sleep disorders in a sample of relatively young patients. Also, the cross-sectional design has limitations in and of itself; an observational study comparing sleep parameters before and after the onset of dialysis (daily and conventional) would allow assessment of other variables along the study period and enable the establishment of individual baseline parameters. Finally, pain, an important variable to be considered for the evaluation of sleep quality, was not addressed in this study. Davison and Jhangri have pointed out that, regardless of treatment modality, about 50% of dialysis patients experience pain and that those with moderate or severe pain experience insomnia more than those reporting mild or no pain do [28].

In summary, contrary to previous studies employing qualitative methods, the present study using actigraphy did not observe differences in sleep parameters between patients undergoing daily or conventional dialysis. Additional research is necessary to elucidate factors that may impair sleep in this population and promote better sleep quality for patients undergoing any of the currently available renal replacement modalities.

Acknowledgments

The authors acknowledge grants from the Brazilian Council for Scientific and Technological Development (CNPq) (no. 400927/2016-0) and from the Foundation for Research Support of the Brazilian Federal District (FAPDF) (no. 193.000.659-2015), both to Einstein Francisco Camargos. The authors wish to thank Dr. Flávio José Dutra de Moura for allowing data acquisition at the Nephron Clinic. They are also thankful for a fellowship for productivity in research to Otávio Toledo Nóbrega (CNPq).

References

[1] A. Gul, N. Aoun, and E. M. Trayner Jr., "Why do patients sleep on dialysis?" *Seminars in Dialysis*, vol. 19, no. 2, pp. 152–157, 2006.

[2] S. C. W. Tang and K. N. Lai, "Sleep disturbances and sleep apnea in patients on chronic peritoneal dialysis," *Journal of Nephrology*, vol. 22, no. 3, pp. 318–325, 2009.

[3] R. M. Elias, C. T. Chan, and T. D. Bradley, "Altered sleep structure in patients with end-stage renal disease," *Sleep Medicine*, vol. 20, pp. 67–71, 2016.

[4] J. K. Leypoldt, A. K. Cheung, C. E. Carroll et al., "Effect of dialysis membranes and middle molecule removal on chronic hemodialysis patient survival," *American Journal of Kidney Diseases*, vol. 33, no. 2, pp. 349–355, 1999.

[5] F. Locatelli, A. Martin-Malo, T. Hannedouche et al., "Effect of membrane permeability on survival of hemodialysis patients," *Journal of the American Society of Nephrology*, vol. 20, no. 3, pp. 645–654, 2009.

[6] J. R. DePalma, E. A. Pecker, and M. H. Maxwell, "A new automatic coil dialyzer system for 'daily' dialysis," *Hemodialysis International*, vol. 8, no. 1, pp. 19–23, 2004.

[7] B. L. Jaber, B. Schiller, J. M. Burkart et al., "Impact of short daily hemodialysis on restless legs symptoms and sleep disturbances," *Clinical Journal of the American Society of Nephrology*, vol. 6, no. 5, pp. 1049–1056, 2011.

[8] R. M. Elias, M. C. M. Castro, E. L. De Queiroz, H. Abensur, J. E. Romão-Junior, and G. Lorenzi-Filho, "Obstructive sleep apnea in patients on conventional and short daily hemodialysis," *American Journal of Nephrology*, vol. 29, no. 6, pp. 493–500, 2009.

[9] M. L. Unruh, B. Larive, P. W. Eggers et al., "The effect of frequent hemodialysis on self-reported sleep quality: Frequent Hemodialysis Network Trials," *Nephrology Dialysis Transplantation*, vol. 31, no. 6, pp. 984–991, 2016.

[10] M. F. Folstein, S. E. Folstein, and P. R. McHugh, ""Mini mental state". A practical method for grading the cognitive state of patients for the clinician," *Journal of Psychiatric Research*, vol. 12, no. 3, pp. 189–198, 1975.

[11] C. Gorenstein, L. Andrade, A. H. Guerra Vieira Filho, T. C. Tung, and R. Artes, "Psychometric properties of the portuguese version of the Beck Depression Inventory on Brazilian college students," *Journal of Clinical Psychology*, vol. 55, no. 5, pp. 553–562, 1999.

[12] M. Rai, T. Rustagi, S. Rustagi, and R. Kohli, "Depression, insomnia and sleep apnea in patients on maintenance hemodialysis," *Indian Journal of Nephrology*, vol. 21, no. 4, pp. 223–229, 2011.

[13] A. Sadeh, "The role and validity of actigraphy in sleep medicine: an update," *Sleep Medicine Reviews*, vol. 15, no. 4, pp. 259–267, 2011.

[14] R. J. Cole, D. F. Kripke, W. Gruen, D. J. Mullaney, and J. C. Gillin, "Automatic sleep/wake identification from wrist activity," *Sleep*, vol. 15, no. 5, pp. 461–469, 1992.

[15] N. T. Fonseca, J. J. Urbano, S. R. Nacif et al., "A systematic review of sleep disorders in patients with chronic kidney disease undergoing hemodialysis," *Journal of Physical Therapy Science*, vol. 28, no. 7, pp. 2164–2170, 2016.

[16] J. P. C. Bastos, R. B. De Sousa, L. A. D. M. Nepomuceno et al., "Sleep disturbances in patients on maintenance hemodialysis: Role of dialysis shift," *Revista da Associacao Medica Brasileira*, vol. 53, no. 6, pp. 492–496, 2007.

[17] M. Sabbatini, B. Minale, A. Crispo et al., "Insomnia in maintenance haemodialysis patients," *Nephrology Dialysis Transplantation*, vol. 17, no. 5, pp. 852–856, 2002.

[18] K. P. Parker, N. G. Kutner, D. L. Bliwise, J. L. Bailey, and D. B. Rye, "Nocturnal sleep, daytime sleepiness, and quality of life in stable patients on hemodialysis," *Health and Quality of Life Outcomes*, vol. 1, article no. 68, 2003.

[19] K. P. Parker, D. L. Bliwise, J. L. Bailey, and D. B. Rye, "Daytime sleepiness in stable hemodialysis patients," *American Journal of Kidney Diseases*, vol. 41, no. 2, pp. 394–402, 2003.

[20] J. Trbojevic-Stankovic, B. Stojimirovic, Z. Bukumiric et al., "Depression and quality of sleep in maintenance hemodialysis patients," *Srpski arhiv za celokupno lekarstvo*, vol. 142, no. 7-8, pp. 437–443, 2014.

[21] G. Merlino, A. Piani, P. Dolso et al., "Sleep disorders in patients with end-stage renal disease undergoing dialysis therapy," *Nephrology Dialysis Transplantation*, vol. 21, no. 1, pp. 184–190, 2006.

[22] M. Novak, C. M. Shapiro, D. Mendelssohn, and I. Mucsi, "Diagnosis and management of insomnia in dialysis patients," *Seminars in Dialysis*, vol. 19, no. 1, pp. 25–31, 2006.

[23] B. C. P. Koch, J. E. Nagtegaal, G. A. Kerkhof, and P. M. Ter Wee, "Circadian sleep-wake rhythm disturbances in end-stage renal disease," *Nature Reviews Nephrology*, vol. 5, no. 7, pp. 407–416, 2009.

[24] L. R. Stow and M. L. Gumz, "The circadian clock in the kidney," *Journal of the American Society of Nephrology*, vol. 22, no. 4, pp. 598–604, 2011.

[25] A. N. Vgontzas, C. Tsigos, E. O. Bixler et al., "Chronic insomnia and activity of the stress system: A preliminary study," *Journal of Psychosomatic Research*, vol. 45, no. 1, pp. 21–31, 1998.

[26] R. M. De Santo, M. Bartiromo, M. C. Cesare, N. G. De Santo, and M. Cirillo, "Sleeping Disorders in Patients With End-Stage Renal Disease and Chronic Kidney Disease," *Journal of Renal Nutrition*, vol. 16, no. 3, pp. 224–228, 2006.

[27] A. A. Sabry, H. Abo-Zenah, E. Wafa et al., "Sleep disorders in hemodialysis patients," *Saudi Journal of Kidney Diseases and Transplantation*, vol. 21, no. 2, pp. 300–305, 2010.

[28] S. N. Davison and G. S. Jhangri, "The impact of chronic pain on depression, sleep, and the desire to withdraw from dialysis in hemodialysis patients," *Journal of Pain and Symptom Management*, vol. 30, no. 5, pp. 465–473, 2005.

18

Prevalence and Risk Factors of Lower Limb Amputation in Patients with End-Stage Renal Failure on Dialysis

Rajit A. Gilhotra, Beverly T. Rodrigues, Venkat N. Vangaveti, and Usman H. Malabu

School of Medicine and Dentistry, James Cook University, Townsville, QLD 4811, Australia

Correspondence should be addressed to Usman H. Malabu; umalabu@gmail.com

Academic Editor: Laszlo Rosivall

Background. Renal dialysis has recently been recognised as a risk factor for lower limb amputation (LLA). However, exact rates and associated risk factors for the LLA are incompletely understood. *Aim.* Prevalence and risk factors of LLA in end-stage renal failure (ESRF) subjects on renal dialysis were investigated from the existing literature. *Methods.* Published data on the subject were derived from MEDLINE, PubMed, and Google Scholar search of English language literature from January 1, 1980, to July 31, 2015, using designated key words. *Results.* Seventy studies were identified out of which 6 full-text published studies were included in this systematic review of which 5 included patients on haemodialysis alone and one included patients on both haemodialysis and peritoneal dialysis. The reported findings on prevalence of amputation in the renal failure on dialysis cohort ranged from 1.7% to 13.4%. Five out of the six studies identified diabetes as the leading risk factor for amputation in subjects with ESRF on renal dialysis. Other risk factors identified were high haemoglobin A1c, elevated c-reactive protein, and low serum albumin. *Conclusions.* This review demonstrates high rate of LLA in ESRF patients receiving dialysis therapy. It has also identified diabetes and markers of inflammation as risk factors of amputation in ESRF subjects on dialysis.

1. Introduction

End-stage renal failure, defined as nonreversible kidney damage requiring replacement therapy [1], is a recognised risk factor for peripheral artery disease leading to nonhealing ulcers and lower limb amputation (LLA) [2–6]. The aetiology of ESRF such as diabetes may be associated with complex vascular dysfunction and widespread organ involvement including cardiovascular and musculoskeletal systems, the two being the most important cause of morbidity and mortality in patients with ESRF on haemodialysis [1, 2, 7].

The prevalence of diabetes globally, as reported by the International Diabetes Federation in 2015, was 415 million (8.3% of the world's adult population) and is projected to alarmingly rise to 642 million by 2040, a significant rise over a small period of time [8, 9]. Diabetes is a leading cause of foot ulcer and renal failure amongst others [10]. In the case of

foot ulcer, the combination of vascular insufficiency and local infection worsens the prognosis resulting in life threatening sepsis, LLA, and death [11–14]. Furthermore, the prevalence of foot complications in general is considerably higher in patients with diabetes and ESRF as compared to patients with diabetes without ESRF [5, 6, 13, 14]. It is known that LLA increases patient disability, decreases quality of life, and contributes to high morbidity, mortality, and health care costs [15–17] yet not much information on the extent of the problems is known worldwide.

Although various studies investigating the outcome of foot complications in patients with diabetes have been reported, prevalence of lower limb amputation in subjects on renal dialysis remains poorly recognised [6, 18]. Furthermore, clinical and biochemical features accounting for the high rate of LLA in subjects on renal dialysis are inconclusive. This systematic review aimed to critically appraise published studies which have assessed LLA as an outcome in patients with ESRF on dialysis and to determine prevalence and risk factors associated with LLA in the study population.

2. Methods

2.1. Protocol and Focus. This systematic review was performed with the standardised written protocol that followed the Preferred Reporting Items for Systematic Reviews and Meta-Analyses (PRISMA) guidelines [25]. The review focuses on studies which assessed the prevalence and identified risk factors for lower limb amputation in patients who have received renal dialysis.

2.2. Search Criteria. A search strategy was formulated to identify studies in which LLA was assessed in patients with ESRF on dialysis. Databases from MEDLINE/PubMed (US National Library of Medicine, Bethesda, MD, USA) and Google Scholar (Google, Mountain View, CA, USA) were searched from January 1, 1980, to July 31, 2015. Keyword sets combined "diabetes" or "diabetic ulcer" or "diabetic foot" and "amputation" and "renal dialysis".

2.3. Eligibility Criteria. To be eligible, studies were required to focus on amputation as an outcome in ESRF patients on renal dialysis. For inclusion, studies had to be published before July 31, 2015. Publications were restricted to human studies and those published in English. There was no restriction on study size. For the inclusion of publications, the studies needed to be full articles which investigated patients on haemodialysis and/or peritoneal dialysis as a cohort and required recording of the prevalence and/or the risk factors associated with amputation as an outcome in this cohort.

Publications were excluded from this systematic review if they were review articles, looked at traumatic/neoplastic, only upper extremity/penile amputation as outcomes, compared prognosis of different interventions, and included only a subgroup of dialysis patients in the study (such as patients with diabetes on renal dialysis and patients on renal dialysis who had peripheral artery bypass).

2.4. Data Extraction. Data from the identified studies was extracted by one author. Any uncertainty was resolved by discussion between authors. Data extraction from eligible literature included information regarding geographical location, sample size, mean age, percentage of male patients, mean time on dialysis, diabetes mellitus, smoking history, hypertension, coronary artery disease, amputation, and risk factors (RR, OR, HR, RH, p values, and confidence intervals). Data was transcribed into an excel data collection sheet.

3. Results

3.1. Search Results. Seventy published studies were identified as per the abovementioned search criteria (Figure 1). Fifty studies were excluded due to various reasons such as lack of investigating lower limb amputation as an outcome, dialysis/renal replacement/renal replacement therapy/end-stage

renal failure/renal failure/end-stage kidney disease/kidney failure not being mentioned in the title, and comparing prognosis and outcomes of various pharmacological and surgical interventions. Abstracts were critically screened for the 20 remaining studies out of which another 14 were excluded due to being review articles (n = 6); being case studies (n = 2); only including a subset of dialysis patients (n = 2); not including dialysis patients (n = 1); assessing vascular changes in amputated limbs as an outcome (n = 1); assessing prognosis of percutaneous transluminal angioplasty as an outcome (n = 1); inability to access full text (n = 1). In all, 6 full-text publications were reviewed as detailed in Figure 1.

3.2. Characteristics of Included Studies and Subjects. Five out of the six studies included patients on haemodialysis [19–23] and one study included both haemodialysis and peritoneal dialysis patients [24]. There was no study that only included peritoneal dialysis patients.

As for the outcomes, two of the studies investigated only amputation in particular [19, 22] and the remaining four explored other outcomes as well such as foot problems, peripheral vascular disease related procedures, myocardial infarction, and mortality [20, 21, 23, 24]. The data related to these outcomes was presented separately in all these studies; therefore, it was possible to assess data specific to amputation by itself. There was marked variation in sample size between studies. All studies included at least 100 subjects (Table 1). Two studies included between 100 and 500 patients (n = 271, n = 232) [20, 21], three studies had between 1000 and 5000 subjects (n = 1513, n = 1041, and n = 3272) [19, 23, 24], and one study had 29838 subjects [22]. Most publications sourced participants from hospital or dialysis clinics, apart from one study that was conducted on patients from a nursing home setting [21]. Three of the studies recruited participants from single centres [20, 21, 23] and three from multiple centres [19, 22, 24]. Populations examined also varied between studies. Three studies focused on American patients [19, 21, 24]. Single studies recruited patients from Japan [23] and Canada [20]. One study included patients from around the world including 12 countries [22]. Three studies extracted data from larger studies such as the Choices for Healthy Outcomes in Caring for End-Stage Renal Disease (CHOICE) [24], Dialysis Outcomes and Practice Patterns Study (DOPPS) [22], and the ESRF Core Indicator/Clinical Performance Measure (CPM) Project [19].

All the studies were consistent in defining their inclusion criteria of patients on dialysis therapy; they all identified that patients with ESRF were placed on renal dialysis as a form of renal replacement therapy, that being either haemodialysis or peritoneal dialysis. The studies defined the endpoint being development of amputation, which could have been performed when uncontrollable limb infection existed even after undergoing revascularization and/or medical treatment. One publication specifically defined nontraumatic lower limb amputation and excluded digital amputation as one of the primary outcomes that were investigated [24]. Only one study specifically defined major amputation as above-the-knee amputation [23].

TABLE 1: Characteristics of studies that assessed amputation in subjects on renal dialysis.

Author	Country	Total cases	Mean age (y)	Male (%)	Time on dialysis	DM	Smoking	HTN	CAD	Amputation (%)
Speckman et al., 2004 [19]	USA	3272 HD	—	53.4%	—	1751 (53.5%)	—	—	1711 (52.3%)	116 (4%)
Locking-Cusolito et al., 2005 [20]	Canada	232 HD	65.1	130 (56%)	—	98 (42.2%)	—	75%	50%	31 (13.4%)
Reddy et al., 2007 [21]	USA	271 HD	70.5 ± 12	127 (47%)	18 ± 27 (m)	176 (65%)	37 (14%)	244 (90%)	146 (54%)	34 (13%)
Combe et al., 2009 [22]	Multinational	29838 HD	61.3 ± 15	57.7%	3.3 ± 5 (y)	11129	17.7%	77.2%	41.6%	6%
Ishii et al., 2012 [23]	Japan	1513 HD	63 ± 13.5	66.7%	—	739	22.6%	74.05%	4.4%	26 (1.7%)
Plantinga et al., 2009 [24]	USA	1041 (767 HD, 274 PD)	57.9 ± 15	54.2%	—	54%	60.6%	—	24.5%	136 (13%)

HTN, hypertension; CAD, coronary artery disease; DM, diabetes mellitus; HD, haemodialysis; PD, peritoneal dialysis; (y), years; (m), months; USA, Unites States of America.

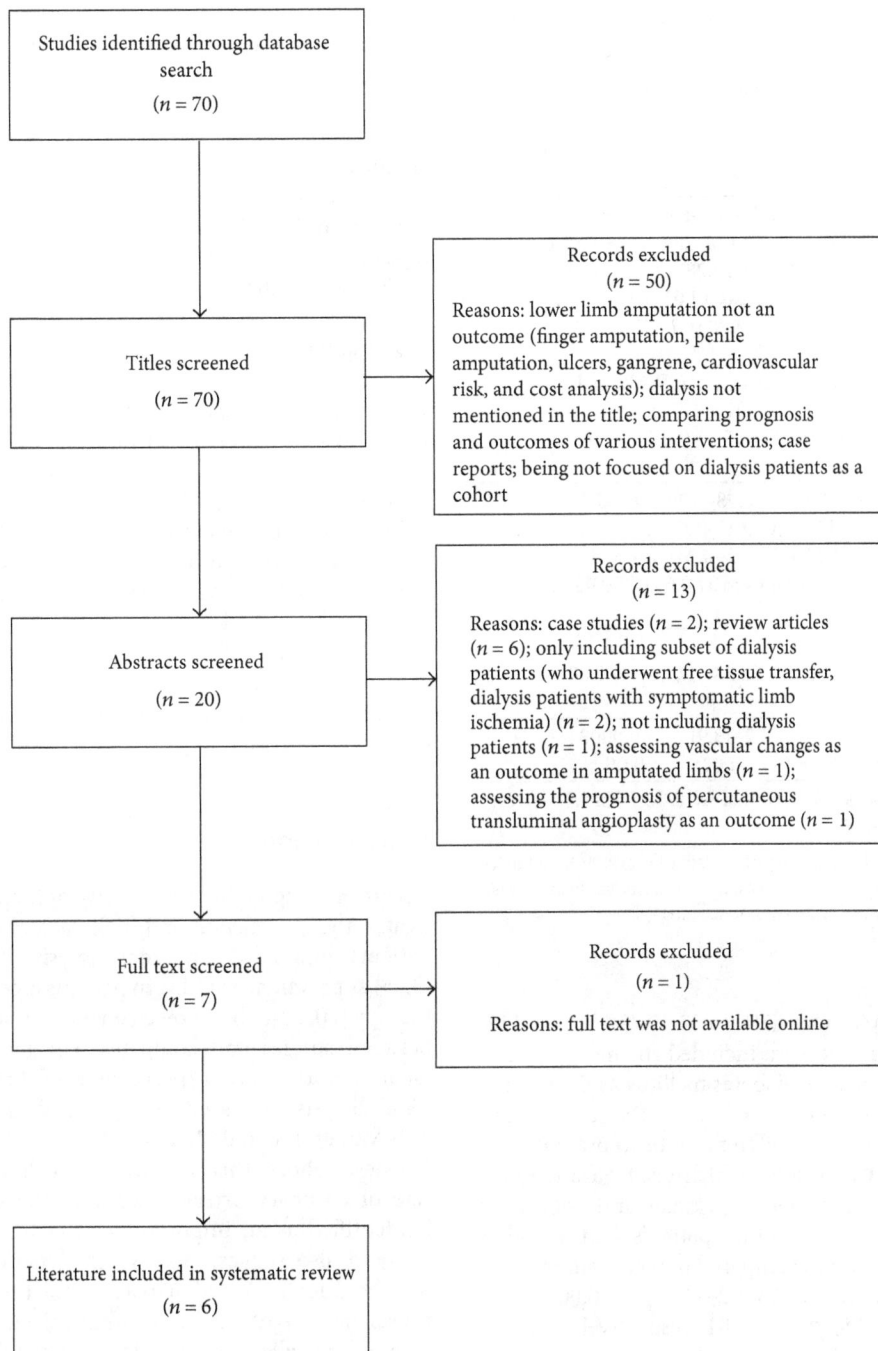

Figure 1: Flow diagram to illustrate the studies identified for this review.

Five of the studies were longitudinal cohort studies, out of which four were retrospectively designed [19, 21, 22, 24] and one of each of prospective longitudinal format [23] and observational case-control study [20], respectively. Although all the studies were investigated for comorbidities in the participant population, there were some variations in the different studies. The prevalence of comorbidities also varied from study to study; for example, only 4.4% [23] of participants in one study had coronary artery disease compared to 54% in another [21]. All the retrospective studies collected their data via databases or medical chart review. Locking-Cusolito and colleagues used a foot assessment instrument which was used in clinics to collect data from patients attending their clinic [20]. The prospective study had a follow-up time period of 96 months over which the data was collected via direct patient contact, medical charts, or telephonic interview.

3.3. Amputation in Subjects on Renal Dialysis. The reported finding on prevalence of amputation in patients with renal

TABLE 2: Summary of studies assessing risk factors of amputation in subjects on renal dialysis.

Author	Risk factors for amputation in all dialysis patients
Speckman et al., 2004 [19]	MUR < 58.5%: HR 2.4 (CI 1.4–4.2), $p < 0.01$ CVD: HR 2.4 (CI 1.6–3.7), $p < 0.001$
Combe et al., 2009 [22]	DM: AOR 5.55 (CI 4.63–6.64), $p < 0.001$ Men: AOR 1.82 (CI 1.61–2.06), $p < 0.001$ Blacks: AOR 1.45 (CI 1.28–1.65), $p < 0.001$ Smoking: AOR 1.22 (CI 1.03–1.43), $p < 0.001$ Retinopathy: AOR 1.78 (CI 1.55–2.04), $p < 0.001$ Peripheral neuropathy: AOR 2.25 (CI 1.98–2.56), $p < 0.001$ Calciphylaxis: AOR 2.37 (CI 1.63–3.45), $p < 0.001$
Plantinga et al., 2009 [24]	DM: RH 4.33 (CI 2.98–6.30), $p < 0.05$ PVD: RH 1.59 (CI 1.17–2.15), $p < 0.05$ CRP: RH 2.7 (CI 1.72–4.23), $p < 0.05$ Albumin < 3.3 g/dL: RH 0.63 (CI 0.42–0.94), $p < 0.05$
Locking-Cusolito et al., 2005 [20]	DM: AOR 10.17 (CI 3.7–27.7), $p < 0.001$
Ishii et al., 2012 [23]	DM: HR 5.29 (CI 2–13.9), $p = 0.0008$ CRP: HR 1.01 (CI 1–1.02), $p < 0.05$
Reddy et al., 2007 [21]	Dialysis > 12 months: AOR 2.74 (CI 1.22–6.16), $p < 0.05$

DM, diabetes mellitus; HR, hazard ratio; RH, relative hazard; AOR, adjusted odds ratio; PVD, peripheral vascular disease; CVD, cardiovascular disease; MUR, mean urea reduction; CI: 95% confidence interval.

failure on renal dialysis was 1.7% to 13.4% (Table 1). Five out of the six studies that were included in the systematic review identified presence of diabetes mellitus as the leading risk factor for amputation ($p < 0.05$) [19, 20, 22–24]. Although all the studies used different ratios to present their findings, there were two studies which used hazard ratios (HR). Ishii and colleagues and Speckman and colleagues reported that diabetic renal failure patients had a higher risk of getting amputation as compared to their counterparts without diabetes, HR 5.29, 95% CI 2–13.9, $p = 0.0008$, and HR 7.4, 95% CI 4.1–13.5, $p < 0.001$, respectively. On the other hand, Reddy and colleagues investigated the association of duration of renal replacement therapy and amputation as an outcome. They found that a higher percentage (19%) of established haemodialysis patients (dialysis for ≥12 months) had to have amputation as compared to new haemodialysis patients (8%) (dialysis for ≤3 months) ($p = 0.01$) [21].

3.4. Risk Factors of Amputation in Subjects on Renal Dialysis. Detailed risk factors are shown in Table 2. Diabetes was reported as a leading risk factor associated with amputation in renal dialysis patients in 5 out of the 6 studies. Two studies compared diabetic and nondiabetic subjects on dialysis showing higher rate of amputation amongst diabetics as shown in Table 3.

Other amputation risk factors reported in subjects on renal dialysis included longer duration of dialysis therapy, HbA1c levels, c-reactive protein (CRP), and low serum albumin. In patients with diabetes, a higher HbA1c level after commencement of dialysis was found to be statistically significant as a risk factor for amputation [20, 23]. Ishii and colleagues established that all patients requiring major amputation ($n = 7$) were found to fall in the highest HbA1c quartile (HbA1c > 6.8%). Overall, 6.1% of all amputees had an HbA1c > 6.8% as compared to only 0.9% of amputees with HbA1c < 5.4%. The association of a higher HbA1c and amputation was also found to be statistically significant: HbA1c > 6.8%, HR 2.99, 95% CI 1.17–7.7, $p = 0.023$. A higher CRP level, as a marker of inflammation, was found to be related to amputation by Ishii and colleagues, HR 1.01, 95% CI 1–1.02, $p = 0.047$, and by Plantinga and colleagues showing relative hazard (RH) 2.7, 95% CI 1.72–4.23, $p < 0.05$ [24]. Subjects on renal dialysis with a low mean serum albumin (<3.3 g/dL) were also found to be at risk of amputation by Speckman and colleagues: HR 1.8, 95% CI 1.1–3, $p < 0.05$. If these subjects had diabetes, the risk was further increased: HR 3.8, 95% CI 1.1–12.5, $p < 0.05$. In the same study, Plantinga et al. reported increased albumin levels were associated with significantly decreased risk of amputation: RH 0.63, 95% CI 0.42–0.94, $p < 0.05$ [24].

4. Discussion

This review highlights the scarcity of literature which investigates the prevalence and risk factors of amputation in patients with ESRF on renal dialysis. It revealed 1.7% to 13.4% as prevalence of LLA in patients receiving renal dialysis therapy [20, 23]. This showed a wide variation in amputation between studies and countries. For instance, study from Japan reported lower prevalence of LLA in subjects on renal dialysis compared to higher rate in USA and Canada. This variation could suggest a better outcome amongst the Japanese cohort. This is in keeping with the finding of lower rate of coronary artery disease in the population, which is identified as an important risk factor for LLA [1, 2, 7]. It could also suggest that North Americans have a lower threshold for LLA. Other reasons for the wide variation in prevalence might be due to multiple factors. For instance, Combe and colleagues conducted a large scale multinational, multicentre study which included a large number of subjects (29838) and investigated various associated risk factors such as age, ethnicity, calciphylaxis, retinopathy, and neuropathy [22]. However, the methodology used to collect the data did not differentiate between types of amputation. Though this study presented an overall worldwide 6% prevalence of amputation in renal dialysis patients, it may have been an overestimation. Plantinga and colleagues on the other hand excluded digital amputation from their data collection; this might have resulted in an underestimation of all amputations in renal dialysis patients [24]. Nevertheless, these findings warrant further studies.

Interestingly, we have identified presence of diabetes as an important single risk factor for LLA, with up to 26.5%

TABLE 3: Summary of studies assessing risk factors of amputation in diabetic and nondiabetic patients on dialysis.

Author	Total patients with DM	DM patients having amputation	Risk factors for amputation in patients with DM	Total non-DM patients	Non-DM patients having amputation	Risk factors for amputation in patients without DM
Speckman et al., 2004 [19]	1751	104 (6%)	CVD: HR 1.7 (CI 1.1–2.6), $p < 0.05$ MUR < 58.5%: HR 2.6 (CI 1.4–4.8), $p < 0.01$	1469	12 (1%)	Increasing age: HR 1.09 (CI 1.02–1.2), $p < 0.01$ Mean serum albumin < 3.5 g/dL: HR 3.8 (CI 1.1–12.5), $p < 0.01$
Combe et al., 2009 [22]	11129	14.2%	Peripheral neuropathy: AOR 2.23 (CI 1.94–2.56), $p < 0.001$ Calciphylaxis: AOR 2.02 (CI 1.32–3.1), $p < 0.001$ Men: AOR 1.69 (CI 1.48–1.94), $p < 0.001$	18203	1.60%	Calciphylaxis: AOR 3.41 (CI 1.74–6.7), $p < 0.001$ Men: AOR 2.56 (CI 1.86–3.51), $p < 0.001$ Blacks: AOR 1.88 (CI 1.23–2.86), $p < 0.001$ Smoking: AOR 1.62 (CI 1.11–2.37), $p < 0.001$

DM, diabetes mellitus; HR, hazard ratio; RH, relative hazard; AOR, adjusted odds ratio; CVD, cardiovascular disease; MUR, mean urea reduction; CI: 95% confidence interval.

of patients with diabetes receiving renal dialysis having amputation [20]. Renal dialysis has been found to increase the risk of foot ulcer in patients with diabetes. This significant temporal association is suggested by a 3 times higher risk of having foot ulcer in the first year of starting dialysis therapy and an almost 32 times higher risk for major amputation in the first year of starting dialysis therapy [26–28]. This risk is further increased in the presence of elevated CRP [23, 24] and low serum albumin [19, 24] as well as high HbA1c level [20, 23] at the onset of dialysis in agreement with recent reports [27, 28], suggesting that acute phase reactants and poor control of diabetes worsen the prognosis further. These findings were suggested from studies which were limited to patients on haemodialysis [19–23]. On the other hand, the only study which included both peritoneal dialysis and haemodialysis [24] reported a high prevalence of limb amputation of 13%; however, the authors did not provide a comparison between patients receiving haemodialysis and those on peritoneal dialysis.

Although studies have shown that peripheral arterial disease is common amongst patients on chronic dialysis therapy, the indication for bypass surgery in these patients is still a controversial topic. This is due to the high morbidity and mortality rates of these patients. Even though PTA is considered a possible procedure to treat critical limb ischemia, there is limited literature available on the prognosis of this intervention. In a 2-year follow-up prospective study on haemodialysis patients with diabetic foot wounds who were treated with PTA and minor amputation, it was found that only 41.9% of patients survived without reamputation with a 2-year postoperative mortality rate of 38.7% [29]. This study

had a small sample size of 31 haemodialysis patients; hence, it is important to explore the prognosis of PTA as treatment and prevention of amputation by doing more studies with a larger sample size. Other aspects of the review include associations between surgical procedures for vascular access and amputation. In patients with and without diabetes, both variables were increased after initiation of haemodialysis therapy. Amputations, which are potentially preventable, were associated with significant mortality amongst haemodialysis patients [30]. Thus, early interventions at primary care level have been found to lower the rate of foot complications and amputation, further stressing the need for multidisciplinary care in order to prevent adverse outcome in this group of population [31].

5. Conclusion

This review has demonstrated the high rate of lower limb amputation in patients with ESRF receiving dialysis therapy. It has also identified the risk factors associated with an adverse outcome, the chief amongst them being presence of diabetes. Other identified risk factors include hypoalbuminemia and elevated CRP. Thus, with early intervention in diabetic subjects, many limbs would likely be salvaged and the overall rate of adverse outcome from LLA would eventually be lowered. However, there is still a limited literature on preventative programs for LLA in subjects on renal dialysis. Furthermore, association between peritoneal dialysis and LLA is scanty as most studies were conducted on haemodialysis subjects. More studies are needed to further characterise findings in these areas.

References

[1] R. G. Luke, "Chronic renal failure—a vasculopathic state," *The New England Journal of Medicine*, vol. 339, no. 12, pp. 841–843, 1998.

[2] A. M. O'Hare, D. V. Glidden, C. S. Fox, and C.-Y. Hsu, "High prevalence of peripheral arterial disease in persons with renal insufficiency: results from the national health and nutrition examination survey 1999-2000," *Circulation*, vol. 109, no. 3, pp. 320–323, 2004.

[3] A. M. O'Hare, P. Bacchetti, M. Segal, C.-Y. Hsu, and K. L. Johansen, "Factors associated with future amputation among patients undergoing hemodialysis: results from the dialysis morbidity and mortality study waves 3 and 4," *American Journal of Kidney Diseases*, vol. 41, no. 1, pp. 162–170, 2003.

[4] B. G. Jaar, B. C. Astor, J. S. Berns, and N. R. Powe, "Predictors of amputation and survival following lower extremity revascularization in hemodialysis patients," *Kidney International*, vol. 65, no. 2, pp. 613–620, 2004.

[5] D. J. Margolis, O. Hofstad, and H. I. Feldman, "Association between renal failure and foot ulcer or lower-extremity amputation in patients with diabetes," *Diabetes Care*, vol. 31, no. 7, pp. 1331–1336, 2008.

[6] A. Ndip, M. K. Rutter, L. Vileikyte et al., "Dialysis treatment is an independent risk factor for foot ulceration in patients with diabetes and stage 4 or 5 chronic kidney disease," *Diabetes Care*, vol. 33, no. 8, pp. 1811–1816, 2010.

[7] F. K. Port, "Morbidity and mortality in dialysis patients," *Kidney International*, vol. 46, no. 6, pp. 1728–1737, 1994.

[8] D. R. Whiting, L. Guariguata, C. Weil, and J. Shaw, "IDF Diabetes Atlas: global estimates of the prevalence of diabetes for 2011 and 2030," *Diabetes Research and Clinical Practice*, vol. 94, no. 3, pp. 311–321, 2011.

[9] IDF, *Diabetes Atlas. Update 2015*, International Diabetes Federation, 7th edition, 2015.

[10] P. A. Lazzarini, J. M. Gurr, J. R. Rogers, A. Schox, and S. M. Bergin, "Diabetes foot disease: the Cinderella of Australian diabetes management?" *Journal of Foot and Ankle Research*, vol. 5, no. 1, article 24, 2012.

[11] H. Stiegler, "Diabetic foot syndrome," *Herz*, vol. 29, no. 1, pp. 104–115, 2004.

[12] B. Bruhn-Olszewska, A. Korzon-Burakowska, M. Gabig-Cimińska, P. Olszewski, A. Wegrzyn, and J. Jakóbkiewicz-Banecka, "Molecular factors involved in the development of diabetic foot syndrome," *Acta Biochimica Polonica*, vol. 59, no. 4, pp. 507–513, 2012.

[13] P. W. Eggers, D. Gohdes, and J. Pugh, "Nontraumatic lower extremity amputations in the Medicare end-stage renal disease population," *Kidney International*, vol. 56, no. 4, pp. 1524–1533, 1999.

[14] H. Al-Thani, A. El-Menyar, V. Koshy et al., "Implications of foot ulceration in hemodialysis patients: a 5-year observational study," *Journal of Diabetes Research*, vol. 2014, Article ID 945075, 6 pages, 2014.

[15] N. Tentolouris, S. Al-Sabbagh, M. G. Walker, A. J. M. Boulton, and E. B. Jude, "Mortality in diabetic and nondiabetic patients after amputations performed from 1990 to 1995: a 5-year follow-up study," *Diabetes Care*, vol. 27, no. 7, pp. 1598–1604, 2004.

[16] R. Sinha, W. J. A. van den Heuvel, and P. Arokiasamy, "Factors affecting quality of life in lower limb amputees," *Prosthetics and Orthotics International*, vol. 35, no. 1, pp. 90–96, 2011.

[17] U. H. Malabu, V. Manickam, G. Kan, S. L. Doherty, and K. S. Sangla, "Calcific uremic arteriolopathy on multimodal

combination therapy: still unmet goal," *International Journal of Nephrology*, vol. 2012, Article ID 390768, 6 pages, 2012.

[18] W. G. Goodman, J. Goldin, B. D. Kuizon et al., "Coronary-artery calcification in young adults with end-stage renal disease who are undergoing dialysis," *The New England Journal of Medicine*, vol. 342, no. 20, pp. 1478–1483, 2000.

[19] R. A. Speckman, D. L. Frankenfield, S. H. Roman et al., "Diabetes is the strongest risk factor for lower-extremity amputation in new hemodialysis patients," *Diabetes Care*, vol. 27, no. 9, pp. 2198–2203, 2004.

[20] H. Locking-Cusolito, L. Harwood, B. Wilson et al., "Prevalence of risk factors predisposing to foot problems in patients on hemodialysis," *Nephrology Nursing Journal*, vol. 32, no. 4, pp. 373–384, 2005.

[21] N. C. Reddy, S. M. Korbet, J. A. Wozniak, S. L. Floramo, and E. J. Lewis, "Staff-assisted nursing home haemodialysis: patient characteristics and outcomes," *Nephrology Dialysis Transplantation*, vol. 22, no. 5, pp. 1399–1406, 2007.

[22] C. Combe, J. M. Albert, J. L. Bragg-Gresham et al., "The burden of amputation among hemodialysis patients in the dialysis outcomes and practice patterns study (DOPPS)," *American Journal of Kidney Diseases*, vol. 54, no. 4, pp. 680–692, 2009.

[23] H. Ishii, Y. Kumada, H. Takahashi et al., "Impact of diabetes and glycaemic control on peripheral artery disease in Japanese patients with end-stage renal disease: long-term follow-up study from the beginning of haemodialysis," *Diabetologia*, vol. 55, no. 5, pp. 1304–1309, 2012.

[24] L. C. Plantinga, N. E. Fink, J. Coresh et al., "Peripheral vascular disease-related procedures in dialysis patients: predictors and prognosis," *Clinical Journal of the American Society of Nephrology*, vol. 4, no. 10, pp. 1637–1645, 2009.

[25] A. Liberati, D. G. Altman, J. Tetzlaff et al., "The PRISMA statement for reporting systematic reviews and meta-analyses of studies that evaluate healthcare interventions: explanation and elaboration," *The British Medical Journal*, vol. 339, Article ID b2700, 2009.

[26] F. L. Game, S. Y. Chipchase, R. Hubbard, R. P. Burden, and W. J. Jeffcoate, "Temporal association between the incidence of foot ulceration and the start of dialysis in diabetes mellitus," *Nephrology Dialysis Transplantation*, vol. 21, no. 11, pp. 3207–3210, 2006.

[27] N. J. Jones, J. Chess, S. Cawley, A. O. Phillips, and S. G. Riley, "Prevalence of risk factors for foot ulceration in a general haemodialysis population," *International Wound Journal*, vol. 10, no. 6, pp. 683–688, 2013.

[28] M. Kaminski, N. Frescos, and S. Tucker, "Prevalence of risk factors for foot ulceration in patients with end-stage renal disease on haemodialysis," *Internal Medicine Journal*, vol. 42, no. 6, pp. e120–e128, 2012.

[29] K. Matsuzaki, A. Miyamoto, N. Hakamata et al., "Diabetic foot wounds in haemodialysis patients: 2-year outcome after percutaneous transluminal angioplasty and minor amputation," *International Wound Journal*, vol. 9, no. 6, pp. 693–700, 2012.

[30] M. Martinez, R. Last, E. I. Agaba et al., "Surgical procedures before and after starting chronic hemodialysis in a predominantly male population with high prevalence of diabetes," *International Journal of Artificial Organs*, vol. 35, no. 9, pp. 648–654, 2012.

[31] T. Pliakogiannis, S. Bailey, S. Cherukuri et al., "Vascular complications of the lower extremities in diabetic patients on peritoneal dialysis," *Clinical Nephrology*, vol. 69, no. 5, pp. 361–367, 2008.

19

Phosphate and Cardiovascular Disease beyond Chronic Kidney Disease and Vascular Calcification

Sinee Disthabanchong ⓘ

Division of Nephrology, Department of Medicine, Faculty of Medicine, Ramathibodi Hospital, Mahidol University, Bangkok, Thailand

Correspondence should be addressed to Sinee Disthabanchong; sineemd@hotmail.com

Academic Editor: Nicolas Verheyen

Phosphate is essential for life but its accumulation can be detrimental. In end-stage renal disease, widespread vascular calcification occurs as a result of chronic phosphate load. The accumulation of phosphate is likely to occur long before the rise in serum phosphate above the normal range since several observational studies in both general population and early-stage CKD patients have identified the relationship between high-normal serum phosphate and adverse cardiovascular outcomes. Consumption of food high in phosphate increases both fasting and postprandial serum phosphate and habitual intake of high phosphate diet is associated with aging, cardiac hypertrophy, endothelial dysfunction, and subclinical atherosclerosis. The decline in renal function and dietary phosphate load can increase circulating fibroblast growth factor-23 (FGF-23) which may have a direct impact on cardiomyocytes. Increased FGF-23 levels in both CKD and general populations are associated with left ventricular hypertrophy, congestive heart failure, atrial fibrillation, and mortality. Increased extracellular phosphate directly affects endothelial cells causing cell apoptosis and vascular smooth muscle cells (VSMCs) causing transformation to osteogenic phenotype. Excess of calcium and phosphate in the circulation can promote the formation of protein-mineral complex called calciprotein particles (CPPs). In CKD, these CPPs contain less calcification inhibitors, induce inflammation, and promote VSMC calcification.

1. Introduction

The discovery of phosphorus occurred by accident in 1669 when a German alchemist named Hennig Brand boiled down 60 buckets of urine in search of the "philosopher's stone," a compound that would turn ordinary metals into gold. The discovered compound glowed in the dark in pale-green color, self-ignited and blew up into flame. He named the compound "phosphorus," which was taken from the Greek word meaning "bearer of light" [1]. Due to the high reactivity, phosphorus is never found as free element. White phosphorus has been used in manufacturing bombs and red phosphorus is used to make the strike plate of match boxes. The common use of phosphorus in the form of phosphoric acid nowadays is in the fertilizer industry.

Phosphorus is essential for life and exists in the body as phosphate. Phosphates are components of RNA, DNA, adenosine triphosphate (ATP), cell membrane, and bone. An average adult contains approximately 700 gram of phosphorus which is the result of an intake and excretion of 1-2 grams per day. Phosphate is excreted mostly in the urine. Only 0.1% of body phosphate circulates in the blood.

Despite its importance, the accumulation of phosphate can produce deleterious effects. Such example can be seen in end-stage renal disease patients when widespread vascular and soft tissue calcifications occur as a result of chronic phosphate accumulation. In early stages of chronic kidney disease (CKD), serum phosphate is normally maintained within the normal range owing to the compensatory increase in fibroblast growth factor-23 (FGF-23) and parathyroid hormone up until the estimated glomerular filtration rate (eGFR) reaching $30 \, \text{mL/min/1.73 m}^2$. Beyond this point hyperphosphatemia begins to develop [2, 3] (Figure 1). However, the accumulation of phosphate occurs long before the rise in serum phosphate above the upper normal limit since several observational studies in both general population and early-stage CKD patients have identified the relationship between high-normal serum phosphate and adverse cardiovascular outcomes. The following review will focus on the role of phosphate accumulation in

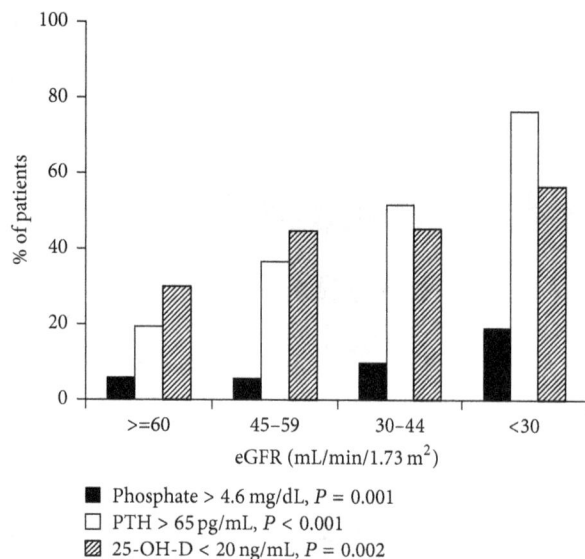

FIGURE 1: *Prevalence of hyperphosphatemia according to kidney function. P values represent the significance of trend. Reuse with permission from Chartsrisak et al. [3].*

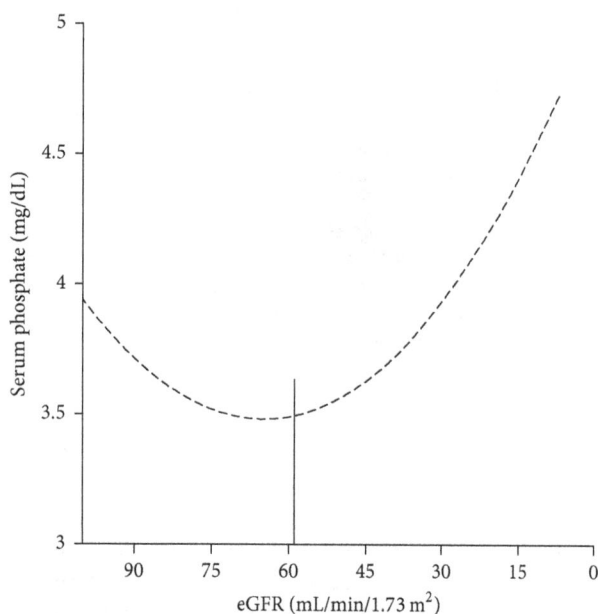

FIGURE 2: *Serum phosphate according to kidney function.* Vertical line represents the change in slope. *Modified from Chartsrisak et al. [3].*

cardiovascular disease (CVD) beyond CKD and vascular calcification.

2. Serum Phosphate and Outcomes

In CKD, the gradual increase in serum phosphate can be observed since the beginning of stage 3 [2] (Figure 2). Several studies in early-stage CKD patients have identified the relationship between increased serum phosphate but still within the normal range with adverse cardiovascular and renal

outcomes and overall survival [5–8]. The reported thresholds of serum phosphate in nondialysis CKD stages 2–5 patients that have been shown to predict adverse outcomes ranged between 3.5 and 4.6 mg/dL (Table 1). These data suggest that phosphate accumulation occurs since early stages of CKD prior to the development of hyperphosphatemia. More interestingly, the relationship between high-normal serum phosphate and adverse outcomes extends beyond CKD population. Among population with preserved renal function (normally defined as eGFR $>=$ 60 mL/min/1.73 m^2), the increase in serum phosphate not only displays a relationship with makers of atherosclerosis, for example, vascular and valvular calcifications, but also predicts atherosclerotic and nonatherosclerotic cardiovascular events and mortality [9–19]. The reported thresholds of serum phosphate for adverse outcomes were lower than CKD population and ranged between 2.5 and 3.8 mg/dL (Table 1). Since two major factors that determine serum phosphate level are dietary phosphate and urinary excretion, it is likely that high dietary phosphate is one of the mediators of such relationship.

3. Dietary Phosphate

The study that included both healthy and CKD subjects revealed a circadian rhythm of serum phosphate after ingestion of phosphate-rich meal (Figure 3) [4]. Serum phosphate is lowest in the morning and highest at 4 pm and midnight. Consumption of 1500 mg/day (normal phosphate diet) and especially 2500 mg/day of phosphate (high phosphate diet) resulted in a higher fasting and peak serum phosphate compared to consumption of 1000 mg/day of phosphate plus lanthanum carbonate (low phosphate diet). This circadian rhythm also presents in CKD patients but is much less pronounced. Another study in both healthy humans and rats with varying degree of kidney function revealed similar findings. A more rapid elevation of serum phosphate was observed in humans and rats with higher levels of kidney function [20]. These data confirmed that high phosphate diet results in a substantial increase in both fasting and postprandial serum phosphate. Therefore, a habitual intake of high dietary phosphate is likely to chronically elevate serum phosphate, eventually resulting in unfavorable outcomes mentioned above. The study that examined a relationship between increased serum and dietary phosphate with biochemical markers of aging revealed significant associations with telomere length, DNA methylation content, and chronological age [21]. In this study, dietary derived phosphate was closely related to the amount of red meat consumption. Moreover, the relationship between serum phosphate (within the normal range) and dietary phosphate with left ventricular mass was observed in early stages of CKD patients as well as in individuals with preserved renal function [22, 23]. In a large cohort of healthy subjects with no known CVD, dietary phosphate intake >1 gram/day was significantly associated with greater left ventricular mass after adjustment for confounders. Acute dietary phosphate load in healthy adult subjects can impair endothelial-dependent flow-mediated dilatation which may predispose to future atherosclerotic CVD [24, 25]. The associations between increased serum

TABLE 1: Thresholds of serum phosphate for cardiovascular events and mortality in early-stage CKD and general populations.

Studies (year)	Populations	Number	Serum phosphate (mg/dL)	Outcomes
Kestenbaum et al. (2005)	Women: Cr ≥ 1.2 mg/dL Men: Cr ≥ 1.5 mg/dL	3490	>=3.5	All-cause mortality
Bellasi et al. (2011)	CKD stages 3–5	1716	>=4.3	Combined ESRD and all-cause mortality
Chartsrisak et al. (2013)	CKD stages 2–4	466	>4.2	Combined ESRD and all-cause mortality
McGovern et al. (2013)	CKD stages 3–5	13292	>=4.6	Combined CV events and all-cause mortality
McGovern et al. (2013)	CKD stages 1-2	20356	>=3.86	Combined CV events and all-cause mortality
McGovern et al. (2013)	eGFR >= 90, no proteinuria	24184	>=3.86	Combined CV events and all-cause mortality
Tonelli et al. (2005)	Previous acute MI, eGFR >= 60 mL/min	4127	>=2.5	All-cause mortality
			>=2.5	Combined fatal and non-fatal CV events
Dhingra et al. (2007)	eGFR >= 60 mL/min	3676	>=3.2	Incident CVD
Foley et al. (2008)	97% has eGFR >= 60 mL/min	13822	>=3.8	All-cause mortality
Larsson et al. (2010)	Men, eGFR >= 60 mL/min	2176	>=2.8	All-cause mortality
Chang and Grams (2014)	95% has eGFR >= 60 mL/min	12984	>3.5	All-cause mortality
			>3.5	CV mortality

CKD = chronic kidney disease; ESRD = end-stage renal disease; CV = cardiovascular; CVD = cardiovascular disease; eGFR = estimated glomerular filtration rate; MI = myocardial infarction.

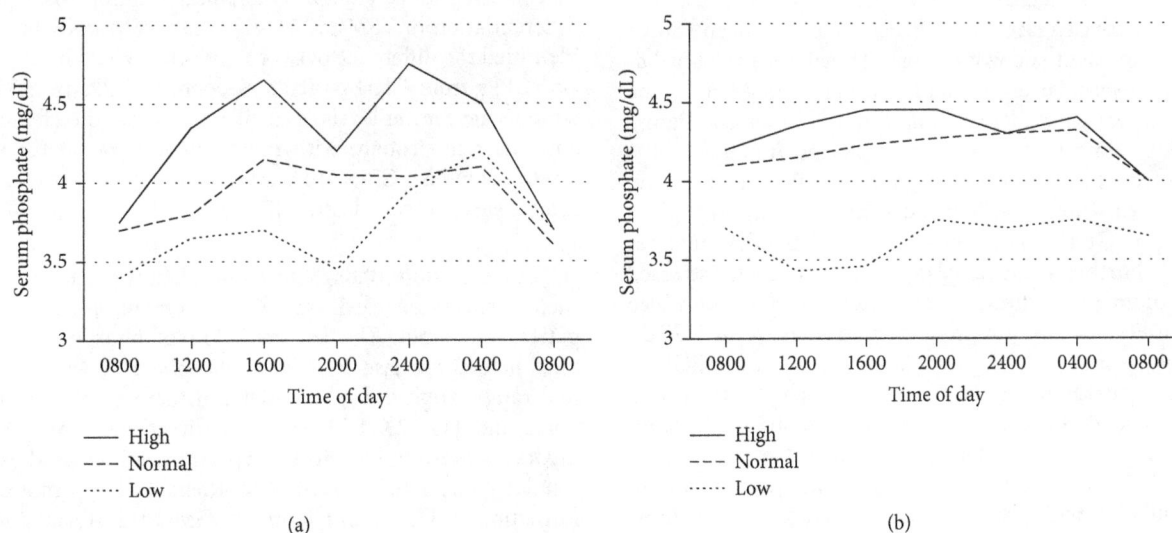

FIGURE 3: *Serum phosphate concentrations throughout the day in healthy controls (a) and CKD patients (b).* High phosphate = 2500 mg/day; normal phosphate = 1500 mg/day; low phosphate = 1000 mg/day plus lanthanum carbonate. Adapted from Ix et al. [4]. Reuse under the copyright license of free access article from American Society of Nutrition. https://nutrition.org/publications/guidelines-and-policies/license/.

phosphate and increased consumption of dietary phosphate additives with carotid intima-media thickness also exist [26, 27] In addition, dietary phosphate load can also increase FGF-23 concentration and the increase in FGF-23 has been linked to cardiac hypertrophy and adverse cardiovascular outcomes [28–30].

4. Fibroblast Growth Factor-23

FGF-23 is produced by osteoblasts and osteocytes in the bone under physiological condition. In the kidney, FGF-23 binds to FGF receptor in the proximal tubule in the presence of coreceptor klotho resulting an inhibition of proximal tubular phosphate reabsorption and a suppression of 1,25-dihydroxy vitamin D synthesis [31]. In CKD, FGF-23 levels increase since stage 2 and continue to rise as CKD progresses. In CKD stages 5-5D, FGF-23 levels are normally several hundred folds above the normal range [2, 32]. In healthy subjects, FGF-23 increases after hours of dietary phosphate load; however, a 4-hour intravenous infusion of phosphate does not alter FGF-23 level at 6 hours, whereas chronic phosphate infusion results in an increase in FGF-23 at 24 hours [28–30, 33, 34]. These data suggest a rather indirect influence of phosphate on FGF-23 secretion. The situation may be somewhat different in CKD when these patients are predisposed to phosphate accumulation due to reduced renal function. To date, the exact relationship between phosphate and FGF-23 in CKD remains unclear. In epidemiological studies, both eGFR and serum phosphate correlate closely with FGF-23 levels [35, 36]. Similar to healthy subjects, dietary phosphate load in subjects with impaired renal function results in an increase in circulating FGF-23 [37]. However, both experimental and epidemiological studies have confirmed the increase in circulating FGF-23 since CKD stage 2 prior to any significant accumulation of phosphate. This early increase in FGF-23 drives a dip in serum phosphate from baseline as a result of heightened urinary phosphate excretion (Figure 2) [2, 38]. These evidences indicate that, initially, the stimuli for FGF-23 secretion is the decline in eGFR followed by the accumulation of phosphate in the later period.

Several studies in populations with preserved renal function and early CKD have linked FGF-23 to left ventricular hypertrophy and decreased left ventricular ejection fraction [39–42]. Increased circulating FGF-23 has also been shown to predict incident and worsening heart failure, atrial fibrillation, cardiovascular events, and mortality [40, 43–55]. One of the important evidences that connects high circulating FGF-23 to abnormal cardiac structure and function is the direct effect of FGF-23 on cardiomyocytes. Pathological level of FGF-23 can induce cardiomyocyte hypertrophy through its binding to FGF receptor-4 in a klotho-independent manner [56, 57]. Further evidence also indicates that the stressed myocardium under pressure or volume overload can also produce FGF-23 resulting in a marked increase in FGF-23 level [58]. These data suggest that the stimuli for FGF-23 secretion include not only diminished renal function and phosphate load but also myocardium under stress. The latter explains the rather consistent relationship between increased FGF-23 levels with cardiac hypertrophy and heart failure in the population with preserved renal function. Furthermore, the antagonistic effect of FGF-23 on 1,25-dihydroxyvitamin D can also trigger renin-angiotensin-aldosterone system resulting in an increase in sodium reabsorption [54, 59]. Recent evidence also suggests that FGF-23 is a negative regulator of erythropoiesis and may promote inflammation [60–62].

5. Extracellular Phosphate and Cytotoxicity

Increased extracellular phosphate can induce vascular smooth muscle cell (VSMC) transformation to osteogenic phenotype [63]. These osteogenic VSMCs can release matrix vesicles in a similar fashion to osteoblasts but with less calcification inhibitor, matrix-gla protein. Dying VSMCs also form apoptotic body. Both matrix vesicles and apoptotic bodies have the ability to concentrate and crystalize calcium and phosphate in the preparation for mineralization [64]. In addition to the effect on VSMCs, increased extracellular phosphate can also induce endothelial cell apoptosis [65]. Recent knowledge on extracellular phosphate and cytotoxicity is derived from works related to the formation of protein-mineral complex or calciprotein particles (CPPs). First, fetuin-A, a naturally occurring calcification inhibitor, binds and sequesters calcium and phosphate forming primary CPPs. Primary CPPs then undergo topological rearrangement to form a more stable structure referred to as secondary CPPs. These CPPs exist as colloids and do not precipitate spontaneously [66]. Serum CPP levels increase as kidney function declines and correlate independently with serum phosphate. CPPs can be detected since early stages of CKD when baseline serum phosphate is still within the normal range [67, 68]. At first, CPPs were believed to play a protective role in sequestering and inhibiting calcium-phosphate crystal growth. However, several observational studies have identified the relationship between increased circulating CPPs, especially secondary CPPs, with inflammation, coronary artery calcification, aortic stiffness, and mortality [68, 69]. It is possible that CPPs are bioactive ligand that can induce cellular toxicity. Indeed, in vitro studies have shown that secondary CPPs (not primary CPPs) can induce inflammation and promote osteogenic differentiation of VSMCs [70, 71]. The recent study has also identified the difference between CPPs from healthy subjects and CPPs from CKD patients. Secondary CPPs from CKD patients have lower levels of calcification inhibitors, fetuin-A, and Gla-rich protein, with increased mineral maturation. These secondary CPPs are readily taken up by VSMCs and induce vascular calcification [72].

In conclusion, phosphate accumulation produces detrimental effects on cardiovascular system resulting in poor patient outcomes. The accumulation of phosphate occurs long before the rise in serum phosphate above the normal range. High phosphate diet can increase serum phosphate and FGF-23. FGF-23 has a direct effect on cardiac myocytes causing myocardial hypertrophy. Increased extracellular phosphate is toxic to endothelial cells, promotes the formation of CPPs, and induces VSMC transformation to osteogenic phenotype.

References

[1] M. E. Weeks, "The discovery of the elements. II. elements known to the alchemists," *Journal of Chemical Education*, vol. 9, no. I, pp. 11–21, 1932.

[2] T. Isakova, P. Wahl, G. S. Vargas et al., "Fibroblast growth factor 23 is elevated before parathyroid hormone and phosphate in

chronic kidney disease," *Kidney International*, vol. 79, no. 12, pp. 1370–1378, 2011.

[3] K. Chartsrisak, K. Vipattawat, M. Assanatham et al., "Mineral metabolism and outcomes in chronic kidney disease stage 2-4 patients," *BMC Nephrology*, vol. 14, no. 1, article no. 14, 2013.

[4] J. H. Ix, C. A. M. Anderson, G. Smits, M. S. Persky, and G. A. Block, "Effect of dietary phosphate intake on the circadian rhythm of serum phosphate concentrations in chronic kidney disease: A crossover study," *American Journal of Clinical Nutrition*, vol. 100, no. 5, pp. 1392–1397, 2014.

[5] B. Kestenbaum, J. N. Sampson, K. D. Rudser et al., "Serum phosphate levels and mortality risk among people with chronic kidney disease," *Journal of the American Society of Nephrology*, vol. 16, no. 2, pp. 520–528, 2005.

[6] A. Bellasi, M. Mandreoli, L. Baldrati et al., "Chronic kidney disease progression and outcome according to serum phosphorus in mild-to-moderate kidney dysfunction," *Clinical Journal of the American Society of Nephrology*, vol. 6, no. 4, pp. 883–891, 2011.

[7] A. P. McGovern, S. de Lusignan, J. van Vlymen et al., "Serum Phosphate as a Risk Factor for Cardiovascular Events in People with and without Chronic Kidney Disease: A Large Community Based Cohort Study," *PLoS ONE*, vol. 8, no. 9, Article ID e74996, 2013.

[8] J. Da, X. Xie, M. Wolf et al., "Serum Phosphorus and Progression of CKD and Mortality: A Meta-analysis of Cohort Studies," *American Journal of Kidney Diseases*, vol. 66, no. 2, pp. 258–265, 2015.

[9] M. Tonelli, F. Sacks, M. Pfeffer, Z. Gao, and G. Curhan, "Relation between serum phosphate level and cardiovascular event rate in people with coronary disease," *Circulation*, vol. 112, no. 17, pp. 2627–2633, 2005.

[10] R. Dhingra, L. M. Sullivan, C. S. Fox et al., "Relations of serum phosphorus and calcium levels to the incidence of cardiovascular disease in the community," *JAMA Internal Medicine*, vol. 167, no. 9, pp. 879–885, 2007.

[11] R. N. Foley, A. J. Collins, A. Ishani, and P. A. Kalra, "Calcium-phosphate levels and cardiovascular disease in community-dwelling adults: The Atherosclerosis Risk in Communities (ARIC) Study," *American Heart Journal*, vol. 156, no. 3, pp. 556–563, 2008.

[12] R. N. Foley, "Phosphate levels and cardiovascular disease in the general population," *Clinical Journal of the American Society of Nephrology*, vol. 4, no. 6, pp. 1136–1139, 2009.

[13] T. E. Larsson, H. Olauson, E. Hagström et al., "Conjoint effects of serum calcium and phosphate on risk of total, cardiovascular, and noncardiovascular mortality in the community," *Arteriosclerosis, Thrombosis, and Vascular Biology*, vol. 30, no. 2, pp. 333–339, 2010.

[14] J. P. Linefsky, K. D. OBrien, R. Katz et al., "Association of serum phosphate levels with aortic valve sclerosis and annular calcification," *Journal of the American College of Cardiology*, vol. 58, no. 3, pp. 291–297, 2011.

[15] S. Shin, K.-J. Kim, H.-J. Chang et al., "Impact of serum calcium and phosphate on coronary atherosclerosis detected by cardiac computed tomography," *European Heart Journal*, vol. 33, no. 22, pp. 2873–2881, 2012.

[16] S. G. Wannamethee, N. Sattar, O. Papcosta, L. Lennon, and P. H. Whincup, "Alkaline phosphatase, serum phosphate, and incident cardiovascular disease and total mortality in older men," *Arteriosclerosis, Thrombosis, and Vascular Biology*, vol. 33, no. 5, pp. 1070–1076, 2013.

[17] A. R. Chang and M. E. Grams, "Serum Phosphorus and mortality in the Third National Health and Nutrition Examination Survey (NHANES III): Effect modification by fasting," *American Journal of Kidney Diseases*, vol. 64, no. 4, pp. 567–573, 2014.

[18] J.-W. Li, C. Xu, Y. Fan, Y. Wang, and Y.-B. Xiao, "Can serum levels of alkaline phosphatase and phosphate predict cardiovascular diseases and total mortality in individuals with preserved renal function? A systemic review and meta-analysis," *PLoS ONE*, vol. 9, no. 7, Article ID e102276, 2014.

[19] W. Bai, J. Li, and J. Liu, "Serum phosphorus, cardiovascular and all-cause mortality in the general population: A meta-analysis," *Clinica Chimica Acta*, vol. 461, pp. 76–82, 2016.

[20] M. E. Turner, C. A. White, W. M. Hopman et al., "Impaired Phosphate Tolerance Revealed With an Acute Oral Challenge," *Journal of Bone and Mineral Research*, vol. 33, no. 1, pp. 113–122, 2018.

[21] R. McClelland, K. Christensen, S. Mohammed et al., "Accelerated ageing and renal dysfunction links lower socioeconomic status and dietary phosphate intake," *AGING*, vol. 8, no. 5, pp. 1135–1149, 2016.

[22] C. D. Chue, N. C. Edwards, W. E. Moody, R. P. Steeds, J. N. Townend, and C. J. Ferro, "Serum phosphate is associated with left ventricular mass in patients with chronic kidney disease: A cardiac magnetic resonance study," *Heart*, vol. 98, no. 3, pp. 219–224, 2012.

[23] K. T. Yamamoto, C. Robinson-Cohen, M. C. De Oliveira et al., "Dietary phosphorus is associated with greater left ventricular mass," *Kidney International*, vol. 83, no. 4, pp. 707–714, 2013.

[24] E. Shuto, Y. Taketani, R. Tanaka et al., "Dietary phosphorus acutely impairs endothelial function," *Journal of the American Society of Nephrology*, vol. 20, no. 7, pp. 1504–1512, 2009.

[25] B. M. Levac, M. A. Adams, and K. E. Pyke, "The impact of an acute oral phosphate load on endothelium dependent and independent brachial artery vasodilation in healthy males," *Applied Physiology, Nutrition, and Metabolism*, vol. 42, no. 12, pp. 1307–1315, 2017.

[26] S. T. Itkonen, H. J. Karp, V. E. Kemi et al., "Associations among total and food additive phosphorus intake and carotid intima-media thickness - A cross-sectional study in a middle-aged population in Southern Finland," *Nutrition Journal*, vol. 12, no. 1, article no. 94, 2013.

[27] A. Ramírez-Morros, M. Granado-Casas, N. Alcubierre et al., "Calcium Phosphate Product Is Associated with Subclinical Carotid Atherosclerosis in Type 2 Diabetes," *Journal of Diabetes Research*, vol. 2017, pp. 1–8, 2017.

[28] S. L. Ferrari, J.-P. Bonjour, and R. Rizzoli, "Fibroblast growth factor-23 relationship to dietary phosphate and renal phosphate handling in healthy young men," *The Journal of Clinical Endocrinology & Metabolism*, vol. 90, no. 3, pp. 1519–1524, 2005.

[29] Y. Nishida, Y. Taketani, H. Yamanaka-Okumura et al., "Acute effect of oral phosphate loading on serum fibroblast growth factor 23 levels in healthy men," *Kidney International*, vol. 70, no. 12, pp. 2141–2147, 2006.

[30] S.-A. M. Burnett, S. C. Gunawardene, F. R. Bringhurst, H. Jüppner, H. Lee, and J. S. Finkelstein, "Regulation of C-terminal and intact FGF-23 by dietary phosphate in men and women," *Journal of Bone and Mineral Research*, vol. 21, no. 8, pp. 1187–1196, 2006.

[31] T. Shimada, H. Hasegawa, Y. Yamazaki et al., "FGF-23 is a potent regulator of vitamin D metabolism and phosphate

homeostasis," *Journal of Bone and Mineral Research*, vol. 19, no. 3, pp. 429–435, 2004.

[32] R. C. Pereira, H. Juppner, C. E. Azucena-Serrano, O. Yadin, I. B. Salusky, and K. Wesseling-Perry, "Patterns of FGF-23, DMP1, and MEPE expression in patients with chronic kidney disease," *Bone*, vol. 45, no. 6, pp. 1161–1168, 2009.

[33] N. Ito, S. Fukumoto, Y. Takeuchi et al., "Effect of acute changes of serum phosphate on fibroblast growth factor (FGF)23 levels in humans," *Journal of Bone and Mineral Metabolism*, vol. 25, no. 6, pp. 419–422, 2007.

[34] N. Arai-Nunota, M. Mizobuchi, H. Ogata et al., "Intravenous phosphate loading increases fibroblast growth factor 23 in uremic rats," *PLoS ONE*, vol. 9, no. 3, Article ID e91096, 2014.

[35] O. Gutierrez, T. Isakova, E. Rhee et al., "Fibroblast growth factor-23 mitigates hyperphosphatemia but accentuates calcitriol deficiency in chronic kidney disease," *Journal of the American Society of Nephrology*, vol. 16, no. 7, pp. 2205–2215, 2005.

[36] D. Fliser, B. Kollerits, U. Neyer et al., "Fibroblast growth factor 23 (FGF23) predicts progression of chronic kidney disease: the Mild to Moderate Kidney Disease (MMKD) Study," *Journal of the American Society of Nephrology*, vol. 18, no. 9, pp. 2600–2608, 2007.

[37] M. Sigrist, M. Tang, M. Beaulieu et al., "Responsiveness of FGF-23 and mineral metabolism to altered dietary phosphate intake in chronic kidney disease (CKD): Results of a randomized trial," *Nephrology Dialysis Transplantation* , vol. 28, no. 1, pp. 161–169, 2013.

[38] H. Hasegawa, N. Nagano, I. Urakawa et al., "Direct evidence for a causative role of FGF23 in the abnormal renal phosphate handling and vitamin D metabolism in rats with early-stage chronic kidney disease," *Kidney International*, vol. 78, no. 10, pp. 975–980, 2010.

[39] O. M. Gutiérrez, J. L. Januzzi, T. Isakova et al., "Fibroblast growth factor 23 and left ventricular hypertrophy in chronic kidney disease," *Circulation*, vol. 119, no. 19, pp. 2545–2552, 2009.

[40] S. Seiler, B. Cremers, N. M. Rebling et al., "The phosphatonin fibroblast growth factor 23 links calciumphosphate metabolism with left-ventricular dysfunction and atrial fibrillation," *European Heart Journal*, vol. 32, no. 21, pp. 2688–2696, 2011.

[41] K. Smith, C. Defilippi, T. Isakova et al., "Fibroblast growth factor 23, high-sensitivity cardiac troponin, and left ventricular hypertrophy in CKD," *American Journal of Kidney Diseases*, vol. 61, no. 1, pp. 67–73, 2013.

[42] I. Agarwal, N. Ide, J. H. Ix et al., "Fibroblast growth factor-23 and cardiac structure and function," *Journal of the American Heart Association*, vol. 3, no. 1, Article ID e000584, 2014.

[43] S. Seiler, B. Reichart, D. Roth, E. Seibert, D. Fliser, and G. H. Heine, "FGF-23 and future cardiovascular events in patients with chronic kidney disease before initiation of dialysis treatment," *Nephrology Dialysis Transplantation* , vol. 25, no. 12, pp. 3983–3989, 2010.

[44] J. Kendrick, A. K. Cheung, J. S. Kaufman et al., "FGF-23 associates with death, cardiovascular events, and initiation of chronic dialysis," *Journal of the American Society of Nephrology*, vol. 22, no. 10, pp. 1913–1922, 2011.

[45] J. H. Ix, R. Katz, B. R. Kestenbaum et al., "Fibroblast growth factor-23 and death, heart failure, and cardiovascular events in community-living individuals: CHS (Cardiovascular Health Study)," *Journal of the American College of Cardiology*, vol. 60, no. 3, pp. 200–207, 2012.

[46] J. S. Mathew, M. C. Sachs, and R. Katz, "Fibroblast growth factor-23 and incident atrial fibrillation: The multi-ethnic study of atherosclerosis (MESA) and the cardiovascular health study (CHS)," *Circulation*, vol. 130, no. 4, pp. 298–307, 2014.

[47] B. Kestenbaum, M. C. Sachs, A. N. Hoofnagle et al., "Fibroblast growth factor-23 and cardiovascular disease in the general population the multi-ethnic study of atherosclerosis," *Circulation: Heart Failure*, vol. 7, no. 3, pp. 409–417, 2014.

[48] J. J. Scialla, H. Xie, M. Rahman et al., "Fibroblast growth factor-23 and cardiovascular events in CKD," *Journal of the American Society of Nephrology*, vol. 25, no. 2, pp. 349–360, 2014.

[49] J. A. Udell, D. A. Morrow, P. Jarolim et al., "Fibroblast growth factor-23, cardiovascular prognosis, and benefit of angiotensin-converting enzyme inhibition in stable ischemic heart disease," *Journal of the American College of Cardiology*, vol. 63, no. 22, pp. 2421–2428, 2014.

[50] S. Seiler, K. S. Rogacev, H. J. Roth et al., "Associations of FGF-23 and sKlotho with cardiovascular outcomes among patients with CKD stages 2–4," *Clinical Journal of the American Society of Nephrology*, vol. 9, no. 6, pp. 1049–1058, 2014.

[51] R. D. Giuseppe, B. Buijsse, F. Hirche et al., "Plasma fibroblast growth factor 23, parathyroid hormone, 25-hydroxyvitamin D3, and risk of heart failure: A prospective, case-cohort study," *The Journal of Clinical Endocrinology & Metabolism*, vol. 99, no. 3, pp. 947–955, 2014.

[52] L. Koller, M. E. Kleber, V. M. Brandenburg et al., "Fibroblast Growth Factor 23 Is an Independent and Specific Predictor of Mortality in Patients With Heart Failure and Reduced Ejection Fraction," *Circulation: Heart Failure*, vol. 8, no. 6, pp. 1059–1067, 2015.

[53] P. L. Lutsey, A. Alonso, E. Selvin et al., "Fibroblast growth factor-23 and incident coronary heart disease, heart failure, and cardiovascular mortality: The atherosclerosis risk in communities study," *Journal of the American Heart Association*, vol. 3, no. 3, Article ID 000936, 2014.

[54] P. Wohlfahrt, V. Melenovsky, M. Kotrc et al., "Association of Fibroblast Growth Factor-23 Levels and Angiotensin-Converting Enzyme Inhibition in Chronic Systolic Heart Failure," *JACC: Heart Failure*, vol. 3, no. 10, article no. 349, pp. 829–839, 2015.

[55] J. M. ter Maaten, A. A. Voors, K. Damman et al., "Fibroblast growth factor 23 is related to profiles indicating volume overload, poor therapy optimization and prognosis in patients with new-onset and worsening heart failure," *International Journal of Cardiology*, vol. 253, pp. 84–90, 2018.

[56] C. Faul, A. P. Amaral, B. Oskouei et al., "FGF23 induces left ventricular hypertrophy," *The Journal of Clinical Investigation*, vol. 121, no. 11, pp. 4393–4408, 2011.

[57] A. Grabner, A. P. Amaral, K. Schramm et al., "Activation of Cardiac Fibroblast Growth Factor Receptor 4 Causes Left Ventricular Hypertrophy," *Cell Metabolism*, vol. 22, no. 6, pp. 1020–1032, 2015.

[58] S. Slavic, K. Ford, M. Modert et al., "Genetic Ablation of Fgf23 or Klotho Does not Modulate Experimental Heart Hypertrophy Induced by Pressure Overload," *Scientific Reports*, vol. 7, no. 1, Article ID 11298, 2017.

[59] M. H. de Borst, M. G. Vervloet, P. M. ter Wee, and G. Navis, "Cross talk between the renin-angiotensin-aldosterone system and vitamin D-FGF-23-klotho in chronic kidney disease," *Journal of the American Society of Nephrology*, vol. 22, no. 9, pp. 1603–1609, 2011.

[60] L. M. Coe, S. V. Madathil, C. Casu, B. Lanske, S. Rivella, and D. Sitara, "FGF-23 is a negative regulator of prenatal and postnatal erythropoiesis," *The Journal of Biological Chemistry*, vol. 289, no. 14, pp. 9795–9810, 2014.

[61] M. Holecki, J. Chudek, A. Owczarek et al., "Inflammation but not obesity or insulin resistance is associated with increased plasma fibroblast growth factor 23 concentration in the elderly," *Clinical Endocrinology*, vol. 82, no. 6, pp. 900–909, 2015.

[62] S. Singh, A. Grabner, C. Yanucil et al., "Fibroblast growth factor 23 directly targets hepatocytes to promote inflammation in chronic kidney disease," *Kidney International*, vol. 90, no. 5, pp. 985–996, 2016.

[63] S. Jono, M. D. McKee, C. E. Murry et al., "Phosphate regulation of vascular smooth muscle cell calcification," *Circulation Research*, vol. 87, no. 7, pp. e10–e17, 2000.

[64] J. L. Reynolds, A. J. Joannides, J. N. Skepper et al., "Human vascular smooth muscle cells undergo vesicle-mediated calcification in response to changes in extracellular calcium and phosphate concentrations: a potential mechanism for accelerated vascular calcification in ESRD," *Journal of the American Society of Nephrology*, vol. 15, no. 11, pp. 2857–2867, 2004.

[65] G. S. Di Marco, M. Hausberg, U. Hillebrand et al., "Increased inorganic phosphate induces human endothelial cell apoptosis in vitro," *American Journal of Physiology-Renal Physiology*, vol. 294, no. 6, pp. F1381–F1387, 2008.

[66] M. Kuro-o, "Klotho, phosphate and FGF-23 in ageing and disturbed mineral metabolism," *Nature Reviews Nephrology*, vol. 9, no. 11, pp. 650–660, 2013.

[67] T. Hamano, I. Matsui, S. Mikami et al., "Fetuin-mineral complex reflects extraosseous calcification stress in CKD," *Journal of the American Society of Nephrology*, vol. 21, pp. 1998–2007, 2010.

[68] E. R. Smith, M. L. Ford, L. A. Tomlinson, C. Rajkumar, L. P. McMahon, and S. G. Holt, "Phosphorylated fetuin-A-containing calciprotein particles are associated with aortic stiffness and a procalcific milieu in patients with pre-dialysis CKD," *Nephrology Dialysis Transplantation* , vol. 27, no. 5, pp. 1957–1966, 2012.

[69] E. R. Smith, M. L. Ford, L. A. Tomlinson et al., "Serum calcification propensity predicts all-cause mortality in predialysis CKD," *Journal of the American Society of Nephrology*, vol. 25, no. 2, pp. 339–348, 2014.

[70] E. R. Smith, E. Hanssen, L. P. McMahon, and S. G. Holt, "Fetuin-A-containing calciprotein particles reduce mineral stress in the macrophage," *PLoS ONE*, vol. 8, no. 4, Article ID e60904, 2013.

[71] P. Aghagolzadeh, M. Bachtler, R. Bijarnia et al., "Calcification of vascular smooth muscle cells is induced by secondary calciprotein particles and enhanced by tumor necrosis factor-α," *Atherosclerosis*, vol. 251, pp. 404–414, 2016.

[72] C. S. Viegas, L. Santos, A. L. Macedo et al., "Chronic Kidney Disease Circulating Calciprotein Particles and Extracellular Vesicles Promote Vascular Calcification: A Role for GRP (Gla-Rich Protein)," *Arteriosclerosis, Thrombosis, and Vascular Biology*, vol. 38, no. 3, pp. 575–587, 2018.

Proteasome Activators, PA28α and PA28β, Govern Development of Microvascular Injury in Diabetic Nephropathy and Retinopathy

Saeed Yadranji Aghdam[1,2] and Ali Mahmoudpour[3]

[1]*Reynolds Institute on Aging, Room No. 4151, 629 Jack Stephens Drive, Little Rock, AR 72205, USA*
[2]*Department of Geriatrics, University of Arkansas for Medical Sciences, Little Rock, AR, USA*
[3]*Norgen Biotek Corp., 3430 Schmon Parkway, Thorold, ON, Canada L2V 4Y6*

Correspondence should be addressed to Saeed Yadranji Aghdam; syaghdam@uams.edu

Academic Editor: Kazunari Kaneko

Diabetic nephropathy (DN) and diabetic retinopathy (DR) are major complications of type 1 and type 2 diabetes. DN and DR are mainly caused by injury to the perivascular supporting cells, the mesangial cells within the glomerulus, and the pericytes in the retina. The genes and molecular mechanisms predisposing retinal and glomerular pericytes to diabetic injury are poorly characterized. In this study, the genetic deletion of proteasome activator genes, PA28α and PA28β genes, protected the diabetic mice in the experimental STZ-induced diabetes model against renal injury and retinal microvascular injury and prolonged their survival compared with wild type STZ diabetic mice. The improved wellbeing and reduced renal damage was associated with diminished expression of Osteopontin (OPN) and Monocyte Chemoattractant Protein-1 (MCP-1) in the glomeruli of STZ-injected PA28α/PA28β double knockout (Pa28$\alpha\beta$DKO) mice and also in cultured mesangial cells and retinal pericytes isolated from Pa28$\alpha\beta$DKO mice that were grown in high glucose. The mesangial PA28-mediated expression of OPN under high glucose conditions was suppressed by peptides capable of inhibiting the binding of PA28 to the 20S proteasome. Collectively, our findings demonstrate that diabetic hyperglycemia promotes PA28-mediated alteration of proteasome activity in vulnerable perivascular cells resulting in microvascular injury and development of DN and DR.

1. Introduction

Diabetic high blood glucose or hyperglycemia causes mortality and morbidity through DN and DR via disrupting the vascular function in the kidney and retina. These pathologies are the major cause of death associated with renal failure and blindness among the type 1 and type 2 diabetes patients [1–3]. Similar molecular pathways appear to govern the development of diabetic renal and retinal microvascular injury. This speculation arises from higher coincidence rates of DN and DR; that is, patients with DN have already developed DR and patients with DR are vulnerable to develop DN [4, 5]. According to the similarities in pathologic background affecting the retina and kidney, it was hypothesized that DN and DR could arise by injuries to perivascular supporting cells in glomeruli and retina. The vulnerable vascular cell types affected by diabetic hyperglycemia are retinal pericytes (RPC) and their analogs within glomeruli are the mesangial cells. In DR, the RPC undergo cell death and disengage from the retinal vasculature, predisposing the retina to neoangiogenesis, vascular leakage, and tractional retinal detachment culminating in reduced vision or terminal blindness [6–8]. DN is characterized by mesangial matrix expansion and the obstruction of the glomerular capillaries within the renal filtration units, the glomeruli [9]. The glomerulopathy in DN is associated with reduced efficiency of renal filtration, and in chronically established cases it triggers end-stage renal failure and mortality [10].

Several biochemical mechanisms and pathways have been described in speculation of the pathogenesis caused by either

DN or DR. These mechanisms include enhanced oxidative stress, enhanced polyol pathway, PKC activation, inflammation, and advanced glycation end product formation [3, 11–13]. The most extensively investigated mechanisms associated with the development of both DN and DR are enhanced oxidative stress and inflammation caused by metabolic alterations. However, a plethora of evidence indicates that immunological and inflammatory mechanisms are important factors in development and progression of DR and DN [14–17]. The recruitment of the activated macrophages and increased generation of inflammatory and proinflammatory mediators (TNF-α, IL-1β, IL-6, MCP-1, and OPN) in retinal and renal milieu is linked to the progression and exacerbation of the DN and DR [17–22]. However, the exact molecular and cellular mechanisms involved have remained elusive.

Oxidative stress is a phenomenon in which the balance between the generation of free oxidizing radicals and the system responsible for their removal in the cell is disturbed leading to enhanced formation of free reactive ions including reactive oxygen species (ROS). The increased ROS levels in cells subjected to diabetic hyperglycemia drive the antioxidant gene expression to protect the cells from oxidative injuries [23]. One of the target genes to be induced following oxidative stress is the NF-E2-related transcription factor 2 (Nrf2). Two of the recently characterized genes that are regulated by the Nrf-2 and provide protection against oxidative stress and stress-adaptation are proteasome activator genes, PA28α and PA28β [24]. It is speculated that PA28 proteins increase the proteasomal degradation activity to clear the oxidized or misfolded proteins [24–26]. The PA28α/β genes were initially identified as components of immunoproteasomes which are induced in response to interferon-γ. PA28α and PA28β proteins form a heptameric complex (4β/3α) acting as the gate opener for the 20S proteasomes, hence stimulating the degradation of the nonubiquitinated short peptides. The well-characterized function for the PA28 proteins is the generation of the antigenic peptides to be presented by the MHC class I molecules [27, 28].

The PA28α/β are upregulated in the cultured RPC under high glucose conditions and also in the intraglomerular capillaries of older type 1 diabetic Akita mice [1]. To understand the role of PA28α/β genes in development of DN and DR, Pa28αβDKO mice were tested and their physiological and biometric indices were compared with STZ-induced diabetic wild type mice. The diabetic Pa28αβDKO mice provided higher survival rate, higher body weight, more efficient renal filtration function, and reduced microvascular damage in their retinae compared to diabetic wild type mice. The glomeruli, mesangial cells, and the RPC isolated from Pa28αβDKO mice had lower levels of OPN and MCP-1 under high glucose conditions. OPN is known as a proinflammatory protein associated with progression of diabetic microvascular injury [19, 22]. The PA28-dependent regulation of OPN expression was stimulated by high glucose and abrogated by synthetic peptides that block the binding of PA28 to 20S proteasomes. Therefore, the findings of this study provide novel insights into the role of the ubiquitin proteasome system (UPS) and specially the PA28 proteins, in regulating the microvascular injury in diabetes.

2. Material and Methods

2.1. Animals. Animal maintenance, genotyping, treatments, and analytical procedures followed the guidelines accredited by Institutional Animal Care and Use Committee of the University of Wisconsin, School of Medicine and Public Health. All the mice used for the experiments were in C57BL/6 background. For cell isolation, 6-week old male immorto mice (stock number 006553) and to study diabetes, Pa28αβDKO male mice (stock number 021202) were used. Diabetes was induced in animals with a single injection of streptozotocin (STZ; 180 mg/kg in citrate buffer, pH 4.2 by ip injection). Three days following the treatment, the blood glucose of all STZ-injected animals was above 400 mg/dL.

2.2. Albumin-to-Creatinine Ratio (ACR) Analysis. For ACR analysis the urine samples were collected by housing each individual mouse in a metabolic cage (Tecniplast, Italy) for 24 hours. Urinary albumin and creatinine levels were measured by ELISA (Albuwell M, Exocell) and the ACR measurements were conducted according to the guidelines provided by the manufacturer.

2.3. Transmission Electron Microscopy (TEM) and Histological Analysis. Mouse kidneys were sliced and immersion-fixed in a solution of 2% paraformaldehyde (PFA) and 2.5% glutaraldehyde in 0.1 M sodium cacodylate buffer, pH 7.4, overnight at 4°C. The tissue was postfixed at room temperature for 2 hours in 1% osmium tetroxide in the same buffer. Subsequently the samples were dehydrated in a graded ethanol series, then dehydrated in propylene oxide, and embedded in Epon epoxy resin. Ultrathin sections were prepared using Leica UC6 Ultramicrotome and mounted on 200-mesh carbon-coated copper grids. Tissue sections were observed with a Philips CM120 electron microscope, and images were captured with a MegaView III side-mounted digital camera.

For PAS and JMS-H&E staining the formalin fixed, paraffin embedded, 5-6 μm tissue sections were deparaffinized in xylene and rehydrated in descending graded percentage of ethanol (100%, 95%, 80%, and 70%) and routinely stained with recommended reagents. Digital images were taken with NA PL APO objectives (10x/0.25 NA, 40x/0.95 NA, and 63x/1.4 NA oil) on a ScanScope XT system using ImageScope version 10 software (Aperio Technologies Inc.).

2.4. Cell Isolation, Culture, and Peptide Transfections. The isolation and culture of the RPC was described before [29]. Briefly, the retinae from one litter (6-7 pups, 6-week old) immorto mice were collected under a dissecting microscope. The collected retinae were rinsed with serum-free Dulbecco's Modified Eagle's Medium (DMEM), pooled, minced, and digested for 45 min with collagenase type II (1 mg/mL, Worthington) with 0.1% BSA in serum-free DMEM at 37°C. Cells were resuspended in equal amount of DMEM containing 10% Fetal Bovine Serum (FBS) and spun for 5 min at 400 ×g. The pelleted cells were resuspended in 4 mL DMEM containing 10% FBS, 2 mM L-glutamine, 100 μg/mL streptomycin, 100 U/mL penicillin, and recombinant murine IFN-γ (R&D

Systems) at 44 U/mL. Cells were evenly divided into 4 wells of a 24-well tissue culture plate and maintained at 33°C with 5% CO_2. Cells were progressively passed to larger plates and maintained and propagated in 60 mm dishes.

The isolation and culture of mouse REC was described elsewhere [30]. The retinae from one litter (6 to 7 pups, 6-week old) of immorto mice were dissected out aseptically under a dissecting microscope and kept in HBSS buffer containing penicillin/streptomycin. Retinae were pooled together, rinsed with HBSS buffer (Life Technologies), minced into small pieces in a 60 mm tissue culture dish using sterile razor blades, and digested in 5 mL of collagenase type I (1 mg/mL in serum-free DMEM, Worthington) for 45 min at 37°C. Following digestion, DMEM with 10% FBS was added and cells were pelleted. The cells were passed through a sterile 40 μm nylon strainer (BD Falcon) and spun at 400 ×g for 10 min to pellet cells, and cells were washed twice with DMEM containing 10% FBS. The cells were resuspended in 1.5 mL medium (DMEM with 10% FBS) and incubated with anti-PECAM-1 antibody-conjugated Dynabeads (Life Technologies). After affinity binding, magnetic beads were rinsed six times with DMEM with 10% FBS and bound cells in endothelial cell growth medium were plated into a single well of a 24-well plate precoated with 2 μg/mL of human fibronectin (BD Biosciences). Endothelial cells were grown in DMEM containing 20% FBS, 2 mM L-glutamine, 2 mM sodium pyruvate, 20 mM HEPES, 1% nonessential amino acids, 100 μg/mL streptomycin, 100 U/mL penicillin, freshly added heparin at 55 U/mL (Sigma), endothelial growth supplement 100 μg/mL (Sigma), and recombinant murine IFN-γ (R&D Systems) at 44 U/mL. Cells were maintained at 33°C with 5% CO_2. Cells were progressively passed to larger plates, maintained, and propagated in 1% gelatin-coated 60 mm dishes.

The glomeruli and mesangial cells were isolated using a standard procedure described before [31]. Briefly, 8×10^7 Dynabeads (Life Technologies) were diluted in 40 mL of phosphate-buffered saline and perfused through the heart of the adult mice. The kidneys were extracted, mechanically minced, digested with type 1 collagenase, and filtered through 100 μm strainer. The glomeruli were collected with a magnet and washed three times to eliminate the nonglomerular cells and debris. The glomeruli were grown in either pericytes growth medium to establish the mesangial cell culture.

The KGEC were isolated from the glomeruli similar to mesangial cell isolation following a procedure described before [32]. The purified glomeruli were seeded and allowed to grow in REC medium on coated 35 mm plates. Upon 80–85% confluency, the cells were incubated with anti-PECAM-1 antibody-conjugated Dynabeads, washed, and enriched similar to REC cultures. The purity of the isolated cells was determined by FACS and immunostaining. The BPC, BEC, KPC, HPC, and LPC were isolated by following a procedure similar to RPC isolation. The peptides (CPC Scientific) and the Chariot transfection reagent (Active Motif) were reconstituted and used according to the manufacturer guidelines.

2.5. Trypsin-Digested Retinal Vascular Preparations. The enucleated eyes were fixed in 4% paraformaldehyde for at least 24 h. The dissected retinae were washed overnight in deionized water and incubated in 3% Trypsin (Difco™ Trypsin 250, Becton Dickinson and Company) prepared in 0.1 M Tris, 0.1 M maleic acid, and pH 7.8 containing 0.2 M NaF for 2 h at 37°C. The neuroretinal tissue was gently brushed away, and the resultant isolated vascular tree was air dried onto a glass microscope slide [33].

2.6. RNA Isolation and Real-Time PCR. Total RNA from cells was extracted by total RNA isolation kit (Norgenbiotek) according to the manufacturer's instructions. Cells were allowed to reach 85–90% confluence, rinsed twice with PBS, scraped off the plates, and transferred to RNase-free microfuge tubes. The RNA was purified using Trizol reagent (Life Technologies). The cDNA synthesis was performed with 1 μg of total RNA. One microliter of 1/10-diluted cDNA was used as real-time PCR template in triplicate groups and reaction was completed using SYBR Green master mix in Mastercycler Realplex (Eppendorf) with the specified primers in Supplemental Experimental Procedures. Thermal cycles were programmed as 95°C for 2 min; 40 cycles of amplification (95°C for 15 s and 60°C for 40 s); and a dissociation curve step (95°C for 15 s, 60°C for 15 s, and 95°C for 15 s). Standard curves were generated from known quantities for each target gene of linearized plasmid DNA. Tenfold diluted series were used for each known target to be amplified by SYBR Green qPCR premix. The linear regression line for ng of DNA was calculated from relative fluorescent units at a threshold fluorescence value (Ct) to quantify amplification targets from cell extracts by comparing the relative fluorescent units at the Ct to the standard curve, normalized by the simultaneous amplification of RpL13A (a housekeeping gene) for all samples.

2.7. Protein Isolation and Western Blot. For protein isolation, the cells in 80% confluent dishes were harvested following adding the lysis buffer (150 mM NaCl, 1% Triton X-100, 20 mM Tris-HCl (pH 7.4), protease inhibitor cocktail (1 mM PMSF, 10 mM Leupeptin, 10 mM Pepstatin)). For western blot analysis, 50 μg cell lysate or conditioned medium proteins were mixed with Laemmli sample buffer and the reduced or nonreduced samples were boiled for 10 min. The boiled samples were loaded into 4–20% Tris Glycine acrylamide gels (Life Technologies) and electrophoresis was performed using SDS running buffer (25 mM Tris, 190 mM glycine, 0.1% SDS, pH 8.3).

2.8. Plasmids and Cell Transfections. Mouse cDNA encoding the PA28α and PA28β were cloned into pLVX-IRES-Hyg and pLVX-IRES-Neo plasmids (Clontech), respectively. The lentiviral particles were prepared by transfecting the Lenti-X 293T cells (Clontech) and collecting the conditioned media. The pBABE-OPN/Puro plasmid and the packaging cells are described elsewhere [34]. Cultured cells were transfected using the FuGENE6 reagent (Promega) according to recommended protocol. After 48 h, Hygromycin B (500 μg/mL; Sigma-Aldrich), Neomycin (750 μg/mL; Life Technologies),

TABLE 1: Blood glucose levels in nondiabetic and STZ-injected diabetic mice.

Wild type		Pa28αβDKO		
No STZ	4 m STZ	No STZ	4 m STZ	6 m STZ
139	473	135	483	527
177	569	123	467	483
164	452	226	504	505
192	527	179	513	539
184	568	146	476	543
150	492	152	535	569
182	480	139	432	476
129	493	182	528	481
164	559	165	542	509

The values represent the measured milligrams of glucose per deciliter of blood (mg/dL) in nine wild type and nine Pa28αβDKO mice before and after four or six months of STZ injection.

and Puromycin (5 μg/mL; Sigma-Aldrich) were added to cell cultures.

2.9. Statistical Analysis. The data are represented as the mean ± SEM. Lifespan analyses were performed using Kaplan-Meier survival analysis. Statistical significance was determined by analysis of variance (ANOVA) and Tukey-Kramer post hoc analysis for multiple comparisons using p value of 0.05 in GraphPad Prism software (San Diego, CA, USA). p values $p < 0.05$ were considered significant.

3. Results and Discussion

3.1. PA28α and PA28β Regulate the Survival Rate and Renal Filtration Efficiency in STZ-Induced Diabetic Mice. The PA28 proteasome regulators were previously shown to be dramatically upregulated in the glomerular capillaries of Akita mouse model with chronic hyperglycemia for 8 months but not in the same age wild type nondiabetic mice [1]. In this study the role of PA28α/β in modulating diabetic microvascular disorders was investigated via streptozotocin (STZ) injection to both wild type and Pa28αβDKO mice. STZ has cytotoxic effects on insulin-secreting pancreatic β-cells and induces type I diabetes in experimental animals [35].

All the Pa28αβDKO/STZ and wild type/STZ mice had blood glucose levels above 450 mg/dL three days after STZ injection and on the day of sacrifice (Table 1). In comparison with Pa28αβDKO/STZ mice, the wild type/STZ mice exhibited significantly reduced survival rates and weight loss by four months of STZ injection. The Pa28αβDKO/STZ mice were protected and had no obvious weight loss or reduced survival after six months of STZ injection (Figures 1(a) and 1(b)). It was assumed that improved renal function was responsible for the observed improvement in the health of the Pa28αβDKO/STZ mice. To test this, the albumin-to-creatinine ratio (ACR) test was used. ACR is a cornerstone assay for the diagnosis of renal filtration disorders [36, 37] and reflects the efficiency of the kidney filtration function. The measured albuminuria was significantly higher in wild

type/STZ (291 ± 8.54 μg/mg) compared to that of non-STZ wild type (25.61 ± 2.18 μg/mg) mice and 28αβDKO/STZ mice (119.6 ± 5.61 μg/mg) (Figure 1(c)).

Next the histological and ultrastructural properties of the glomeruli in the non-STZ and STZ-injected mice were assessed. Renal histology in kidney sections was evaluated using the combined Jones Methenamine Silver- (JMS-) Hematoxylin and Eosin (H&E) staining and also Periodic Acid Schiff (PAS) staining. The JMS and PAS staining is routinely used to detect the mesangial matrix increase and changes in the glomerular basement membrane (GBM) [38]. There were no discernible alterations in the appearance of GBMs, the adjacent tubules, and also the mesangial or endothelial cells in different animal groups (Figure 2(a)).

Similar to light microscopic analysis, TEM analysis did not show any significant difference in the thickness of GBM in wild type/STZ and Pa28αβDKO/STZ mice. The lack of visible diabetic glomerular pathology in TEM test despite the reduced renal filtration efficiency (determined by ACR test) in mice studied here is likely due to the resistance of the C57BL/6 mouse line against morphological changes in GBM (Figures 2(b) and 2(c)). However, there was a significant reduction in the relative number of intraglomerular endothelial fenestrae in four-month STZ-injected wild type mice compared to those of Pa28αβDKO/STZ mice (47.5 ± 1.74 versus 60.3 ± 0.67) (Figure 2(d)). Similarly, the six-month STZ-injected Pa28αβDKO mice provided higher endothelial fenestrae compared with four-month STZ-injected wild type mice (56 ± 0.93 versus 47.5 ± 1.74) (Figure 2(d)). Since the inflammatory mediators OPN and MCP-1 have been shown to be closely associated with the development and progression of the DN and DR, we investigated their levels using real-time PCR in the glomerular mRNA isolated from STZ-injected and nondiabetic wild type and Pa28αβDKO mice. The qPCR analyses did not provide any differences in the levels of IL-1β and TNF-α mRNA among wild type and Pa28αβDKO mice under both normal and STZ- injected conditions (not shown). However, the mRNA for OPN and MCP-1 showed significant increase in wild type/STZ versus nondiabetic wild type glomeruli (Figures 3(a) and 3(b)). Interestingly, unlike the wild type/STZ glomeruli, in Pa28αβDKO/STZ glomeruli the expression of OPN and MCP-1 was not altered significantly. These data demonstrate that PA28α and PA28β regulate the diabetic glomerular vascular injuries most likely through regulating the expression of proinflammatory agents.

3.2. Cultured Pa28αβDKO Mesangial Cells Express Reduced Quantities of OPN and MCP-1 under High Glucose Conditions. To understand how PA28α and PA28β genes promote glomerular injuries during diabetes, as an in vitro model, the mesangial cells from wild type and Pa28αβDKO mice were isolated for further characterizations [29, 31, 39]. Since the mRNA levels for OPN and MCP-1 in Pa28αβDKO/STZ glomeruli were lower than those of wild type/STZ mice and the expression of these proteins has been linked to the development of DN and DR, we investigated whether higher glucose concentrations in vitro could induce the expression of

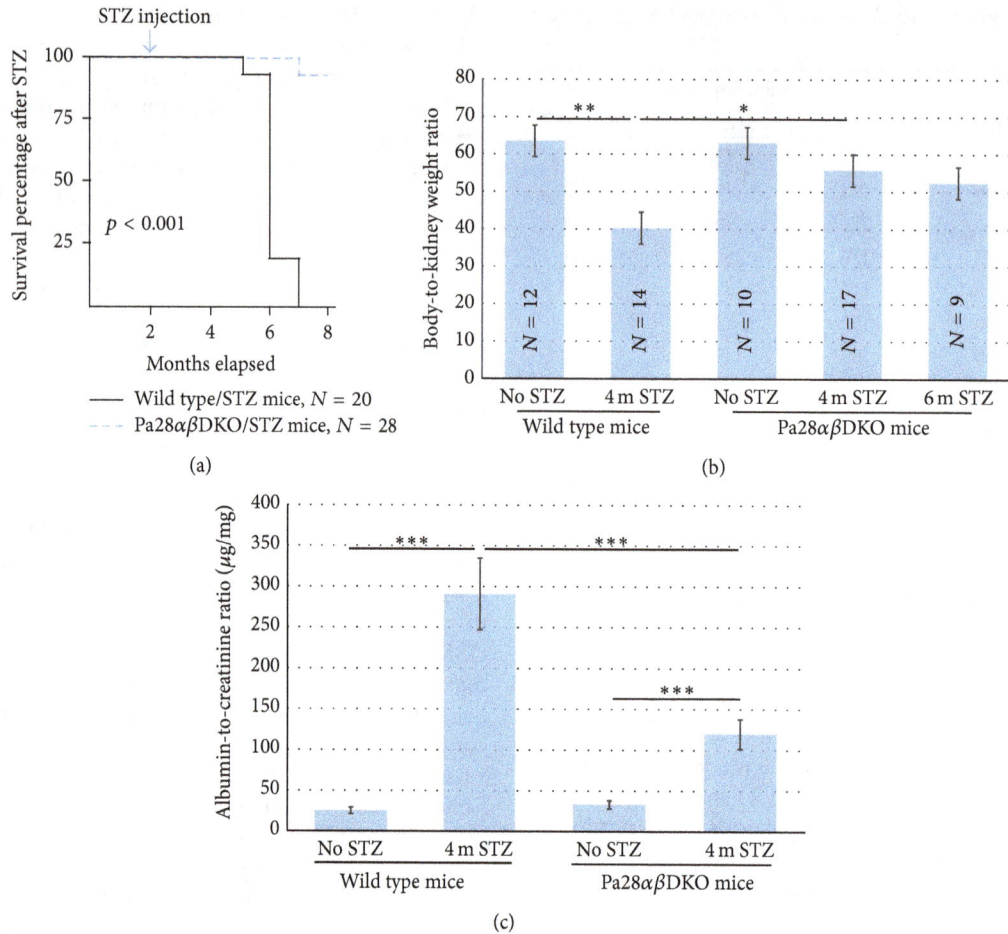

FIGURE 1: Pa28αβDKO/STZ mice provide higher survival rate and better renal filtration efficiency than wild type/STZ mice. (a) Survival rate of wild type and Pa28αβDKO mice following STZ injection. N represents the number of animals in each experimental group. (b) Body-to-kidney weight ratio in wild type and Pa28αβDKO mice before and after STZ injection for four and six months. (c) Albumin-to-creatinine ratio in urine samples of wild type and Pa28αβDKO mice before and after four months of STZ injection. Results presented as mean ± SEM. $^*p < 0.05$, $^{**}p < 0.01$, and $^{***}p < 0.001$.

OPN and MCP-1 genes in isolated mesangial cells. Western blot and qPCR analysis of these genes were performed following three days of treatment with either normal (5 mM D-glucose), high glucose (25 mM or 40 mM D-glucose), or osmolarity control (5 mM D-glucose plus 20 mM L-glucose). Western blot analysis of the conditioned medium provided robust induction of OPN expression in wild type but not in Pa28αβDKO mesangial cells following treatment with high glucose (Figure 4(a)). The qPCR analysis of wild type and Pa28αβDKO cells also confirmed the upregulation of OPN expression in wild type but not in Pa28αβDKO mesangial cells treated with high glucose (Figure 4(b)). Because MCP-1 protein could not be detected by western blot (not shown), we used qPCR to evaluate changes in MCP-1 transcript levels in cultured mesangial cells under normal and high glucose conditions. Consistent with the qPCR data for OPN, the MCP-1 transcripts were significantly increased in the wild type mesangial cells grown under high glucose conditions, whereas the Pa28αβDKO cells had markedly lower levels of MCP-1 transcripts at the same conditions (Figure 4(c)).

It was next tested whether lentiviral-mediated reexpression of the PA28α and PA28β individually or simultaneously restored the OPN expression in Pa28αβDKO mesangial cells. The reexpression of PA28α alone or PA28α and PA28β together restored the OPN release from Pa28αβDKO cells under both normal and high glucose conditions (Figure 4(d)). The overexpression of PA28α resulted in less vigorous expression of OPN compared to simultaneous overexpression of both PA28α and PA28β. This effect could be attributed to the ability of the PA28α subunits to form an active homoheptameric proteasome regulatory complex that has not been reported for PA28β monomers [28].

3.3. Pa28αβDKO/STZ Mice Provide Lower Number of Retinal Acellular Capillaries.

DR is another microvascular complication of diabetes attributed to the diminution of pericytes in retinal microvessels and subsequent death of endothelial cells. In retina, such obsolete blood vessels will appear as thinner entities known as acellular capillaries [40]. Therefore, we

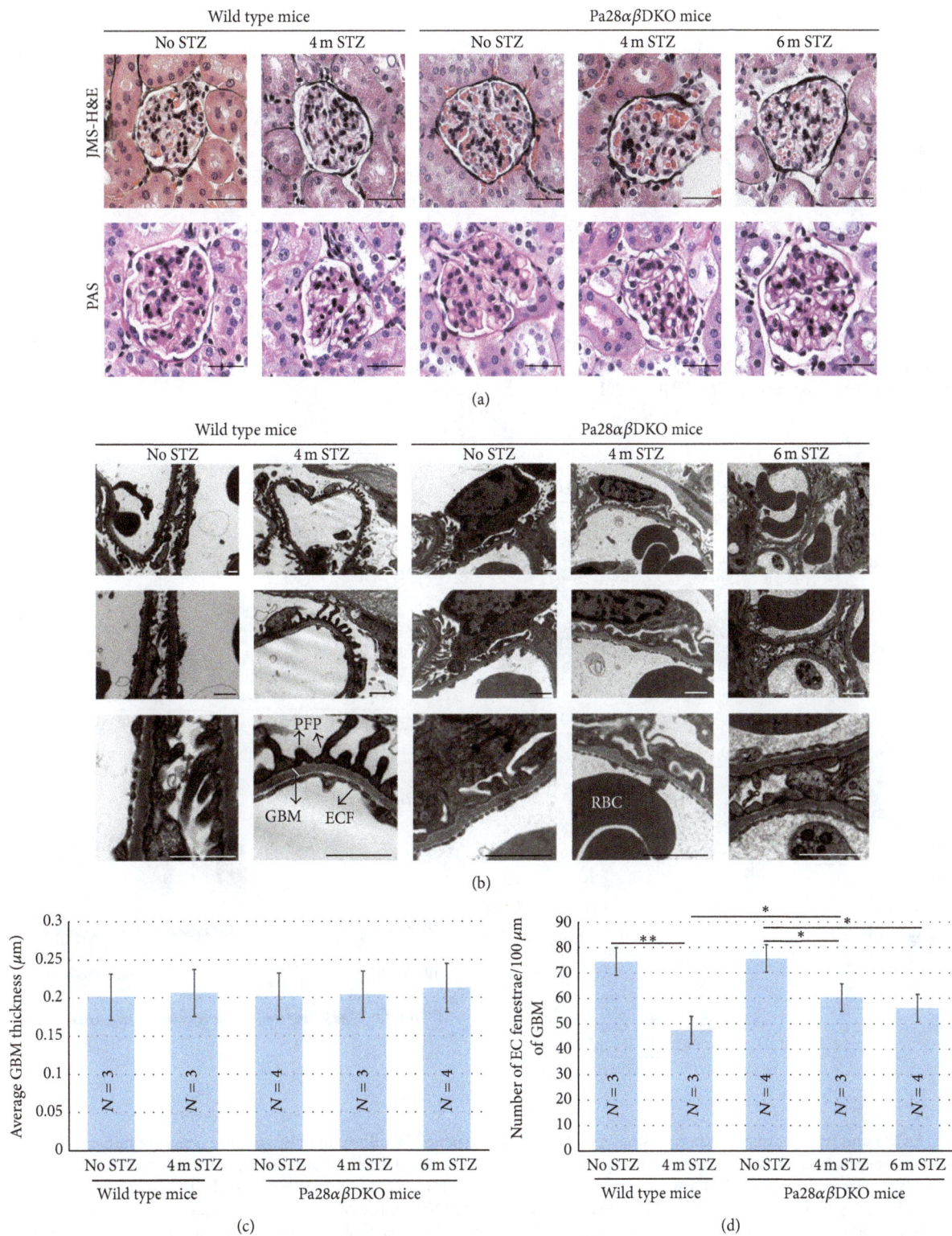

(a)

(b)

(c)

(d)

FIGURE 2: Light microscopic and TEM analysis of the glomeruli. (a) JMS-H&E and PAS staining of the nondiabetic and STZ-diabetic wild type and Pa28αβDKO glomeruli. Scale bars, 30 μm. (b) Ultrastructure of the glomeruli in wild type and Pa28αβDKO mice before and after STZ injection for indicated time points. Glomerular basement membrane (GBM), podocyte foot processes (PFP), endothelial cell fenestrae (ECF), and red blood cell (RBC) are shown. Scale bars, 1 μm. (c) Quantitation of the GBM thickness in TEM images of wild type and Pa28αβDKO glomeruli. (d) Quantitation of the average number of the EC fenestrae in TEM images of wild type and Pa28αβDKO glomeruli. N represents the number of animals in each experimental group. Results presented as mean ± SEM. $^*p < 0.05$, $^{**}p < 0.01$.

(a)

(b)

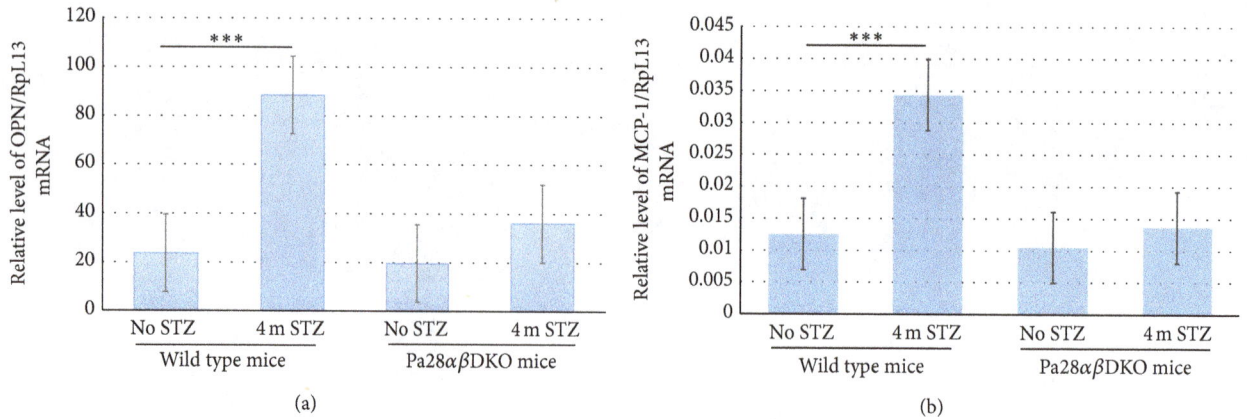

FIGURE 3: Deletion of the PA28α and PA28β genes suppresses the glomerular expression of OPN and MCP-1 in STZ-injected mice. (a) qPCR analysis of OPN and (b) MCP-1 mRNA in wild type and Pa28$\alpha\beta$DKO glomeruli without or with four months of STZ injection. $n = 3$ per group. Results presented as mean ± SEM. ***$p < 0.001$.

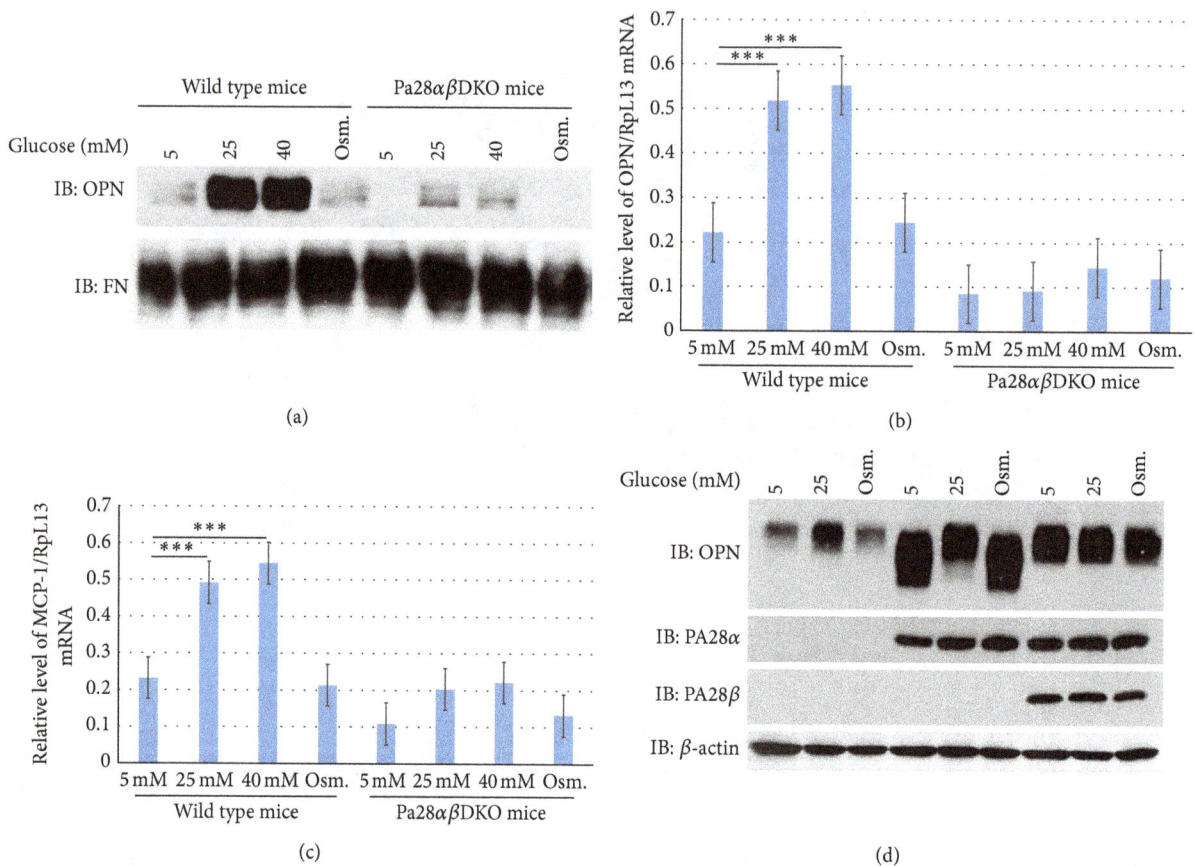

(a)

(b)

(c)

(d)

FIGURE 4: PA28α and PA28β regulate the expression of OPN in cultured mesangial cells under high glucose concentrations. (a) Western blot analysis of the conditioned media of cultured wild type and Pa28$\alpha\beta$DKO mesangial cells under different glucose conditions and osmolarity treatment. OPN: Osteopontin and FN: Fibronectin. (b) qPCR analysis of OPN and (c) MCP-1 mRNA in wild type and Pa28$\alpha\beta$DKO mesangial cells under different glucose concentrations. (d) Western blot analysis for OPN in the conditioned media and PA28α, PA28β, and β-actin in the cell lysate following lentiviral reexpression of PA28α and PA28α/PA28β in Pa28$\alpha\beta$DKO mesangial cells. Results presented as mean ± SEM. ***$p < 0.001$.

investigated to test in respect of protection against glomerular microvascular injury in Pa28$\alpha\beta$DKO/STZ mice whether these mice were similarly protected against microvascular injury in the retina. Compared with four-month STZ-injected wild type mice, the prepared retinal flat mounted microvessels of Pa28$\alpha\beta$DKO mice showed remarkable reduction in the number of acellular capillaries after four months (8.71±0.43 versus 4.43±0.45) and six months of STZ injection (8.71 ± 0.43 versus 5.07 ± 0.28), respectively (Figures 5(a) and 5(b)).

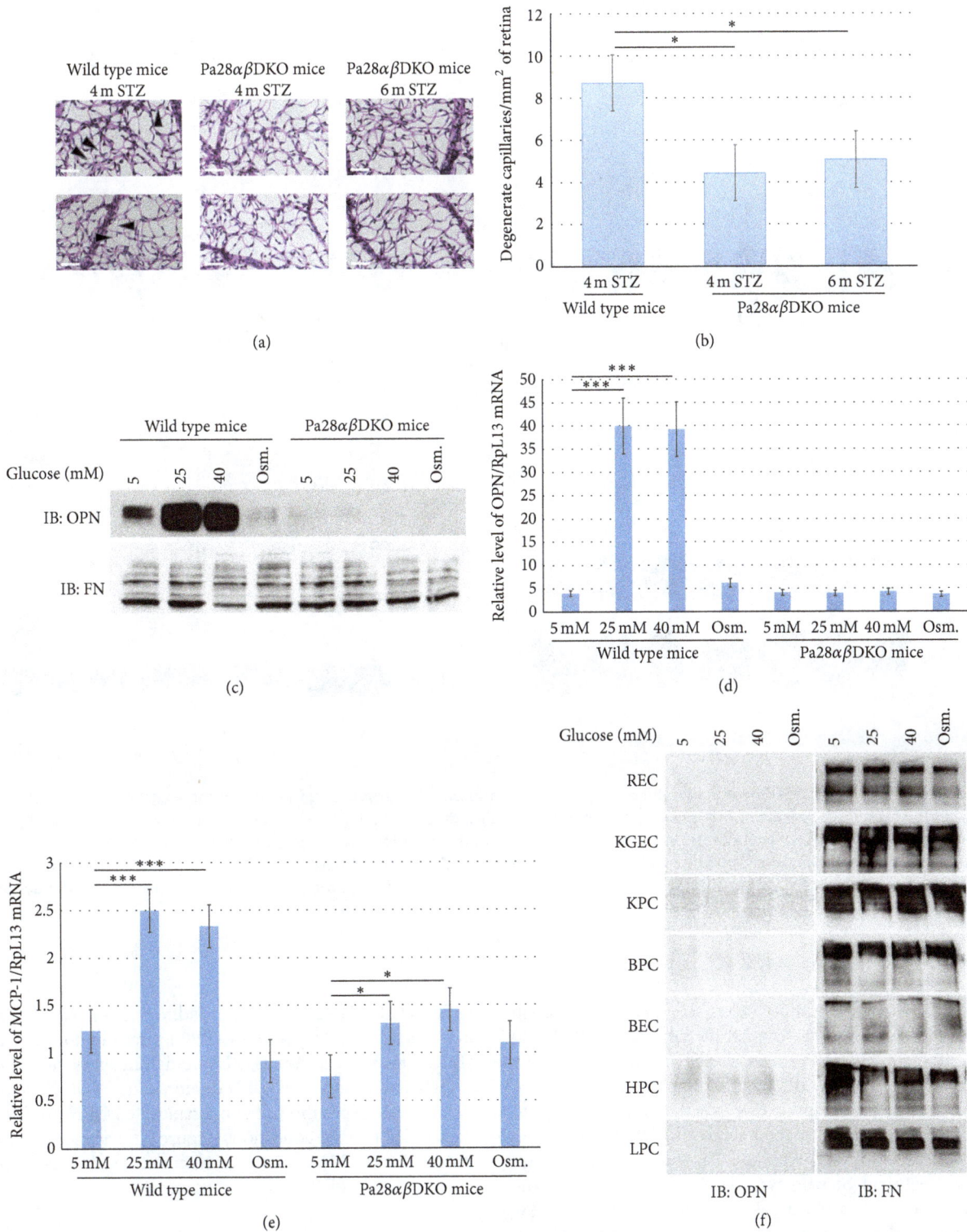

(a)

(b)

(c)

(d)

(e)

(f)

FIGURE 5: PA28α and PA28β regulate the diabetic retinal microvascular injury. (a) Light microscopic images of the flat mounted retinae from wild type and Pa28αβDKO mice following four or six months of STZ injection. The arrowheads point to the degenerate capillaries. Scale bars, 10 μm. (b) Quantitation of the number of degenerate capillaries in wild type/STZ and Pa28αβDKO/SZT mice. (c) Western blot analysis of the conditioned media of cultured wild type and Pa28αβDKO RPC under different glucose conditions and osmolarity treatment. (d) qPCR analysis of OPN and (e) MCP-1 mRNA in wild type and Pa28αβDKO RPC under different glucose concentrations. (f) Western blot analysis of OPN and FN in the conditioned media obtained from various vascular and perivascular cell types under different glucose conditions. Results presented as mean ± SEM. $^*p < 0.05$, $^{***}p < 0.001$.

(a)

(b)

(c)

(d)

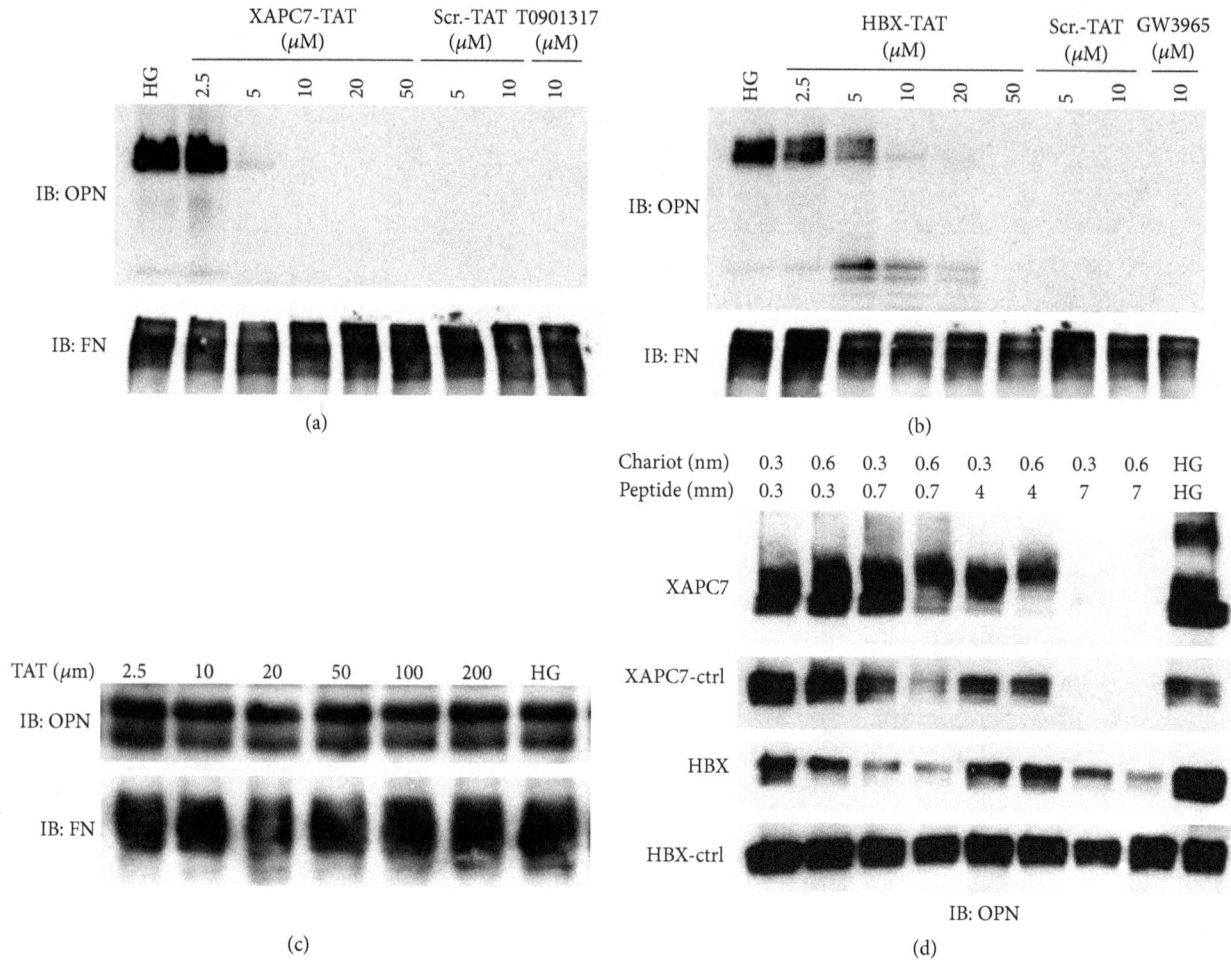

FIGURE 6: The XAPC7 and HBX peptides inhibit the high glucose-induced OPN production in cultured mesangial cells. (a) Western blot analysis of the conditioned media of cultured wild type mesangial cells treated with XAPC7-TAT and scrambled XAPC7-TAT or (b) HBX-TAT and scrambled HBX-TAT peptides under high glucose (HG, 25 mM) conditions. (c) Western blot analysis of the conditioned media of cultured wild type mesangial cells treated with TAT peptide under high glucose (25 mM) conditions. (d) Western blot analysis of the conditioned media of cultured wild type mesangial cells treated with Chariot/XAPC7, Chariot/HBX, and Chariot/scramble peptides under high glucose conditions (25 mM).

Reduction in the number of the acellular capillaries in Pa28$\alpha\beta$DKO/STZ retinae demonstrated that loss of PA28α/β genes protected the RPC against cell death triggered by hyperglycemia. To assay the effect of high glucose treatment on cultured RPC and investigate whether they respond to high glucose the same as to mesangial cells, RPC were isolated and cultured from wild type and Pa28$\alpha\beta$DKO mice. High glucose treatment of wild type RPC robustly induced the expression of OPN and MCP-1 while the Pa28$\alpha\beta$DKO RPC treated with high glucose did not manifest such increase in OPN and MCP-1 expression (Figures 5(c)–5(e)). Next it was tested whether increased expression of OPN in response to high glucose was uniquely restricted to RPC and mesangial cells or other vascular cell types also responded similarly. For this purpose, different mouse endothelial and perivascular cell types were isolated from various organs and exposed to high glucose similar to RPC and mesangial cells. These cells included retinal endothelial cells (REC), kidney glomerular

endothelial cells (KGEC), total kidney nonglomerular pericytes (KPC), brain pericytes (BPC), brain endothelial cells (BEC), heart pericytes (HPC), and lung pericytes (LPC). Western blot analyses of OPN demonstrated that any of these vascular cell types did not contain elevated OPN production under high glucose conditions (Figure 5(f)). Hence, increased production of OPN under high glucose conditions is a unique characteristic of RPC and mesangial cells.

3.4. The XAPC7 and HBX Peptides Inhibit the OPN Release from Cultured Mesangial Cells under High Glucose Conditions. To investigate if the OPN release from mesangial cells exposed to high glucose was caused by the binding of Pa28α/β proteins to the 20S proteasomes, we examined peptides capable of disrupting the association of Pa28α/β with the 20S proteasome. The PA28-inhibitory peptides fused to TAT domain of the HIV virus were used for this assay

[41]. TAT sequence was added to the XAPC7 and HBX peptides to promote the transduction of the cultured cells. The XAPC7-TAT and HBX-TAT peptides as well as scrambled control peptides fused to TAT were used to transfect the cultured mesangial cells for three days under high glucose condition to promote OPN release. Western blot analyses of conditioned media provided strong inhibition of OPN release after treatment with XAPC7-TAT and HBX-TAT at 5 μM and 10 μM concentrations, respectively (Figures 6(a) and 6(b)). Treatment with the liver X receptor (LXR) agonists, T0901317 and GW3965, was shown to inhibit OPN release and ameliorate the severity of DN [42]. Hence, as positive control for our peptide treatment experiments and suppression of OPN release, we used LXR agonists in cotreatment of the mesangial cells with high glucose. As a result, almost both T0901317 and GW3965 completely inhibited the OPN release at 10 μM concentrations (Figures 6(a) and 6(b)). Interestingly, the TAT-fused scrambled peptides also suppressed OPN release in response to high glucose. TAT peptide had been previously demonstrated to inhibit the PA28 binding to the 20S proteasomes [43, 44]. Therefore, the inhibitory effect of the TAT-scrambled peptides could be attributed to the TAT domain of the peptides. However, treatment of the mesangial cells with TAT-only peptide even at 200 μM concentration did not inhibit the OPN release (Figure 6(c)). The failure of the TAT-only peptide in inhibiting the OPN release under high glucose conditions suggests that TAT requires fusion to a juxtaposing peptide to inhibit PA28 binding to the 20S proteasome. In order to exclude the inhibitory effect of the TAT domain, XAPC7 and HBX peptides without TAT domain were synthesized and delivered to the mesangial cells using Chariot transfection reagent. Treatment with XAPC7 and its scrambled control resulted in complete dose-dependent inhibition of the OPN release (Figure 6(d)). This effect of control peptide is possibly caused by the shorter size and positive charge of these peptides compared with HBX peptide. The HBX showed marked reduction in OPN release at various concentrations but this inhibition was less potent than XAPC7. The scrambled HBX peptide did not markedly affect the OPN release from the mesangial cells (Figure 6(d)). Collectively, these findings demonstrate that high glucose-induced binding of Pa28α and Pa28β to 20S proteasomes in RPC and mesangial cells regulates OPN production.

Taking advantage of the Pa28αβDKO mice, the mesangial cells, and RPC isolated from Pa28αβDKO mice it was demonstrated in this study that PA28α and PA28β genes are key determinants of diabetic microvascular injuries. Evidence is provided for the involvement of PA28 proteasome regulators in exacerbating the pathogenesis of DN by demonstrating that, compared with wild type/STZ mice, the Pa28αβDKO/STZ mice do not develop severe albuminuria. Further testing provided that, compared to wild type, the OPN and MCP-1 inflammatory mediators are markedly suppressed in the Pa28αβDKO/STZ glomeruli, mesangial cells, and RPC under high glucose conditions. OPN secretion was regulated by Pa28α/β and, among different vascular cell types, was only detectable in cultured RPC and mesangial cells exposed to high glucose. This is consistent with the higher sensitivity of RPC and mesangial cells to the cytotoxic

effects of high glucose compared to other vascular cell types including the REC, KGEC, BPC, and BEC. These findings have strong implications in addressing why the trigger for the development of diabetic microvascular complications lies in the RPC and mesangial cells. The cell injury and death of these perivascular supporting cells in the retina and kidney caused by hyperglycemia precede the development of DR and DN. The increased OPN expression is reportedly associated with the development of DN and DR and pharmacological reagents capable of inhibiting OPN release provide protection against DN and DR [21, 42, 45]. OPN has macrophage chemoattractive function and the progression of DN and DR is facilitated by the recruitment of the macrophages and monocytes into retina and kidney. OPN release by perivascular cells in diabetic kidney and retina might regulate the local inflammatory cues to increase macrophage recruitment and activation. The novel function of PA28α and PA28β proteins in regulating OPN expression and diabetic microvascular injury demonstrates that, apart from their antigen processing properties, these proteins possess unexplored functions in sensing and responding to metabolic changes in a certain subset of vascular cells. Importantly, the increased expression of OPN following exposure to high glucose exclusively in RPC and mesangial cells that are main targets of diabetic hyperglycemia injury demonstrates a cell-specific function for PA28α and PA28β in sensing and responding to altered glucose levels.

Similar to LXR agonists, T0901317 and GW3965, that inhibit OPN expression and the severity of DN in STZ diabetic mice [42], the delivery of peptides that inhibit PA28 binding to 20S proteasomes, the XAPC7, HBX, and TAT-conjugated peptides inhibited OPN release from mesangial cells under high glucose conditions. This suggests that OPN expression under high glucose conditions from mesangial cells is regulated by PA28α and PA28β binding to the 20S proteasome. In agreement with the role of PA28α and PA28β in regulating the OPN expression, the reexpression of PA28α alone or PA28α and PA28β together in Pa28αβDKO mesangial cells restored the OPN expression. Interestingly the expression of PA28α alone also stimulated the OPN release from the Pa28αβDKO mesangial cells. This observation can be explained by the exceptional ability of the PA28α monomers to form an active regulatory complex capable of binding and activating the 20S proteasomes. Presently, it is unclear whether the reduced expression of OPN or MCP-1 alone is accountable for the ameliorated diabetic microvascular injury in Pa28αβDKO mice or other pathways are also involved. Nevertheless, since other groups showed that proteasome inhibition in mice attenuates the development of DN [46–48], the relative inhibition of the proteasomes in Pa28αβDKO RPC and mesangial cells would also provide a suitable explanation for their protection against diabetic renal and retinal injury. This can be supported by previous study in which the PA28 proteins were shown to be upregulated in RPC and also in diabetic glomeruli where expression level of PA28 proteins correlated with the severity of diabetic renal injury [1, 49]. It therefore appears that excessive activation or deregulation of the proteasomes by upregulated PA28 proteins could possibly result in microvascular damage in the retinal and glomerular vasculature.

Other investigators have shown that high glucose treatment of RPC and mesangial cells induces oxidative stress [50, 51]. The PA28α and PA28β were demonstrated to play key role in the clearance of misfolded and oxidized proteins and adaptation to oxidative stress in cultured cardiomyocytes [26]. Similarly, in RPC and mesangial cells, the PA28α and PA28β proteins could assist the RPC and mesangial cells in their adaptation to oxidative stress caused by high glucose. For instance, it was shown that RPC have lower proteasomal degradational capacity compared to other vascular cell types such as REC [1]. Therefore, PA28-α/-β proteins could assist the degradation of proteins damaged by exposure of RPC to high glucose but overt activation of the proteasomes in RPC and mesangial cells provokes tragic consequences.

4. Conclusions

This study provides major insights into the role of PA28α and PA28β genes in promoting diabetic renal and retinal microvascular injury. First of all, deletion of PA28α and PA28β genes protected diabetic animals against DN. Secondly, the expression of MCP-1 and OPN as important mediators of DN or DR was shown to be regulated by PA28α and PA28β in RPC and mesangial cells grown under high glucose. Thirdly, Pa28$\alpha\beta$DKO mice showed reduced severity of DR reflected by reduced number of acellular capillaries in their retinae. Lastly, the suppressive effect of PA28-inhibitory peptides on OPN release by mesangial cells grown in high glucose was demonstrated. Therefore, modulating the degradational activity of ubiquitin proteasome system mediated by PA28α and PA28β proteins offers a suitable candidate for the development of future treatments for microvascular complications of diabetes particularly in the retina and kidney.

Acknowledgments

The authors thank M. Slesarev, V. Rogness, and N. Sheibani for scientific suggestions and technical assistance and also H. Rao for preparing the viral transfection material. They also thank Drs. A. Sijts (University of Utrecht) and K. Tanaka (University of Tokyo) for providing the PA28α and PA28β overexpressing plasmids and also the Pa28$\alpha\beta$DKO mouse. This work was supported by Grants EY016995, EY021357, and P30-EY016665 from the National Institutes of Health.

References

[1] S. Y. Aghdam, Z. Gurel, A. Ghaffarieh, C. M. Sorenson, and N. Sheibani, "High glucose and diabetes modulate cellular proteasome function: implications in the pathogenesis of diabetes complications," *Biochemical and Biophysical Research Communications*, vol. 432, no. 2, pp. 339–344, 2013.

[2] W. T. Cade, "Diabetes-related microvascular and macrovascular diseases in the physical therapy setting," *Physical Therapy*, vol. 88, no. 11, pp. 1322–1335, 2008.

[3] C. Rask-Madsen and G. L. King, "Vascular complications of diabetes: mechanisms of injury and protective factors," *Cell Metabolism*, vol. 17, no. 1, pp. 20–33, 2013.

[4] R. Klein, B. Zinman, R. Gardiner et al., "The relationship of diabetic retinopathy to preclinical diabetic glomerulopathy lesions in type 1 diabetic patients: The Renin-Angiotensin System Study," *Diabetes*, vol. 54, no. 2, pp. 527–533, 2005.

[5] A. Kofoed-Enevoldsen, T. Jensen, K. Borch-Johnsen, and T. Deckert, "Incidence of retinopathy in type I [insulin-dependent] diabetes: association with clinical nephropathy," *Journal of Diabetic Complications*, vol. 1, no. 3, pp. 96–99, 1987.

[6] H.-P. Hammes, J. Lin, O. Renner et al., "Pericytes and the pathogenesis of diabetic retinopathy," *Diabetes*, vol. 51, no. 10, pp. 3107–3112, 2002.

[7] T. S. Kern, J. Tang, M. Mizutani et al., "Response of capillary cell death to aminoguanidine predicts the development of retinopathy: comparison of diabetes and galactosemia," *Investigative Ophthalmology & Visual Science*, vol. 41, no. 12, pp. 3972–3978, 2000.

[8] M. Mizutani, T. S. Kern, and M. Lorenzi, "Accelerated death of retinal microvascular cells in human and experimental diabetic retinopathy," *Journal of Clinical Investigation*, vol. 97, no. 12, pp. 2883–2890, 1996.

[9] M. W. Steffes, R. Østerby, B. Chavers, and S. M. Mauer, "Mesangial expansion as a central mechanism for loss of kidney function in diabetic patients," *Diabetes*, vol. 38, no. 9, pp. 1077–1081, 1989.

[10] M. E. Molitch, A. I. Adler, A. Flyvbjerg et al., "Diabetic kidney disease: a clinical update from kidney disease: improving global outcomes," *Kidney International*, vol. 87, no. 1, pp. 20–30, 2015.

[11] Z. J. Fu, S.-Y. Li, N. Kociok, D. Wong, S. K. Chung, and A. C. Y. Lo, "Aldose reductase deficiency reduced vascular changes in neonatal mouse retina in oxygen-induced retinopathy," *Investigative Ophthalmology & Visual Science*, vol. 53, no. 9, pp. 5698–5712, 2012.

[12] N. Kashihara, Y. Haruna, V. K. Kondeti, and Y. S. Kanwar, "Oxidative stress in diabetic nephropathy," *Current Medicinal Chemistry*, vol. 17, no. 34, pp. 4256–4269, 2010.

[13] K. Shikata and H. Makino, "Microinflammation in the pathogenesis of diabetic nephropathy," *Journal of Diabetes Investigation*, vol. 4, no. 2, pp. 142–149, 2013.

[14] M. A. Attawia and R. C. Nayak, "Circulating antipericyte autoantibodies in diabetic retinopathy," *Retina*, vol. 19, no. 5, pp. 390–400, 1999.

[15] A. Kuhad and K. Chopra, "Attenuation of diabetic nephropathy by tocotrienol: involvement of NFkB signaling pathway," *Life Sciences*, vol. 84, no. 9-10, pp. 296–301, 2009.

[16] Y. Li, D. Smith, Q. Li et al., "Antibody-mediated retinal pericyte injury: implications for diabetic retinopathy," *Investigative Ophthalmology & Visual Science*, vol. 53, no. 9, pp. 5520–5526, 2012.

[17] H. Schmid, A. Boucherot, Y. Yasuda et al., "Modular activation of nuclear factor-κB transcriptional programs in human diabetic nephropathy," *Diabetes*, vol. 55, no. 11, pp. 2993–3003, 2006.

[18] J. Bidwell, L. Keen, G. Gallagher et al., "Cytokine gene polymorphism in human disease: on-line databases," *Genes & Immunity*, vol. 1, no. 1, pp. 3–19, 1999.

[19] D. Gordin, C. Forsblom, N. M. Panduru et al., "Osteopontin is a strong predictor of incipient diabetic nephropathy, cardiovascular disease, and all-cause mortality in patients with type 1 diabetes," *Diabetes Care*, vol. 37, no. 9, pp. 2593–2600, 2014.

[20] S. K. Jain, J. Rains, J. Croad, B. Larson, and K. Jones, "Curcumin supplementation lowers TNF-α, IL-6, IL-8, and MCP-1 secretion in high glucose-treated cultured monocytes and blood levels of TNF-α, IL-6, MCP-1, glucose, and glycosylated hemoglobin in diabetic rats," *Antioxidants and Redox Signaling*, vol. 11, no. 2, pp. 241–249, 2009.

[21] S. Kase, M. Yokoi, W. Saito et al., "Increased osteopontin levels in the vitreous of patients with diabetic retinopathy," *Ophthalmic Research*, vol. 39, no. 3, pp. 143–147, 2007.

[22] S. B. Nicholas, J. Liu, J. Kim et al., "Critical role for osteopontin in diabetic nephropathy," *Kidney International*, vol. 77, no. 7, pp. 588–600, 2010.

[23] Q. Ma, "Role of Nrf2 in oxidative stress and toxicity," *Annual Review of Pharmacology and Toxicology*, vol. 53, pp. 401–426, 2013.

[24] A. M. Pickering, R. A. Linder, H. Zhang, H. J. Forman, and K. J. A. Davies, "Nrf2-dependent induction of proteasome and Pa28αβ regulator are required for adaptation to oxidative stress," *The Journal of Biological Chemistry*, vol. 287, no. 13, pp. 10021–10031, 2012.

[25] T. J. A. Höhn and T. Grune, "The proteasome and the degradation of oxidized proteins: part III-redox regulation of the proteasomal system," *Redox Biology*, vol. 2, no. 1, pp. 388–394, 2014.

[26] J. Li, S. R. Powell, and X. Wang, "Enhancement of proteasome function by PA28α overexpression protects against oxidative stress," *The FASEB Journal*, vol. 25, no. 3, pp. 883–893, 2011.

[27] K. Ahn, M. Erlander, D. Leturcq, P. A. Peterson, K. Früh, and Y. Yang, "*In vivo* characterization of the proteasome regulator PA28," *The Journal of Biological Chemistry*, vol. 271, no. 30, pp. 18237–18242, 1996.

[28] A. Ciechanover and A. L. Schwartz, "The ubiquitin-proteasome pathway: the complexity and myriad functions of proteins death," *Proceedings of the National Academy of Sciences of the United States of America*, vol. 95, no. 6, pp. 2727–2730, 1998.

[29] E. A. Scheef, C. M. Sorenson, and N. Sheibani, "Attenuation of proliferation and migration of retinal pericytes in the absence of thrombospondin-1," *American Journal of Physiology—Cell Physiology*, vol. 296, no. 4, pp. C724–C734, 2009.

[30] X. J. Su, C. Sorenson, and N. Sheibani, "Isolation and characterization of murine retinal endothelial cells," *Molecular Vision*, vol. 9, pp. 171–178, 2003.

[31] M. Takemoto, L. Q. He, J. Norlin, K. Tryggvason, and C. Betsholtz, "A new method for large scale isolation of kidney glomeruli from mice-toward transcriptional profiling of mouse kidney glomerulus," *Journal of the American Society of Nephrology*, vol. 14, no. 2, pp. 367a–368a, 2003.

[32] N. Akis and M. P. Madaio, "Isolation, culture, and characterization of endothelial cells from mouse glomeruli," *Kidney International*, vol. 65, no. 6, pp. 2223–2227, 2004.

[33] R. A. Feit-Leichman, R. Kinouchi, M. Takeda et al., "Vascular damage in a mouse model of diabetic retinopathy: relation to neuronal and glial changes," *Investigative Ophthalmology and Visual Science*, vol. 46, no. 11, pp. 4281–4287, 2005.

[34] D. Leali, P. Dell'Era, H. Stabile et al., "Osteopontin (Eta-1) and fibroblast growth factor-2 cross-talk in angiogenesis," *Journal of Immunology*, vol. 171, no. 2, pp. 1085–1093, 2003.

[35] A. A. Rossini, A. A. Like, W. E. Dulin, and G. F. Cahill Jr., "Pancreatic beta cell toxicity by streptozotocin anomers," *Diabetes*, vol. 26, no. 12, pp. 1120–1124, 1977.

[36] J. M. Ginsberg, B. S. Chang, R. A. Matarese, and S. Garella, "Use of single voided urine samples to estimate quantitative proteinuria," *The New England Journal of Medicine*, vol. 309, no. 25, pp. 1543–1546, 1983.

[37] S. J. Schwab, R. L. Christensen, K. Dougherty, and S. Klahr, "Quantitation of proteinuria by the use of protein-to-creatinine ratios in single urine samples," *Archives of Internal Medicine*, vol. 147, no. 5, pp. 943–944, 1987.

[38] K. J. Henriksen, S. M. Meehan, and A. Chang, "Nonneoplastic kidney diseases in adult tumor nephrectomy and nephroureterectomy specimens: common, harmful, yet underappreciated," *Archives of Pathology & Laboratory Medicine*, vol. 133, no. 7, pp. 1012–1025, 2009.

[39] K. Katsuya, E. Yaoita, Y. Yoshida, Y. Yamamoto, and T. Yamamoto, "An improved method for primary culture of rat podocytes," *Kidney International*, vol. 69, no. 11, pp. 2101–2106, 2006.

[40] H.-P. Hammes, J. Lin, P. Wagner et al., "Angiopoietin-2 causes pericyte dropout in the normal retina: evidence for involvement in diabetic retinopathy," *Diabetes*, vol. 53, no. 4, pp. 1104–1110, 2004.

[41] R. Stohwasser, H.-G. Holzhütter, U. Lehmann, P. Henklein, and P.-M. Kloetzel, "Hepatitis B virus HBx peptide 116–138 and proteasome activator PA28 compete for binding to the proteasome α4/MC6 subunit," *Biological Chemistry*, vol. 384, no. 1, pp. 39–49, 2003.

[42] H. Tachibana, D. Ogawa, Y. Matsushita et al., "Activation of liver X receptor inhibits osteopontin and ameliorates diabetic nephropathy," *Journal of the American Society of Nephrology*, vol. 23, no. 11, pp. 1835–1846, 2012.

[43] E. Jankowska, M. Gaczynska, P. Osmulski et al., "Potential allosteric modulators of the proteasome activity," *Biopolymers*, vol. 93, no. 5, pp. 481–495, 2010.

[44] J. Witkowska, P. Karpowicz, M. Gaczynska, P. A. Osmulski, and E. Jankowska, "Dissecting a role of a charge and conformation of Tat2 peptide in allosteric regulation of 20S proteasome," *Journal of Peptide Science*, vol. 20, no. 8, pp. 649–656, 2014.

[45] S. Hazra, A. Rasheed, A. Bhatwadekar et al., "Liver X receptor modulates diabetic retinopathy outcome in a mouse model of streptozotocin-induced diabetes," *Diabetes*, vol. 61, no. 12, pp. 3270–3279, 2012.

[46] C. Gao, K. Aqie, J. Zhu et al., "MG132 ameliorates kidney lesions by inhibiting the degradation of smad7 in streptozotocin-induced diabetic nephropathy," *Journal of Diabetes Research*, vol. 2014, Article ID 918396, 8 pages, 2014.

[47] W. Huang, C. Yang, Q. Nan et al., "The proteasome inhibitor, MG132, attenuates diabetic nephropathy by inhibiting SnoN degradation *in vivo* and *in vitro*," *BioMed Research International*, vol. 2014, Article ID 684765, 11 pages, 2014.

[48] Z.-F. Luo, W. Qi, B. Feng et al., "Prevention of diabetic nephropathy in rats through enhanced renal antioxidative

capacity by inhibition of the proteasome," *Life Sciences*, vol. 88, no. 11-12, pp. 512–520, 2011.

[49] S. Y. Aghdam and N. Sheibani, "The ubiquitin-proteasome system and microvascular complications of diabetes," *Journal of Ophthalmic & Vision Research*, vol. 8, no. 3, pp. 244–256, 2013.

[50] M. A. Catherwood, L. A. Powell, P. Anderson, D. McMaster, P. C. Sharpe, and E. R. Trimble, "Glucose-induced oxidative stress in mesangial cells," *Kidney International*, vol. 61, no. 2, pp. 599–608, 2002.

[51] T. S. Devi, K.-I. Hosoya, T. Terasaki, and L. P. Singh, "Critical role of TXNIP in oxidative stress, DNA damage and retinal pericyte apoptosis under high glucose: implications for diabetic retinopathy," *Experimental Cell Research*, vol. 319, no. 7, pp. 1001–1012, 2013.

21

Renal Dysfunction and Recovery following Initial Treatment of Newly Diagnosed Multiple Myeloma

Benjamin A. Derman ⓘ,[1] **Jochen Reiser** ⓘ,[2] **Sanjib Basu,**[3] **and Agne Paner**[3]

[1]Section of Hematology/Oncology, University of Chicago, 5841 S. Maryland Ave, M/C 2115, Chicago, IL 60637, USA
[2]Department of Medicine, Rush University Medical Center, Chicago, IL, USA
[3]Division of Hematology/Oncology, Rush University Medical Center, Chicago, IL, USA

Correspondence should be addressed to Benjamin A. Derman; bderman@medicine.bsd.uchicago.edu

Academic Editor: Anil K. Agarwal

Introduction. Renal insufficiency (RI) in Multiple Myeloma (MM) portends a higher tumor burden and worse prognosis. Reversal of RI in newly diagnosed MM (NDMM) improves patient outcomes, but it is unknown if there is a disparity in renal recovery in NDMM between African Americans (AA) and non-African Americans. *Methods.* A retrospective chart review was conducted of 690 patients with NDMM at Rush University Medical Center from 2005 to 2016. 118 patients (59 AA and 59 non-AA) with NDMM and an estimated glomerular filtration rate (eGFR) < 90 mL/min/1.73 m^2 at the time of diagnosis were identified and analyzed. The time to best renal response and best eGFR achieved during initial myeloma therapy were tabulated. *Results.* Median eGFR at the time of diagnosis was similar between the AA and non-AA groups (47.89 versus 51.95, p=0.56). Median absolute change in eGFR after initial therapy was significantly higher in the AA (+33.64) versus the non-AA group (+21.07, p=0.00183). This difference remained whether the baseline eGFR at diagnosis was <90 or <60 mL/min/1.73 m^2. *Discussion.* AA patients with NDMM treated in the era of novel agents have greater improvement in renal function in comparison to non-AA patients, regardless of myeloma response. The biological underpinnings for this disparity require further investigation.

1. Introduction

Renal insufficiency (RI) is present in roughly 20% of newly diagnosed multiple myeloma (NDMM) patients and over 50% of multiple myeloma (MM) patients will experience RI at some point during the course of their disease [1–3]. RI in multiple myeloma has been defined by the Internal Myeloma Working Group (IMWG) as a serum creatinine > 2 mg/dL or as an estimated glomerular filtration rate (eGFR) < 40 mL/min/1.73 m^2 as calculated by the Modification of Diet in Renal Disease (MDRD) formula [4].

RI in MM portends a higher tumor burden and worse prognosis [5–8]. Survival appears to be tightly linked to the stage of chronic kidney disease (CKD), with survival decreasing in parallel with a decline in eGFR. In particular, those with an eGFR < 30 mL/min/1.73 m^2 appear to have the worst prognosis [9]. Recent clinical trials have demonstrated that patients treated with "novel" agents, particularly proteasome inhibitors, are more likely to experience renal recovery. However, there is conflicting evidence as to whether reversal of RI in MM in the era of novel agents can improve overall survival. Of those studies that did show a survival difference, the prevailing theory is that reversal of RI in NDMM improves patient outcomes, but it remains inferior to patients whose renal function was normal at diagnosis [9–12].

The majority of patients in these trials were Caucasian, which may limit the external validity of the studies when considering a disease with a twofold predilection for African Americans (AA) and when addressing a population with a higher proportion of AA patients [13]. Moreover, AAs have a 5-times higher rate of stage 4 CKD and end stage renal disease (ESRD) in the United States compared to Caucasians. The cause for this disparity is multifactorial: less access to healthcare, higher incidence of causal diseases such as diabetes and hypertension, and differences in genetic factors

TABLE 1: Renal response criteria∗.

Renal Response	Baseline eGFR (mL/min/1.73m^2)	Best CrCl Response
Complete Response	< 50	≥ 60 mL/min
Partial Response	< 15	30-59 mL/min
Minor Response	< 15	15-39 mL/min
	15-29	30-59 mL/min

∗Adapted from the IMWG consensus statement on renal insufficiency in newly diagnosed multiple myeloma.

(*APOL1* gene variants in AA populations) [14–17]. Recent insights suggest that APOL1 risk for kidney disease depends on the plasma levels of soluble urokinase receptor, an immune derived signaling molecule whose level is associated with lifestyle, infections, and even certain types of cancers [18].

Monitoring renal response has been standardized by IMWG's consensus statement on RI in MM (see Table 1). The eGFR, as calculated by the MDRD equation, can be used as a suitable substitute for creatinine clearance [4, 5]. The more recent CKD-EPI (Chronic Kidney Disease Epidemiology Collaboration) equation has been shown to be more accurate for estimating eGFR in the range of 60 to 90 mL/min/1.73 m^2; however, the initial validation set was limited by lesser numbers of the elderly and of racial minorities [19].

Given the dearth of evidence regarding renal recovery in AAs receiving therapy for NDMM, the goal of this study is to compare renal recovery between AA and non-AA patients following initial treatment for NDMM.

2. Materials and Methods

A retrospective chart review was performed of patients with NDMM at Rush University Medical Center from January 1, 2005, to August 1, 2016. 690 charts were selected and reviewed through a myeloma registry; patients who were on hemodialysis for alternative reasons prior to diagnosis, had an eGFR > 90 mL/min/1.73 m^2, or for whom records were incomplete were excluded via a thorough chart audit. The eGFR was calculated using the MDRD equation and confirmed using the CKD-EPI equation to ensure accurate eGFR assessment in the 60-90 mL/min/1.73 m^2 range. 118 patients with NDMM and an eGFR < 90 mL/min/1.73 m^2 (corresponding to National Kidney Foundation's chronic kidney disease stage 2 or worse) at the time of diagnosis were identified. Time to best renal response and the best eGFR achieved during initial myeloma therapy were recorded. MM response was recorded using the updated 2016 IMWG consensus criteria [20]. Continuous variables were compared between the two groups using the Mann-Whitney U test, and binary variables were compared using Fisher's exact test. The design of this study was approved by the hospital Institutional Review Board and is compliant with the Helsinki Declaration.

3. Results

3.1. Baseline Characteristics. A total of 118 patient records were reviewed, with 59 AA and 59 non-AA individuals with RI at the time of NDMM. The baseline patient characteristics at the time of diagnosis of multiple myeloma can be seen in Table 2. Both groups were comparable by age, gender, baseline eGFR, revised International Staging System for myeloma (R-ISS) and by anti-myeloma therapies received. The AA patient group presented with a higher incidence of hypertension, a greater degree of anemia, and a larger M-protein on serum protein electrophoresis compared to the non-AA group. There was a nonsignificant difference in the quantity of proteinuria at the time of diagnosis; proteinuria data was only available in 24 of the AA group and in 26 of the non-AA group. Cytogenetics by fluorescence in situ hybridization were evaluated from bone marrow biopsy samples in all patients. There was no significant difference in the cytogenetic risk as determined from the IMWG consensus on risk stratification [21]. In the AA group, there were 12 patients classified as having adverse risk cytogenetics compared to 14 patients in the non-AA group (p=0.825).

3.2. Renal Function at Diagnosis and after Recovery. Although median eGFR at the time of diagnosis of MM was similar between the AA and non-AA groups (47.89 versus 51.95 mL/min/1.73 m^2, p=0.56), the median absolute change in eGFR after initial therapy was significantly higher in the AA group (+33.64 mL/min/1.73 m^2) versus the non-AA group (+21.07 mL/min/1.73 m^2, p=0.00183). This difference remained whether the baseline eGFR at diagnosis was <90 or <60 mL/min/1.73 m^2 (Table 3). There was no significant difference in the median time to best renal response between the two groups (91 days in the AA group versus 79 days in the non-AA group, p=0.383). When substituting the CKD-EPI equation for the MDRD equation, 4 patients in the non-AA were reclassified as having a GFR > 90 mL/min/1.73 m^2 and 0 patients in the AA group were reclassified. This did not have an appreciable effect on any of the eGFR variables.

3.3. Myeloma Response. The majority of patients were treated with a bortezomib-based regimen (86.4% for the AA group and 84.7% for the non-AA group, p=1). MM response rates to induction therapy were similar: very good partial response (VGPR) or better was achieved in 44.1% of AA and 35.6% of non-AA (p=0.452). There was not a significant difference in the percentage decrease in the involved-to-uninvolved serum free light chain ratio between the groups (87.39% in the AA group versus 92.88% in the non-AA group, *p*=0.103). 45.8% of AA individuals underwent autologous stem cell transplant (ASCT) compared to 64.4% of non-AA (p=0.0637). 80% of AA and 88% of non-AA patients received bisphosphonates (p=0.317, see Table 4).

TABLE 2: Baseline data and patient characteristics.

	AA (n=59)	Non-AA (n=59)	p-value
Age (median)	67.21	64.4	p=0.372
Gender			
Male	23	32	p=0.140
Female	36	27	
Comorbidities			
Hypertension	46	31	p=0.0064
Diabetes Mellitus	18	11	p=0.1991
Human Immunodeficiency Virus	1	0	p=1
Hepatitis C Virus	1	0	p=1
Systemic Lupus Erythematosus	1	1	p=1
Congestive Heart Failure	10	8	p=0.799
Chronic Kidney Disease	9	6	p=0.582
Laboratory Data (median)			
Hemoglobin (g/dL)	9	10.6	p<0.001
Platelets (10^9/L)	194	206	p=0.126
eGFR (MDRD, mL/min/1.73 m^2)	47.89	51.95	p=0.522
Myeloma Parameters (median)			
Protein Gap (g/dL)	5.9	4.15	p=0.00241
Lactate Dehydrogenase (U/L)	216	182.5	p=0.400
Beta2-Microglobulin (mg/L)	5.15	4.98	p=0.742
Urine Protein (mg/24 hrs)	279.5	1218	p=0.192
Serum Free Light Chain Ratio (Involved/Uninvolved)	70.37	164.96	p=0.103
M-protein (g/dL)	3.2	2	p=0.0139
% Bone Marrow Plasmacytosis	50	40	p=0.053
Light Chain only	12	13	p=0.841
Adverse Risk Cytogenetics*	12	14	P=0.825
Concurrent Amyloid	4	2	p=0.679
R-ISS Stage			
1	4	10	p=0.153
2	35	39	p=0.568
3	20	10	p=0.056
Criteria for Treatment			
Hypercalcemia (Calcium > 11 mg/dL)	13	13	p=1
eGFR <60 mL/min/1.73 m^2	45	37	p=0.161
eGFR 60-90 mL/min/1.73 m^2	14	22	
Anemia (Hemoglobin < 10 g/dL)	32	17	p=0.0086
Bone disease	31	29	p=0.854
Therapy Received			
Triplet	24	27	p=0.71
Doublet	31	31	p=1
Other	4	1	p=0.364
Bortezomib-based	50	50	p=1
Bortezomib/Dexamethasone	24	23	p=0.884
Bortezomib/Lenalidomide/Dexamethasone	12	17	p=0.353
Cyclophosphamide/Bortezomib/Dexamethasone	11	6	p=0.225
Other	3	4	p=0.705
Bisphosphonate	47	52	p=0.317

*Includes deletion 17p, t(4;14), t(14;20), t(14;16), and/or 1q21 gain. Triplet = 3-drug combination consisting of a corticosteroid and 2 other antimyeloma therapies. Doublet = 2-drug combination consisting of a corticosteroid and another antimyeloma agent.

TABLE 3: Renal response following initial therapy for newly diagnosed multiple myeloma.

For eGFR <90 mL/min/1.73 m^2 (MDRD)	AA (n=59)	Non-AA (n=59)	p-value
eGFR at diagnosis (median)	47.89	51.95	p=0.56
Change in eGFR (median)	33.64	21.07	p=0.00183
Time to best eGFR (median days)	91	79	p=0.383
For eGFR < 60 mL/min/1.73 m^2 (MDRD)	AA (n=45)	Non-AA (n=37)	
eGFR at diagnosis (median)	34.09	31.29	p=0.597
Change in eGFR (median)	35.64	21.83	p=0.0278
Time to best eGFR (median days)	97.5	102	p=0.983
Required HD	6	6	p=1

TABLE 4: Multiple myeloma response following initial therapy.

Myeloma Response	AA (n=59)	Non-AA (n=59)	p-value
Complete Response	11	8	p=0.617
Very Good Partial Response	15	13	p=0.829
Partial Response	27	28	p=1
Minimal Response	6	6	p=1
Stable Disease	0	4	p=0.119
Light Chain Response (median)			
% Decrease in Involved/Uninvolved Serum Free Light Chain Ratio	87.39	92.88	p=0.187
Proceeded to ASCT	27	38	p=0.0637

ASCT = autologous stem cell transplant.

4. Discussion

This is the first study to analyze disparities in renal dysfunction and recovery between AA and non-AA individuals with newly diagnosed multiple myeloma (NDMM). We demonstrate that, in our institution, AA patients with NDMM treated in the era of novel agents have greater improvement in renal function in comparison to non-AA patients, irrespective of myeloma response.

Prior studies examining renal recovery during treatment for NDMM have shown a positive correlation with overall survival; however, they have had limited external validity as they have primarily investigated Caucasian subjects. Our present work raises the question of whether there may be some biologic underpinning that accounts for the difference in renal recovery between AAs and non-AAs.

It is important to note that the IMWG diagnostic criteria for MM and the consensus statement on RI in MM are limited as they pertain to renal function in MM. Renal insufficiency in MM is defined as a creatinine clearance <40 mL/minute or serum creatinine >2 mg/dL. However, this cutoff is far below what is required to make the diagnosis of chronic kidney disease (CKD). This represents a key missed opportunity: early identification (and possibly treatment) of patients with renal insufficiency and MM. We argue that it is both reasonable and prudent to include patients with an eGFR <90 mL/min/1.73 m^2, corresponding to patients with stage 2 CKD or worse. We have included a subanalysis of patients with a GFR <60 mL/min/1.73 m^2 as well, corresponding to patients with stage 3 CKD or worse. In that same vein, we have eschewed the use of the IMWG renal response criteria

and used the absolute change in eGFR from baseline in order to best quantify the renal response in our patients. The weaknesses of both the renal insufficiency criteria for MM and the renal response criteria must be readdressed in future guideline statements to more accurately assess renal response in MM.

This single-institution retrospective study is limited by its lack of power to investigate the effect of renal recovery on overall survival amongst the two groups and whether there is an association between myeloma response and renal response. Few renal biopsies were performed on patients in this data set, which limits the ability to attribute MM as the root cause of renal disease. Though serial serum free light chain measurements were performed reliably, the same cannot be said for serial proteinuria assessments which were missing. Delineating acute kidney injury from CKD in the setting of MM has historically been a challenge, owing to the overlapping contributions to renal injury by light chain cast nephropathy, volume depletion, radiologic contrast media, hypercalcemia, and non-steroidal anti-inflammatory agents used for bone pain prior to diagnosis [22]. It is possible that changes in muscle mass or dietary intake could have accounted for changes in the calculated eGFR over time. The median time to achieving best eGFR in this study (79-102 days) makes this less likely to have had an effect. Serum cystatin-C may be superior to creatinine in evaluating early renal dysfunction, and could be considered for future studies [23]. Moreover, nearly all MM patients undergo several lines of therapy during the course of their disease; our study only investigates renal recovery after the initial therapy modality.

5. Conclusion

Given that renal recovery in NDMM is known to impact overall survival, our findings suggest that further studies should be done to elucidate the differences in the epidemiology and disease biology that could account for the racial disparities in renal dysfunction and recovery. A promising explanation may lie in the interplay between *APOL1* gene expression and circulating soluble urokinase plasminogen activator receptor (suPAR) [24]. The *APOL1* G1 and G2 gene variants, which are prevalent in individuals with recent African ancestry and absent in Caucasians, are known risk factors for developing CKD and progression to ESRD in AAs [25]. Furthermore, it has been shown recently that APOL1-related decline in renal function is dependent on circulating suPAR levels, [24] which itself has been implicated in the onset and progression of CKD [26]. A murine model has been identified with "bone marrow immature myeloid cells (Sca-1^{lo}Gr-1^{lo}) as cellular sources of suPAR"; however, the human correlate has not yet been determined [27]. Myeloid lineage cells make up the bone marrow tumor microenvironment in MM and have clearly been shown to "promote [MM] cell survival, proliferation, and chemoresistance." [28] Based on this evidence and the data that we present here, we speculate that the myeloid cells in the MM microenvironment may cause suPAR levels to rise and that antimyeloma therapies may act by altering this environment and lead to a resultant decrease in suPAR levels. This would provide an additional pathway for renal dysfunction and recovery in MM and might explain the racial differences in renal recovery described here. This presents an exciting potential mechanism that requires further investigation. In summary, our study suggests that AA patients with MM and renal disease experience greater recovery in kidney function with initial therapy. The biology underlying this interesting finding requires further study.

Disclosure

An earlier abstract-only version of this work was made available as part of the 2016 American Society of Hematology 'Abstracts & Meeting Program'.

Authors' Contributions

Benjamin Derman contributed to study design, data collection, manuscript drafting, and revisions. Jochen Reiser helped in data analysis and abstract and manuscript drafting and revisions. Sanjib Basu assisted in data analysis and abstract drafting. Agne Paner contributed to study design, abstract drafting, and manuscript revisions.

References

[1] L. M. Knudsen, E. Hippe, M. Hjorth, E. Holmberg, and J. Westin, "Renal function in newly diagnosed multiple myeloma — A demographic study of 1353 patients," *European Journal of Haematology*, vol. 53, no. 4, pp. 207–212, 1994.

[2] R. A. Kyle, M. A. Gertz, T. E. Witzig et al., "Review of 1027 patients with newly diagnosed multiple myeloma," *Mayo Clinic Proceedings*, vol. 78, no. 1, pp. 21–33, 2003.

[3] M. R. Gaballa, J. P. Laubach, R. L. Schlossman et al., "Management of myeloma-associated renal dysfunction in the era of novel therapies," *Expert Review of Hematology*, vol. 5, no. 1, pp. 51–68, 2012.

[4] M. A. Dimopoulos, P. Sonneveld, N. Leung et al., "International Myeloma working group recommendations for the diagnosis and management of Myeloma-Related Renal Impairment," *Journal of Clinical Oncology*, vol. 34, no. 13, pp. 1544–1557, 2016.

[5] M. A. Dimopoulos, E. Terpos, A. Chanan-Khan et al., "Renal impairment in patients with multiple myeloma: A consensus statement on behalf of the International Myeloma Working Group," *Journal of Clinical Oncology*, vol. 28, no. 33, pp. 4976–4984, 2010.

[6] K. C. Abbott and L. Y. Agodoa, "Multiple myeloma and light chain-associated nephropathy at end-stage renal disease in the United States: Patient characteristics and survival," *Clinical Nephrology*, vol. 56, no. 3, pp. 207–210, 2001.

[7] V. Sakhuja, V. Jha, S. Varma et al., "Renal involvement in multiple myeloma: A 10-year study," *Renal Failure*, vol. 22, no. 4, pp. 465–477, 2000.

[8] L. M. Knudsen, M. Hjorth, and E. Hippe, "Renal failure in multiple myeloma: Reversibility and impact on the prognosis," *European Journal of Haematology*, vol. 65, no. 3, pp. 175–181, 2000.

[9] K. Uttervall, A. D. Duru, J. Lund et al., "The use of novel drugs can effectively improve response, delay relapse and enhance overall survival in multiple myeloma patients with renal impairment," *PLoS ONE*, vol. 9, no. 7, 2014.

[10] R. Khan, S. Apewokin, M. Grazziutti et al., "Renal insufficiency retains adverse prognostic implications despite renal function improvement following Total Therapy for newly diagnosed multiple myeloma," *Leukemia*, vol. 29, no. 5, pp. 1195–1201, 2015.

[11] W. I. Gonsalves, N. Leung, S. V. Rajkumar et al., "Improvement in renal function and its impact on survival in patients with newly diagnosed multiple myeloma," *Blood Cancer Journal*, vol. 5, no. 3, article no. e296, 2015.

[12] M. A. Dimopoulos, M. Roussou, M. Gkotzamanidou et al., "The role of novel agents on the reversibility of renal impairment in newly diagnosed symptomatic patients with multiple myeloma," *Leukemia*, vol. 27, no. 2, pp. 423–429, 2013.

[13] A. J. Waxman, P. J. Mink, S. S. Devesa et al., "Racial disparities in incidence and outcome in multiple myeloma: A population-based study," *Blood*, vol. 116, no. 25, pp. 5501–5506, 2010.

[14] Q. Zhang and D. Rothenbacher, "Prevalence of chronic kidney disease in population-based studies: systematic review," *BMC Public Health*, vol. 8, article no. 117, 2008.

[15] W. W. Williams and M. R. Pollak, "Health disparities in kidney disease - Emerging data from the human genome," *The New England Journal of Medicine*, vol. 369, no. 23, pp. 2260–2261, 2013.

[16] M. E. Grams, E. K. H. Chow, D. L. Segev, and J. Coresh, "Lifetime Incidence of CKD stages 3-5 in the United States," *American Journal of Kidney Diseases*, vol. 62, no. 2, pp. 245–252, 2013.

[17] S. Rosset, S. Tzur, D. M. Behar, W. G. Wasser, and K. Skorecki, "The population genetics of chronic kidney disease: Insights from the MYH9-APOL1 locus," *Nature Reviews Nephrology*, vol. 7, no. 6, pp. 313–326, 2011.

[18] C.-A. A. Hu, E. I. Klopfer, and P. E. Ray, "Human apolipoprotein L1 (ApoL1) in cancer and chronic kidney disease," *FEBS Letters*, vol. 586, no. 7, pp. 947–955, 2012.

[19] A. S. Levey, L. A. Stevens, C. H. Schmid et al., "A new equation to estimate glomerular filtration rate," *Annals of Internal Medicine*, vol. 150, no. 9, pp. 604–612, 2009.

[20] S. Kumar, B. Paiva, K. C. Anderson et al., "International Myeloma Working Group consensus criteria for response and minimal residual disease assessment in multiple myeloma," *Lancet Oncol*, vol. 17, pp. e328–e346, 2016.

[21] W. J. Chng, A. Dispenzieri, C.-S. Chim et al., "IMWG consensus on risk stratification in multiple myeloma," *Leukemia*, vol. 28, no. 2, pp. 269–277, 2014.

[22] K. Basnayake, S. J. Stringer, C. A. Hutchison, and P. Cockwell, "The biology of immunoglobulin free light chains and kidney injury," *Kidney International*, vol. 79, no. 12, pp. 1289–1301, 2011.

[23] E. Terpos, E. Katodritou, E. Tsiftsakis et al., "Cystatin-C is an independent prognostic factor for survival in multiple myeloma and is reduced by bortezomib administration," *Haematologica*, vol. 94, no. 3, pp. 372–379, 2009.

[24] S. S. Hayek, K. H. Koh, M. E. Grams et al., "A tripartite complex of suPAR, APOL1 risk variants and $\alpha v\beta 3$ integrin on podocytes mediates chronic kidney disease," *Nature Medicine*, vol. 23, pp. 945–953, 2017.

[25] M. C. Foster, J. Coresh, M. Fornage et al., "APOL1 variants associate with increased risk of CKD among African Americans," *Journal of the American Society of Nephrology*, vol. 24, no. 9, pp. 1484–1491, 2013.

[26] S. S. Hayek, S. Sever, Y. A. Ko et al., "Soluble urokinase receptor and chronic kidney disease," *The New England Journal of Medicine*, vol. 373, no. 20, pp. 1916–1925, 2015.

[27] E. Hahm, C. Wei, I. Fernandez et al., "Bone marrow-derived immature myeloid cells are a main source of circulating suPAR contributing to proteinuric kidney disease," *Nature Medicine*, vol. 23, no. 1, pp. 100–106, 2017.

[28] S. E. Herlihy, C. Lin, and Y. Nefedova, "Bone marrow myeloid cells in regulation of multiple myeloma progression," *Cancer Immunology, Immunotherapy*, vol. 66, no. 8, pp. 1007–1014, 2017.

22

Glomerulonephritis Pattern at a Jordanian Tertiary Care Center

Randa I. Farah ⓘ

Department of Internal Medicine, School of Medicine, University of Jordan, Amman, Jordan

Correspondence should be addressed to Randa I. Farah; r.farah@ju.edu.jo

Academic Editor: Jaime Uribarri

Aim. To determine the prevalence and frequency of different pathological patterns of glomerulonephritis (GN) in adolescent (age ≥ 11 years) and adult Jordanian patients. *Materials and Methods.* A retrospective analysis of all clinical and pathological reports of Jordanian patients who had native renal biopsies at the University of Jordan hospital between January 2007 and March 2018 to assess the prevalence and pathological pattern of GN. The data were analyzed statistically using descriptive statistics, the chi-squared test, and Fisher's exact tests. The level of significance was set at $P < 0.05$. *Results.* Two hundred and nine patients (88 males and 121 females) had native kidney biopsies diagnosed as having GN; the mean age at the time of biopsy was 36.0 ± 14.9 years. Primary GN (51.2%) was more common than secondary GN (48.8%). The most common GN was lupus nephritis (LN) (33.5%), followed by membranous nephropathy (MGN) (15.3%), and diabetic nephropathy (DN) (11.0%). Furthermore, IgA nephropathy was noted in 8.1% of cases. LN was the most common among the secondary GN and occurred in 49.6% of females; MGN was the most common primary GN and occurred in 22.7% of males. There was a statistically significant difference between males and females in the prevalence of LN and MGN ($P < .001$ and $P = .011$, respectively). LN was also dominant in all age groups expect for the ≥60 years group, which tended to exhibit DN (40%). *Conclusion.* LN is the most common GN type in Jordan, followed by MGN and DN. MGN is the predominant primary GN with a higher prevalence among males; LN is the predominant secondary GN and tends to occur in Jordanian females. The GN patterns in this study shifted from membranoproliferative GN to MGN in Jordan, which revealed a shift towards similar patterns exhibited in developed countries. Furthermore, DN is the most frequent GN in the elderly.

1. Introduction

Glomerulonephritis (GN) is a generic term for glomeruli injuries, which may range from massive inflammatory injuries that largely destroy the glomerulus to the injuries that can only be detected using sensitive techniques such as electron microscopy. GN is one of the main causes of chronic kidney disease and end-stage renal disease (ESRD) worldwide, which are responsible for major morbidity and mortality worldwide [1]. To establish a definitive diagnosis of GN and specify the pattern of glomerular injury, a histopathological and immunohistochemical analysis of the tissues typically obtained from patient's kidney via renal biopsy is necessary. Each type of GN has a specific histopathological pattern but does not have a specific clinical entity [2].

Glomerulonephritis can be classified into primary glomerular disease (primary GN) when there is no associated disease and secondary glomerular disease (secondary GN) when glomeruli involvement is part of a systemic disease such as connective tissue diseases, systemic lupus erythematosus, systemic vasculitis, and infective endocarditis. However, the mechanisms of glomerular injury are still not fully understood [3].

The incidence and period prevalence of GN resulting in death and ESRD in Jordan are unknown. A careful study of the incidence of different histopathological patterns of GN is necessary to establish the patterns and trends of glomerular diseases in a specific geographical area [4]. This will improve our ability to monitor disease trends, to formulate policies for an early detection of disease, and to take appropriate preventive and interventional measures.

Unfortunately, there are no recent data on the incidence of different histopathological patterns of GN in Jordan. Therefore, the aim of this cross-sectional study was to determine the prevalence and incidence of different histopathological patterns of GN in adolescent and adult patients in Jordan.

TABLE 1: Distribution of glomerular diseases based on incidence and patients' sex.

Diagnosis	Number (%)	Male (%)	Female (%)	P value
Primary Glomerulonephritis				
MGN	32 (15.3%)	20 (22.7%)	12 (9.9%)	0.018*
IgAN	17 (8.1%)	9 (10.2%)	8 (6.6%)	0.244
FSGS	12 (5.7%)	8 (9.1%)	4 (3.3%)	0.071
MCD	10 (4.8%)	6 (6.8%)	4 (3.3%)	0.198
MesPGN	9 (4.3%)	5 (5.7%)	4 (3.3%)	0.309
MPGN	9 (4.3%)	2 (2.3%)	7 (5.8%)	0.189
Chronic GN	9 (4.3%)	7 (8.0%)	2 (1.7%)	0.189
Post infectious GN	4 (1.9%)	3 (3.4%)	1 (0.8%)	0.202
Alport disease	1 (0.5%)	1 (1.1%)	0	0
CGN	4 (1.9%)	2 (2.3%)	2 (1.7%)	1
Secondary Glomerulonephritis				
Lupus nephritis	70 (33.5%)	10 (11.4%)	60 (49.6%)	< .001*
Diabetic nephropathy	23 (11.0%)	11 (12.5%)	12 (9.9%)	0.355
Fibrillary	5 (2.4%)	2 (2.3%)	3 (2.5%)	0.647
Renal amyloidosis	4 (1.9%)	3 (3.4%)	1 (0.8%)	0.202
Total	209 (100%)	88 (42.1%)	121 (57.9%)	

*Statistically significant difference. FSGS: focal and segmental glomerulosclerosis; MGN: membranous glomerulonephritis; IgAN: IgA nephropathy; MPGN: membranoproliferative glomerulonephritis; CGN: crescentic glomerulonephritis; MCD: minimal change disease; MesPGN: mesangioproliferative glomerulonephritis; GN: glomerulonephritis.

2. Materials and Methods

The pathological reports of native kidney biopsies, completed between January 2007 and March 2018, of 315 patients aged >11 years were retrieved from digital archives of the pathology department of Jordan University Hospital and were reviewed retrospectively. Indications for kidney biopsy were nephrotic proteinuria, nonnephrotic proteinuria with or without hematuria, unexplained acute kidney injury, unexplained chronic kidney disease, isolated glomerular hematuria, and systemic lupus erythromatous with evidence of renal involvement. All biopsies had been conducted percutaneously using real-time ultrasound guidance by a nephrologist or interventional radiologist. The specimens were prepared and examined in the hospital's pathological laboratory using light microscopy and immunofluorescence techniques. A few samples were processed (fixed and stained) and examined under electron microscopy.

The reports of kidney transplant biopsies, in addition to biopsies that revealed nonglomerular pathologies, including renal malignancies, tubulointerstitial diseases, and those with "no detectable abnormality" or "non-specific changes," were excluded from the study. The pathological reports of the remaining 209 patients with GN-diagnosed biopsies were investigated further, and their medical records, including biochemistry and urinalysis results, histopathological findings, and clinical indications of biopsy, were collected. The clinical indication was reported. The demographic information including patient sex, age at the time of biopsy, and nationality was also recorded. Repeat biopsies for the same patients during the study period were considered if they had a different clinical indication or pathological finding.

This study was conducted in accordance with the World Medical Association Declaration of Helsinki principles, and ethical approval was obtained as per the university hospital protocols.

2.1. Statistical Analysis. All analyses were performed using SPSS version 20 (IBM Corp., Chicago, IL, USA). P values less than 0.05 indicated statistical significance. Data are presented as means, standard deviations, frequencies, and percentages. We used the chi-squared test for association or Fisher's exact test (when the expected cell frequencies were less than 5) to investigate the statistically significant relationships between patients' sex and different histopathological patterns of GN.

2.2. Results. The records of native kidney biopsies of 209 patients were included and analyzed in this study. The mean age of patients at the time of biopsy was 36.0 ± 14.9 years (range: 11–77 years); 88 (42.11%) patients in the cohort were male, and 121 (57.9%) were female. One hundred and seventy-one patients (81.8%) were aged 19–59 years, 23 (11.0%) patients were aged ≤18 years, and 15 (7.2%) patients were aged ≥60 years. There were 107 patients (51.2%) with primary GN and 102 (48.8%) patients with secondary GN. The most common type of GN was lupus nephritis (33.5%), followed by membranous nephropathy (15.3%), and diabetic nephropathy (11.0%); the least common types of GN were Alport syndrome with an incidence of less than 1% and amyloidosis, crescentic GN, and postinfectious GN with an incidence of 4 (1.9%) each (Table 1, Figure 1). The four cases of crescentic GN were reported within the primary GN supgroup because there were

TABLE 2: Distribution of glomerular diseases based on etiology.

Diagnosis / Gender	Primary Glomerulonephritis	Secondary Glomerulonephritis	P value
Female No./ (%)	45 (42.1%)	76 (74.5%)	< .001[*]
Male No. /(%)	62 (57.9%)	26 (25.5%)	
TOTAL	107 (51.2%)	102 (48.8%)	

[*]Statistically significant difference.

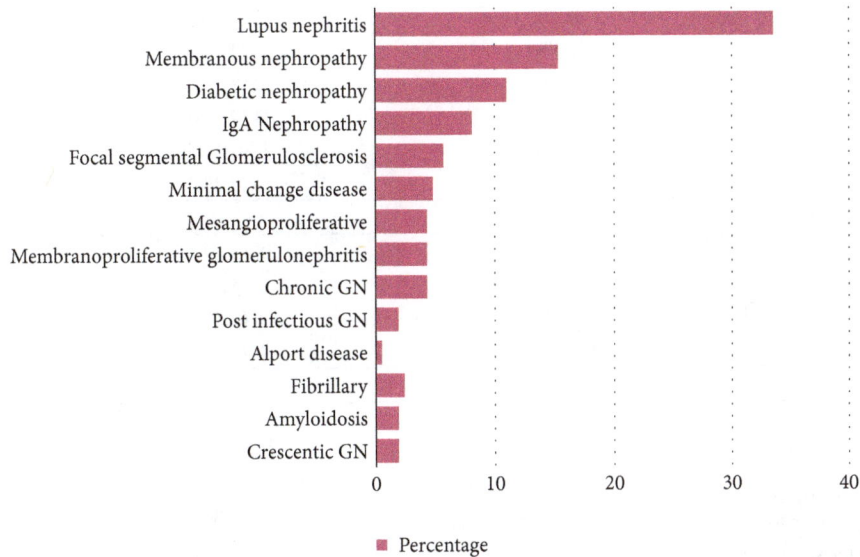

FIGURE 1: Incidence of different histopathological patterns of glomerulonephritis in the study population.

no signs of involvement by immunological or other systemic disease in these cases.

Roughly three quarters (74.5%) of patients who presented secondary GN were females; 57.9% of primary GN biopsies were from males (Table 2). There was a statistically significant association between patients' sex and histopathological presentation of GN (primary or secondary) (χ^2 (1) = 22.563, P < .001) with a moderate strength association (φ = 0.329, P < .001). The most common type of GN in male patients was membranous nephropathy (22.7%) followed by diabetic nephropathy (12.5%). In female patients, the most common type was lupus nephritis (49.6%) followed by membranous nephropathy and diabetic nephropathy (9.9% each). There was a statistically significant difference between male and female patients in terms of the prevalence of lupus nephritis (P < 0.001; Table 1).

Lupus nephritis was the most common histopathological pattern in young patients aged ≤18 years (43.5%) and in patients aged 19–59 years (33.9%). Diabetic nephropathy was the most common histopathological pattern in patients older than 60 years (40.0%; Table 3).

Lupus nephritis was the most common among secondary GN (68.6%), followed by diabetic nephropathy (22.5%); membranous nephropathy was the most common primary GN (30.0%), followed by IgA nephropathy (16.6%) (Figure 2).

2.3. Discussion. In this study, I reported the incidence of different histopathological patterns of GN in an adult patient population at Jordan University Hospital. This hospital is a tertiary care university-based hospital in the center of Amman, Jordan, with a capacity of approximately 600 beds [5]. It receives a large number of patients from all parts of Jordan, thus providing a good representative sample for our study, and all subjects in our study were Jordanians. I studied the incidence of different histopathological patterns of GN in Jordan between January 2007 and March 2018 and the changes in glomerular disease distribution that were associated with patients' age and sex. We compared our results with similar data reported previously from Jordan and other countries.

The prevalence of GN varies worldwide with time and location depending on the genetic profile and environmental exposure of populations [6]. Assessing changes of the glomerular disease pattern is important for an optimal allocation of resources and to focus our research on improving disease outcomes in the future.

Jordan has one of the youngest populations in the world; people aged under 55 years constitute 92% of the population, and the median age is 22.5 years [7]. Most of our patients were younger than 59 years (92%) with a median age of 36 years, and the proportion of elderly patients was quite low (7.5%).

Three studies reporting different histopathological patterns of glomerular disease and representing three different decades have been reported in Jordan [8–10]. The first of these was published by Ghnaimat et al. in 1999, which analyzed the biopsy reports of 191 adult patients from 1994 to 1997. In

TABLE 3: Distribution of glomerular diseases based on patients' age.

Diagnosis	Adolescent ≤18 years (%)	Adult 19–59 years (%)	Elderly ≥ 60 years (%)
Primary Glomerulonephritis			
MGN	2 (8.7%)	27 (15.8%)	3 (20.0%)
IgAN	1 (4.3%)	16 (9.4%)	0 (0%)
FSGS	3 (13.0%)	9 (5.3%)	0 (0%)
MCD	4 (17.4%)	6 (3.5%)	0 (0%)
MesPGN	2 (8.7%)	7 (4.1%)	0 (0%)
MPGN	1 (4.3%)	8 (4.7%)	0 (0%)
Chronic GN	0 (0%)	8 (4.7%)	1 (6.7%)
Post infectious GN	0 (0%)	4 (2.3%)	0 (0%)
Alport disease	0 (0%)	1 (0.58%0	0 (0%)
CGN	0 (0%)	4 (2.3%)	0 (0%)
Secondary Glomerulonephritis			
Lupus nephritis	10 (43%)	58 (33.9%)	2 (13.3%)
Diabetic nephropathy	0 (0%)	17 (9.9%)	6 (40%)
Fibrillary	0 (0%)	4 (2.3%)	1 (6.7%)
Renal amyloidosis	0 (0%)	2 (1.2%)	2 (13.3%)
Total	23 (11.0%)	171 (81.8%)	15 (7.2%)

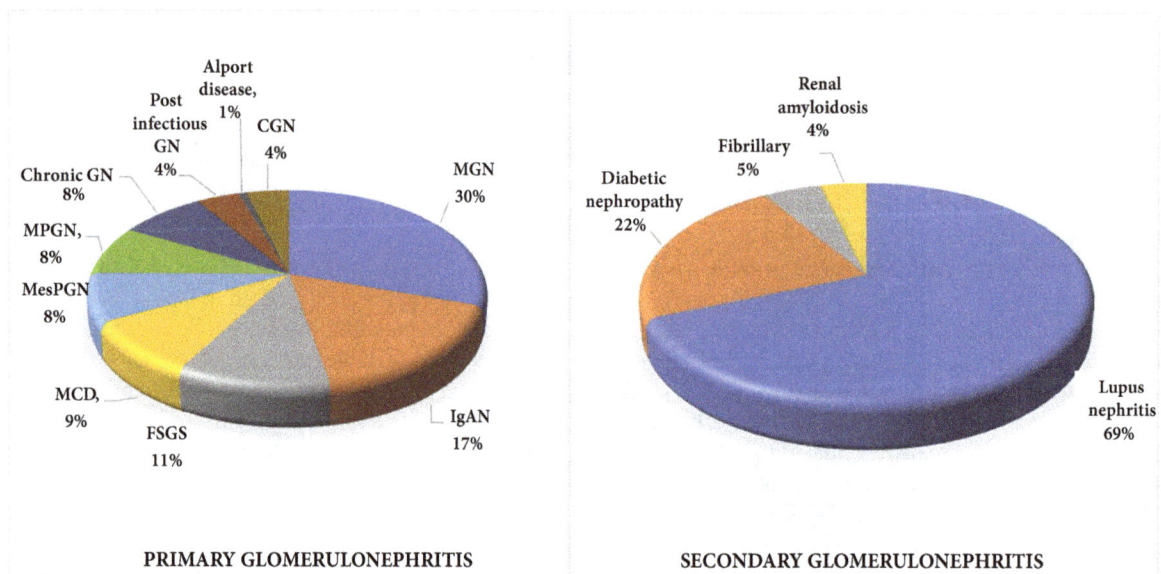

FIGURE 2: Different histopathological patterns of glomerulonephritis within the subgroup of primary and secondary GN.

this study, membranoproliferative GN (MPGN) was the most common histopathological pattern of glomerular disease that was reported in 25% of the patients, and the second most common type was focal segmental glomerulosclerosis (FSGS) that was reported in 22% of the patients [10]. The second study published by Said R et al. in 2000 analyzed the biopsy reports of 350 patients during two periods, i.e., from 1986 to 1989 and from 1997 to 1999. According to this study, MPGN was the most common type of primary glomerular disease that was reported in 18% of the patients, and FSGS was the second most common type reported in 13% of the patients [9]. The latest report was published by Wahbeh et al. in 2008 that included data on 64 patients from 2002 to 2006. According to this study, lupus nephritis was the most

common type of glomerular disease reported in 26.5% of the patients, and FSGS was the second most common type of primary glomerular disease reported in 17.2% of the patients [8].

In this cross-sectional study, data were collected for 209 patients from 2007 to 2018. Lupus nephritis was the most common type of glomerular disease reported in 33.5% of the patients; membranous nephropathy was the most commonly observed primary glomerular lesion reported in 15.3% of the patients and 30% of the patients with primary GN (Figure 2); and MPGN was reported in 4.3% of all patients with GN.

Although biopsy-based estimates are subject to selection bias due to clinical criteria used for kidney biopsy indication, the difference between our study and previous three studies may reflect the actual change in histopathological patterns of glomerular diseases. Jordan has changed in terms of social, environmental, and other factors including changes in living and other conditions. These changes may explain the differences in histopathological patterns of glomerular diseases over a period of time [6].

Membranous nephropathy has a high prevalence in Western countries, and there has been a rise in its incidence in different countries [6]. According to this study, changes in the patterns of primary GN (membranous nephropathy is the most common) can be attributed to social and economic factors as well as other factors such as better housing facility, higher standard of living, reduced exposure to infections, and improved healthcare [1]. These factors are also responsible for changing trends in Jordan towards being a more developed and industrialized country [7].

Lupus nephritis is the most common glomerular disease in Jordan. Among all types of GN, lupus nephritis has the highest incidence at 33.5% of the GN cases in Jordan (68.6% of the cases with secondary GN) and is considered to have the highest prevalence in the age group of 19-59 years, with a higher prevalence in female patients ($P < 0.05$) and a male/female ratio of around 1:6; these data are similar to those reported in the United States of America [11]. Contrary to the earlier studies, there is a trend towards an increase in the incidence of lupus nephritis over decades. Ghnaimat et al. and Said et al. [9, 10] reported low incidences of lupus nephritis in their studies at 9.4% and 8%, retrospectively. On the contrary, Wahbeh's [8] and our studies showed a high incidence of lupus nephritis at 26.5% and 33.5%, retrospectively. This can be related to a complex interplay of genetic, hormonal, environmental, and socioeconomic factors [12, 13].

The high incidence of lupus nephritis has been reported in most biopsy-based studies [14, 15]. In the countries neighboring Jordan, lupus nephritis is the most common type of secondary GN, and it is most likely related to the same environmental and genetic factors. For instance, in Oman, lupus nephritis affects 36.15% of the GN cases [13]; in Bahrain, 38.9% of the secondary GN cases [16]; in Egypt, 28.57% of the secondary GN cases [17]; and in Kuwait, 23.4% of secondary GN. The estimated total incidence of lupus nephritis as per the Saudi Arabia registry in 2000 had reached 57% of the secondary GN cases [18].

In this study, diabetic nephropathy was the second most common type of secondary GN reported in 22.5% of the secondary GN cases and 11% of the GN cases, and this is compatible with the data related to the high prevalence of diabetes in Jordan [19] and other countries; however, it may cause an underestimated true incidence of diabetic nephropathy in our population, especially because kidney biopsies are performed in patients with diabetes only if there is suspicion of nephropathy or if there is clinical indication of kidney biopsy. As noted in our study, the high-grade proteinuria with or without renal impairment was the clinical indication of kidney biopsy. Among the neighboring countries of Jordan, Qatar has a diabetic nephropathy prevalence of 50% of secondary GN [20], and Dubai has a diabetic nephropathy prevalence of 14% of secondary GN and 4.4% of GN [21].

MPGN and mesangial proliferative GN were each reported in 4.3% of our patients, and these were less prevalent in our cohort compared with that in earlier studies [8–10] owing to an improved infection control; similar results have been reported in recent data from Saudi Arabia [22] and Dubai [21].

FSGS was reported as the predominant pattern of GN in a previous report from Jordan [8]; however, it was less prevalent in our study. It is still the most common type of primary GN in Saudi Arabia [22] and Iran [23] and the second most common type of primary GN in the United States of America [11]. FSGS prevalence was underestimated in our study because of the clinical indications of kidney biopsy, changes in nephrologist's practice with advanced renal impairment in the presence of proteinuria and hypertension, and absence of renal disease screening strategies.

The incidence of immunoglobulin A nephropathy (IgAN) was slightly higher in our cohort compared to that in earlier studies. It was the second most common type of primary GN, reported in 8.1% of all cases and 18.2% of the primary GN cases [8–10]. IgAN is regarded as the most common type of GN in the world and is most prevalent in Asia (30–40%) and relatively less prevalent in Europe (20%) and North America (10%) [11]; however, it still has a much lower prevalence than that in other countries. These changes may be influenced by clinical indication of kidney biopsy and changes in nephrologist's practice in regard to performing kidney biopsy.

The prevalence of membranous nephropathy in our study was almost twice (6.3% vs. 15.3%) that reported in the earlier studies in Jordan [8], and it was significantly higher in male patients ($P < 0.05$) with a male/female ratio of 1.7:1, which is consistent with its typical racial distribution. All cases of membranous nephropathy in this study were idiopathic with a median age of 38 years. Membranous nephropathy is the most common type of primary GN in Western Saudi Arabia and has a high prevalence in countries such as Iran [23], Italy [24], and the United Arab Emirates [6].

In this study, the incidence of primary GN was slightly more than that of secondary GN (51.2% vs. 48.8%), which is consistent with the global reports and previous reports from Jordan [8–10], but there was a slightly higher incidence of secondary GN compared to that reported in previous studies in Jordan and the neighboring countries. This may be related to a significant increase in the incidence of lupus nephritis and diabetic nephropathy in our population.

The changing patterns of GN in Jordan could be related to the economic changes in the population as 91.0% of the total population is urban, and the annual rate of urbanization is reported as 2.43% [7]. This trend reflects improvement in housing facilities and standards of living with more frequent vaccination and less exposure to infections.

This study had a few limitations. First, this was a single-center study that lacked the data on Jordanian registry for GN. Second, the sample size was limited, which made it difficult to interpret the age- and sex-related differences in several subgroups of this study. Therefore, we recommend that a multicenter study with a larger sample size should be conducted to allow a more comprehensive interpretation of our results among the different subgroups of GN.

3. Conclusion

The data presented in this study will help to shed light on the epidemiology of GN in Jordan in the past 10 years. Our results show that lupus nephritis is the most common GN type in Jordan followed by membranous nephropathy and diabetic nephropathy. Membranous nephropathy is the most common type of primary GN with a higher prevalence in the male patient population. Lupus nephritis is the most common type of secondary GN with a higher prevalence in the female patient population. Secondary GN is slightly less common than primary GN. Furthermore, diabetic nephropathy is the most common type of GN in the elderly. The histopathological patterns of GN in this study shifted from MPGN to membranous nephropathy. These results differ notably from those of previous studies conducted in Jordan and reveal a shift towards similar patterns exhibited in developed countries, which indicate that there are fewer cases of GN associated with infections and more cases of GN associated with autoimmune diseases, antigen exposure, ageing, and obesity.

References

[1] A. Schieppati and G. Remuzzi, "Chronic renal diseases as a public health problem: epidemiology, social, and economic implications," *Kidney International Supplements*, vol. 68, no. 98, pp. S7–S10, 2005.

[2] P. W. Mathieson, "Glomerulonephritis," *Seminars in Immunopathology*, vol. 29, no. 4, pp. 315-316, 2007.

[3] H. L. Abbate, D. Macconi, and G. Remuzzi, "Mechanisms of glomerular injury," in *Toxicology of the Kidney*, J. B. Hook and R. S. Goldstein, Eds., pp. 153–200, Raven Press Ltd, New York, NY, USA, 1993.

[4] U. Das, K. V. Dakshinamurty, and A. Prayaga, "Pattern of biopsy-proven renal disease in a single center of south India: 19 years experience," *Indian Journal of Nephrology*, vol. 21, no. 4, pp. 250–257, 2011.

[5] "University of Jordan hospital. Annual report. Illustrations about the hospital," March 2012.

[6] K.-T. Woo, C. M. Chan, Y. M. Chin et al., "Global evolutionary trend of the prevalence of primary glomerulonephritis over the past three decades," *Nephron Clinical Practice*, vol. 116, no. 4, pp. c337–c346, 2010.

[7] The world factbook, "Washington (DC): Central Intelligence Agency (CIA)," 2018, https://www.cia.gov/library/publications/the-world-factbook/geos/jo.html.

[8] A. M. Wahbeh, M. H. Ewais, and M. E. Elsharif, "Spectrum of glomerulonephritis in adult Jordanians at Jordan university hospital." *Saudi journal of kidney diseases and transplantation : an official publication of the Saudi Center for Organ Transplantation, Saudi Arabia*, vol. 19, no. 6, pp. 997-1000, 2008.

[9] R. Said, Y. Hamzeh, and M. Tarawneh, "The Spectrum of Glomerulopathy in Jordan," *Saudi Journal of Kidney Disease and Transplantation*, vol. 11, no. 3, pp. 430–433, 2000.

[10] M. Ghnaimat, N. Akash, and M. El-Lozi, "Kidney biopsy in jordan: complications and histopathological findings," *Saudi Journal of Kidney Disease and Transplantation*, vol. 10, no. 2, pp. 152-156, 1999.

[11] C. H. Feldman, L. T. Hiraki, J. Liu et al., "Epidemiology and sociodemographics of systemic lupus erythematosus and lupus nephritis among US adults with Medicaid coverage, 2000-2004," *Arthritis & Rheumatology*, vol. 65, no. 3, pp. 753–763, 2013.

[12] G. S. Cooper, M. A. Dooley, E. L. Treadwell, E. W. St. Clair, C. G. Parks, and G. S. Gilkeson, "Hormonal, environmental, and infectious risk factors for developing systemic lupus erythematosus," *Arthritis & Rheumatology*, vol. 41, no. 10, pp. 1714–1724, 1998.

[13] D. Al Riyami, K. Al Shaaili, Y. Al Bulushi, A. Al Dhahli, and A. Date, "The spectrum of glomerular diseases on renal biopsy: Data from a single tertiary center in Oman," *Oman Medical Journal*, vol. 28, no. 3, pp. 213–215, 2013.

[14] P. Malafronte, G. Mastroianni-Kirsztajn, G. N. Betônico et al., "Paulista registry of glomerulonephritis: 5-year data report," *Nephrology Dialysis Transplantation*, vol. 21, no. 11, pp. 3098–3105, 2006.

[15] S. Murugapandian, I. Mansour, M. Hudeeb et al., "Epidemiology of glomerular disease in southern Arizona review of 10-year renal biopsy data," *Medicine (United States)*, vol. 95, no. 18, p. e3633, 2016.

[16] A. Al Arrayed, S. M. George, A. K. Malik et al., "The spectrum of glomerular diseases in the Kingdom of Bahrain: An epidemiological study based on renal biopsy interpretation," *Transplantation Proceedings*, vol. 36, no. 6, pp. 1792–1795, 2004.

[17] S. Ibrahim, A. Fayed, S. Fadda, and D. Belal, "A five-year analysis of the incidence of glomerulonephritis at Cairo University Hospital-Egypt." *Saudi journal of kidney diseases and transplantation : an official publication of the Saudi Center for Organ Transplantation, Saudi Arabia*, vol. 23, no. 4, pp. 866–870, 2012.

[18] S. Huraib, A. Al Khader, and F. A. Shaheen, "The spectrum of glomerulonephritis in Saudi Arabia: the results of the Saudi registry," *Saudi Journal of Kidney Disease and Transplantation*, vol. 11, no. 3, pp. 434–441, 2000.

[19] K. Ajlouni, Y. S. Khader, A. Batieha, H. Ajlouni, and M. El-Khateeb, "An increase in prevalence of diabetes mellitus in Jordan over 10 years," *Journal of Diabetes and its Complications*, vol. 22, no. 5, pp. 317–324, 2008.

[20] W. Mubarak, A. Awad, and W. Jafery, "Renal Diseases: Analysis of the Renal Biopsy Service in a Single National Institute. Poster session presented at," in *Proceedings of the European Congress of Radiology*, Vienna, Austria, 2015.

[21] A. Alhadari, F. Alalawi, A. Seddik et al., "Pattern of acute glomerulonephritis in adult population in Dubai: A single-center experience," *Saudi Journal of Kidney Diseases and Transplantation*, vol. 28, no. 3, p. 571, 2017.

[22] K. I. Almatham, A. F. Alfayez, R. A. Alharthi et al., "Glomerulonephritis disease pattern at saudi tertiary care center," *Saudi Medical Journal*, vol. 38, no. 11, pp. 1113–1117, 2017.

[23] H. Mohammadhoseiniakbari, N. Rezaei, A. Rezaei, S. K. Roshan, and Y. Honarbakhsh, "Pattern of glomerulonephritis in Iran: A preliminary study and brief review," *Medical Science Monitor*, vol. 15, no. 9, pp. PH109–PH114, 2009.

[24] P. Stratta, G. P. Segoloni, C. Canavese et al., "Incidence of biopsy-proven primary glomerulonephritis in an Italian province," *American Journal of Kidney Diseases*, vol. 27, no. 5, pp. 631–639, 1996.

23

Projecting the Burden of Chronic Kidney Disease in a Developed Country and its Implications on Public Health

L. Y. Wong⬛,[1] A. S. T. Liew,[2] W. T. Weng,[2] C. K. Lim,[3] A. Vathsala,[4] and M. P. H. S. Toh[1,5]

[1]*Chronic Disease Epidemiology, Population Health, National Healthcare Group, Singapore*
[2]*Renal Medicine, Tan Tock Seng Hospital, Singapore*
[3]*Clinical Services, National Healthcare Group Polyclinics, Singapore*
[4]*Nephrology, National University Hospital, Singapore*
[5]*Population Health, National Healthcare Group, Singapore*

Correspondence should be addressed to L. Y. Wong; lai_yin_wong@nhg.com.sg

Academic Editor: Franca Anglani

Background. Chronic Kidney Disease (CKD) is a major public health problem worldwide. There is limited literature on a model to project the number of people with CKD. This study projects the number of residents with CKD in Singapore by 2035 using a Markov model. *Methods.* A Markov model with nine mutually exclusive health states was developed according to the clinical course of CKD, based on a discrete time interval of 1 year. The model simulated the transition of cohorts across different health states from 2007 to 2035 using prevalence, incidence, mortality, disease transition, and disease detection rates. *Results.* From 2007 to 2035, the number of residents with CKD is projected to increase from 316,521 to 887,870 and the prevalence from 12.2% to 24.3%. Patients with CKD stages 1-2 constituted the largest proportion. The proportion of undiagnosed cases will decline from 72.1% to 56.4%, resulting from faster progression to higher CKD stages and its eventual detection. *Conclusion.* By 2035, about one-quarter of the Singapore residents are expected to have CKD. National policies need to focus on primary disease prevention and early disease detection to avoid delayed treatment of CKD which eventually leads to end-stage renal disease.

1. Introduction

Chronic Kidney Disease (CKD) is a major public health problem worldwide. The prevalence of CKD in Singapore was reported to be 15.6% [1] in 2007. This was considered excessive compared to countries with higher incidence of end-stage renal disease (ESRD) such as USA [2], Korea [3], Japan [4], and Taiwan [5]. Although the definition of CKD used in the estimation of prevalence for these countries was inconsistent and made cross-country comparison challenging, the prevalence of CKD in Singapore remained relatively high even after adjustments were made to allow for comparison across these countries [2–5].

Previous literature [6] reported high prevalence of cardiovascular diseases in individuals with CKD, and likewise, CKD had been recognized as an independent risk factor of cardiovascular disease outcomes. CKD is associated with elevated risks of all-cause mortality and increased healthcare utilization [7–9]. The hazard ratios of death among individuals with CKD stages 3-5 vis-à-vis those without CKD ranged between 1.2 and 5.9 [7, 10]. In addition, individuals with CKD were 1.6 - 2.2 times more likely to be hospitalized [9]. Consequently, the unadjusted annual incremental direct all-cause healthcare costs associated with CKD among cohorts with (a) diabetes only, (b) hypertension only, and (c) both diabetes and hypertension were USD11,814, USD8,412, and USD10,625, respectively [11]. Patients with CKD were also reported to have compromised quality of life (QoL), with progressively lower QoL scores as CKD advances [12]. Thus, the burden of CKD to both the healthcare providers and patients is heavy and overwhelming.

Notwithstanding that earlier CKD stages, if treated early, may prevent the progression to ESRD [13, 14], the rate of diagnosis and public awareness of CKD remain low [2, 5, 15, 16]. Many people with CKD present in late stages with some presenting only during ESRD requiring dialysis or renal transplantation. From 2011 to 2014, Singapore had consistently ranked as one of the top five countries with the highest ESRD incidence rates in the world [17]. Consequently, as the prevalence of CKD increases, the impact on the ESRD burden will become increasingly significant. By 2030, 20.5% of Singapore's population is estimated to be elderly (age more than 65 years) [18]. With an ageing population, the prevalence of CKD is expected to increase considerably as kidney function declines even with normal ageing [19]. Therefore, projecting the future prevalence of CKD, especially for the population in whom the condition is undiagnosed, would quantify the magnitude of its burden with insights on disease progression. This can influence policy-making to address public health concerns and develop preventive interventions to retard CKD progression.

Currently, there is limited literature on a model to project the number of people with CKD and undiagnosed cases. The aim of this study is to project the number of Singapore residents who are aged 21+ years and have CKD in 2035 using a Markov model.

2. Methods

2.1. Markov Model and Health States. A Markov model, which assumes that an individual is always in one of a finite number of discrete health states, is commonly used to project the number of persons with mutually exclusive health states [20–22]. It offers a dynamic forecasting approach by simulating the progression of individuals from one health state to another at discrete time intervals (i.e., cycles) based on time-dependent transition probabilities, $Pij\ (0,\ t)$, which is the probability of an individual who is in state i at time 0, who will transit to be in state j at time t.

In this study, we projected the number of residents with CKD stages 1 to 5 between 2007 and 2035 using a Markov cohort simulation based on a discrete time interval of 1 year (i.e., 28 one-year cycles). We developed a Markov model with nine mutually exclusive health states according to the clinical course of CKD: (i) Non-CKD; (ii) stages 1-2 (undetected); (iii) stages 1-2 (detected); (iv) stage 3 (undetected); (v) stage 3 (detected); (vi) stage 4 (undetected); (vii) stage 4 (detected); (viii) stage 5; and (ix) death (Figure 1).

Transition between health states occurs on a one-year cycle. During the 28 one-year cycles, population growth in each health state occurs through entry of new population (i.e., net migrants and live births) and cohort transition from one health state to another during each cycle. Subjects who start at the "normal" health state may stay in the same state or progress to CKD stages 1-2 (with proteinuria) or CKD 3 (without proteinuria) during the year ahead. If they progress to CKD stages 1-2 and are screened, they will move to the "detected CKD stages 1-2" state in the next cycle. If they progress to CKD stages 1-2 and are not screened, they will move to "undetected CKD stages 1-2" instead. If they do not progress, they will remain at the state of "normal". Similarly, those who start at "detected CKD stages 1-2" may progress to CKD stage 3. If they were screened, they will move to "detected CKD stage 3" in the next cycle; otherwise, they will move to "undetected CKD stage 3". However, if they do not

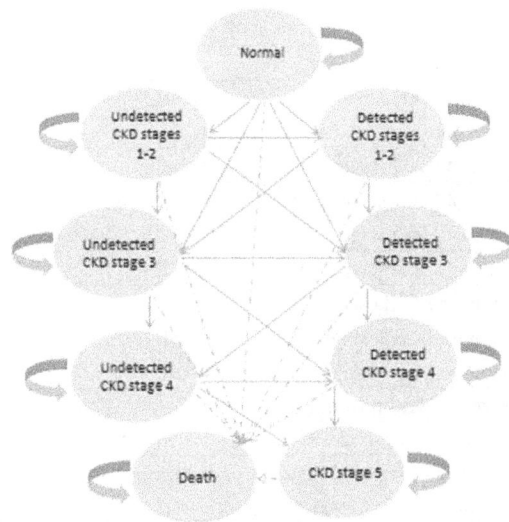

FIGURE 1: Markov state transition model for the progression of CKD.

progress, they will remain at the state of "detected CKD stages 1-2" regardless of whether screening is performed.

2.2. Data Sources. In 2007, the National Healthcare Group (NHG) launched an enterprise-wide chronic disease registry, Chronic Disease Management System (CDMS), to deliver comprehensive and continuous care for patients with chronic diseases [23]. The CDMS links administrative and clinical information of patients who seek care at NHG, which includes three acute care public hospitals and nine primary care clinics. The integrated data enables information access and longitudinal tracking of patient outcomes across different care settings from inpatient, emergency department and specialist outpatient clinics to primary care clinics. Despite the unavailability of private healthcare utilization records, CDMS was able to capture 69% of all detected diabetes and 73% of all detected prediabetes in Singapore [20]. Thus, CDMS is representative of the patient population in Singapore.

Input values for the base year in this study were shown in Table 1.

2.3. Definition of CKD in the CDMS. The definition of CKD in CDMS follows the Kidney Disease: Improving Global Outcomes (KDIGO) 2012 CKD Guidelines [25]. In CDMS, earlier CKD stages (stages 1 and 2) are defined based on both estimated Glomerular Filtration Rate (eGFR) level and marker of kidney damage such as Urinary Albumin-to-Creatinine Ratio (UACR) and Urinary Protein-to-Creatinine Ratio (UPCR), whilst moderate to severe CKD stages are defined primarily by eGFR level (Table 2).

For simplicity, patients with eGFR 30-59 mls/min/1.73m2 were defined to have CKD stage 3. The eGFR in the CDMS was estimated using Modification of Diet in Renal Disease (MDRD) equation.

2.4. Estimating the Coverage of CDMS for CKD. The national numbers of patients with CKD stages 1 to 3 were computed

TABLE 1: Input values for the base year.

Parameter (aged 21+ years)	Value	Source(s)
Demographic variables		
Prevalence of non-CKD, 2007 (unadjusted)	84.4%	Sabanayagam et al., 2010 [1]
Prevalence of CKD stages 1-2, 2007 (unadjusted)	10.0%	Sabanayagam et al., 2010 [1]
Prevalence of CKD stage 3, 2007 (unadjusted)	5.3%	Sabanayagam et al., 2010 [1]
Prevalence of CKD stage 4, 2007 (unadjusted)	0.2%	Sabanayagam et al., 2010 [1]
Prevalence of CKD stage 5, 2007 (unadjusted)	0.01%	Sabanayagam et al., 2010 [1]
% undiagnosed CKD stages 1-2, 2007 (adjusted)	85.3%	Sabanayagam et al., 2010 [1] and CDMS (with assumption)
% undiagnosed CKD stage 3, 2007 (adjusted)	66.9%	Sabanayagam et al., 2010 [1] and CDMS (with assumption)
% undiagnosed CKD stage 4, 2007 (adjusted)	47.3%	Sabanayagam et al., 2010 [1] and CDMS (with assumption)
Singapore resident population		
Singapore resident population, 2007	2,603,628	Population Trends 2014 [24]
Mortality rates (per 1000 resident population)		
Mortality rate, 2007	6.50	Population Trends 2014 [24]

CDMS: Chronic Disease Management System; CKD: Chronic Kidney Disease.

TABLE 2: Definition of CKD in the CDMS.

Stages of CKD	eGFR	Marker of kidney damage in CDMS
Early (Stages 1-2)	≥ 60 ml/min/1.73 m^2	Any 1 of the following: (i) Two UACR lab tests ≥ 2.5 mg/mmol (male), 90 days apart (ii) Two UACR lab tests ≥ 3.5 mg/mmol (female), 90 days apart (iii) Two UACR lab tests > 30mg/g, 90 days apart (iv) Two UPCR lab tests ≥ 20mg/mmol, 90 days apart (v) Two UPCR lab tests > 0.2mg/mg, 90 days apart (vi) Two Urine Protein lab tests ≥ 0.2 g/day, 90 days apart
Moderate (Stage 3A)	45-59 ml/min/1.73 m^2	With or without kidney damage
Moderate (Stage 3B)	30-44 ml/min/1.73 m^2	With or without kidney damage
Severe (Stage 4)	15-29 ml/min/1.73 m^2	With or without kidney damage
Severe (Stage 5)	<15ml/min/1.73 m^2	With or without kidney damage

based on the national prevalence of each CKD stage estimated from a local population-based study [1]. The CDMS coverage for CKD stages 1 to 3 were derived by taking the prevalent numbers of patients in each stage in the CDMS as a proportion of the national numbers of patients in the respective CKD stage.

The yearly national incidence of CKD stage 5 was available from the National Registry Disease Office (NRDO). The CDMS coverage for stage 5 was estimated based on the proportion of stage 5 incident cases in the CDMS divided by the national CKD stage 5 incidence. As the NRDO does not report incidence of CKD stages 1 to 4, the CDMS coverage for stage 4 was estimated by taking the average of CDMS coverage for stages 3 and 5, based on the assumption that the CDMS coverage rises with CKD severity as a result of higher healthcare utilization by those with more severe conditions.

To attenuate the risk of underestimating the CDMS coverage for each CKD stage for base year (i.e., 2007, the same

year the CDMS was launched), the CDMS coverage for 2010 was also computed by assuming that the data captured in CDMS would be stabilized after 3 years. The average CDMS coverage of years 2007 and 2010 was estimated for each CKD stage and was used in this study.

2.5. National Prevalence of CKD in the Base Year. The prevalence of CKD in 2007 was estimated from a study by Sabanayagam et al. [1] which was a local population-based epidemiological study conducted in 2007. The authors used objective measurements to determine the presence of CKD among multiethnic groups (Chinese, Malay, and Indians) in Singapore. Hence 2007 was used as the base year to build the model in our study.

Sabanayagam et al. [1] reported the national prevalence of CKD stages 1-2, 3, 4, and 5 to be 10.0%, 5.3%, 0.2%, and 0.01%, respectively. CKD stages 1-2 were defined as eGFR ≥ 60 ml/min/1.73 m^2 with the presence of albuminuria. However, as the KDIGO defined kidney damage as persistent abnormality in albumin-creatinine ratio or other markers for more than 3 months [25], the use of a single UACR measurement by Sabanayagam et al. [1] to define albuminuria could have overestimated the prevalence of CKD stages 1-2. In this study, we estimated the proportion of individuals with persistent albuminuria among the people with stages 1-2 based on percentages reported in the literature [26–28] and adjusted the pertinent prevalence reported by Sabanayagam et al. [1] to 5.6%.

The prevalence of CKD stages 4 and 5 reported by Sabanayagam et al. [1] was low, as the survey could have been underrepresented by those with severe CKD. Hence, we estimated the respective prevalence using the CDMS coverage. We divided the numbers of prevalent patients in the CDMS by the CDMS coverage to derive the national numbers of individuals with stages 4 and 5 and further divide these numbers by the number of Singapore residents to yield the national prevalence of CKD stages 4 and 5. No adjustment was made to the prevalence of CKD stage 3 reported by Sabanayagam et al. [1].

2.6. National Prevalence of Detected CKD in the Base Year. For simplicity, we assumed the coverage of the CDMS for detected CKD to be 70%, similar to the rate for detected diabetes (69%) and prediabetes (73%) at national level [20]. We derived the national numbers of detected CKD stages 1 to 4 based on this assumption and the respective numbers of prevalent CKD patients in the CDMS. Further comparison of the national numbers of detected CKD stages 1 to 4 with the respective national numbers of CKD (both detected and undetected) yielded the detection rates for the four stages. We multiplied the CKD prevalence rates with detection rates to obtain the prevalence of detected CKD for each stage.

2.7. Annual Transition and Detection Probabilities. Movement of individuals between health states over time was tracked using transition probabilities. The historical transition probabilities of each CKD stage were derived primarily from the CDMS based on the annual incidence of each CKD stage. Historical CKD detection probabilities were determined by specifying an equation representing sources of detected CKD incident cohorts and equated this equation with the historical observed data. Detection probabilities from this equation were derived based on the assumption that ratio of detection probabilities of individuals at a higher (e.g., CKD stage 3) to lower (e.g., CKD stages 1-2) disease continuum was equal to their mortality rate ratio.

To forecast future time-dependent transition and detection probabilities between 2015 and 2035, we computed the base transition and detection probabilities by averaging the respective probabilities from 2010 to 2014 and elevated these base probabilities for CKD stages 1 to 4 using an ageing index. The ageing index is a product of the yearly proportion of elderly residents (aged 65+ years) and the yearly increase in the proportion of the elderly from the reference rate (5-year average elderly proportion in 2010-14). Elevation of transition

and detection probabilities using the aging index aims to address the forthcoming population ageing in Singapore, given that kidney function declines with ageing [19] and the elderly has higher healthcare utilization [29], thus translating into higher CKD incidence and detection rates.

The ageing index was not applied to the transition probabilities from stage 4 to stage 5 as it was found that there were higher competing risks of death among the elderly patients [30, 31]. For stage 5, we assumed 100% detection rate in this study as the NRDO captures the incidence of renal failure at national level.

2.8. Historical and Forecast Mortality Rates. The mortality risks of individuals with CKD were found to be higher than those without CKD [32]; thus we assumed the mortality rate of individuals with CKD was equal to the product of the relative risk of death for people with CKD and the mortality rate of those without CKD as in the following equation:

$$MR_{it} = RR_{it} \times MR_t \tag{1}$$

where MR_{it} is the mortality rate of individuals with CKD stage i at time t; MR_t is the mortality rate of individuals without CKD at time t; RR_{it} is the relative risk of death for individuals with CKD stage i versus without CKD at time t

2.8.1. Historical Mortality Rates. For individuals with CKD, we estimated their historical mortality rates at different CKD stages (ie. MR_{it}) using both hospital deaths and national deaths recorded in the CDMS. For those without CKD, the historical mortality rate at time t (i.e., MR_t) was derived using (2), where the historical number of deaths at time t at national level (i.e., MV_t) was available from public source [33]:

$$MV_t = MR_{12t} \times CKD_{12t} + MR_{3t} \times CKD_{3t} + MR_{4t}$$
$$\times CKD_{4t} + MR_{5t} \times CKD_{5t} + MR_t \times NCKD_t \tag{2}$$

where MV_t is the total number of deaths at time t; MR_{it} is the mortality rate of individuals with CKD stage i at time t; MR_t is the mortality rate of individuals without CKD at time t; CKD_{it} is the estimated number of individuals with CKD stage i at time t; $NCKD_t$ is the estimated number of individuals without CKD at time t.

Based on MR_{it} and MR_t, we derived historical RR_{it} using (1) and estimated the 5-year average (2010 to 2014) relative risk of death for individuals with CKD stage i versus without CKD (i.e., RR_i) based on RR_{it}.

2.8.2. Forecast Mortality Rates. Future mortality rates of individuals without CKD were forecast based on (3). Detailed methodologies on the forecasts of national residents and residents' mortality (i.e., MV_t) have been published elsewhere [20]. In short, we projected future population growth using compounded annual growth rates and forecast future MV_t for those aged 21+ years at national level after we forecast (i) life expectancy; (ii) number of deaths of all ages; and (iii) number of deaths of people aged <21 years.

$$MR_t = \frac{MV_t}{\left(RR_{12} \times CKD_{12t} + RR_3 \times CKD_{3t} + RR_4 \times CKD_{4t} + RR_5 \times CKD_{5t} + NCKD_t\right)} \tag{3}$$

The forecast mortality rates of those without CKD were used as input values to forecast mortality rates of individuals with CKD using the following equation:

$$MR_{it} = RR_i \times MR_t \tag{4}$$

2.9. Other Assumptions. We assumed individuals will reside in a health state for a minimum of one cycle (i.e., 1 year) before progressing to the next and the CKD progression was one-way without regression to the previous state.

2.10. Approval. Approval to conduct this study was obtained from the NHG Ethics Review Board (Domain-Specific Review Board).

3. Results

3.1. Forecasting the Prevalence and Number of CKD Individuals. After adjustments to CKD prevalence using estimates from Sabanayagam et al. [1], we estimated there were 145,803, 137,992, 24,293, and 8,434 cases of CKD stages 1-2, 3, 4, and 5, respectively, in 2007. By 2035, the Markov model projected the numbers to be 383,122 (95% CI: 322,402 - 435,781), 337,779 (95% CI: 310,663 - 365,407), 118,821 (95% CI: 106,048 - 131,950), and 48,148 (95% CI: 33,271 - 66,070), respectively. The total number of individuals with CKD in 2035 is almost triple that in 2007 and the prevalence is projected to increase from 12.2% in 2007 to 24.3% (95% CI: 21.2% - 27.4%) in 2035 (Figure 2). Throughout the 28 years, stages 1-2 constituted the largest proportion of CKD cases, followed by stages 3, 4, and 5. During this period, the proportion of people with stages 4 and 5 is estimated to increase from 7.7% to 13.4% and from 2.7% to 5.4%, respectively. Number of individuals with stage 5 is expected to increase by 5-fold from 8,434 in 2007 to 48,148 in 2035.

The overall prevalence of undiagnosed CKD was 8.8% (stages 1-2: 4.8%; stage 3: 3.5%; stage 4: 0.4%) in 2007. This is projected to increase to 13.7% (stages 1-2: 7.5%; stage 3: 5.0%; stage 4: 1.2%) by 2035. The proportion of undiagnosed cases is expected to decline from 72.1% in 2007 to 56.4% in 2035. The increase in the detection rates is postulated to be fuelled by the faster progression to the higher CKD stages as part of population ageing. As older patients and those with higher CKD stages are more likely to have routine visits to healthcare, we expect them to have laboratory tests as part of their regular care thus increasing the likelihood of detecting CKD. Throughout the 28 years, CKD stages 1-2 remained the main sources of undiagnosed cases as these contributed more than half of such cases (Figure 3).

3.2. Sensitivity Analysis. The sensitivity analysis showed that an annual 1% reduction in the incident CKD stages 1-2

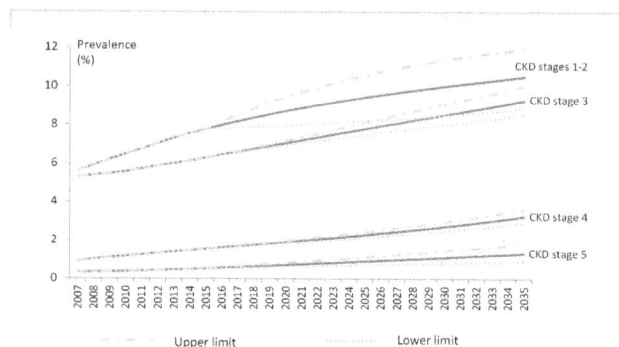

FIGURE 2: Prevalence of CKD by stage, with projection till 2035.

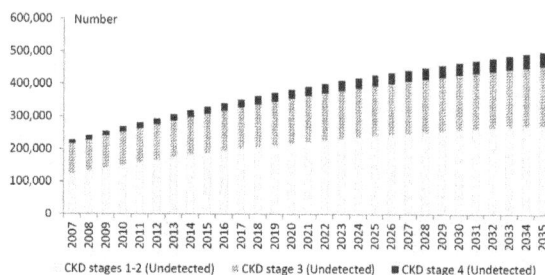

FIGURE 3: Number of undiagnosed cases of CKD by stage, with projection till 2035.

between 2007 and 2035 could prevent 5,197 CKD cases from the baseline forecast of 887,870. Similarly, an annual 1% increase in detection rate for stages 1-2 would reduce 942 undetected CKD cases over baseline forecast, whilst an annual 1% increase in detection rate for stage 4 would reduce 208 cases. Thus, a steady 1% increase in detection rate annually for CKD stages 1-2 vis-à-vis CKD stage 4 would reduce undetected cases by 734.

4. Discussion

This study projected that the number of individuals with CKD will reach 887,870 in 2035, almost triple that in 2007, whilst the number of undiagnosed CKD cases is forecast to be 500,600, more than double that in 2007. One of the main drivers behind the surge in CKD prevalence could be the increase in incidence of diabetes and hypertension. In Singapore, the prevalence of diabetes and hypertension in 2010 was 11.3% and 23.5%, respectively [34]. This represents 56% and 7% increases in the numbers of people with diabetes and hypertension, respectively, over 6 years from 2004 [34]. By 2035, the prevalence of diabetes among Singapore residents is projected to be 1 in 5 [20]. Although the forecast of the prevalence of hypertension is unavailable, it is expected to rise in tandem with that of diabetes as both conditions share common pathophysiologic pathways [35]. Apart from this, population growth and the longer life expectancy of Singapore residents are other potential drivers leading to increase in the prevalence of CKD. The life expectancy at birth in Singapore had increased steadily from 65.8 years in 1970 to 82.7 years in 2015 [33]. The upward trend is expected to continue and projected to reach 87.7 years by 2035 [20]. The ageing population is postulated to increase the CKD cases as renal impairment is common in the elderly.

Previous literature [36, 37] raised concerns on the use of a universal GFR threshold of 60 ml/min/1.73m^2 to define CKD, in particular among the elderly, as decline in "normal" GFR with ageing in the absence of kidney damage marker is physiologic and the associated mortality risk of those with eGFR of 45-59 ml/min/1.73m^2 was found to be trivial. Various suggestions had been made in the literature to revise the CKD classification, including lowering the eGFR threshold to below 45 ml/min/1.73m^2 for stage 3 definition [38] and introducing age- and gender-specific qualifying levels of GFR [39, 40]. If we revised our projection by excluding the elderly aged 65+ years whose eGFR was 45-59 ml/min/1.73m^2 but without proteinuria, the adjusted number of CKD individuals in 2035 is estimated to be reduced by one-quarter from the baseline forecast of 887,870 to 668,987. This study used MDRD equation to define CKD stage. Our forecast of CKD numbers may be different if CKE-EPI was used as it more accurately estimates GFR and categorized ESRD risk than the MDRD equation [41]. CKD-EPI classified fewer individuals as having CKD [41] and thus our forecast of CKD prevalence would be lower if CKD-EPI was used. Nevertheless, we are unable to estimate the magnitude of the reduction as identification of individuals with CKD using CKD-EPI is currently not configured in the CDMS.

With the expected rise in CKD in the coming years, more extensive health resources including ambulatory, hospitalization, and dialysis care would be required. In Singapore, the prevalence of ESRD increased from 1,405 per million residents in 2006 to 2,076 per million residents in 2016, representing 47.8% increase in a decade [42]. Our healthcare expenditure had increased from 4% of GDP expenditure in 2005 to 4.9% in 2014 [43]. The health system would need to be prepared for the significant surge in demand for health services in the next decades. However, CKD is often undiagnosed, largely due to its asymptomatic nature. Our CKD detection rate in the base year was low at 27.9%. In countries with the highest ESRD incidence rates in the world such as USA, Thailand, and Taiwan, the CKD awareness rates among those with CKD were even lower (USA: 6% [44]; Thailand: 1.9% [45]; Taiwan: 3.5% [5]). In USA, despite the efforts to increase CKD awareness among the nephrologists, general physicians, and the public via dissemination of KDOQI guidelines, setting up of CKD education programmes, and offering free screening to the public, there was merely marginal improvement in awareness rates [44]. In Thailand, the low awareness could be attributed to the underdiagnosis of CKD as only serum creatinine was widely available and used by the local healthcare professionals to assess kidney

function, instead of eGFR prediction equation such as MDRD equation [45]. Similarly, the eGFR prediction equation based on calibrated creatinine was not commonly used in Taiwan, leading to underdiagnosis of CKD and low awareness among the patients [5]. Our detection rate was relatively high compared to the awareness rates in USA, Thailand, and Taiwan. This could be due to the fundamental differences in definitions and methodologies used to estimate the CKD detection and awareness rates. Whilst our CKD detection rate was derived from the CDMS using MDRD prediction equation, the awareness rates reported by the overseas studies [5, 44, 45] were ascertained from patient surveys using generic questions such as whether they had ever been told to have (i) kidney disease in general (which could have included urinary tract infection or urinary stones) [5] or (ii) weak or failing kidneys (excluding kidney stones, bladder infections, or incontinence) [44]. Both the low detection rate in our study and the low awareness rates reported by the overseas studies [5, 44, 45] suggest that underdiagnosis and lack of awareness of CKD are common global issues. As CKD is treatable, low disease awareness and detection would need to be addressed. The use of equations for prediction of eGFR by healthcare professionals needs to be encouraged to increase the detection of CKD cases.

Delaying the progression of CKD to later stages, or even primary prevention of CKD, is possible through pharmacological intervention or lifestyle modification. Lifestyle modification [46] such as having regular physical activity, healthy diet, BMI≤25, moderate or less alcohol consumption, and being a nonsmoker are beneficial for primary prevention of CKD, possibly through the prevention of diabetes and hypertension as the three conditions have common pathway in disease development. Combined effect of the healthy lifestyle factors is reported to significantly reduce risks of cardiovascular diseases and CKD, and there was a dose-response relationship between the number of healthy lifestyle factors attained and magnitude of disease risk reduction [46]. Thus, leading a healthy lifestyle could play a major role in the war against CKD. For individuals with CKD, pharmacological intervention, such as the use of inhibitors of the renin-angiotensin system to control hypertension and proteinuria, has also been found to be effective in delaying the CKD progression [47]. Regression of proteinuric CKD is achievable particularly in patients without diabetes [48]. Ricardo et al. found that, among persons with CKD, nonsmokers and BMI≥25 were associated with lower risk of CKD progression, whilst having regular physical activity, nonsmoking, and BMI≥30 were associated with reduced all-cause mortality. In the general population, elevated BMI is associated with an increased risk of cardiovascular events; however, in individuals with CKD, BMI was found to have an inverse relationship with CKD progression or mortality [49, 50]. Reasons for the paradoxical association are unclear to date; some proposed explanations included higher BMI signaled nutritional adequacy [51] and more stable hemodynamic status [52]. Recently, there is emerging evidence on the role of diet in kidney health. Snelson et al. [53] reported that imposing dietary constraints and optimizing diet quality could complement therapies for CKD prevention or retarding CKD progression, as diet is implicated in the kidney health via modification of gut homeostasis or through haemodynamic effects [53]. Currently, patients with CKD are recommended to restrict sodium, potassium, and protein intake [53]. Whilst McMahon et al. [54] reported that restriction on salt consumption in patients with later CKD stages was effective for reducing blood pressure, albuminuria, and proteinuria, Adrogué et al. [55] found that the salt-sensitivity in patients with CKD might be abolished by the consumption of diet high in potassium which is believed to be antihypertensive, thus slowing the progression of CKD to later stages. There is also emerging evidence [53] that maintaining protein balance with adequate prevention of protein energy wasting by shifting from animal to plant-based protein intake may improve renal outcomes. More studies are needed before changes are made to the current recommendations.

Our study was limited by the lack of demographic specific national prevalence of detected CKD at base year and the forecast mortality rates. Thus we could not stratify the projections of individuals with CKD by subpopulations. This may underestimate the disease burden especially with the expectant ageing population in Singapore. To overcome this problem, we used an ageing index to elevate the transition and detection probabilities to compensate for the effect of population ageing. Although this might not fully capture the complexities of age on the changes in the transition and detection probabilities, elevation of the two probabilities using the ageing index could partially address the forthcoming population ageing that may potentially cause a rise in number of individuals with CKD.

This study assumed that the CKD progression was one-way without regression to the previous state. However, mild CKD, in particular CKD stages 1 and 2, is reversible. Previous study [56] found that 30%-54% of individuals with diabetes had regressed from moderate albuminuria to normo-albuminuria. Our assumption on one-way disease progression will inevitably result in overestimation of the number of individuals with more advanced CKD state in 2035. This study did not model the progression of each CKD stage based on the presence or absence of proteinuria due to incomplete data. As proteinuria is a strong predictor of an increased risk of disease progression [57], the lack of complete data signals that our transition probabilities estimated from the CDMS for each CKD stage are biased by sampling variations. Our projections could also be affected by future migration trends as susceptibility to diseases among the foreign-born residents could be different from the local population and these would impact the stability of the disease transition probabilities. Future ethnicity ratio is unlikely to significantly affect our results as the ethnic distribution in Singapore is likely to remain stable in the next two decades.

Despite these limitations, this study was conducted using robust methodology. We simulated the disease progression based on time-dependent probabilities and rates and sys-

tematically projected the number of individuals with CKD in each stage according to the clinical course. We estimated the number of undiagnosed cases to quantify the magnitude of the disease burden so that early interventions could be formulated. Whilst our findings may be artifacts of the projection methodologies, we are unaware of any local CKD study that can provide evidence to support or contradict our projections and findings. To the best of our knowledge, this is the first study on the projection of number of individuals with CKD in Singapore, with insights into undiagnosed CKD burden. Thus further research is warranted.

By 2035, about one-quarter of the Singapore residents aged 21+ years are expected to have CKD. Of these, more than half remain undiagnosed and majority of these undiagnosed cases are contributed by the CKD stages 1-2. National policies need to focus on primary disease prevention and early disease detection to avoid delayed treatment of CKD leading to ESRD. The forecast of future burden of CKD and the number of undiagnosed cases in this study can aid in the planning of future healthcare resources and manpower, which in turn translates into improvement in the healthcare system, better preventive care, and favourable patient outcomes.

Acknowledgments

The authors thank Mr. Abdul Zaidi Bin Abdul Hamid Khan for his support in data extraction from the Chronic Disease Management System as well as the Population Registry, National Healthcare Group, Singapore; and Ms. Samantha Ong Shih Hui from the Nephrology Division, National University Hospital, Singapore, for her support in this study. They also express appreciation to the NHG and IHIS colleagues who build and maintain the NHG Chronic Disease Management System. The study was performed as part of the corresponding author's employment by the National Healthcare Group.

References

[1] C. Sabanayagam, S. C. Lim, T. Y. Wong, J. Lee, A. Shankar, and E. S. Tai, "Ethnic disparities in prevalence and impact of risk factors of chronic kidney disease," *Nephrology Dialysis Transplantation* , vol. 25, no. 8, pp. 2564–2570, 2010.

[2] United States Renal Data System, "Chronic Kidney Disease (CKD) in the United States. CKD in the General Population," 2014, https://www.usrds.org/2014/view/.

[3] S. Kim, C. S. Lim, D. C. Han et al., "The prevalence of chronic kidney disease (CKD) and the associated factors to CKD in Urban Korea: A population-based cross-sectional epidemiologic study," *Journal of Korean Medical Science*, vol. 24, no. 1, pp. S11–S21, 2009.

[4] E. Imai, M. Horio, T. Watanabe et al., "Prevalence of chronic kidney disease in the Japanese general population," *Clinical & Experimental Nephrology*, vol. 13, no. 6, pp. 621–630, 2009.

[5] C. P. Wen, T. Y. D. Cheng, M. K. Tsai et al., "All-cause mortality attributable to chronic kidney disease: a prospective cohort study based on 462 293 adults in Taiwan," *The Lancet*, vol. 371, no. 9631, pp. 2173–2182, 2008.

[6] M. J. Sarnak, A. S. Levey, A. C. Schoolwerth et al., "Kidney disease as a risk factor for development of cardiovascular disease: a statement from the American Heart Association Councils on Kidney in Cardiovascular Disease, High Blood Pressure Research, Clinical Cardiology, and Epidemiology and Prevention," *Hypertension*, vol. 42, no. 5, pp. 1050–1065, 2003.

[7] A. S. Go, G. M. Chertow, D. Fan, C. E. McCulloch, and C. Hsu, "Chronic kidney disease and the risks of death, cardiovascular events, and hospitalization," *The New England Journal of Medicine*, vol. 351, no. 13, pp. 1296–1305, 2004.

[8] M. F. Yuyun, K.-T. Khaw, R. Luben et al., "Microalbuminuria independently predicts all-cause and cardiovascular mortality in a British population: The European Prospective Investigation into Cancer in Norfolk (EPIC-Norfolk) population study," *International Journal of Epidemiology*, vol. 33, no. 1, pp. 189–198, 2004.

[9] D. H. Smith, C. M. Gullion, G. Nichols, D. S. Keith, and J. B. Brown, "Cost of Medical Care for Chronic Kidney Disease and Comorbidity among Enrollees in a Large HMO Population," *Journal of the American Society of Nephrology*, vol. 15, no. 5, pp. 1300–1306, 2004.

[10] P. Sharma, K. McCullough, G. Scotland et al., "Does stage-3 chronic kidney disease matter?: A systematic literature review," *British Journal of General Practice*, vol. 60, no. 575, pp. 266–276, 2010.

[11] F. Laliberté, B. K. Bookhart, F. Vekeman et al., "Direct all-cause health care costs associated with chronic kidney disease in patients with diabetes and hypertension: A managed care perspective," *Journal of Managed Care Pharmacy*, vol. 15, no. 4, pp. 312–322, 2009.

[12] E. Zimbudzi, C. Lo, S. Ranasinha et al., "Predictors of health-related quality of life in patients with co-morbid diabetes and chronic kidney disease," *PLoS ONE*, vol. 11, no. 12, Article ID e0168491, 2016.

[13] National Kidney Foundation, "K/DOQI clinical practice guidelines for chronic kidney disease: evaluation, classification, and stratification," *American Journal of Kidney Diseases*, vol. 39, pp. S1–S266, 2002.

[14] T. H. Jafar, C. H. Schmid, M. Landa et al., "Angiotensin-converting enzyme inhibitors and progression of nondiabetic renal disease. A meta-analysis of patient-level data," *Annals of Internal Medicine*, vol. 135, no. 2, pp. 73–87, 2001.

[15] L. G. Glynn, J. Anderson, D. Reddan et al., "Chronic kidney disease in general practice: prevalence, diagnosis, and standards of care," *Irish Medical Journal*, vol. 102, no. 9, pp. 285–288, 2009.

[16] J. Coresh, D. Byrd-Holt, B. C. Astor et al., "Chronic kidney disease awareness, prevalence, and trends among U.S. adults, 1999 to 2000," *Journal of the American Society of Nephrology*, vol. 16, no. 1, pp. 180–188, 2005.

[17] United States Renal Data System, "End-stage Renal Disease (ESRD) in the United States. International Comparisons. 2016," https://www.usrds.org/2016/view/Default.aspx.

[18] Ministry of Health, "Action plan for successful ageing. 2016".

[19] RJ. Glassock and C. Winearls, "Ageing and the glomerular filtration rate: truths and consequences," *Transactions of the American Clinical and Climatological Association*, vol. 120, pp. 419–428, 2009.

[20] L. Y. Wong, M. P. H. S. Toh, and L. W. C. Tham, "Projection of prediabetes and diabetes population size in Singapore using a dynamic Markov model," *Journal of Diabetes*, vol. 9, no. 1, pp. 65–75, 2017.

[21] A. A. Honeycutt, J. P. Boyle, K. R. Broglio et al., "A dynamic Markov model for forecasting diabetes prevalence in the United States through 2050," *Health Care Management Science*, vol. 6, no. 3, pp. 155–164, 2003.

[22] Y. Murakami and Y. Ohashi, "Projected number of diabetic renal disease patients among insulin-dependent diabetes mellitus children in Japan using a Markov model with probabilistic sensitivity analysis," *International Journal of Epidemiology*, vol. 30, no. 5, pp. 1078–1083, 2001.

[23] M. P. Toh, H. S. Leong, and B. K. Lim, "Development of a diabetes registry to improve quality of care in the National Healthcare Group in Singapore," *ANNALS Academy of Medicine Singapore*, vol. 38, no. 6, p. 546, 2009.

[24] Department of Statistics Singapore, "Population Trends 2014," 2014, https://www.singstat.gov.sg/.

[25] "Kidney Disease: Improving Global Outcomes (KDIGO) CKD Work Group. KDIGO 2012 clinical practice guideline for the evaluation and management of chronic kidney disease," *Kidney International Supplements*, vol. 3, pp. 1–150, 2013.

[26] J. Coresh, E. Selvin, L. A. Stevens et al., "Prevalence of chronic kidney disease in the United States," *Journal of the American Medical Association*, vol. 298, no. 17, pp. 2038–2047, 2007.

[27] L. Zhang, P. Zhang, F. Wang et al., "Prevalence and factors associated with CKD: a population study from Beijing," *American Journal of Kidney Diseases*, vol. 51, no. 3, pp. 373–384, 2008.

[28] M. J. Bottomley, A. Kalachik, C. Mevada, M. O. Brook, T. James, and P. N. Harden, "Single estimated glomerular filtration rate and albuminuria measurement substantially overestimates prevalence of chronic kidney disease," *Nephron Clinical Practice*, vol. 117, no. 4, pp. c348–c352, 2011.

[29] L. Y. Wong, B. H. Heng, J. T. S. Cheah, and C. B. Tan, "Using spatial accessibility to identify polyclinic service gaps and volume of under-served population in Singapore using Geographic Information System," *International Journal of Health Planning and Management*, vol. 27, no. 3, pp. e173–e185, 2012.

[30] B. O. Eriksen and O. C. Ingebretsen, "The progression of chronic kidney disease: A 10-year population-based study of the effects of gender and age," *Kidney International*, vol. 69, no. 2, pp. 375–382, 2006.

[31] L. S. Dalrymple, R. Katz, B. Kestenbaum et al., "Chronic kidney disease and the risk of end-stage renal disease versus death," *Journal of General Internal Medicine*, vol. 26, no. 4, pp. 379–385, 2011.

[32] M. Tonelli, N. Wiebe, B. Culleton et al., "Chronic kidney disease and mortality risk: a systematic review," *Journal of the American Society of Nephrology*, vol. 17, no. 7, pp. 2034–2047, 2006.

[33] Department of Statistics Singapore, "Population Trends 2016," 2016, https://www.singstat.gov.sg/.

[34] Ministry of Health. National Health Survey 2010 Singapore Epidemiology and Disease Control Division. 2010.

[35] B. M. Y. Cheung and C. Li, "Diabetes and hypertension: is there a common metabolic pathway?" *Current Atherosclerosis Reports*, vol. 14, no. 2, pp. 160–166, 2012.

[36] A. Denic, R. J. Glassock, and A. D. Rule, "Structural and functional changes with the aging kidney," *Advances in Chronic Kidney Disease*, vol. 23, no. 1, pp. 19–28, 2016.

[37] P. Delanaye, RJ. Glassock, and H. Pottel, "An age-calibrated definition of chronic kidney disease: rationale and benefits," *The Clinical Biochemist Reviews*, vol. 37, no. 1, pp. 17–26, 2016.

[38] R. J. Glassock and C. Winearls, "An epidemic of chronic kidney disease: Fact or fiction?" *Nephrology Dialysis Transplantation*, vol. 23, no. 4, pp. 1117–1121, 2008.

[39] C. Bauer, M. L. Melamed, and T. H. Hostetter, "Staging of chronic kidney disease: Time for a course correction," *Journal of the American Society of Nephrology*, vol. 19, no. 5, pp. 844–846, 2008.

[40] R. J. Glassock and C. Winearls, "The global burden of chronic kidney disease: How valid are the estimates?" *Nephron Clinical Practice*, vol. 110, no. 1, pp. c39–c46, 2008.

[41] K. Matsushita, B. K. Mahmoodi, M. Woodward et al., "Comparison of risk prediction using the CKD-EPI equation and the MDRD study equation for estimated glomerular filtration rate," *JAMA*, vol. 307, no. 18, pp. 1941–1951, 2012.

[42] Health Promotion Board Singapore. Singapore renal registry annual report, 1999 - 2016. 2018.

[43] World Health Organisation, "Singapore statistics," http://www.who.int/countries/sgp/en/.

[44] L. C. Plantinga, L. E. Boulware, J. Coresh et al., "Patient awareness of chronic kidney disease: Trends and predictors," *JAMA Internal Medicine*, vol. 168, no. 20, pp. 2268–2275, 2008.

[45] A. Ingsathit, A. Thakkinstian, A. Chaiprasert et al., "Prevalence and risk factors of chronic kidney disease in the Thai adult population: Thai SEEK study," *Nephrology Dialysis Transplantation*, vol. 25, no. 5, pp. 1567–1575, 2010.

[46] M. Wakasugi, J. J. Kazama, S. Yamamoto, K. Kawamura, and I. Narita, "A combination of healthy lifestyle factors is associated with a decreased incidence of chronic kidney disease: A population-based cohort study," *Hypertension Research*, vol. 36, no. 4, pp. 328–333, 2013.

[47] G. Remuzzi, P. Ruggenenti, and N. Perico, "Chronic renal diseases: renoprotective benefits of renin-angiotensin system inhibition," *Annals of Internal Medicine*, vol. 136, no. 8, pp. 604–615, 2002.

[48] P. Ruggenenti, E. Perticucci, P. Cravedi et al., "Role of remission clinics in the longitudinal treatment of CKD," *Journal of the American Society of Nephrology*, vol. 19, no. 6, pp. 1213–1224, 2008.

[49] AC. Ricardo, CA. Anderson, W. Yang et al., "Healthy lifestyle and risk of kidney disease progression, atherosclerotic events, and death in CKD: findings from the Chronic Renal Insufficiency Cohort (CRIC) Study," *American Journal of Kidney Diseases*, vol. 65, no. 3, pp. 412-24, 2015.

[50] J. D. Kopple, Z. Xiaofei, L. Nancy L, and E. G. Lowrie, "Body weight-for-height relationships predict mortality in maintenance hemodialysis patients," *Kidney International*, vol. 56, no. 3, pp. 1136–1148, 1999.

[51] S. D. Navaneethan, J. D. Schold, S. Arrigain, J. P. Kirwan, and J. V. Nally, "Body mass index and causes of death in chronic kidney disease," *Kidney International*, vol. 89, no. 3, pp. 675–682, 2016.

[52] C. P. Kovesdy, J. E. Anderson, and K. Kalantar-Zadeh, "Paradoxical association between body mass index and mortality in men with CKD not yet on dialysis," *American Journal of Kidney Diseases*, vol. 49, no. 5, pp. 581–591, 2007.

[53] M. Snelson, R. E. Clarke, and M. T. Coughlan, "Stirring the pot: Can dietary modification alleviate the burden of CKD?" *Nutrients*, vol. 9, no. 3, article no. 265, 2017.

[54] E. J. McMahon, J. D. Bauer, C. M. Hawley et al., "A randomized trial of dietary sodium restriction in CKD," *Journal of the American Society of Nephrology*, vol. 24, no. 12, pp. 2096–2103, 2013.

[55] H. J. Adrogué and N. E. Madias, "Sodium and potassium in the pathogenesis of hypertension," *The New England Journal of Medicine*, vol. 356, no. 19, pp. 1966–1978, 2007.

[56] P. Vijayakumar, A. Hoyer, R. G. Nelson, R. Brinks, and M. E. Pavkov, "Estimation of chronic kidney disease incidence from prevalence and mortality data in American Indians with type 2 diabetes," *PLoS ONE*, vol. 12, no. 2, Article ID e0171027, 2017.

[57] B. R. Hemmelgarn, B. J. Manns, A. Lloyd et al., "Relation between kidney function, proteinuria, and adverse outcomes," *Journal of the American Medical Association*, vol. 303, no. 5, pp. 423–429, 2010.

24

Urinary Markers of Tubular Injury in Early Diabetic Nephropathy

Temesgen Fiseha and Zemenu Tamir

Department of Clinical Laboratory Science, College of Medicine and Health Sciences, Wollo University, Dessie, Ethiopia

Correspondence should be addressed to Temesgen Fiseha; temafiseha@gmail.com

Academic Editor: Franca Anglani

Diabetic nephropathy (DN) is a common and serious complication of diabetes associated with adverse outcomes of renal failure, cardiovascular disease, and premature mortality. Early and accurate identification of DN is therefore of critical importance to improve patient outcomes. Albuminuria, a marker of glomerular involvement in early renal damage, cannot always detect early DN. Thus, more sensitive and specific markers in addition to albuminuria are needed to predict the early onset and progression of DN. Tubular injury, as shown by the detection of tubular injury markers in the urine, is a critical component of the early course of DN. These urinary tubular markers may increase in diabetic patients, even before diagnosis of microalbuminuria representing early markers of normoalbuminuric DN. In this review we summarized some new and important urinary markers of tubular injury, such as neutrophil gelatinase associated lipocalin (NGAL), kidney injury molecule-1 (KIM-1), liver-type fatty acid binding protein (L-FABP), N-acetyl-beta-glucosaminidase (NAG), alpha-1 microglobulin (A1M), beta 2-microglobulin (B2-M), and retinol binding protein (RBP) associated with early DN.

1. Introduction

Diabetic nephropathy (DN) is a common and serious complication of diabetes associated with adverse outcomes of renal failure, cardiovascular disease, and premature mortality [1–3]. It is also the leading cause of end-stage renal disease (ESRD), requiring costly renal replacement therapy in the form of dialysis or transplantation [4]. Early and accurate identification of DN is therefore of critical importance to improve clinical outcomes. Clinically, the appearance of pathological albuminuria, microalbuminuria, is considered a hallmark of early onset of DN. However, a substantial proportion of renal impairment occurs among normoalbuminuric diabetic patients and is associated with more advanced diabetic glomerular lesions and increased risk of progression [5–7]. Moreover, since microalbuminuria is diagnosed once significant glomerular damage has occurred, changes in albuminuria are being increasingly recognized as complementary rather than obligatory manifestations of DN [8, 9].

Recently, changes in the renal tubules, which may be termed diabetic tubulopathy, are increasingly implicated in the development of progressive diabetic kidney disease [10, 11]. It has been reported that, in addition to the glomeruli, the renal tubules are heavily involved in the pathogenesis of DN [12, 13]. In line with this, several glomerular and tubular biomarkers predicting onset or progression of DN have been identified and are becoming increasingly important in clinical diagnostics. The urinary concentrations of these damage markers (both glomerular and tubular) are elevated in diabetic patients and are associated with the severity of DN [14]. Interestingly, some of these markers already are elevated in normoalbuminuric diabetic patients with normal estimated glomerular filtration rate (eGFR) [14]. Therefore, more sensitive and specific markers in addition to albuminuria are needed to predict the development and progression of DN in diabetics even at the very early stage (normoalbuminuric DN).

Tubular injury, as shown by the detection of tubular damage markers in the urine, is a critical component of the early course of DN and has been suggested to contribute in a primary way, rather than a secondary manner, to the development of early DN [15, 16]. Urinary excretion of these tubular markers could, therefore, be useful for assessing an initial malfunction or damage of the renal tubules in the early stage of potentially progressive DN. Several tubular damage markers recently have been discovered and have clinical implications as markers for the development and progression of DN. Some studies have demonstrated that these tubular damage markers increase in patients with diabetes, even before diagnosis of microalbuminuria representing early markers of normoalbuminuric DN with a good sensitivity and specificity [17–19]. This review article summarizes some new and important urinary markers of tubular injury associated with early DN.

2. Neutrophil Gelatinase Associated Lipocalin

Neutrophil gelatinase associated lipocalin (NGAL) is a small, 25-kDa, protein that belongs to the lipocalin protein family released from neutrophils and many epithelial cell types including kidney tubular cells. It is representative of the functioning tubular mass and produced as a response to tubular injury [20]. Urinary NGAL levels were found to be markedly elevated in patients with diabetes when compared with nondiabetic control subjects [14, 21–27] and to correlate negatively with eGFR and positively with serum Cystatin C (CysC), serum creatinine (SCr), proteinuria, albuminuria, and urinary albumin excretion (UAE) and albumincreatinine ratio (UACR), indicating the possible clinical application of urinary NGAL as a complementary marker for early detection of DN [19, 25–29]. It is also significantly correlated with the duration of diabetes, glycemic control (HbA1c), and urinary interleukin-18 (IL-18: proinflammatory biomarker) and angiotensinogen (renin-angiotensin system biomarker), suggesting urinary NGAL as a useful noninvasive tool for the evaluation of renal involvement in diabetes [21, 23, 25, 28, 29].

In diabetics, urinary excretion of NGAL was significantly higher in microalbuminuric in comparison with normoalbuminuric patients and controls and correlated positively with UACR, indicating diabetic tubular damage at the early stage of DN [18, 23, 25, 26, 30]. Urine levels of NGAL were significantly higher in microalbuminuria group compared to normoalbuminuria and were positively correlated to UACR in both diabetes and prediabetes, which suggested that tubular damage may play major role in the development of nephropathy in prediabetes [30]. It was also suggested that NGAL might play an important role in the pathophysiology of renal adaptation to diabetes, and its measurement might become a useful and noninvasive tool for the evaluation of renal involvement in these patients as well as for the early diagnosis of incipient DN [26]. In addition, urinary NGAL showed better area under curve (AUC; diagnostic accuracy) for estimating microalbuminuria, demonstrating its value as a more suitable and sensitive marker for detecting the onset of DN [25, 30].

Higher urinary levels of NGAL have been found in diabetics compared to controls, even in normoalbuminuric patients, indicating that diabetic tubular damage may develop before the stage of microalbuminuria [14, 17, 22, 23, 26, 31, 32]. The urinary NGAL level (1.5-fold) already was significantly

elevated in normoalbuminuric patients with diabetes compared with nondiabetic controls and was significantly associated with albuminuria [14]. Mean urinary NGAL and NGAL/creatinine ratio (NGAL/Cr) levels in both microalbuminuric and nonmicroalbuminuric diabetic patients were found to be higher than those in the controls, indicating that tubular involvement may precede glomerular involvement, as urinary NGAL levels are increased in the very early phase of diabetes before microalbuminuria develops [24].

The increased levels of urinary NGAL in diabetic patients, with or without albuminuria, point to early tubular damage and can be used as an early sensitive marker in detecting DN [14, 22, 27, 31]. In addition, urinary NGAL levels were increased in diabetic patients with normal or mildly increased albuminuria, which indicated that tubular and glomerular injuries may be occurring even at the earliest stage of diabetic kidney disease and urinary NGAL could be an early marker of renal dysfunction in diabetic patients without current evidence of nephropathy [19, 31].

NGAL increases in diabetic patients, even before diagnosis of microalbuminuria representing an early marker of "normoalbuminuric" DN, and could be used for the evaluation of early renal involvement in the course of diabetes [17]. Urine NGAL was significantly increased in diabetic patients, even normoalbuminuric, and was positively correlated with HbA1c, duration of diabetes, and urine ACR, suggesting that urinary NGAL could have the potential to be an earlier marker of DN, in normoalbuminuric patients, as a supplement to albuminuria [23]. In addition, urinary levels of NGAL were higher in normoalbuminuric patients with diabetes than in control subjects and increased with increasing categories of albuminuria [14, 29].

Because levels of urinary NGAL were significantly different according to the degree of albuminuria and increased in parallel with the severity of renal disease, reaching higher levels in patients with manifest DN, urinary NGAL levels expresses the degree of renal impairment in DN and, together with albuminuria, it could be used as a sensitive and specific markers for predicting the progression of DN [14, 17, 19, 22, 26, 31]. Furthermore, baseline levels of urinary NGAL were significantly elevated and correlated with the severity of albuminuria in patients with diabetes and were observed to be significantly correlated with a rapid decline in the eGFR [33]. Elevated levels of urinary NGAL are also predictive of decline in eGFR in type 2 diabetic patients with micro- or macroalbuminuria [34]. Another study also found that urinary concentrations of NGAL were associated with progression to ESRD and death in type 2 diabetes, even after adjustment for baseline albuminuria and GFR, indicating the potential importance of urinary NGAL for the identification of persons most likely to progress to ESRD or to premature death [35].

3. Kidney Injury Molecule-1

Kidney injury molecule-1 (KIM-1) is a transmembrane protein and its expression is not measurable in normal proximal tubule cells but is markedly upregulated with injury/dedifferentiation [36]. It has been suggested that its presence in the urine is highly specific for kidney injury and may serve as a useful biomarker for renal proximal tubule injury facilitating the early diagnosis of the disease [36, 37]. Renal tubular damage, as evidenced by increased levels of urinary KIM-1, is evident even prior to the development of diabetes and overt kidney disease [38].

Urinary levels of KIM-1 were significantly higher in patients with diabetes when compared with nondiabetic control subjects and correlated with urinary albumin, UACR, SCr, blood urea, and BUN, indicating the possible clinical application of urinary KIM-1 as a complementary marker for early detection of DN [14, 18, 21, 22, 27, 39]. Urinary KIM-1 levels have also been found to be correlated with the urinary IL-18 and angiotensinogen, body mass index, duration of diabetes, glycemic control, and systolic and diastolic blood pressures (BP), which may reflect the role of Kim-1 as a marker for diagnosis and prognosis of DN among diabetic patients taking into account other risk factors [19, 21, 39–41]. In addition, urinary KIM-1 levels were significantly increased both in subgroups of DN and in chronic kidney disease (CKD) compared with controls [41]. In this study, urinary KIM-1 levels, along with urinary albumin excretion and the duration of diabetes, were found to be independent risk factors associated with low GFRs [41].

Urinary levels of KIM-1 were found significantly elevated in diabetic patients with microalbuminuria, in comparison with diabetics with normoalbuminuria and nondiabetic healthy controls, demonstrating the existence of diabetic tubular damage at the early stage of DN [16, 18, 21, 39, 41]. In one study, urinary Kim-1 levels were elevated significantly (10-fold) in type 2 diabetic microalbuminuric patients (whose SCr level was <2 mg/dL) as compared to the controls and normoalbuminuric patients, indicating its potential value in the identification of diabetics with nephropathy at the early stage [39]. Urinary KIM-1 was also significantly increased in early detected inflamed kidney of diabetic patients compared to controls and was positively associated with degree of kidney inflammation [42]. The highest level of KIM-1 was found in the DN patients compared to the kidney inflammation state alone, suggesting that urinary KIM-1 excretion could help differentiate kidney inflammation versus DN [42]. In addition, urinary KIM-1 levels were increased in type 2 diabetic patients with normal or mildly increased albuminuria, indicating that tubular and glomerular injuries may coexist at the earliest stage of diabetic kidney disease and KIM-1 could be potential marker of early DN [19].

Urinary KIM-1 excretion is elevated in diabetic patients compared to controls, even before they develop microalbuminuria, indicating that diabetic tubular involvement may precede glomerular involvement and, by measuring KIM-1, this "tubular phase" of renal damage could be detected before albuminuria becomes pathologically elevated [14, 16, 18, 22, 32, 41]. Urinary KIM-1 levels seems to predict renal injury secondary to DN in early period independent of albuminuria, because urinary KIM-1 was elevated despite normal urinary albumin excretion in the normoalbuminuric subgroup [41]. It has been suggested that increased renal biomarkers, such as urinary KIM-1 in diabetics, are early sensitive and specific markers of DN, even preceding the development

of microalbuminuria, denoting that they can be used as early and sensitive markers for early detection of DN [18].

In type 2 diabetes, urinary KIM-1 was markedly increased compared with the controls and its levels increased from the normoalbuminuria to the last macroalbuminuria group, predicting the progression of DN [27]. Urinary Kim-1 also was high in normoalbuminuric diabetics before reduction in GFR, indicating early diabetic kidney injury [32]. Furthermore, higher levels of urinary KIM-1 were associated with a faster decline in kidney function and an increased risk of mortality during 4 years of follow-up [40]. Another follow-up study among type 2 diabetic patients with various degrees of incipient or established DN also found that higher levels of urinary KIM-1 were associated with a faster decline in eGFR [34]. Moreover, low baseline levels of urinary KIM-1 were strongly associated with regression of microalbuminuria independent of clinical characteristics [16]. In another study, Irbesartan treatment significantly reduced levels of the tubular marker urinary KIM-1 in patients with type 2 diabetes and microalbuminuria, indicating the role of KIM-1 in monitoring treatment effect in DN [43].

4. Liver-Type Fatty Acid Binding Protein

Liver-type fatty acid binding protein (L-FABP) is a low molecular weight (15 kDa) intracellular carrier protein that is expressed in the renal proximal tubule and liver. In renal disease L-FABP gene expression in the kidney was upregulated and its urinary excretion was found to correlate with the severity of tubulointerstitial injury, reflecting stresses on the proximal tubules [44]. A study in CKD showed that serum L-FABP levels do not influence the urinary L-FABP level, which suggested that the measured L-FABP in urine originates primarily from tubular cells [45]. Urinary L-FABP was significantly higher in diabetic patients compared with healthy controls and correlated with albumin excretion rate and creatinine clearance (CrCl) [46]. Urinary L-FABP levels were significantly higher in diabetic patients with nephropathy than in healthy subjects and correlated positively with urinary albumin, UACR, and albuminuria and inversely with GFR, indicating its possible clinical application as a complementary marker of DN [47–49].

Urinary L-FABP levels were significantly increased in macroalbuminuric patients compared with microalbuminuric and currently normoalbuminuric patients [46]. In one study from type 2 diabetes mellitus patients, elevated levels of urinary L-FABP were evident from the microalbuminuric stage, indicating tubular damage at the early stage of DN [50]. According to this study, urinary excretion of L-FABP levels in the microalbuminuric group was significantly correlated with systolic BP, fasting plasma glucose, and HbA1c, which indicated that urinary L-FABP could be most sensitive marker for detecting glomerular and tubular dysfunction at the early stage of DN [50].

Additionally, urinary levels of L-FABP in patients with microalbuminuria were significantly higher than in those with normoalbuminuria [18, 47, 51]. Increased urinary L-FABP excretion has been also found in the micro- and macroalbuminuric patients compared with the patients with persistent normoalbuminuria [52]. Urinary L-FABP levels were also elevated in patients with reduced eGFR and showed a positive correlation with systolic BP and protein/Cr ratio, suggesting the importance of tubular damage in the development of DN and urinary L-FABP excretion in the assessment of tubular dysfunction in early DN [50].

Urinary L-FABP excretion is higher in diabetic patients compared to healthy controls, including in patients without current evidence of nephropathy (normoalbuminuria), indicating its value in detecting DN even before the appearance of pathological albuminuria, the earlier measurable sign of renal diabetic involvement [18, 48, 53, 54]. Urinary levels of L-FABP were significantly higher in the patients with type 2 diabetes who had normoalbuminuria than in normal control subjects and progressively increased in subjects with normo-, micro-, or macroalbuminuria and further increased in patients with ESRD [54]. The levels of urinary L-FABP in each DN group were significantly different from the levels in all of the other groups and significantly increased according to the severity of DN [47, 49, 54]. Levels of urinary L-FABP were elevated in normoalbuminuric patients than in the controls and were further increased with increasing levels of albuminuria, indicating its value in accurately reflecting severity of tubular damage in the early stage of DN [48]. In the prospective study, high urinary L-FABP levels were associated with the increase in albuminuria, progression to ESRD, or induction of hemodialysis [54]. Surprisingly, even in the subgroup of patients without renal dysfunction, higher urinary levels of L-FABP were associated with the progression of DN, demonstrating the usefulness of urinary L-FABP as a marker for predicting the progression of DN in the early stage [54].

Urinary L-FABP was elevated at an early stage, even before any clinical signs of glomerular damage are detectable, and independently predicted the development of microalbuminuria and death, suggesting its value as a useful marker for the detection of tubular damage early in the course of diabetes and for the prediction of DN and death [52]. In addition, urinary concentrations of L-FABP were associated with progress to ESRD in patients with type 2 diabetes, even after adjustment for baseline albuminuria and GFR, indicating the potential importance of urinary L-FABP in identification of persons most likely to progress to ESRD [35]. A long term observational study on type 2 diabetic patients without advanced nephropathy revealed that higher urinary levels of L-FABP were associated with deteriorating renal function and a higher incidence rate of CVD. This association was markedly observed even in patients with normoalbuminuria, which indicated its potential role as a marker for predicting future renal dysfunction and incidence of CVD in diabetic patients with an early stage of nephropathy, independently of albuminuria [51].

5. N-Acetyl-beta-D-glucosaminidase

N-acetyl-beta-D-glucosaminidase (NAG) is a hydrolytic lysosomal enzyme found predominantly in proximal tubule. It has been demonstrated as a useful marker of renal tubular impairment in various conditions involved with renal injury or dysfunction [55]. Urinary activities of NAG are elevated in patients with diabetes when compared with nondiabetic control subjects and showed a significant positive correlation with serum Cys C, SCr, UAE, and UACR and an inverse correlation with measured and estimated CrCl in all patients, indicating the possible clinical application of urinary NAG as a complementary marker for early detection of DN [14, 25, 56-60]. It is also correlated positively with disease duration and poor glycemic control (HbA1c) [25, 57, 59, 60]. In diabetic patients with poor metabolic control (HbA1c > 8%), a statistically significant increase in urinary NAG was found compared with the diabetic patients with good metabolic control [25, 60].

In diabetics, urine NAG level was significantly higher in microalbuminuric patients compared to both normoalbuminuric patients and controls, suggesting that tubular dysfunction is already present in this period [16, 25, 56, 57, 59-61]. Urinary NAG excretion was significantly higher in all patients with type 2 diabetes than in controls and in microalbuminuric than in normoalbuminuric patients, representing early marker of incipient DN [25]. The ROC curve analysis of the above study showed that urinary NAG is the most sensitive marker of microalbuminuria and early renal damage with sensitivity of 83.3% and specificity of 77.8% [25].

It was also suggested that NAG had higher sensitivity as urinary marker in early detection of tubular and glomerular lesions in diabetic patients and could be used as screening test for early diagnosis of DN [56]. In another study, urinary NAG and microalbuminuria in the diabetic patients were significantly increased compared to those in the controls and urinary NAG showed the highest sensitivity and specificity (100% and 87.5%, resp.) as compared to sensitivity and specificity of SCr, CrCl, and microalbuminuria (25% and 24.9%, 50% and 58.3%, and 25% and 75%, resp.) [60]. The investigators from this study suggested that measuring urinary NAG excretion could be useful for the assessment of renal failure in patients with diabetes and confirmed the use of this enzyme as a routine screening test [60].

Compared to healthy controls, urinary NAG excretion is higher in diabetic patients, even before they develop microalbuminuria [14, 25, 56, 59, 61-64]. Urinary NAG activity was within the normal ranges in the healthy control groups and significantly increased over the upper reference limit in the groups of patients with normoalbuminuria, indicating the great importance of NAG in discovering the renal tubule cells damage, especially at the early stage before the appearance of microalbuminuria [65]. On the other hand urinary NAG already showed 9-fold increase in the normoalbuminuric patients compared with the controls, whereas albuminuria (and eGFR) in these patients was comparable with controls, which demonstrated the potential value of urinary NAG as sensitive marker of DN as its level increases before other traditional markers become pathologically elevated [14, 62]. Thus, values of the urinary NAG were elevated before microalbuminuria was observed, with the highest values detected in the group of patients with microalbuminuria, indicating that increased excretion of urinary NAG points to early tubular damage and can be used as the most sensitive marker in the early detection of DN [61, 66].

In a more recent study, urinary NAG excretion gradually increases with the increase in duration of diabetes and appeared much before the microalbuminuria, decreased eGFR, and increased SCr. In this study, the urinary NAG activity increased 16- and 18-fold in moderately increased albuminuria and DN patients, respectively, without any change in non-DN patients. A cutoff value of 3 U/L of urinary NAG has demonstrated a sensitivity of 96.1% and a specificity of 100% discriminating healthy controls from patients with microalbuminuria (AUC 0.999) and DN (AUC 1.000), and the investigators concluded that the urinary NAG may be considered as a potential site-specific early tubular damage marker leading to DN [67]. In addition, significantly increased levels of urinary NAG were found in diabetic patients with varying degree of albuminuria and this increase was parallel to the severity of renal involvement expressed with the level of albuminuria [14, 56, 59, 60, 68]. Urinary levels of NAG were higher in patients with diabetes than in controls and increased with increasing categories of albuminuria, suggesting that it could be used as a useful marker reflecting the degree of renal impairment in DN [14, 59].

Urinary NAG activities tended to be higher in diabetic patients with and without albuminuria than in control subjects and differences among the diabetic groups were statistically significant, which implies that this enzyme is a more sensitive marker of tubular damage and could be used as a biomarker for the detection of early stage of DN, even in normoalbuminuric patients. Furthermore, baseline urinary excretion of NAG and rising NAG excretion across time predict both microalbuminuria and macroalbuminuria, which suggested that early NAG excretion may be a marker of susceptibility to DN and combining AER and NAG in repeated measures may help to identify individuals susceptible to DN [69]. Also, low baseline concentrations of urinary NAG were significantly associated with the regression of microalbuminuria over the subsequent 2 years, indicating that tubular dysfunction is a critical component of the early course of DN and urinary NAG can be used as an early marker of normoalbuminuric DN [16].

6. Alpha-1 Microglobulin

Alpha-1 microglobulin (A1M) is a small molecular weight protein (27 kDa) present in various body fluids. In the healthy kidney, it passes freely through the glomerular membranes, and about 99% is reabsorbed and catabolized by the proximal tubular cells. Increased A1M in urine can therefore be an early sign of renal damage, primarily on the proximal tubules [70]. The level of urinary A1M was significantly increased in the group of diabetic patients as compared to the level of normal subjects [71]. Urinary A1M levels were markedly elevated in diabetic patients when compared with control subjects [61, 72–74] and correlated directly with urinary albumin excretion, UACR, and serum CysC and negatively with eGFR [72–76], indicating the possible clinical application of urinary A1M as a complementary marker for early detection of DN. It also correlates with urinary advanced glycation end-products, diabetes duration, HbA1c, fasting, and postprandial blood glucose [72, 73]. Urinary A1M level was higher in the patients with poor glucose control (HbA1c > 8.5%) and directly related to albuminuria [61]. Urinary A1M was also related to the duration, severity, and control of diabetes, indicating that it is a good marker of the severity of renal impairment in type 2 diabetic subjects [75].

A proteomic based study among microalbuminuric diabetic patients showed the early and coappearance of A1M with albumin, demonstrating that urinary A1M can be used as markers for specific and accurate clinical analysis of DN [77]. The concentration of A1M during the development of albuminuria also showed a very strong positive correlation [61]. In addition, the urinary excretion of A1M was significantly higher in microalbuminuric in comparison with normoalbuminuric patients and controls, indicating tubular damage at an early stage of DN [61, 72, 78]. It also demonstrated the importance of tubular dysfunction, as an early and integral component of the DN in diabetic patients [73]. A1M is a marker of tubular dysfunction in diabetic patients and hyperglycemia was the most important risk factor associated with A1M urinary excretion, emphasizing the value of tight glycemic control in slowing the progress of tubular dysfunction in diabetic patients [73, 79].

In a sample of community treated type 2 diabetic subjects, 45.2% had elevated A1M urinary excretion, 32.7% had micro/macroalbuminuria, and 27.2% had a GFR < 60 mL/min, indicating tubular dysfunction and nonalbuminuric renal disease in patients with diabetes [79]. In addition to albuminuria measuring glomerular dysfunction, urinary A1M estimating proximal tubular dysfunction is useful for the early detection of nephropathy in diabetes [75]. It was also suggested that urinary A1M provides a noninvasive and inexpensive diagnostic alternative for the early detection of tubular disorders of DN [71].

Urinary A1M is a sensitive biomarker in detecting tubular dysfunction in early DN, even in normoalbuminuric patients, demonstrating that tubular injury is an early event in diabetes [61, 76, 80–83]. Diabetic patients with normoalbuminuria excreted significantly higher levels of urinary A1M compared with healthy individuals, while there was no significant difference between the patients and controls in respect to serum/urine Cr [61]. In another study, urinary A1M was increased in 27.9% normoalbuminuric type 2 diabetic patients, indicating that urinary A1M precedes the onset of albuminuria and may serve as a marker in early DN [80]. Elevated levels of urinary A1M in normoalbuminuric patients with diabetes showed that proximal tubule dysfunction may develop before the stage of microalbuminuria and that A1M is a significant biomarker for incipient DN [81]. A1M also correctly identified normoalbuminuric diabetics from healthy controls with accuracy of 89.0%, sensitivity of 86.3%, and specificity of 94.2% [83]. Urinary A1M levels also significantly increased with severity of albuminuria, indicating its value in predicting progression of DN as suggested by increasing albuminuria [75].

7. Beta 2-Microglobulin

Beta (β) 2-microglobulin (B2-M) is a low molecular weight protein (11.8 kDA), produced by all cells expressing major histocompatibility complex class I antigen. It is readily filtered through the glomerulus and almost completely reabsorbed and catabolized by the renal proximal tubules. Increase in urinary B2-M indicates tubular dysfunction, and measurement of B2-M in urine is a sensitive and reliable assay for detecting tubular injury [84]. The level of B2-M in urine of the patients with diabetes was higher than normal [85, 86] and showed significant correlation with urinary albumin excretion and 2-hour postprandial blood sugar [85]. Urine B2-M in the children with type 1 diabetes was significantly increased compared to the controls and correlated positively with disease duration and glycemic control [87].

In type 2 diabetes, significant correlation was found between level of microalbumin and urine B2-M with length of diabetes and serum and urine Cr [86]. Urinary B2-M excretion is elevated in the patients with a poor metabolic control (HbA1c > 8.0%) compared to those with a good one [61]. Urinary B2-M levels were higher in diabetic patients with macro- and/or microvascular complications, indicating that increased urinary B2-M excretion was associated with more severe disease in these patients [85, 88]. In addition, they appear to be useful in early detection of DN with positive correlation with the duration of type 1 diabetes and glycemic control (HbA1c) [87]. Most importantly, urine B2-M was able to reliably identify biopsy-proven DN, indicating the potential clinical application of urinary B2-M as a marker for early DN in diabetic patients [89].

Urinary B2-M exhibited a significant positive correlation with urinary albumin levels and negative correlation with GFR and serum B2-M in type 2 DN [90]. This study also found that diabetic kidney damage exhibits an initial increase in urinary B2-M levels, as compared with nondiabetic kidney damage, and renal dysfunction aggravated as urinary B2-M levels gradually increased [90]. In addition, urinary B2-M excretion is significantly higher in the patients with microalbuminuria than normoalbuminuria and in the controls, indicating the presence of tubular injury in early DN as characterised by increased B2-M excretion [61, 78, 85]. In patients with type 2 diabetes and biopsy-proven DN, urinary excretion of B2-M was significantly correlated with the severity of tubulointerstitial injury, demonstrating the usefulness of B2-M as marker of tubular dysfunction in early DN [91]. A urinary proteomic analysis study found high amounts of B2-M in the urine of diabetic patients with macro- or microalbuminuria compared with controls and patients without micro- or macroalbuminuria [92].

Increased excretion of B2-M was found in early course while albumin excretion was still in normal range in the urine of diabetic patients, which indicated that the increase in urinary B2-M precedes the stage of albuminuria and that early DN is related to proximal tubule dysfunction [80–82]. Urinary B2-M was increased in 23.5% of normoalbuminuric patients with type 2 diabetes, suggesting that proximal tubule dysfunction may be responsible for early DN independently of preceding glomerular endothelial dysfunction and urinary B2-M may be used as sensitive marker in the diagnosis of early DN [80]. In addition, the urinary excretion of B2-M increased progressively from normoalbuminuria to macroalbuminuria, indicating its value in predicting progression of DN at early stage [85].

8. Retinol Binding Protein

Retinol binding protein (RBP) is another low molecular weight protein (21 kDa) which is freely filtered at the glomerulus and then almost completely reabsorbed in the proximal tubule. Both serum and urine levels have been shown to be elevated in patients with diabetes [85, 93, 94]. RBP showed significant positive correlations with triglyceride, systolic BP, and log urinary albumin excretion [93]. Urinary RBP excretion has been found to be increased in diabetic subjects compared with healthy controls [87, 95–97] and to correlate with UAE, serum and urine Cr, CrCl, and 24 h urine protein, indicating its potential clinical application as a marker of early DN [85, 95, 97]. It has been also shown to correlate closely with duration of diabetes and glycemic control (HbA1c) [87, 94, 95, 97].

Urinary RBP4 levels were higher in subjects with prediabetes or type 2 diabetes than in subjects with normal glucose tolerance and correlated strongly with fasting glucose, triglycerides, BP, eGFR, and UACR [98]. In addition, urinary excretion of RBP was higher in patients with macro- and/or microvascular complications of diabetes compared to those without, which confirmed the utility of RBP as a renal biomarker for predicting diabetic complications [85, 88]. Urinary RBP was also a predictor of the risk of dialysis, doubling of SCr, or death in diabetic patients with macroalbuminuric DN, suggesting that RBP may serve as a marker to follow-up clinical monitoring of diabetics with DN [99].

Levels of urinary RBP were significantly higher in microalbuminuric diabetics when compared with normoalbuminuric and normal controls, indicating impaired proximal renal tubular function in early stage of DN [85, 95, 97]. In one study, diabetic patients with microalbuminuria had concomitant renal tubular disorder indicated by high urinary RBP in 90.9% of them, which suggested that elevated urinary RBP might be a useful marker of renal injury in early DN [95]. Furthermore, urinary RBP4 was highly predictive of microalbuminuria, even after adjustment for other metabolic parameters. In this study, urinary RBP4 concentration showed a stronger association with urinary ACR than serum RBP4 concentration for microalbuminuria and combined micro- and macroalbuminuria. The AUC (diagnostic accuracy) for urinary RBP4 to detect the presence of microalbuminuria was 0.80±0.02 with sensitivity of 80.18% and specificity of 64.03%; urinary RBP4 may therefore be used as early stage marker for predicting of diabetic renal damage [98].

Urinary RBP excretion is higher in diabetic patients compared to healthy controls, even before the diagnosis of microalbuminuria [95, 96]. In the above study, urinary RBP excretion was significantly higher in normoalbuminuric patients than controls and showed a significant correlation with urinary NAG and HbA1c in these patients [95]. Among these normoalbuminuric patients, 82% had raised urinary excretion of RBP, which suggested that proximal tubular dysfunction may occur independently of glomerular alteration

[95]. In normoalbuminuric diabetics, the excretion rate of RBP was significantly higher compared to control subjects and correlated to the excretion rate of NAG and albumin [100].

Among type 2 diabetic patients, 50% were positive for urinary RBP, while 28% and 6% of them were positive for micro- and macroalbuminuria, respectively [85]. The increase in the urinary excretion of RBP4 in diabetics is highly specific for tubular disease, which occurs earlier than glomerular (albumin) affection, as urinary RBP4 excretion is increased in early DN and might even be a marker of early renal damage preceding microalbuminuria [96]. Furthermore, the urinary excretion of RBP increased progressively from normoalbuminuria to macroalbuminuria, indicating progression of DN at the early stage [85].

9. Conclusions

Tubular injury, as shown by increased urinary tubular damage markers at the microalbuminuria stage of diabetes, is a critical component of the early course of DN. Urinary excretion of these tubular markers is significantly higher in diabetics compared to healthy controls, even before the diagnosis of microalbuminuria, supporting the hypotheses that tubular injury is an early event in diabetes. The tubular markers discriminate between healthy subjects and diabetics in early stages of nephropathy and might also serve as a marker of the efficacy of renal protective agents. Urinary markers of tubular injury are early, sensitive, and specific markers of DN, even preceding the development of microalbuminuria, denoting that they can be used as early and sensitive markers for early detection of DN. Despite the promise of these new tubular injury markers, further large, multicenter prospective studies are still needed to confirm their clinical utility as urinary markers in early DN for everyday practice.

Abbreviations

A1M: Alpha- (α-) 1 microglobulin
B2-M: Beta (β) 2-microglobulin
DN: Diabetic nephropathy
eGFR: Estimated glomerular filtration rate
KIM-1: Kidney injury molecule-1
L-FABP: Liver-type fatty acid binding protein
NAG: N-Acetyl-beta-glucosaminidase
NGAL: Neutrophil gelatinase associated lipocalin
RBP: Retinol binding protein
UACR: Urinary albumin-creatinine ratio.

Acknowledgments

The authors would like to acknowledge all work leading to this paper.

References

[1] T. Ninomiya, V. Perkovic, B. E. de Galan et al., "Albuminuria and kidney function independently predict cardiovascular and renal outcomes in diabetes," *Journal of the American Society of Nephrology*, vol. 20, no. 8, pp. 1813–1821, 2009.

[2] P.-H. Groop, M. C. Thomas, J. L. Moran et al., "The presence and severity of chronic kidney disease predicts all-cause mortality in type 1 diabetes," *Diabetes*, vol. 58, no. 7, pp. 1651–1658, 2009.

[3] G. Targher, G. Zoppini, M. Chonchol et al., "Glomerular filtration rate, albuminuria and risk of cardiovascular and all-cause mortality in type 2 diabetic individuals," *Nutrition, Metabolism and Cardiovascular Diseases*, vol. 21, no. 4, pp. 294–301, 2011.

[4] R. C. Atkins and P. Zimmet, "Editorial: Diabetic kidney disease: act now or pay later," *Kidney International*, vol. 77, no. 5, pp. 375–377, 2010.

[5] K. Walczak, M. Sodolska, I. Materek, A. Krysicka, and D. Moczulski, "Impaired renal function in type 2 diabetes patients in the absence of increased urine albumin excretion rate," *Diabetologia Doświadczalna i Kliniczna*, vol. 8, no. 4, pp. 165–168, 2008.

[6] M. L. Caramori, P. Fioretto, and M. Mauer, "Low glomerular filtration rate in normoalbuminuric type 1 diabetic patients: an indicator of more advanced glomerular lesions," *Diabetes*, vol. 52, no. 4, pp. 1036–1040, 2003.

[7] P. Budhiraja, B. Thajudeen, and M. Popovtzer, "Absence of albuminuria in type 2 diabetics with classical diabetic nephropathy: clinical pathological study," *Journal of Biomedical Science and Engineering*, vol. 6, no. 5, pp. 20–25, 2013.

[8] J. Barratt and P. Topham, "Urine proteomics: the present and future of measuring urinary protein components in disease," *Canadian Medical Association Journal*, vol. 177, no. 4, pp. 361–368, 2007.

[9] R. J. MacIsaac and G. Jerums, "Diabetic kidney disease with and without albuminuria," *Current Opinion in Nephrology and Hypertension*, vol. 20, no. 3, pp. 246–257, 2011.

[10] M. C. Thomas, W. C. Burns, and M. E. Cooper, "Tubular changes in early diabetic nephropathy," *Advances in Chronic Kidney Disease*, vol. 12, no. 2, pp. 177–186, 2005.

[11] S. C. W. Tang and K. N. Lai, "The pathogenic role of the renal proximal tubular cell in diabetic nephropathy," *Nephrology Dialysis Transplantation*, vol. 27, no. 8, pp. 3049–3056, 2012.

[12] D. M. Gibb, P. A. Tomlinson, N. R. Dalton, C. Turner, V. Shah, and T. M. Barratt, "Renal tubular proteinuria and microalbuminuria in diabetic patients," *Archives of Disease in Childhood*, vol. 64, no. 1, pp. 129–134, 1989.

[13] S. C. W. Tang, J. C. K. Leung, and K. N. Lai, "Diabetic tubulopathy: an emerging entity," *Diabetes and the Kidney*, vol. 170, pp. 124–134, 2011.

[14] F. L. Nauta, W. E. Boertien, S. J. L. Bakker et al., "Glomerular and tubular damage markers are elevated in patients with diabetes," *Diabetes Care*, vol. 34, no. 4, pp. 975–981, 2011.

[15] J. V. Bonventre, "Can we target tubular damage to prevent renal function decline in diabetes?" *Seminars in Nephrology*, vol. 32, no. 5, pp. 452–562, 2012.

[16] V. S. Vaidya, M. A. Niewczas, L. H. Ficociello et al., "Regression of microalbuminuria in type 1 diabetes is associated with lower levels of urinary tubular injury biomarkers, kidney injury molecule-1, and N-acetyl-β-D-glucosaminidase," *Kidney International*, vol. 79, no. 4, pp. 464–470, 2011.

[17] A. Lacquaniti, V. Donato, B. Pintaudi et al., "'Normoalbuminuric' diabetic nephropathy: tubular damage and NGAL," *Acta Diabetologica*, vol. 50, no. 6, pp. 935–942, 2013.

[18] S. Abd El Dayem, A. E. El Bohy, and A. El Shehaby, "Value of the intrarenal arterial resistivity indices and different renal biomarkers for early identification of diabetic nephropathy in type 1 diabetic patients," *Journal of Pediatric Endocrinology and Metabolism*, vol. 29, no. 3, pp. 273–279, 2015.

[19] J. A. de Carvalho, E. Tatsch, B. S. Hausen et al., "Urinary kidney injury molecule-1 and neutrophil gelatinase-associated lipocalin as indicators of tubular damage in normoalbuminuric patients with type 2 diabetes," *Clinical Biochemistry*, vol. 49, no. 3, pp. 232–236, 2016.

[20] K. Mori and K. Nakao, "Neutrophil gelatinase-associated lipocalin as the real-time indicator of active kidney damage," *Kidney International*, vol. 71, no. 10, pp. 967–970, 2007.

[21] S. S. Kim, S. H. Song, I. J. Kim et al., "Clinical implication of urinary tubular markers in the early stage of nephropathy with type 2 diabetic patients," *Diabetes Research and Clinical Practice*, vol. 97, no. 2, pp. 251–257, 2012.

[22] S. E. Nielsen, K. J. Schjoedt, A. S. Astrup et al., "Neutrophil gelatinase-associated lipocalin (NGAL) and kidney injury molecule 1 (KIM1) in patients with diabetic nephropathy: a cross-sectional study and the effects of lisinopril," *Diabetic Medicine*, vol. 27, no. 10, pp. 1144–1150, 2010.

[23] M. H. Hafez, F. A. F. El-Mougy, S. H. Makar, and S. S. Abd El Shaheed, "Detection of an earlier tubulopathy in diabetic nephropathy among children with normoalbuminuria," *Iranian Journal of Kidney Diseases*, vol. 9, no. 2, pp. 126–131, 2015.

[24] Z. Yürük Yıldırım, A. Nayır, A. Yılmaz, A. Gedikbaşı, and R. Bundak, "Neutrophil gelatinase-associated lipocalin as an early sign of diabetic kidney injury in children," *Journal of Clinical Research in Pediatric Endocrinology*, vol. 7, no. 4, pp. 274–279, 2015.

[25] H. S. Assal, S. Tawfeek, E. A. Rasheed, D. El-Lebedy, and E. H. Thabet, "Serum cystatin C and tubular urinary enzymes as biomarkers of renal dysfunction in type 2 diabetes mellitus," *Clinical Medicine Insights: Endocrinology and Diabetes*, vol. 6, pp. 7–13, 2013.

[26] D. Bolignano, A. Lacquaniti, G. Coppolino et al., "Neutrophil gelatinase-associated lipocalin as an early biomarker of nephropathy in diabetic patients," *Kidney and Blood Pressure Research*, vol. 32, no. 2, pp. 91–98, 2009.

[27] W.-J. Fu, S.-L. Xiong, Y.-G. Fang et al., "Urinary tubular biomarkers in short-term type 2 diabetes mellitus patients: a cross-sectional study," *Endocrine*, vol. 41, no. 1, pp. 82–88, 2012.

[28] J. Zachwieja, J. Soltysiak, P. Fichna et al., "Normal-range albuminuria does not exclude nephropathy in diabetic children," *Pediatric Nephrology*, vol. 25, no. 8, pp. 1445–1451, 2010.

[29] A. A. Al-Refai, S. I. Tayel, A. Ragheb, A. G. Dala, and A. Zahran, "Urinary neutrophil gelatinase associated lipocalin as a marker of tubular damage in type 2 diabetic patients with and without albuminuria," *Open Journal of Nephrology*, vol. 4, no. 1, pp. 37–46, 2014.

[30] V. Garg, M. Kumar, H. S. Mahapatra, A. Chitkara, A. K. Gadpayle, and V. Sekhar, "Novel urinary biomarkers in pre-diabetic nephropathy," *Clinical and Experimental Nephrology*, vol. 19, no. 5, pp. 895–900, 2015.

[31] K. Demir, A. Abaci, T. Küme, A. Altincik, G. Çatli, and E. Böber, "Evaluation of neutrophil gelatinase-associated lipocalin in normoalbuminuric normotensive type 1 diabetic adolescents," *Journal of Pediatric Endocrinology and Metabolism*, vol. 25, no. 5-6, pp. 517–523, 2012.

[32] A. Ucakturk, B. Avci, G. Genc, O. Ozkaya, and M. Aydin, "Kidney injury molecule-1 and neutrophil gelatinase associated lipocalin in normoalbuminuric diabetic children," *Journal of Pediatric Endocrinology and Metabolism*, vol. 29, no. 2, pp. 145–151, 2015.

[33] J. Wu, Y. Ding, C. Zhu et al., "Urinary TNF-α and NGAL are correlated with the progression of nephropathy in patients with type 2 diabetes," *Experimental and Therapeutic Medicine*, vol. 6, no. 6, pp. 1482–1488, 2013.

[34] S. E. Nielsen, H. Reinhard, D. Zdunek et al., "Tubular markers are associated with decline in kidney function in proteinuric type 2 diabetic patients," *Diabetes Research and Clinical Practice*, vol. 97, no. 1, pp. 71–76, 2012.

[35] G. D. Fufaa, E. J. Weil, R. G. Nelson et al., "Association of urinary KIM-1, L-FABP, NAG and NGAL with incident end-stage renal disease and mortality in American Indians with type 2 diabetes mellitus," *Diabetologia*, vol. 58, no. 1, pp. 188–198, 2015.

[36] J. V. Bonventre, "Kidney injury molecule-1 (KIM-1): a urinary biomarker and much more," *Nephrology Dialysis Transplantation*, vol. 24, no. 11, pp. 3265–3268, 2009.

[37] W. K. Han, V. Bailly, R. Abichandani, R. Thadhani, and J. V. Bonventre, "Kidney Injury Molecule-1 (KIM-1): a novel biomarker for human renal proximal tubule injury," *Kidney International*, vol. 62, no. 1, pp. 237–244, 2002.

[38] A. C. Carlsson, M. Calamia, U. Risérus et al., "Kidney injury molecule (KIM)-1 is associated with insulin resistance: results from two community-based studies of elderly individuals," *Diabetes Research and Clinical Practice*, vol. 103, no. 3, pp. 516–521, 2014.

[39] N. E. El-Ashmawy, E. A. El-Zamarany, N. F. Khedr, A. I. Abd El-Fattah, and S. A. Eltoukhy, "Kidney injury molecule-1 (Kim-1): an early biomarker for nephropathy in type II diabetic patients," *International Journal of Diabetes in Developing Countries*, vol. 35, no. S3, pp. 431–438, 2015.

[40] B. R. Conway, D. Manoharan, D. Manoharan et al., "Measuring urinary tubular biomarkers in type 2 diabetes does not add prognostic value beyond established risk factors," *Kidney International*, vol. 82, no. 7, pp. 812–818, 2012.

[41] B. K. Tekce, H. Tekce, G. Aktas, and M. Sit, "Evaluation of the urinary kidney injury molecule-1 levels in patients with diabetic nephropathy," *Clinical and Investigative Medicine*, vol. 37, no. 6, pp. E377–E383, 2014.

[42] S. A. Ahmed and M. A. Hamed, "Kidney injury molecule-1 as a predicting factor for inflamed kidney, diabetic and diabetic nephropathy Egyptian patients," *Journal of Diabetes and Metabolic Disorders*, vol. 14, no. 1, article 6, 2015.

[43] S. E. Nielsen, K. Rossing, G. Hess et al., "The effect of RAAS blockade on markers of renal tubular damage in diabetic nephropathy: U-NGAL, u-KIM1 and u-LFABP," *Scandinavian Journal of Clinical and Laboratory Investigation*, vol. 72, no. 2, pp. 137–142, 2012.

[44] A. Kamijo, T. Sugaya, A. Hikawa et al., "Urinary excretion of fatty acid-binding protein reflects stress overload on the proximal tubules," *American Journal of Pathology*, vol. 165, no. 4, pp. 1243–1255, 2004.

[45] A. Kamijo, T. Sugaya, A. Hikawa et al., "Urinary liver-type fatty acid binding protein as a useful biomarker in chronic kidney disease," *Molecular and Cellular Biochemistry*, vol. 284, no. 1-2, pp. 175–182, 2006.

[46] M. Von Eynatten, M. Baumann, U. Heemann et al., "Urinary L-FABP and anaemia: distinct roles of urinary markers in type 2 diabetes," *European Journal of Clinical Investigation*, vol. 40, no. 2, pp. 95–102, 2010.

[47] T. Nakamura, T. Sugaya, Y. Kawagoe, Y. Ueda, S. Osada, and H. Koide, "Effect of pitavastatin on urinary liver-type fatty acid–binding protein levels in patients with early diabetic nephropathy," *Diabetes Care*, vol. 28, no. 11, pp. 2728–2732, 2005.

[48] S. E. Nielsen, T. Sugaya, L. Tarnow et al., "Tubular and glomerular injury in diabetes and the impact of ACE inhibition," *Diabetes Care*, vol. 32, no. 9, pp. 1684–1688, 2009.

[49] K. Suzuki, T. Babazono, H. Murata, and Y. Iwamoto, "Clinical significance of urinary liver-type fatty acid-binding protein in patients with diabetic nephropathy," *Diabetes Care*, vol. 28, no. 8, pp. 2038–2039, 2005.

[50] V. Viswanathan, S. Sivakumar, V. Sekar, D. Umapathy, and S. Kumpatla, "Clinical significance of urinary liver-type fatty acid binding protein at various stages of nephropathy," *Indian Journal of Nephrology*, vol. 25, no. 5, pp. 269–273, 2015.

[51] S.-I. Araki, M. Haneda, D. Koya et al., "Predictive effects of urinary liver-type fatty acid-binding protein for deteriorating renal function and incidence of cardiovascular disease in type 2 diabetic patients without advanced nephropathy," *Diabetes Care*, vol. 36, no. 5, pp. 1248–1253, 2013.

[52] S. E. Nielsen, T. Sugaya, P. Hovind, T. Baba, H.-H. Parving, and P. Rossing, "Urinary liver-type fatty acid-binding protein predicts progression to nephropathy in type 1 diabetic patients," *Diabetes Care*, vol. 33, no. 6, pp. 1320–1324, 2010.

[53] N. M. Panduru, C. Forsblom, M. Saraheimo et al., "Urinary liver-type fatty acid-binding protein and progression of diabetic nephropathy in type 1 diabetes," *Diabetes Care*, vol. 36, no. 7, pp. 2077–2083, 2013.

[54] A. Kamijo-Ikemori, T. Sugaya, T. Yasuda et al., "Clinical significance of urinary liver-type fatty acid-binding protein in diabetic nephropathy of type 2 diabetic patients," *Diabetes Care*, vol. 34, no. 3, pp. 691–696, 2011.

[55] S. Skálová, "The diagnostic role of urinary N-acetyl-beta-D-glucosaminidase (NAG) activity in the detection of renal tubular impairment," *Acta Medica*, vol. 48, no. 2, pp. 75–80, 2005.

[56] S. Uslu, B. Efe, Ö. Alataş et al., "Serum cystatin C and urinary enzymes as screening markers of renal dysfunction in diabetic patients," *Journal of Nephrology*, vol. 18, no. 5, pp. 559–567, 2005.

[57] B. R. Bouvet, C. V. Paparella, S. M. M. Arriaga, A. L. Monje, A. M. Amarilla, and A. M. Almará, "Evaluation of urinary N-acetyl-beta-D-glucosaminidase as a marker of early renal damage in patients with type 2 diabetes mellitus," *Arquivos Brasileiros de Endocrinologia e Metabologia*, vol. 58, no. 8, pp. 798–801, 2014.

[58] F. P. Udomah, U. E. Ekrikpo, E. Effa, B. Salako, A. Arije, and S. Kadiri, "Association between urinary N-acetyl-beta-D-glucosaminidase and microalbuminuria in diabetic black Africans," *International Journal of Nephrology*, vol. 2012, Article ID 235234, 5 pages, 2012.

[59] G. Sheira, N. Noreldin, A. Tamer, and M. Saad, "Urinary biomarker N-acetyl-β-D-glucosaminidase can predict severity of renal damage in diabetic nephropathy," *Journal of Diabetes and Metabolic Disorders*, vol. 14, article 4, 2015.

[60] A. Mohammadi-Karakani, S. Asgharzadeh-Haghighi, M. Ghazi-Khansari, and R. Hosseini, "Determination of urinary enzymes as a marker of early renal damage in diabetic patients," *Journal of Clinical Laboratory Analysis*, vol. 21, no. 6, pp. 413–417, 2007.

[61] G. Nikolov, M. Boncheva, T. Gruev, S. Biljali, O. Stojceva-Taneva, and E. Masim-Spasovska, "Urinary biomarkers in the early diagnosis of renal damage in diabetes mellitus patients," *Scripta Scientifica Medica*, vol. 45, no. 3, pp. 58–64, 2013.

[62] W. K. Gatua, J. N. Makumi, E. M. Njagi, C. S. Kigondu, S. O. Mcligeyo, and S. K. Waithaka, "Evaluation of urinary tubular enzymes as screening markers of renal dysfunction in patients suffering from diabetes mellitus," *Asian Journal of Medical Sciences*, vol. 3, no. 3, pp. 84–90, 2011.

[63] R. Bansal, D. Lahon, B. B. Thakur, and A. Saikia, "A study of urinary enzymes as a marker of early renal damage in patients suffering from diabetes mellitus," *Indian Journal of Basic & Applied Medical Research*, vol. 4, no. 4, pp. 768–776, 2015.

[64] V. Ambade, P. Singh, B. L. Somani, and D. Basannar, "Urinary N-acetyl beta glucosaminidase and gamma glutamyl transferase as early markers of diabetic nephropathy," *Indian Journal of Clinical Biochemistry*, vol. 21, no. 2, pp. 142–148, 2006.

[65] V. Vlatković, B. Stojimirović, and R. Obrenović, "Damage of tubule cells in diabetic nephropathy type 2: urinary N-acetyl-β-D-glucosaminidasis and γ-glutamil-transferasis," *Vojnosanitetski Pregled*, vol. 64, no. 2, pp. 123–127, 2007.

[66] V. Vlatković, B. Stojimirović, R. Obrenović, and S. Nogić, "Damage to proximal tubular epithelial cells in type 2 diabetes mellitus," *Medicinski pregled*, vol. 60, no. 5-6, pp. 272–276, 2007.

[67] D. N. Patel and K. Kalia, "Efficacy of urinary N-acetyl-β-D-glucosaminidase to evaluate early renal tubular damage as a consequence of type 2 diabetes mellitus: a cross-sectional study," *International Journal of Diabetes in Developing Countries*, vol. 35, no. 3, supplement, pp. 449–457, 2015.

[68] A. Piwowar, M. Knapik-Kordecka, I. Fus, and M. Warwas, "Urinary activities of cathepsin B, N-acetyl-β-D-glucosaminidase, and albuminuria in patients with type 2 diabetes mellitus," *Medical Science Monitor*, vol. 12, no. 5, pp. CR210–CR214, 2006.

[69] E. F. O. Kern, P. Erhard, W. Sun, S. Genuth, and M. F. Weiss, "Early urinary markers of diabetic kidney disease: a nested case-control study from the diabetes Control and Complications Trial (DCCT)," *American Journal of Kidney Diseases*, vol. 55, no. 5, pp. 824–834, 2010.

[70] O. Bakoush, A. Grubb, B. Rippe, and J. Tencer, "Urine excretion of protein HC in proteinuric glomerular diseases correlates to urine IgG but not to albuminuria," *Kidney International*, vol. 60, no. 5, pp. 1904–1909, 2001.

[71] N. Shore, R. Khurshid, and M. Saleem, "Alpha-1 microglobulin: a marker for early detection of tubular disorders in diabetic nephropathy," *Journal of Ayub Medical College*, vol. 22, no. 4, pp. 53–55, 2010.

[72] L. Petrica, A. Vlad, G. Gluhovschi et al., "Glycated peptides are associated with proximal tubule dysfunction in type 2 diabetes mellitus," *International Journal of Clinical and Experimental Medicine*, vol. 8, no. 2, pp. 2516–2525, 2015.

[73] A. Saif and N. Soliman, "Urinary α_1-microglobulin and albumin excretion in children and adolescents with type 1 diabetes," *Journal of Diabetes*, 2016.

[74] E. Korpinen, A.-M. Teppo, L. Hukkanen, H. K. Åkerblom, C. Grönhagen-Riska, and O. Vaarala, "Urinary transforming growth factor-β1 and α1-microglobulin in children and adolescents with type 1 diabetes," *Diabetes Care*, vol. 23, no. 5, pp. 664–668, 2000.

[75] C.-Y. Hong, K. Hughes, K.-S. Chia, V. Ng, and S.-L. Ling, "Urinary α1-microglobulin as a marker of nephropathy in type

2 diabetic Asian subjects in Singapore," *Diabetes Care*, vol. 26, no. 2, pp. 338–342, 2003.

[76] L. Petrica, A. Vlad, G. Gluhovschi et al., "Proximal tubule dysfunction is associated with podocyte damage biomarkers nephrin and vascular endothelial growth factor in type 2 diabetes mellitus patients: a cross-sectional study," *PLoS ONE*, vol. 9, no. 11, Article ID e112538, 2014.

[77] S. Jain, A. Rajput, Y. Kumar, N. Uppuluri, A. S. Arvind, and U. Tatu, "Proteomic analysis of urinary protein markers for accurate prediction of diabetic kidney disorder," *Journal of Association of Physicians of India*, vol. 53, pp. 513–520, 2005.

[78] A. Kalansooriya, I. Holbrook, P. Jennings, and P. H. Whiting, "Serum cystatin C, enzymuria, tubular proteinuria and early renal insult in type 2 diabetes," *British Journal of Biomedical Science*, vol. 64, no. 3, pp. 121–123, 2007.

[79] M. L. Robles-Osorio and E. Sabath, "Tubular dysfunction and non-albuminuric renal disease in subjects with type 2 diabetes mellitus," *Revista de Investigacion Clinica*, vol. 66, no. 3, pp. 234–239, 2014.

[80] L. Petrica, M. Petrica, A. Vlad et al., "Proximal tubule dysfunction is dissociated from endothelial dysfunction in normoalbuminuric patients with type 2 diabetes mellitus: a cross-sectional study," *Nephron Clinical Practice*, vol. 118, no. 2, pp. c155–c164, 2011.

[81] L. Petrica, M. Petrica, A. Vlad et al., "Nephro- and neuroprotective effects of rosiglitazone versus glimepiride in normoalbuminuric patients with type 2 diabetes mellitus: a randomized controlled trial," *Wiener Klinische Wochenschrift*, vol. 121, no. 23-24, pp. 765–775, 2009.

[82] L. Petrica, A. Vlad, M. Petrica et al., "Pioglitazone delays proximal tubule dysfunction and improves cerebral vessel endothelial dysfunction in normoalbuminuric people with type 2 diabetes mellitus," *Diabetes Research and Clinical Practice*, vol. 94, no. 1, pp. 22–32, 2011.

[83] D. A. Brott, S. T. Furlong, S. H. Adler et al., "Characterization of renal biomarkers for use in clinical trials: effect of preanalytical processing and qualification using samples from subjects with diabetes," *Drug Design, Development and Therapy*, vol. 9, pp. 3191–3198, 2015.

[84] X. Zeng, D. Hossain, D. G. Bostwick, G. A. Herrera, B. Ballester, and P. L. Zhang, "Urinary β2-microglobulin is a sensitive indicator for renal tubular injury," *Scholarena Journal (SAJ) of Case Reports*, vol. 1, no. 1, pp. 1–6, 2014.

[85] C. Y. Hong, K. S. Chia, and S. L. Ling, "Urine protein excretion among Chinese patients with type 2 diabetes mellitus," *The Medical Journal of Malaysia*, vol. 55, no. 2, pp. 220–229, 2000.

[86] N. Aghamohammadzadeh, A. A. Abolfathi, A. Alizadeh, and H. Ghasemi, "Evaluation of microalbuminuria and urine beta 2 microglobulin in patients with type 1 and 2 diabetes," *International Journal of Current Research and Academic Review*, vol. 3, no. 6, pp. 451–462, 2015.

[87] M. A. Fathy, M. M. Elkady, H. A. Fathy, S. A. Awad, and A. A. Elmenshawy, "Estimation of renal tubular markers for predicting early stage diabetic nephropathy in Egyptian children with type I dibetes mellitus," *Research Journal of Medical Sciences*, vol. 4, no. 2, pp. 207–211, 2009.

[88] C. Y. Hong, K. S. Chia, and S. L. Ling, "Urinary protein excretion in Type 2 diabetes with complications," *Journal of Diabetes and its Complications*, vol. 14, no. 5, pp. 259–265, 2000.

[89] M. Papale, S. Di Paolo, R. Magistroni et al., "Urine proteome analysis may allow noninvasive differential diagnosis of diabetic nephropathy," *Diabetes Care*, vol. 33, no. 11, pp. 2409–2415, 2010.

[90] X. Rao, M. Wan, C. Qiu, and C. Jiang, "Role of cystatin C in renal damage and the optimum cut-off point of renal damage among patients with type 2 diabetes mellitus," *Experimental and Therapeutic Medicine*, vol. 8, no. 3, pp. 887–892, 2014.

[91] K. Mise, J. Hoshino, T. Ueno et al., "Prognostic value of tubulointerstitial lesions, urinary N-acetyl-β-D-glucosaminidase, and urinary β2-microglobulin in patients with type 2 diabetes and biopsy-proven diabetic nephropathy," *Clinical Journal of the American Society of Nephrology*, vol. 11, no. 4, pp. 593–601, 2016.

[92] H. Dihazi, G. A. Müller, S. Lindner et al., "Characterization of diabetic nephropathy by urinary proteomic analysis: identification of a processed ubiquitin form as a differentially excreted protein in diabetic nephropathy patients," *Clinical Chemistry*, vol. 53, no. 9, pp. 1636–1645, 2007.

[93] K. Takebayashi, M. Suetsugu, S. Wakabayashi, Y. Aso, and T. Inukai, "Retinol binding protein-4 levels and clinical features of type 2 diabetes patients," *Journal of Clinical Endocrinology and Metabolism*, vol. 92, no. 7, pp. 2712–2719, 2007.

[94] E. Novery, S. Susanah, and D. Rachmadi, "The correlation of urine retinol binding protein-4 and serum HbA1c with glomerular filtration rate in type 1 (insulin-dependent) diabetic children: a perspective on the duration of diabetes," *Open Journal of Pediatrics*, vol. 5, no. 2, pp. 134–140, 2015.

[95] M. A. K. Salem, S. A. El-Habashy, O. M. Saeid, M. M. K. El-Tawil, and P. H. Tawfik, "Urinary excretion of n-acetyl-β-D-glucosaminidase and retinol binding protein as alternative indicators of nephropathy in patients with type 1 diabetes mellitus," *Pediatric Diabetes*, vol. 3, no. 1, pp. 37–41, 2002.

[96] A. A. S. Abdallah, K. A. El-Shamy, W. M. Morcos, T. H. Mikhail, and N. N. Fadl, "Early marker for renal impairment and angiopathy in diabetic Egyptian children," *Life Science Journal*, vol. 8, no. 3, pp. 358–366, 2011.

[97] N. Zahra, M. A. Javad, and N. Aboalfazl, "Detection of early stage renal disease by elevation of certain low molecular Weight proteins in urine of diabetes patients," *International Journal of Biological Sciences and Applications*, vol. 1, no. 1, pp. 15–18, 2014.

[98] S. E. Park, N. S. Lee, J. W. Park et al., "Association of urinary RBP4 with insulin resistance, inflammation, and microalbuminuria," *European Journal of Endocrinology*, vol. 171, no. 4, pp. 443–449, 2014.

[99] S. M. Titan, J. M. Vieira Jr., W. V. Dominguez et al., "Urinary MCP-1 and RBP: independent predictors of renal outcome in macroalbuminuric diabetic nephropathy," *Journal of Diabetes and its Complications*, vol. 26, no. 6, pp. 546–553, 2012.

[100] C. Catalano, P. H. Winocour, S. Parlongo, I. Gibb, S. Gillespie, and K. G. M. M. Alberti, "Measures of tubular function in normoalbuminuric insulin-dependent diabetic patients and their relationship with sodium lithium countertransport activity," *Nephron*, vol. 73, no. 4, pp. 613–618, 1996.

25

Erythropoietin Dose and Mortality in Hemodialysis Patients: Marginal Structural Model to Examine Causality

Elani Streja,[1] Jongha Park,[1,2] Ting-Yan Chan,[1] Janet Lee,[1] Melissa Soohoo,[1] Connie M. Rhee,[1] Onyebuchi A. Arah,[3] and Kamyar Kalantar-Zadeh[1,3,4]

[1] Harold Simmons Center for Kidney Disease Research and Epidemiology, School of Medicine, University of California, Irvine, Orange, CA, USA
[2] Division of Nephrology, Ulsan University Hospital, University of Ulsan College of Medicine, Ulsan, Republic of Korea
[3] Department of Epidemiology, UCLA Fielding School of Public Health, Los Angeles, CA, USA
[4] Division of Nephrology and Hypertension, School of Medicine, University of California, Irvine, Orange, CA, USA

Correspondence should be addressed to Kamyar Kalantar-Zadeh; kkz@uci.edu

Academic Editor: Jochen Reiser

It has been previously reported that a higher erythropoiesis stimulating agent (ESA) dose in hemodialysis patients is associated with adverse outcomes including mortality; however the causal relationship between ESA and mortality is still hotly debated. We hypothesize ESA dose indeed exhibits a direct linear relationship with mortality in models of association implementing the use of a marginal structural model (MSM), which controls for time-varying confounding and examines causality in the ESA dose-mortality relationship. We conducted a retrospective cohort study of 128 598 adult hemodialysis patients over a 5-year follow-up period to evaluate the association between weekly ESA (epoetin-α) dose and mortality risk. A MSM was used to account for baseline and time-varying covariates especially laboratory measures including hemoglobin level and markers of malnutrition-inflammation status. There was a dose-dependent positive association between weekly epoetin-α doses ≥18 000 U/week and mortality risk. Compared to ESA dose of <6 000 U/week, adjusted odds ratios (95% confidence interval) were 1.02 (0.94–1.10), 1.08 (1.00–1.18), 1.17 (1.06–1.28), 1.27 (1.15–1.41), and 1.52 (1.37–1.69) for ESA dose of 6 000 to <12 000, 12 000 to <18 000, 18 000 to <24 000, 24 000 to <30 000, and ≥30 000 U/week, respectively. High ESA dose may be causally associated with excessive mortality, which is supportive of guidelines which advocate for conservative management of ESA dosing regimen in hemodialysis patients.

1. Introduction

Over the past 20 years, erythropoiesis stimulating agents (ESAs) have been a mainstay in anemia treatment in chronic kidney disease (CKD) and end-stage renal disease (ESRD) patients. Although anemia treatment improves survival in this population, correction of hemoglobin (Hb) to a normal range using ESAs did not demonstrate an additional benefit in previous randomized trials [1–4]. Furthermore, two of these trials unexpectedly showed worse outcomes in patients randomized to achieve higher Hb targets above 13 g/dL [3, 4]. In those studies, the mean ESA dose was greater in the high Hb target arm than in the lower Hb target arm. It has been debated whether high ESA dose mediates the excess observed mortality risk.

As ESA dose and other markers of nutrition and inflammation change over time, the ESA-mortality association remains vulnerable to biases that would arise using conventional survival models [5]. A marginal structural model (MSM) is a type of analysis which can address time-varying covariates that may simultaneously act as a confounder and intermediate variable [6–8]. Notably, Hb level fits this description as it is a critical time-varying confounder that is affected by the previous ESA dose, and it influences the future ESA dose and survival, upon evaluating ESA dose-mortality associations. Furthermore, time-varying ESA dose and nutritional markers may be associated with a greater likelihood of informed censoring. The MSM method attempts to account for these potential time-varying biases by creating

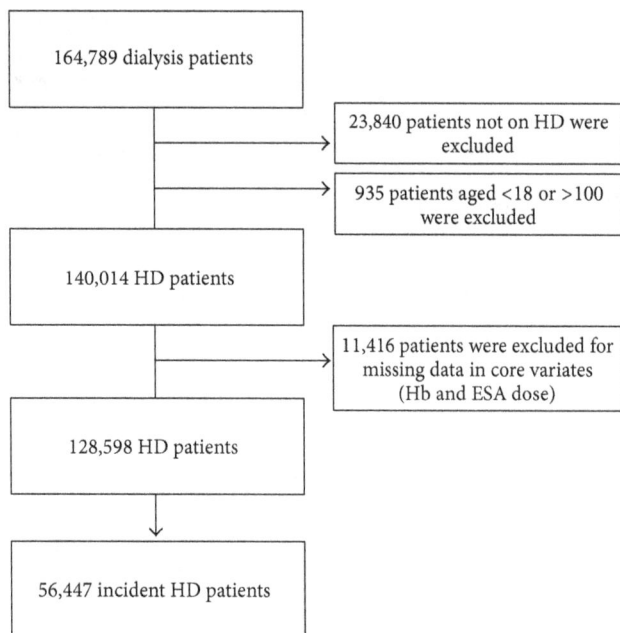

FIGURE 1: Flowchart of patient selection.

weights for each patient at each time interval. These weights estimate the inverse probability of a patient being at his or her exposure (ESA) level for that time interval, and them not having been censored at a prior time interval. The weights are constructed according to baseline and time-varying covariates and attempts to address time-varying confounding leading to ESA dose fluctuations (changes in exposure level) or informative censoring (ESA dose leading to a higher probability of kidney transplant). Holding particular assumptions true in the use of MSM, associations found from MSM are believed to have a causal interpretation. Thus using a MSM and a large cohort of hemodialysis (HD) patients, we aimed to examine the causal effects of weekly epoetin-α dose levels and mortality.

2. Materials and Methods

2.1. Study Cohort. Among a total of 164 789 ESRD patients receiving dialysis treatment from July 1, 2001, through June 30, 2006, in any one of the outpatient facilities of a large dialysis organization (DaVita Healthcare Partners) in the United States, we examined data from 128 598 patients who met the following inclusion criteria: being of age ≥18 years, having underwent HD for at least 90 days, and having had complete data on the main exposure and core covariate (ESA dose and Hb level) (Figure 1). In sensitivity analyses, we restricted analyses to an incident HD cohort, defined as patients whose HD duration at cohort entry was less than 6 months. The institutional review committees of Los Angeles Biomedical Research Institute at Harbor-UCLA, University of California, Irvine, and DaVita Clinical Research approved this study. Given the large sample size, anonymity of the patients studied and nonintrusive nature of the research, the requirement for consent was waived.

2.2. Dose of Erythropoiesis Stimulating Agent. The primary exposure was weekly epoetin-α dose (U/week), which was calculated and averaged for every 3-month interval (calendar quarter) in order to minimize measurement variability. ESA dose was divided into 6 preselected ordinal categories: <6 000 U/week (reference), 6 000 to <12 000 U/week, 12 000 to <18 000 U/week, 18 000 to <24 000 U/week, 24 000 to <30 000 U/week, and ≥30 000 U/week. ESA <6 000 U/week was designated as the reference group. ESA dose during hospitalization was not available in this cohort. The in-hospital ESA dose was imputed using the most recent ESA dose prior to hospitalization.

2.3. Study Outcomes. The primary outcome was all-cause mortality, and the secondary outcomes were cardiovascular (CV) or infectious mortality (see Supplement Table 1 in Supplementary Materials available online at http://dx.doi.org/10.1155/2016/6087134). Detailed information on cause of death was obtained from the US Renal Data System (USRDS) "CDeath" codes, which are derived from the ESRD Death Notification Form (CMS-2746) provided by ESRD networks to the USRDS. Cause of death was categorized as cardiovascular, infectious, or others by clinician decision according to these "CDeath" codes. Patients were followed until the time of death or the end of study period (June 30, 2007). Patients were censored at the time of renal transplantation, change of dialysis modality, that is, HD to peritoneal dialysis, or transfer to a non-DaVita facility.

2.4. Covariates of Interest. Demographic covariates included baseline age, sex, race/ethnicity (Caucasian, African American, Hispanic, Asian, and others), marital status (married, divorced, single, and widowed), primary insurance (Medicare, Medicaid, private insurance, and others), comorbid conditions (see below), calendar quarter of cohort entry, and dialysis vintage (<6 months, 6 months to <24 months, 2 to <5 years, and ≥5 years), for which information was obtained from the USRDS. The following comorbidities were considered: diabetes mellitus, hypertension, ischemic heart disease, congestive heart failure, cerebrovascular disease, peripheral vascular disease, chronic obstructive pulmonary disease, malignancy, nonambulatory state, and current smoking status. Dialysis duration was defined as the duration of time between the first day of dialysis treatment and the first day that patients entered the cohort.

Time-varying lab covariates, also averaged over a successive 3-month (calendar quarter) interval, included Hb level, serum albumin, creatinine, calcium, phosphorus, bicarbonate, total iron binding capacity, ferritin, white blood cell count, lymphocyte percentage, normalized protein nitrogen appearance (a metric of dietary protein intake), dialysis adequacy (single-pool Kt/V), and body mass index. Hb level was measured approximately twice per month. Most laboratory data were measured monthly, except for serum ferritin level that was measured at least quarterly. Blood samples were drawn before HD using uniform techniques in all dialysis clinics and were transported to the central laboratory, usually within 24 hours (DaVita Laboratory, Deland, FL). All laboratory values were measured via automated and standardized methods. Post-HD body weight was used to calculate body mass index.

2.5. Statistical Analysis. Inverse probabilities of treatment weights (IPTWs) were created on the basis of the inverse of the predicted probability of a patient receiving the treatment that was actually received (the above-mentioned ESA dose categories), given the baseline and time-varying covariates. We used ordinal logistic regression to calculate IPTWs at baseline and for each subsequent quarter of follow-up [9]. IPTWs can result in excessively large weights when there is an atypical treatment decision or data error. Hence, stabilized IPTWs have been applied to reduce the potential for extreme IPTWs. In the stabilized IPTWs, the numerator is the calculated probability of the observed treatment (ESA dose) given the previous ESA dose and baseline patient characteristics, while the denominator is the calculated probability of ESA dose, previous ESA dose, and both baseline and time-varying covariates. Baseline covariates included age, gender, race, insurance, marital status, comorbidities, and baseline lab values, while time-varying covariates included time-updated quarterly lab values and their respective lag (previous quarter) values. Estimated weights were then truncated at the 1st and 99th percentile values and used in the analyses [10].

To address informative censoring, we fitted logistic regression models to calculate the inverse probability of censoring weights (IPCWs) at each time interval. As done with IPTWs, we used the same covariates for the numerator and denominator of the stabilized IPCW modeling the calculated probability of observed censorship. As large censoring weights were not observed, truncation was not performed for IPCW values. The final stabilized weights were calculated as the product of the stabilized IPTWs and stabilized IPCWs.

We estimated the odds ratio (OR) using a generalized estimating equation that included ESA dose category and the final stabilized weights on the basis of all baseline covariates. The ESA dose category of <6 000 U/week was treated as the reference group. Missing values for baseline covariates were imputed using multiple imputation with 5 iterations. In both the overall and incident study populations, data were missing for less than 5% and 1%, respectively. To further impute missing time-varying covariates in each time window, we used last-value carried forward. All analyses were conducted using SAS version 9.3 (SAS Institute Inc., Cary, NC).

3. Results

3.1. Patient's Characteristics. Baseline characteristics of the overall patient cohort and stratified across ESA categories are summarized in Table 1. During the baseline quarter, there were 6 644 (5%), 23 314 (18%), 26 852 (21%), 21 487 (17%), 15 278 (12%), and 35 023 (27%) patients receiving a weekly ESA dose of <6 000, 6 000 to <12 000, 12 000 to <18 000, 18 000 to <24 000, 24 000 to <30 000, and ≥30 000 U/week. The mean ± standard deviation (SD) age was 62 ± 15 years, 55% of the patients were women, 32% and 14% were African American and Hispanic, respectively, and 57% were diabetic. The baseline mean ± SD Hb level was 12.1 ± 1.0 g/dL, and the median (interquartile range, IQR) duration of follow-up

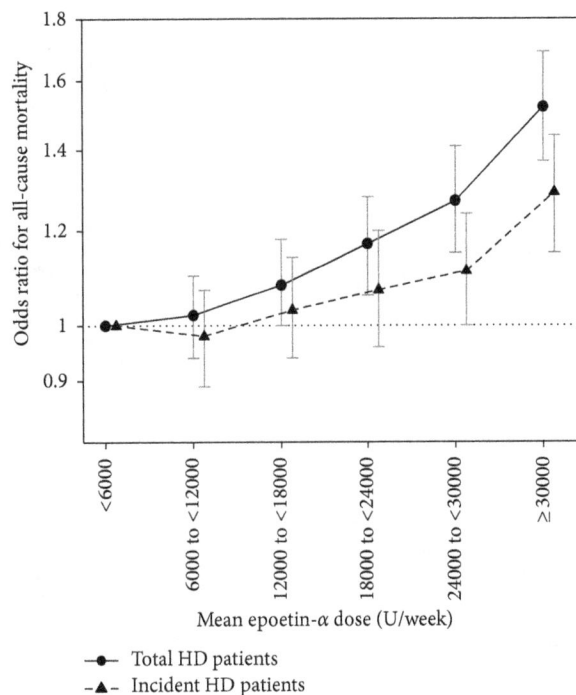

FIGURE 2: Adjusted mortality risk for all-cause mortality by weekly epoetin-α dose estimated by marginal structural model.

was 2.2 (1.2–3.6) years. Patients receiving a higher ESA dose tended to be African American and male and had lower albumin and lymphocyte percentage.

3.2. Distribution of Weights. The distribution of the weights is displayed in Table 2. Stabilized weights had a maximum value of 80.9 and 78.9 in the overall and incident patient cohorts, respectively. The mean stabilized weights were 0.84 and 0.88, respectively.

3.3. Weekly ESA Dose and All-Cause Mortality. Weekly ESA doses ≥18 000 U/week were associated with higher risks of death as compared with a weekly epoetin-α dose of <6 000 U/week. Furthermore, a dose-response relationship was also observed (Figure 2). Weekly ESA doses of 18 000 to <24 000, 24 000 to <30 000, and ≥30 000 U/week showed 17%, 27%, and 52% higher risk of mortality, respectively (Table 3).

3.4. Weekly ESA Dose and Cardiovascular/Infectious Mortality. Weekly ESA dose also showed a strong relationship with CV mortality risk (Table 3). Weekly ESA doses of 6 000 to <12 000, 12 000 to <18 000, 18 000 to <24 000, 24 000 to <30 000, and ≥30 000 U/week showed 13%, 21%, 23%, 35%, and 44% higher risks of CV mortality, respectively. Risk of infectious death was only significantly increased in weekly ESA dose of ≥30 000 U/week (Table 3), while ESA levels <30,000 U/week exhibited a trend toward higher risk of infectious death, compared to reference.

3.5. Sensitivity Analyses. In incident patients ($n = 56\,447$), the relationship between weekly ESA dose and mortality risk

TABLE 1: Patient characteristics by weekly epoetin-α dose categories.

	Total		Averaged weekly epoetin-α dose during follow-up period (U/week)				
		<6000	6000 to <12000	12000 to <18000	18000 to <24000	24000 to <30000	≥30000
n (%)	128 598 (100)	6644 (5)	23 314 (18)	26 852 (21)	21 487 (17)	15 278 (12)	35 023 (27)
Age (yr)	62 ± 15	62 ± 16	63 ± 15	62 ± 15	62 ± 15	62 ± 15	60 ± 15
Female (%)	70 309 (55)	4191 (63)	13 107 (56)	14 604 (54)	11 541 (54)	8153 (53)	18 713 (53)
Dialysis vintage (mo)	3 (1,28)	16 (2,39)	7 (1,30)	4 (1,27)	2 (1,26)	2 (1,25)	2 (1,26)
Race (%)							
Caucasian	55 107 (43)	3181 (48)	10 057 (43)	11 026 (41)	9072 (42)	6460 (42)	15 311 (44)
African American	41 257 (32)	1678 (25)	6286 (27)	8104 (30)	6775 (32)	5173 (34)	13 241 (38)
Hispanic	18 409 (14)	968 (15)	4032 (17)	4384 (16)	3336 (16)	2116 (14)	3573 (10)
Asian	3887 (3)	218 (3)	885 (4)	1002 (4)	675 (3)	436 (3)	671 (2)
Other	9938 (8)	599 (9)	2054 (9)	2336 (9)	1629 (8)	1093 (7)	2227 (6)
Insurance (%)							
Medicare	81 230 (63)	4357 (66)	14 881 (64)	17 062 (64)	13 497 (63)	9645 (63)	21 788 (62)
Medicaid	6777 (5)	194 (3)	989 (4)	1358 (5)	1225 (6)	897 (6)	2114 (6)
Private	12 156 (9)	623 (9)	2344 (10)	2718 (10)	2138 (10)	1414 (9)	2919 (8)
Other	28 435 (22)	1470 (22)	5100 (22)	5714 (21)	4627 (22)	3322 (22)	8202 (23)
Marital status (%)							
Married	51 385 (40)	3057 (46)	9942 (43)	10 888 (41)	8368 (39)	5934 (39)	13 196 (38)
Divorced	8725 (7)	434 (7)	1462 (6)	1778 (7)	1470 (7)	1055 (7)	2526 (7)
Single	29 615 (23)	1482 (22)	4939 (21)	5701 (21)	4873 (23)	3536 (23)	9084 (26)
Widowed	16 521 (13)	823 (12)	3186 (14)	3641 (14)	2783 (13)	1990 (13)	4098 (12)
Comorbidities (%)							
DM	73 847 (57)	3353 (50)	12 972 (56)	15 550 (58)	12 787 (60)	9147 (60)	20 038 (57)
HTN	96 852 (79)	4986 (81)	17 714 (80)	20 485 (80)	16 337 (80)	11 560 (80)	25 770 (78)
IHD	26 062 (21)	1287 (21)	4777 (22)	5549 (22)	4470 (22)	3192 (22)	6787 (20)
CHF	33 534 (28)	1475 (24)	5663 (26)	7005 (27)	5691 (28)	4249 (29)	9451 (28)
PVD	13 820 (11)	669 (11)	2404 (11)	2842 (11)	2373 (12)	1770 (12)	3762 (11)
CVA	9015 (7)	482 (8)	1628 (7)	1928 (8)	1632 (8)	1025 (7)	2320 (7)
COPD	6904 (6)	377 (6)	1140 (5)	1365 (5)	1135 (6)	887 (6)	2000 (6)
Malignancy	5538 (5)	209 (3)	829 (4)	1019 (4)	879 (4)	622 (4)	1980 (6)
Current smoking	5854 (5)	345 (6)	978 (4)	1134 (4)	971 (5)	650 (4)	1776 (5)
BMI (kg/m²)	26.6 ± 6.7	26.7 ± 6.5	26.2 ± 6.0	26.4 ± 6.4	26.7 ± 6.5	26.8 ± 6.9	27.1 ± 7.4
Laboratory parameters							
Hemoglobin (g/dL)	12.1 ± 1.0	12.6 ± 0.8	12.4 ± 0.7	12.3 ± 0.8	12.2 ± 0.8	12.0 ± 0.9	11.5 ± 1.2
Creatinine (mg/dL)	8.2 ± 3.0	8.4 ± 3.2	8.4 ± 3.0	8.4 ± 3.0	8.3 ± 3.0	8.1 ± 3.0	8.0 ± 3.1
Albumin (g/dL)	3.7 ± 0.4	3.9 ± 0.3	3.9 ± 0.3	3.8 ± 0.4	3.7 ± 0.4	3.7 ± 0.4	3.5 ± 0.5
TIBC (mg/dL)	203 ± 41	215 ± 36	211 ± 36	206 ± 37	203 ± 39	201 ± 40	194 ± 46
Calcium (mg/dL)	9.3 ± 0.6	9.4 ± 0.6	9.4 ± 0.6	9.3 ± 0.6	9.3 ± 0.6	9.2 ± 0.6	9.1 ± 0.7
Phosphorus (mg/dL)	5.6 ± 1.3	5.4 ± 1.2	5.4 ± 1.1	5.5 ± 1.2	5.6 ± 1.3	5.6 ± 1.3	5.7 ± 1.4
WBC (×10³/mm³)	7.4 ± 2.4	7.4 ± 2.2	7.4 ± 2.0	7.4 ± 2.1	7.4 ± 2.2	7.5 ± 2.4	7.5 ± 2.9
Lymphocyte (%)	20.3 ± 7.3	22.3 ± 7.4	21.7 ± 7.2	21.0 ± 7.2	20.3 ± 7.2	19.6 ± 7.2	18.8 ± 7.4
Ferritin (ng/mL)	515 (314,742)	572 (377,777)	554 (362,755)	532 (341,741)	509 (313,728)	491 (291,730)	473 (265,737)
Single-pool Kt/V	1.6 ± 0.3	1.7 ± 0.3	1.7 ± 0.3	1.6 ± 0.3	1.6 ± 0.3	1.6 ± 0.3	1.5 ± 0.3
nPNA (g/kg/day)	1.0 ± 0.2	1.0 ± 0.2	1.0 ± 0.2	1.0 ± 0.2	1.0 ± 0.2	1.0 ± 0.2	0.9 ± 0.2

Note: categorical variables are expressed as frequency (percentage). Continuous variables are given as mean ± SD or median (interquartile range) as appropriate. Conversion factors for units: hemoglobin and albumin in g/dL to g/L ×10; creatinine in mg/dL to μmol/L ×88.4; calcium in mg/dL to mmol/L ×0.2495; and phosphorus in mg/dL to mmol/L ×0.3229. No conversion necessary for ferritin in ng/mL and μg/L and WBC count in 10³/μL and 10⁹/L. DM = diabetes mellitus, HTN = hypertension, IHD = ischemic heart disease, CHF = congestive heart failure, PVD = peripheral vascular disease, CVA = cerebrovascular accident, COPD = chronic obstructive pulmonary disease, BMI = body mass index, TIBC = total iron binding capacity, WBC = white blood cell, and nPNA = normalized protein nitrogen appearance.

TABLE 2: Weight distribution for marginal structural model across 3-month time intervals.

Percentile	Overall (prevalent + incident) patients			Incident patients		
	Stabilized IPTW	Stabilized IPCW	Stabilized weight	Stabilized IPTW	Stabilized IPCW	Stabilized weight
Maximum	82.6	3.66	80.9	83.9	3.74	78.7
99th	6.55	1.31	6.28	6.26	1.27	6.10
95th	2.24	1.02	2.17	2.23	1.01	2.18
90th	1.43	1.00	1.40	1.43	1.00	1.41
75th	0.92	0.99	0.92	0.94	0.99	0.93
50th (Median)	0.68	0.97	0.67	0.75	0.98	0.74
25th	0.31	0.94	0.29	0.39	0.96	0.38
10th	0.11	0.90	0.10	0.16	0.93	0.15
5th	0.05	0.86	0.05	0.09	0.90	0.08
1st	0.01	0.78	0.01	0.03	0.83	0.03
Minimum	0.0003	0.076	0.0003	0.0008	0.22	0.0008
Mean	0.86	0.97	0.84	0.90	0.98	0.88

IPTW = inverse probability of treatment weight. IPCW = inverse probability of censoring weight.

TABLE 3: Adjusted odds ratios (95% confidence interval) for mortality by weekly epoetin-α doses in overall patient cohort.

Epoetin-α (U/wk)	All-cause	Cardiovascular	Infectious
<6 000	Reference	Reference	Reference
6 000 to <12 000	1.02 (0.94–1.10)	**1.13 (1.05–1.23)**	1.12 (1.00–1.25)
12 000 to <18 000	1.08 (1.00–1.18)	**1.21 (1.10–1.32)**	1.11 (0.98–1.26)
18 000 to <24 000	**1.17 (1.06–1.28)**	**1.23 (1.12–1.36)**	1.14 (1.00–1.30)
24 000 to <30 000	**1.27 (1.15–1.41)**	**1.35 (1.22–1.50)**	1.13 (0.99–1.29)
≥30 000	**1.52 (1.37–1.69)**	**1.44 (1.29–1.59)**	**1.28 (1.11–1.48)**

Note: bold font indicates statistically significant odds ratios.

was less apparent compared to the overall cohort, which included prevalent patients (Figure 2 and Table 4). Only a weekly ESA dose ≥30 000 U/week was significantly associated with higher mortality compared to a weekly ESA dose of <6 000 U/week (OR: 1.29, 95% confidence interval (CI): 1.15–1.44).

Based on our observation that a weekly ESA dose of ≥30 000 U/week was associated with a higher risk of mortality in both the overall and incident patient cohorts, we dichotomized weekly ESA dose with cutoffs at 30 000 U/week. Also, using a MSM, we then reexamined mortality risk of weekly ESA doses ≥30 000 versus <30 000 U/week (reference) in various subgroups: men versus women, age ≥65 versus <65 years, race/ethnicity (Caucasian versus African American versus Hispanic), diabetic versus nondiabetic, prior history versus no history of ischemic heart disease, body mass index ≥23 versus <23 kg/m^2, and serum albumin level ≥3.8 versus <3.8 g/dL. Among all subgroups, adjusted ORs were significantly higher in weekly ESA dose of ≥30 000 U/week than in that of <30 000 U/week (Figure 3).

4. Discussion

In this study, we used a MSM to evaluate the relationship between ESA dose and mortality in a large cohort of HD patients. We observed a dose-dependent relationship as higher ESA dose was associated with a higher risk of mortality.

After recent randomized trials showed worse outcomes in patients randomized to higher Hb targets [3, 4], the US Food and Drug Administration recommended a more conservative ESA dosing regimen for the treatment of patients with CKD [11]. However, the causal relationship between ESA dose and mortality has still been debated and the ideal ESA dosing regimen remains unknown. The examination of the causal effect of ESA is challenging due to the strong relationship between patient's comorbidity and ESA requirements and especially with the presence of time-dependent confounding of Hb in observational studies. The current ESA dose is influenced by previous ESA dose and Hb and affects future ESA dose and Hb. In addition, Hb itself may affect patient's outcome simultaneously. However, an increase in Hb independent of ESA dose may not be associated with higher mortality risk [12]. In presence of this type of complex confounding, traditional survival models are limited in their capacity to estimate unbiased exposure effect [5]. We used a MSM to control this time-dependent confounding [6, 7, 10, 13]. We observed significantly higher OR estimates in ESA doses over 18 000 U/week as compared to that of <6 000 U/week. Weekly ESA dose ≥30 000 U/week showed a 52% increased mortality risk.

Previous studies have tried to control time-dependent confounding using MSM, but they have reported conflicting results. Zhang et al. reported no harmful effect of median cumulative ESA dose over 30 000 U/week in elderly (≥65 years old) HD patients [14]. However, an additional study by

TABLE 4: Adjusted odds ratio (95% confidence interval) for mortality by weekly epoetin-α doses in incident patients.

Epoetin-α dose (U/wk)	All-cause	Cardiovascular	Infectious
<6 000	Reference	Reference	Reference
6 000 to <12 000	0.98 (0.89–1.07)	1.06 (0.96–1.18)	1.08 (0.93–1.25)
12 000 to <18 000	1.03 (0.94–1.14)	1.07 (0.95–1.19)	1.10 (0.93–1.29)
18 000 to <24 000	1.07 (0.96–1.20)	**1.14 (1.01–1.30)**	1.18 (0.99–1.40)
24 000 to <30 000	1.11 (1.00–1.24)	**1.16 (1.02–1.31)**	1.11 (0.93–1.33)
≥30 000	**1.29 (1.15–1.44)**	**1.23 (1.09–1.40)**	1.18 (1.00–1.40)

Note: incident patient was defined as having a dialysis vintage of less than 6 months at cohort entry. Bold font indicates statistically significant odds ratios.

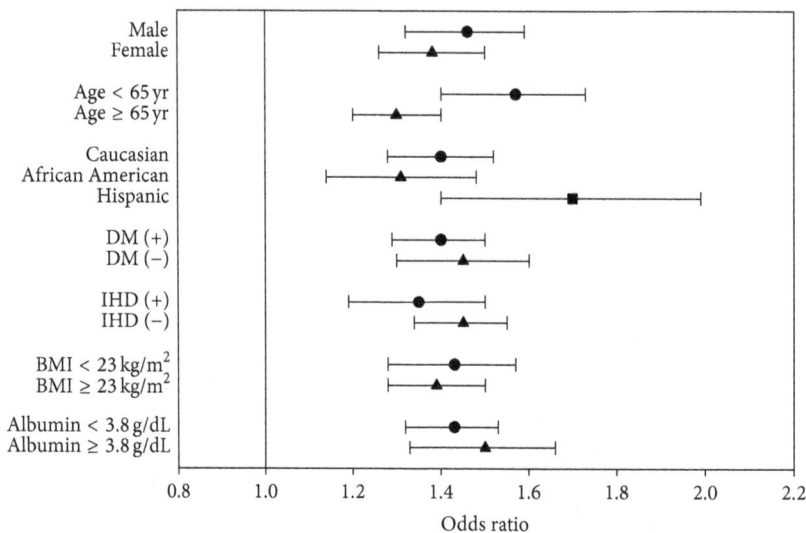

FIGURE 3: Adjusted mortality risk of weekly epoetin-α dose ≥30 000 versus <30 000 U/week (reference) among various subgroups. DM = diabetes mellitus, IHD = ischemic heart disease, and BMI = body mass index.

the same group investigating a larger cohort later reported a 32% increased risk of mortality with ESA dose greater than 40 000 U/week compared with 20 000 to 30 000 U/week especially in diabetic elderly patients [15]. Wang et al. reported a mortality hazard ratio for the highest ESA doses (>49 000 U/2 weeks) of 0.98 (95% CI: 0.76–1.74) compared with ESA dose ≤14 000 U/2 weeks. They concluded that there is appreciable confounding by indication at higher ESA doses and that ESA dose was not associated with increased mortality in analysis using MSM [9]. Recently, in a European cohort, Suttorp et al. reported that the excess mortality risk for patients with high ESA dose did not fully disappear within analysis using the MSM approach. The MSM estimated a hazard ratio of 1.54 (95% CI: 1.08–2.18) for patients with ESA dose above 6 000 U/week compared to the counterpart of less than 6 000 U/week, which is in line with our results [16].

Our results should be interpreted carefully. The MSM estimates what would happen if a patient is always exposed to higher doses of ESA, which is difficult to interpret in clinical practice but nonetheless begs the question if a patient treated with a lower dose of ESA would benefit more from treatment than with a higher ESA dose. In addition, our results could be interpreted causally under the fundamental assumptions of MSM. An important assumption is "positivity," the condition that there are both exposed and unexposed individuals at

every level of the confounders. A relatively large study may have zero proportion for particular exposure and covariate histories as the number of covariates increases. Estimated weights with a mean far from one or very extreme values are indicative of nonpositivity or misspecification of the weight model. In our study, it could be debated whether the mean of the stabilized weights of 0.84 in overall patients and 0.88 in incident patients is close enough to one to justify the conclusion that models were well specified. However, there is a tradeoff between reducing confounding bias and increasing bias/variance due to nonpositivity [10]. The distribution of weights in our study is comparable to that of other MSM studies although the mean of weights in our study is smaller [9, 16].

Thin evidence for biologic plausibility also dampens a conclusive consensus of a causal relationship between ESA dose and mortality. Considering that the most common cause of death in CKD patients is related to CV disease, a harmful effect of high ESA dose, if any, would likely be mediated by an adverse effect due to CV disease. The treatment with exogenous erythropoietin is distinctly different from the normal biology. There is a very rapid rise and supraphysiologic peak in serum concentration of erythropoietin after injection, followed by a rapid decline [17, 18]. Repetitive supraphysiologic stimulation could disorder cardiac modeling, increase vulnerability to stress, or impair the ability of higher Hb to diminish left ventricular hypertrophy [18–20]. Another hypothesis is that iron depletion, increased platelet reactivity and platelet numbers [21], and associated relative thrombocytosis might contribute to increased CV events upon administering a high ESA dose [22]. Moreover, high ESA dose may directly lead to thrombocytosis [23]. A 2014 review summarized additional potential mechanisms, including ESA effect on arterial blood pressure via increasing blood viscosity and vasoconstriction [24]. In our study, estimated ORs for CV death were greater than those for all-cause mortality, although the differences were small (Tables 3 and 4). Further investigations are warranted to validate biologic plausibility.

The association between ESA dose and mortality was observed even in incident patients, but the strength of association was weaker than in the overall cohort, which additionally included prevalent patients. This may be due to the relatively small number of patients or the cumulative effect of ESA exposure. Prevalent patients receiving a high ESA dose during the study period tend to have greater cumulative exposure to ESA prior to enrollment. This observation may not be present in incident HD patients because ESA dose administered during the predialysis CKD stages is usually lower compared to the dose administered during maintenance HD. If a cumulative effect of ESA exposure exists, estimated ORs may be augmented in the overall cohort compared to that of the incident cohort [25]. Another speculation is that, in the early period after HD initiation, other mortality risk factors are more dominant than ESA dose. Survivor bias is more likely to affect studies of prevalent patients opposed to incident patients.

Our study has several limitations. First, the validity of our analysis depends on the assumption that we have adjusted for all confounders (exchangeability). Given the detailed level of information on a variety of demographics, laboratory parameters, and dialysis adequacy in our data, we believe that we have controlled for the most important confounding. However, the possibility of residual confounding or confounding by indication cannot be completely excluded. Although we included serum albumin, white blood cell counts, and lymphocyte percentage in the models [26], we did not have data for other inflammatory markers, such as C-reactive protein [27, 28]. It might be interpreted as a high OR estimate for infectious mortality with ESA dose over 30 000 U/week in our results. Considering that there is no evidence to date that ESA causes infectious complications, a small effect on infectious mortality could indicate residual confounding. Second, the estimates for our MSM could be affected by the level of weight truncation, which is reflective of the tradeoff between control of confounding and precision of our effect estimates [10]. Third, our data did not contain information on ESA dose during hospitalization. We imputed ESA doses assuming thrice-weekly dosing using the prehospitalization dose. Although this approach may not reflect actual in-hospital ESA dosing exactly, it may be an alternative solution to address this missing ESA data problem. Despite these limitations, our cohort is one of the largest ones to investigate the ESA-mortality association and is nationally representative of the United States adult HD population.

Furthermore, our cohort was followed up for an extended period of time, giving sufficient power in this analysis.

In conclusion, estimating the causal relationship between ESA dose and mortality is complex due to the strong relationship between comorbidity, ESA requirements, and time-dependent confounding of Hb. Using a MSM, we observed a possible causal relationship between higher ESA dose and excess mortality risk in HD patients. It supports the current conservative ESA dosing regimen which balances the benefit of anemia correction and a potential harm of higher ESA dose. Further studies (including biological and prospective studies) are warranted to establish the ideal ESA dosing algorithm in CKD and ESRD patients and to further unveil the complex pathophysiological relationship between ESA dose and mortality.

Acknowledgments

The authors thank DaVita Clinical Research (DCR) for providing the clinical data for this research project and Dr. Steven M. Brunelli (Brigham and Women's Hospital, Boston, MA) kindly helped in statistical programming and analyzing data.

References

[1] A. Besarab, W. K. Bolton, J. K. Browne et al., "The effects of normal as compared with low hematocrit values in patients with cardiac disease who are receiving hemodialysis and epoetin," *The New England Journal of Medicine*, vol. 339, no. 9, pp. 584–590, 1998.

[2] T. B. Drüeke, F. Locatelli, N. Clyne et al., "Normalization of hemoglobin level in patients with chronic kidney disease and anemia," *The New England Journal of Medicine*, vol. 355, no. 20, pp. 2071–2084, 2006.

[3] A. K. Singh, L. Szczech, K. L. Tang et al., "Correction of anemia with epoetin alfa in chronic kidney disease," *The New England Journal of Medicine*, vol. 355, no. 20, pp. 2085–2098, 2006.

[4] M. A. Pfeffer, E. A. Burdmann, C.-Y. Chen et al., "A trial of darbepoetin alfa in type 2 diabetes and chronic kidney disease," *The New England Journal of Medicine*, vol. 361, no. 21, pp. 2019–2032, 2009.

[5] B. D. Bradbury, M. A. Brookhart, W. C. Winkelmayer et al., "Evolving statistical methods to facilitate evaluation of the causal association between erythropoiesis-stimulating agent dose and mortality in nonexperimental research: strengths and limitations," *American Journal of Kidney Diseases*, vol. 54, no. 3, pp. 554–560, 2009.

[6] J. M. Robins, M. Á. Hernán, and B. Brumback, "Marginal structural models and causal inference in epidemiology," *Epidemiology*, vol. 11, no. 5, pp. 550–560, 2000.

[7] M. L. Petersen, S. G. Deeks, J. N. Martin, and M. J. van der Laan, "History-adjusted marginal structural models for estimating time-varying effect modification," *American Journal of Epidemiology*, vol. 166, no. 9, pp. 985–993, 2007.

[8] M. A. Hernán and J. M. Robins, "Estimating causal effects from epidemiological data," *Journal of Epidemiology and Community Health*, vol. 60, no. 7, pp. 578–586, 2006.

[9] O. Wang, R. D. Kilpatrick, C. W. Critchlow et al., "Relationship between epoetin alfa dose and mortality: findings from a marginal structural model," *Clinical Journal of the American Society of Nephrology*, vol. 5, no. 2, pp. 182–188, 2010.

[10] S. R. Cole and M. A. Hernán, "Constructing inverse probability weights for marginal structural models," *American Journal of Epidemiology*, vol. 168, no. 6, pp. 656–664, 2008.

[11] FDA, "Drug safty communication: modified dosing recommendations to improve the safe use of erythropoiesis-stimulating agents (ESAs) in chronic kidney disease," http://www.fda.gov/Drugs/DrugSafety/ucm259639.htm.

[12] A. Shah, M. Z. Molnar, L. R. Lukowsky, J. J. Zaritsky, C. P. Kovesdy, and K. Kalantar-Zadeh, "Hemoglobin level and survival in hemodialysis patients with polycystic kidney disease and the role of administered erythropoietin," *American Journal of Hematology*, vol. 87, no. 8, pp. 833–836, 2012.

[13] M. Á. Hernán, B. Brumback, and J. M. Robins, "Marginal structural models to estimate the causal effect of zidovudine on the survival of HIV-positive men," *Epidemiology*, vol. 11, no. 5, pp. 561–570, 2000.

[14] Y. Zhang, M. Thamer, D. J. Cotter, J. Kaufman, and M. A. Hernán, "Estimated effect of epoetin dosage on survival among elderly hemodialysis patients in the United States," *Clinical Journal of the American Society of Nephrology*, vol. 4, no. 3, pp. 638–644, 2009.

[15] Y. Zhang, M. Thamer, J. S. Kaufman, D. J. Cotter, and M. A. Hernán, "High doses of epoetin do not lower mortality and cardiovascular risk among elderly hemodialysis patients with diabetes," *Kidney International*, vol. 80, no. 6, pp. 663–669, 2011.

[16] M. M. Suttorp, T. Hoekstra, M. Mittelman et al., "Treatment with high dose of erythropoiesis-stimulating agents and mortality: analysis with a sequential Cox approach and a marginal structural model," *Pharmacoepidemiology and Drug Safety*, vol. 24, no. 10, pp. 1068–1075, 2015.

[17] A. J. Erslev, "Erythropoietin," *The New England Journal of Medicine*, vol. 324, no. 19, pp. 1339–1344, 1991.

[18] S. Fishbane and A. Besarab, "Mechanism of increased mortality risk with erythropoietin treatment to higher hemoglobin targets," *Clinical Journal of the American Society of Nephrology*, vol. 2, no. 6, pp. 1274–1282, 2007.

[19] H. Wu, S. H. Lee, J. Gao, X. Liu, and M. L. Iruela-Arispe, "Inactivation of erythropoietin leads to defects in cardiac morphogenesis," *Development*, vol. 126, no. 16, pp. 3597–3605, 1999.

[20] A. Anagnostou, Z. Liu, M. Steiner et al., "Erythropoietin receptor mRNA expression in human endothelial cells," *Proceedings of the National Academy of Sciences of the United States of America*, vol. 91, no. 9, pp. 3974–3978, 1994.

[21] P. J. Stohlawetz, L. Dzirlo, N. Hergovich et al., "Effects of erythropoietin on platelet reactivity and thrombopoiesis in humans," *Blood*, vol. 95, no. 9, pp. 2983–2989, 2000.

[22] E. Streja, C. P. Kovesdy, S. Greenland et al., "Erythropoietin, iron depletion, and relative thrombocytosis: a possible explanation for hemoglobin-survival paradox in hemodialysis," *American Journal of Kidney Diseases*, vol. 52, no. 4, pp. 727–736, 2008.

[23] N. D. Vaziri, "Thrombocytosis in EPO-treated dialysis patients may be mediated by EPO rather than iron deficiency," *American Journal of Kidney Diseases*, vol. 53, no. 5, pp. 733–736, 2009.

[24] A. Lund, C. Lundby, and N. V. Olsen, "High-dose erythropoietin for tissue protection," *European Journal of Clinical Investigation*, vol. 44, no. 12, pp. 1230–1238, 2014.

[25] I. Koulouridis, M. Alfayez, T. A. Trikalinos, E. M. Balk, and B. L. Jaber, "Dose of erythropoiesis-stimulating agents and adverse outcomes in CKD: a metaregression analysis," *American Journal of Kidney Diseases*, vol. 61, no. 1, pp. 44–56, 2013.

[26] K. Kalantar-Zadeh, G. H. Lee, J. E. Miller et al., "Predictors of hyporesponsiveness to erythropoiesis-stimulating agents in hemodialysis patients," *American Journal of Kidney Diseases*, vol. 53, no. 5, pp. 823–834, 2009.

[27] B. D. Bradbury, C. W. Critchlow, M. R. Weir, R. Stewart, M. Krishnan, and R. H. Hakim, "Impact of elevated C-reactive protein levels on erythropoiesis- stimulating agent (ESA) dose and responsiveness in hemodialysis patients," *Nephrology Dialysis Transplantation*, vol. 24, no. 3, pp. 919–925, 2009.

[28] J. W. Adamson, "Hyporesponsiveness to erythropoiesis stimulating agents in chronic kidney disease: the many faces of inflammation," *Advances in Chronic Kidney Disease*, vol. 16, no. 2, pp. 76–82, 2009.

26

Low, rather than High, Body Mass Index is a Risk Factor for Acute Kidney Injury in Multiethnic Asian Patients

Allen Yan Lun Liu (ID),[1] **Jiexun Wang,**[2] **Milind Nikam,**[3] **Boon Cheok Lai,**[1] and **Lee Ying Yeoh**[1]

[1]*Division of Renal Medicine, Department of General Medicine, Khoo Teck Puat Hospital, Singapore*
[2]*Clinical Research Unit, Khoo Teck Puat Hospital, Singapore*
[3]*Fresenius Medical Care Pte. Ltd., Singapore*

Correspondence should be addressed to Allen Yan Lun Liu; liu.allen.yl@alexandrahealth.com.sg

Academic Editor: Frank Park

Background. Acute kidney injury (AKI) is common in hospitalised patients. The relationship between body mass index (BMI) and the risk of having AKI for patients in the acute hospital setting is not known, particularly in the Asian population. *Methods.* This was a retrospective, single-centre, observational study conducted in Singapore, a multiethnic population. All patients aged ≥21 years and hospitalised from January to December 2013 were recruited. *Results.* A total of 12,555 patients were eligible for the analysis. A BMI of <18.5 kg/m^2 was independently associated with the development of AKI in hospitalised patients (odds ratio (OR): 1.23 [95% confidence interval [CI]: 1.04–1.44, $P = 0.01$]) but not for overweight and obesity. Subgroup analysis further revealed that underweight patients aged ≥75 and repeated hospitalisation posed a higher risk of AKI (OR: 1.25 [CI: 1.01–1.56], $P = 0.04$; OR: 1.23 [CI: 1.04–1.44], $P = 0.01$, resp.). Analyses by interactions between different age groups and BMI using continuous or categorised variables did not affect the overall probability of developing AKI. *Conclusions.* Underweight Asian patients are susceptible to AKI in acute hospital settings. Identification of this novel risk factor for AKI allows us to optimise patient care by prevention, early detection, and timely intervention.

1. Introduction

Acute kidney injury (AKI) is common in hospitalised patients. Depending on the definitions used and populations under study, 10–30% of hospitalised patients are admitted for or with AKI [1]. The use of AKI definitions from the Kidney Disease: Improving Global Outcomes (KDIGO) clinical practice guideline provided consensus for researchers to identify and stratify populations at risk [2].

The proportion of hospitalised patients with high body mass index (BMI, calculated as kg/m^2) is increasing (up to 30% in developed countries) [3]. High BMI or obesity in the general population is notorious for its negative impact on morbidity and mortality. Obesity is associated with multiple comorbidities; hence, obese patients are postulated to have a higher risk of developing AKI. In fact, previous studies focusing on postsurgery and critically ill patients demonstrated that obese patients were more likely to develop AKI [4–8]. On the contrary, recent reports suggested an inverse or "U" shaped relationship between BMI and mortality in AKI patients [6, 7]. These studies highlighted that malnutrition especially in Asians, which is commonly associated with underweight, was independently associated with increased risks of AKI, morbidity, and mortality [9–11].

No observational studies have yet been specifically designed to explore the association between BMI and AKI in the acute care setting. The current literature has limited information on the Asian-specific BMI classification and its association with AKI risk [12, 13]. Therefore, we conducted this study to address the association between BMI and AKI risk in patients in acute hospital settings from multiethnic

Asian backgrounds and to elucidate its biological plausibility for potential early interventions and treatment.

2. Materials and Methods

This was a single-centre, retrospective cohort study. All patients aged ≥21 years who were hospitalised at Khoo Teck Puat Hospital (a 550-bed regional general hospital) in Singapore, a multiethnic Asian country, from January to December 2013, were recruited for analysis. The study was approved by the National Health Group Domain Specific Review Board (DSRB) of Singapore with adherence to the Declaration of Helsinki. These patients were identified from the hospital's electronic medical records. Data collection included baseline demographics, BMI (calculated from height and weight recorded on hospital admission before any AKI occurrence), primary diagnoses for admission (by the International Classification of Diseases, Ninth Revision [ICD-9] codes), background diagnoses, surgical procedures, laboratory data, hospitalisation length of stay, and survival status within 90 days upon discharge. We excluded individuals with pregnancy and end stage renal failure requiring either maintenance dialysis or renal transplantation. We also excluded patients without measurement of BMI or those with seemingly erroneous measurements (height <70 cm or >250 cm; weight >200 kg). We used an enzymatic colorimetric assay from Custom Biotech, Roche®, for measurement of serum creatinine. AKI was defined by the serum creatinine based KDIGO classification system [2], whereby AKI is defined as a ≥1.5-fold increase in serum creatinine within the previous 7 days, or ≥26.5 μmol/l (≥0.3 mg/dl) increase from baseline within 48 hours. Baseline creatinine was defined as the median of all creatinine values obtained within 12 months preceding the occurrence of AKI for the index admission. If no previous serum creatinine was available, or only one serum creatinine result was known during hospital stay, the baseline creatinine was estimated by backward calculation from the simplified Modification of Diet in Renal Disease (MDRD) formula (assuming a glomerular filtration rate [GFR] of 75 ml/min per 1.73 m^2) [14]. The median time from baseline creatinine measurement to hospitalisation was 71 days. A median of 4 creatinine measurements was used for the determination of the baseline value in our cohort (Tables 1 and 3). We determined the severity of AKI according to the KDIGO criteria. The AKI stages were calculated using serum creatinine with reference to baseline creatinine levels, or using estimated GFR. In order to validate our findings from estimated GFR by MDRD formula, we performed sensitivity analysis for a different AKI definition based on baseline creatinine. Cohen's kappa measured the degree of agreement by these two definitions of AKI, and the result was interpreted by Landis et al.'s guidelines [15, 16]. When we tested the agreement of AKI status between the use of creatinine based on MDRD estimations (if baseline creatinine was not known) and that based on true baseline creatinine values, we had 275 AKI patients (17.1% of the AKI group) accounting for the discordance, giving rise to a Cohen's kappa of 0.674. The agreement was good according to Landis et al.'s

guidelines [15, 16]. We did not use urine output as part of the definition of AKI as the information was not available from the electronic records. The BMI was categorised based on the World Health Organisation (WHO) recommendations for Asians [12] (underweight [BMI < 18.5 kg/m^2], normal [18.5–23 kg/m^2], overweight [23–27.5 kg/m^2], and obese [>27 kg/m^2]). The incidence of AKI was then calculated for each group of the BMI. We used multivariate linear and nonlinear regression analyses for risk factor identification. We also tested for interactions among different variables against BMI to determine any existence of effect modifiers influencing the relationship between AKI and BMI.

3. Statistical Analysis

Continuous variables were summarised as means and standard deviations if normally distributed, and medians and quartiles if distributions were skewed. Categorical variables were presented as frequencies and percentages. We compared clinical and baseline characteristics of patients with and without AKI by using Chi-square test or Fisher's exact test for categorical variables. Student's t-test and Mann–Whitney U test were used for continuous variables with and without normal distribution, respectively (some continuous variables, e.g., age, were expressed as categorical variables with reference to previous published study designs and recommendations) [17, 18]. Statistically significant variables were considered as potential risk factors associated with the patients' AKI status. The bootstrap method is one of the popular methods for selecting the best subset of variables and developing parsimonious prediction models [19]. We referred to a previous study of similar recruitment scale and randomly generated 200 bootstrap datasets with the same size (N = 12,555) from the original data [20]. For each dataset, we performed multivariable logistic regression with a stepwise procedure to select independent risk factors associated with AKI status as the outcome. Variables that were selected in at least 90% of the bootstrap procedures were the best subset of potential risk factors and were included in the final multivariable logistic regression. We used Hosmer-Lemeshow's test for evaluating model goodness of fit. The model fitted the data well if P value ≥ 0.05. We further constructed sets of logistic regression models and performed comparison by the Chi-square test with the primary model if interactions were suspected among different variables which had confounding effects not detected by the primary model.

To delineate the relationship between AKI and BMI, if an assumption of nonlinear relation between continuous BMI and log odds of having AKI was made instead of categorisation, we further developed different models by means of restricted cubic splines (RCS) as a continuous natural spline regression. Model fitness of RCS regression was determined by choice of the number of knots (k) in comparison to cutoffs by BMI categories [21, 22]. We used k = 5 which was considered as adequate with a sample size of more than a hundred [23]. The advantage of RCS regression was that it modeled a wide range of possible nonlinear relations between BMI and AKI while keeping a

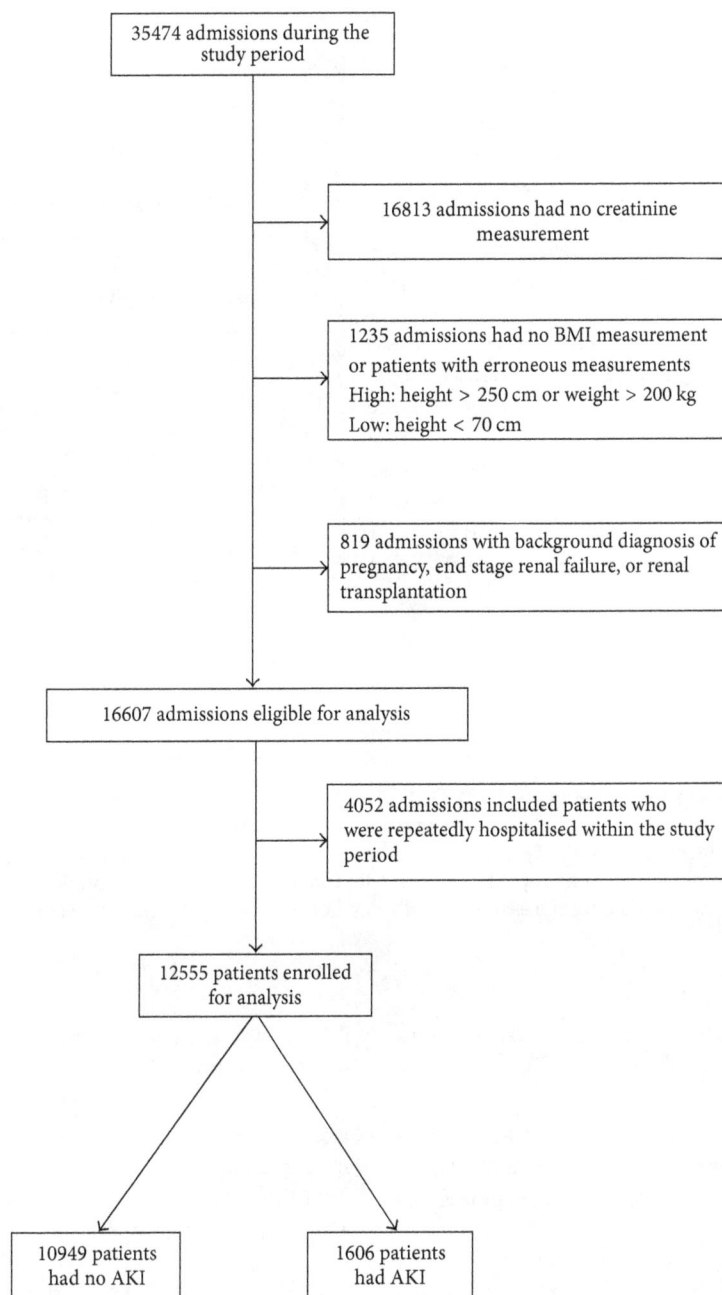

FIGURE 1: Flowchart of patient selection.

good balance between model goodness of fit and simplicity (i.e., model parsimony) [23].

A *P* value of < 0.05 was considered statistically significant. All statistical analyses were performed with R Version 3.3.1 and SPSS® Version 22 (IBM® Corporation).

4. Results

A total of 35,474 admissions were recorded during the study period. The patients with repeated admissions during the study period that had their admissions with the highest AKI staging were selected. As a result, 12,555 patients were

eligible for analysis. Figure 1 shows the flowchart of patient selection for data analysis. *Baseline characteristics of excluded patients are presented in the Supplementary Material* (available here). In our cohort, 61.9% were of a Chinese ethnicity and 53.8% were men. The median age was 64 years (interquartile range [IQR]: 51–77). Seventy-five percent of the patients were hospitalised under the care of general medical units or related specialties, namely, cardiology, nephrology, geriatrics, endocrinology, respiratory medicine, and gastroenterology. ICU admissions comprised 13% of the cohort, while 7.9% of the cohort succumbed to death within 90 days of hospital admission. The most common background diagnosis was

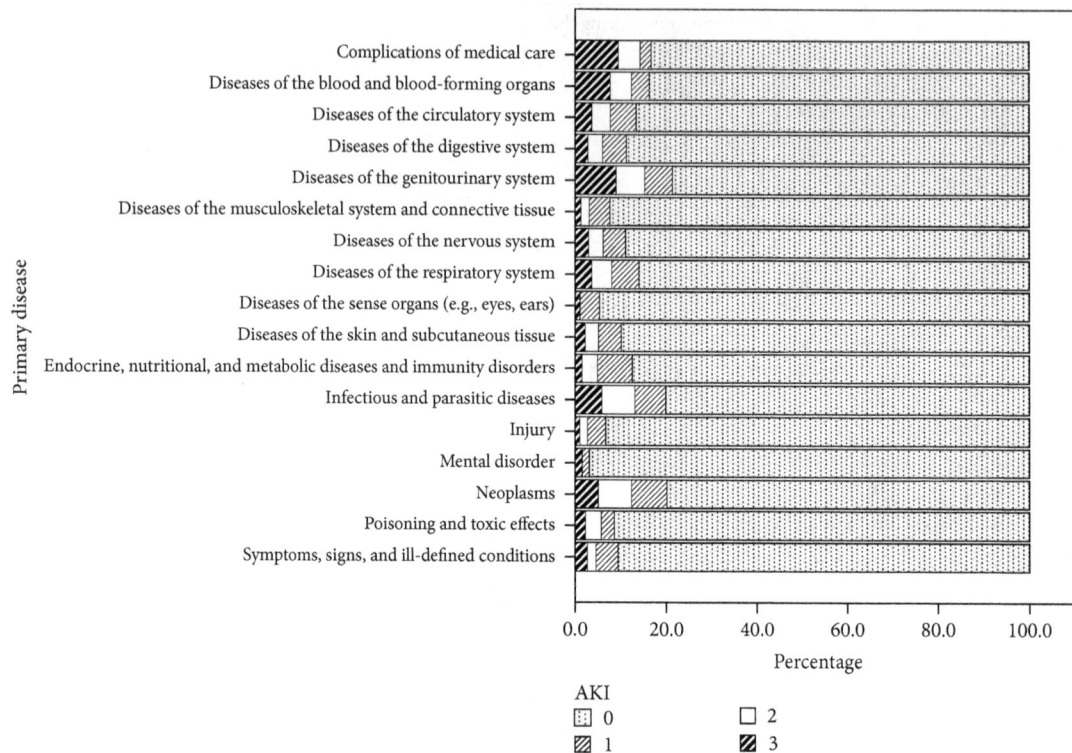

FIGURE 2: Acute kidney injury categories according to KDIGO classification by percentages according to the primary diagnosis by ICD-9 codes. AKI: acute kidney injury, defined as a ≥1.5-fold increase in serum creatinine within the previous 7 days, or ≥26.5 μmol/l (≥0.3 mg/dl) increase from baseline within 48 hours; AKI1: 1.5–1.9-fold increase in serum creatinine within the previous 7 days, or ≥26.5 μmol/l (≥0.3 mg/dl) increase from baseline within 48 hours; AKI2: 2.0–2.9-fold increase in serum creatinine within the previous 7 days; AKI3: 3-fold or higher increase in serum creatinine from baseline within 7 days, or the need for dialysis, or when serum creatinine ≥ 353.6 μmol/l (≥4.0 mg/dl).

hypertension (39%), followed by dyslipidemia (31%), diabetes mellitus (26.2%), and cardiovascular disease (20%).

4.1. The Incidence of AKI for Each Category of BMI.

1,606 patients developed AKI in our cohort (incidence of 12.8%). The severity of AKI was defined as per the KDIGO guidelines (AKI stage 1 (AKI1), defined as a 1.5–1.9-fold increase in serum creatinine within the previous 7 days, or ≥26.5 μmol/l (≥0.3 mg/dl) increase from baseline within 48 hours, comprised 5.5% of the cohort (or 42.7% of the AKI group); AKI stages 2 (AKI2) and 3 (AKI3), defined as 2.0–2.9-fold and ≥3-fold increase in serum creatinine from baseline within 7 days, or the need for dialysis, or when serum creatinine ≥353.6 μmol/l (≥4.0 mg/dl), resp., had an incidence of 3.8% and 3.5% for the whole cohort or 29.6% and 27.7% for the AKI group, resp.). The patients who had recurrent admissions over the 12-month period comprised 33% of the cohort.

4.2. Characteristics among Different BMI Categories.

Baseline characteristics, length of stay, need for intensive care, 90-day mortality, time from baseline creatinine measurement to hospitalisation, and number of creatinine measurements within 12 months before hospitalisation are shown in Table 1 according to BMI categorisation. More obese patients compared to normal BMI patients required ICU admissions ($P <$

0.0001). On the contrary, patients with low BMI had higher mortality within 90 days of admission ($P < 0.0001$).

4.3. Factors Associated with AKI.

The primary diagnoses in our cohort with or without AKI are listed in Table 2. Two important contributing causes for AKI were infection and neoplasm. Figure 2 shows further categorisation of AKI according to ICD-9 codes, among which AKI severity varied with different primary diagnoses. Baseline characteristics, length of stay, need for intensive care, 90-day mortality, time from baseline creatinine measurement to hospitalisation, and number of creatinine measurements within 12 months before hospitalisation are shown in Table 3 according to AKI status. With reference to normal BMI (18.5–23 kg/m^2), the unadjusted odds ratio (OR) for the risk of AKI in patients with BMI < 18.5 kg/m^2 was 1.27 (95% confidence interval [CI]: 1.08–1,48; $P = 0.003$).

4.4. Association between AKI and BMI.

Table 4 shows the variables selected from the bootstrap method for multivariate logistic regression modeling (except for age, gender, ethnicity, and BMI). We identified several traditional background diagnoses that were independently associated with the risk of AKI (diabetes mellitus, cardiovascular disease, and CKD). History of hepatobiliary disease and psychiatric illness was

TABLE 1: Baseline characteristics in relation to body mass index categories according to the World Health Organisation (WHO) classification on Asians.

	Total	BMI, kg/m²			
		<18.5	18.5–23	23–27.5	>27.5
Number of patients	12555	1727	4339	3902	2587
Demographics					
Age, year	63 ± 18.5	70 ± 19.4	63 ± 19.5	62 ± 17.3	57 ± 15.9
Gender, men (%)	6755 (53.8)	856 (49.6)	2329 (53.7)	2264 (58.0)	1306 (50.5)
Ethnicity (%)					
Chinese	7776 (61.9)	1257 (72.8)	2942 (67.8)	2424 (62.1)	1153 (44.6)
Malay	2360 (18.8)	230 (13.3)	626 (14.4)	721 (18.5)	783 (30.3)
Indian	1485 (11.8)	146 (8.5)	458 (10.6)	460 (11.8)	421 (16.3)
Others	934 (7.4)	94 (5.4)	313 (7.2)	297 (7.6)	230 (8.9)
Specialty (%)					
Medicine	6353 (50.6)	871 (50.4)	2175 (50.2)	1977 (50.1)	1330 (51.4)
Surgery	1679 (13.4)	173 (10.0)	631 (14.5)	548 (14.0)	327 (12.6)
Geriatrics	1591 (12.7)	427 (24.7)	637 (14.7)	399 (10.2)	128 (4.9)
Cardiology	1479 (11.8)	111 (6.4)	417 (9.6)	503 (12.9)	448 (17.3)
Orthopedic surgery	1147 (9.1)	121 (7.0)	391 (9.0)	360 (9.3)	275 (10.6)
Urology	248 (2.0)	17 (1.0)	73 (1.7)	94 (2.4)	64 (2.4)
Otolaryngology	41 (0.3)	5 (0.3)	9 (0.2)	14 (0.4)	13 (0.5)
Ophthalmology	17 (0.1)	2 (0.1)	6 (0.1)	7 (0.2)	2 (0.1)
Background diagnosis (%)					
Hypertension	4895 (39.0)	653 (37.8)	1579 (36.4)	1519 (38.9)	1144 (44.2)
Dyslipidemia	3896 (31.0)	435 (25.2)	1229 (28.3)	1271 (32.6)	961 (37.1)
Diabetes mellitus	3289 (26.2)	341 (19.7)	1039 (23.9)	1072 (27.5)	837 (32.4)
Cardiovascular disease	2515 (20.0)	349 (20.2)	878 (20.2)	771 (19.8)	517 (20.0)
Orthopedic related disease	1402 (11.2)	262 (15.2)	470 (10.8)	397 (10.2)	273 (10.6)
Cerebrovascular disease	1314 (10.5)	256 (14.8)	485 (11.2)	392 (10.0)	181 (7.0)
Neurological disease	1219 (9.7)	283 (16.4)	496 (11.4)	307 (7.9)	133 (5.1)
Respiratory disease	1030 (8.2)	199 (11.5)	292 (6.7)	257 (6.6)	282 (10.9)
Hematological disease	955 (7.6)	230 (13.3)	380 (8.8)	226 (5.8)	119 (4.6)
Gastrointestinal disease	936 (7.5)	221 (12.2)	324 (7.5)	243 (6.2)	158 (6.1)
Chronic kidney disease	857 (6.8)	111 (6.4)	270 (6.2)	286 (7.3)	190 (7.3)
Psychiatric illness	760 (6.1)	172 (10.0)	290 (6.7)	205 (5.3)	93 (3.6)
Urological disease	595 (4.7)	120 (6.9)	238 (5.5)	157 (4.0)	80 (3.1)
Underlying malignancy	584 (4.7)	140 (8.1)	234 (5.4)	148 (3.8)	62 (2.4)
Hepatobiliary disease	463 (3.7)	64 (3.7)	155 (3.6)	147 (3.8)	97 (3.7)
Procedures (%)					
Endoscopy	2355 (18.8)	363 (21.0)	853 (19.7)	673 (17.2)	466 (18.0)
Orthopedic surgery	1222 (9.7)	170 (9.8)	413 (9.5)	368 (9.4)	271 (10.5)
Cardiology related procedures (non-open-heart surgery)	584 (4.7)	32 (1.9)	156 (3.6)	219 (5.6)	177 (6.8)
Excision of skin lesions	851 (6.8)	64 (3.7)	259 (6.0)	195 (7.6)	233 (9.0)
Open laparotomy	579 (4.6)	77 (4.5)	231 (5.3)	182 (4.7)	89 (3.4)
Urology related surgery	510 (4.1)	61 (3.5)	169 (3.9)	161 (4.1)	119 (4.6)
Laparoscopic surgery (intra-abdominal)	265 (2.1)	23 (1.3)	85 (2.0)	81 (2.1)	75 (2.9)
Neurosurgery	159 (1.3)	19 (1.1)	68 (1.6)	50 (1.3)	22 (0.9)
Otolaryngology related surgery	149 (1.2)	26 (1.5)	55 (1.3)	33 (0.8)	35 (1.4)
Vascular surgery, open	57 (0.5)	8 (0.5)	15 (0.3)	25 (0.6)	9 (0.3)
Laparoscopic assisted bariatric bypass surgery	12 (0.18)	0 (0)	0 (0)	5 (0.1)	7 (0.3)

TABLE 1: Continued.

	Total	<18.5	BMI, kg/m² 18.5–23	23–27.5	>27.5
Hospitalisation characteristics					
ICU admission (%)	1638 (13.0)	155 (9.0)	490 (11.3)	571 (14.7)	421 (16.3)
Mortality within 90 days of admission (%)	997 (7.9)	256 (14.8)	414 (9.5)	239 (6.1)	88 (3.4)
Length of stay (d, IQR)	5 (3–9)	7 (4–14)	5 (3–10)	4 (3–8)	4 (2–7)
Creatinine measurements					
Time from baseline measurement to hospitalisation (d, IQR)	71 (29–147)	62 (30–140)	69 (28–140.8)	69 (26–148.8)	79 (32–159)
Number of measurements within 365 days before hospitalisation (*n*, IQR)	4 (2–6)	4 (3–6)	4 (2–6)	4 (2–7)	2 (2–6)

AKI: acute kidney injury; ICU: intensive care unit; BMI: body mass index; IQR: interquartile range.

TABLE 2: Primary diagnosis of hospitalised patients with acute kidney injury according to ICD-9 codes and KDIGO classification.

Primary diagnosis	Total	No acute kidney injury (%)	Acute kidney injury (%)	P value
Total number	12555	10949	1606	
Diseases of the respiratory system	1625 (12.9)	1398 (12.8)	227 (14.1)	0.128
Symptoms, signs, and ill-defined conditions	1547 (12.3)	1404 (12.8)	144 (8.9)	<0.001
Diseases of the circulatory system	1505 (12.0)	1305 (11.9)	202 (12.5)	0.538
Diseases of the digestive system	1423 (11.3)	1263 (11.5)	160 (10.0)	0.063
Diseases of the musculoskeletal system and connective tissue	1104 (8.8)	1020 (9.3)	84 (5.2)	<0.001
Diseases of the nervous system	1029 (8.2)	915 (8.4)	114 (7.1)	0.086
Diseases of the genitourinary system	966 (7.7)	760 (6.9)	206 (12.8)	<0.001
Infectious and parasitic diseases	925 (7.4)	742 (6.8)	183 (11.4)	<0.001
Diseases of the skin and subcutaneous tissue	645 (5.1)	581 (5.3)	65 (4.0)	0.025
Endocrine, nutritional, and metabolic diseases and immunity disorders	536 (4.3)	469 (4.3)	67 (4.2)	0.836
Neoplasm	438 (3.5)	350 (3.2)	88 (5.5)	<0.001
Injury	303 (2.4)	283 (2.6)	20 (1.2)	0.001
Poisoning and toxic effects	177 (1.4)	162 (1.5)	15 (0.9)	0.083
Diseases of the blood and blood-forming organs	129 (1.0)	108 (1.0)	21 (1.3)	0.233
Diseases of the sense organs (e.g., eyes, ears)	95 (0.8)	90 (0.8)	5 (0.3)	0.027
Mental disorders	66 (0.5)	64 (0.6)	2 (0.1)	0.017
Complications of medical care	42 (0.3)	35 (0.3)	7 (0.4)	0.451
Complications of pregnancy, childbirth, and the puerperium	0 (0)	0 (0)	0 (0)	-
Congenital anomalies	0 (0)	0 (0)	0 (0)	-
Certain conditions originating in the perinatal period	0 (0)	0 (0)	0 (0)	-

TABLE 3: Baseline characteristics in relation to acute kidney injury categories according to KDIGO classification.

	Total	No AKI	AKI
Number of patients	12555	10949	1606
Demographics			
Age, year	63 ± 18.5	61 ± 18.8	69 ± 15.3
Gender, men (%)	6755 (53.8)	5932 (54.2)	8273 (51.2)
BMI, kg/m^2	23.9 ± 5.7	24.0 ± 5.6	23.4 ± 6.0
BMI, kg/m^2 by categories (%)			
<18.5	1727 (13.8)	1452 (13.3)	275 (17.1)
18.5–23	4339 (34.6)	3775 (34.5)	564 (35.1)
23–27.5	3902 (31.1)	3414 (31.2)	488 (30.4)
>27.5	2587 (20.6)	2308 (21.1)	279 (17.4)
Ethnicity (%)			
Chinese	7776 (61.9)	6755 (61.7)	1021 (63.4)
Malay	2360 (18.8)	2033 (18.6)	327 (20.4)
Indian	1485 (11.8)	1334 (12.2)	151 (9.4)
Others	934 (7.4)	827 (7.6)	107 (6.7)
Specialty (%)			
Medicine	6353 (50.6)	5524 (50.4)	829 (51.6)
Surgery	1679 (13.4)	1478 (13.5)	201 (12.5)
Geriatrics	1591 (12.7)	1302 (11.9)	289 (18.0)
Cardiology	1479 (11.8)	1301 (11.9)	178 (11.0)
Orthopedic surgery	1147 (9.1)	1084 (9.9)	63 (3.9)
Urology	248 (2.0)	205 (1.9)	43 (2.7)
Otolaryngology	41 (0.3)	39 (0.4)	2 (0.1)
Ophthalmology	17 (0.1)	16 (0.1)	1 (0.1)
Background diagnosis (%)			
Hypertension	4895 (39.0)	4045 (36.9)	850 (52.9)
Dyslipidemia	3896 (31.0)	3255 (29.7)	641 (39.9)
Diabetes mellitus	3289 (26.2)	2644 (24.1)	645 (40.2)
Cardiovascular disease	2515 (20)	2004 (18.3)	511 (31.8)
Orthopedic related disease	1402 (11.2)	1146 (10.5)	256 (15.9)
Cerebrovascular disease	1314 (10.5)	1053 (9.6)	261 (16.3)
Neurological disease	1219 (9.7)	1003 (9.2)	216 (13.4)
Respiratory disease	1030 (8.2)	899 (8.2)	131 (8.2)
Hematological disease	955 (7.6)	739 (6.7)	216 (13.4)
Gastrointestinal disease	936 (7.5)	787 (7.2)	149 (9.3)
Chronic kidney disease	857 (6.8)	615 (5.6)	242 (15.1)
Psychiatric illness	760 (6.1)	626 (5.7)	134 (8.3)
Urological disease	595 (4.7)	465 (4.2)	130 (8.1)
Underlying malignancy	584 (4.7)	459 (4.2)	125 (7.8)
Hepatobiliary disease	463 (3.7)	350 (3.2)	113 (7.0)

Table 3: Continued.

	Total	No AKI	AKI
Procedures (%)			
Endoscopy	2355 (18.8)	1941 (17.7)	414 (25.8)
Orthopedic surgery	1222 (9.7)	1072 (9.8)	150 (9.3)
Cardiology related procedures (non-open-heart surgery)	584 (4.7)	538 (4.9)	46 (2.9)
Excision of skin lesions	851 (6.8)	734 (6.7)	117 (7.3)
Open laparotomy	579 (4.6)	468 (4.3)	111 (6.9)
Urology related surgery	510 (4.1)	406 (3.7)	105 (6.5)
Laparoscopic surgery (intra-abdominal)	265 (2.1)	243 (2.2)	22 (1.4)
Neurosurgery	159 (1.3)	131 (1.2)	28 (1.7)
Otolaryngology related surgery	149 (1.2)	112 (1.0)	37 (2.3)
Vascular surgery, open	57 (0.5)	49 (4)	8 (0.5)
Laparoscopic assisted bariatric bypass surgery	12 (0.18)	11 (0.1)	1 (0.1)
Hospitalisation characteristics			
ICU admission (%)	1638 (13.0)	1204 (11.0)	434 (27.0)
Mortality within 90 days of admission (%)	997 (7.9)	572 (5.2)	425 (26.5)
Length of stay (d, IQR)	5 (3–9)	4 (3–8)	11 (5–21)
Creatinine measurements			
Time from baseline measurement to hospitalisation (d, IQR)	71 (29.3–147)	67 (26–144)	79 (37.3–155.5)
Number of measurements within 365 days before hospitalisation (*n*, IQR)	4 (2–6)	4 (2–6)	5 (3–8)

AKI: acute kidney injury; ICU: intensive care unit; BMI: body mass index; IQR: interquartile range.

TABLE 4: Multivariate logistic regression models using bootstrap method for the risk of acute kidney injury in hospitalised patients.

	Odds ratio	95% CI	P value
Age (reference: <55)			
55–75	1.91	1.64–2.24	<0.001
>75	2.24	1.89–2.65	<0.001
Gender (reference: female)			
Male	0.96	0.85–1.07	0.43
Ethnicity (reference: Chinese)			
Indian	0.81	0.67–0.98	0.03
Malay	1.18	1.02–1.36	0.02
Background diagnoses			
Cardiovascular disease	1.53	1.35–1.75	<0.001
Chronic kidney disease	2.01	1.73–2.45	<0.001
Diabetes mellitus	1.60	1.42–1.80	<0.001
Hepatobiliary disease	1.71	1.36–2.15	<0.001
Psychiatric illness	1.40	1.14–1.72	<0.001
Gastrointestinal disease	0.83	0.68–1.00	0.058
Primary diagnoses			
Infectious and parasitic diseases	2.08	1.72–2.49	<0.001
Neoplasm	1.53	1.17–1.98	0.002
Diseases of the genitourinary system	1.93	1.62–2.30	<0.001
Diseases of the musculoskeletal system and connective tissue	0.69	0.54–0.88	0.002
Symptoms, signs, and ill-defined conditions	0.63	0.51–0.76	<0.001
Procedures			
Otolaryngology related surgery	2.91	1.94–4.28	<0.001
Endoscopy	1.30	1.13–1.48	<0.001
Open laparotomy	1.56	1.23–1.97	<0.001
Cardiology related percutaneous procedures	0.64	0.46–0.87	0.007

BMI: body mass index; CI: confidence interval. The P value of Hosmer-Lemeshow's goodness-of-fit test is 0.35.

Variable	OR	95% CI	P value	
BMI group (reference: 18.5–23)				
<18.5	1.23	[1.04, 1.44]	0.01	
23–27.5	1.00	[0.87, 1.14]	0.95	
>27.5	0.90	[0.76, 1.06]	0.20	

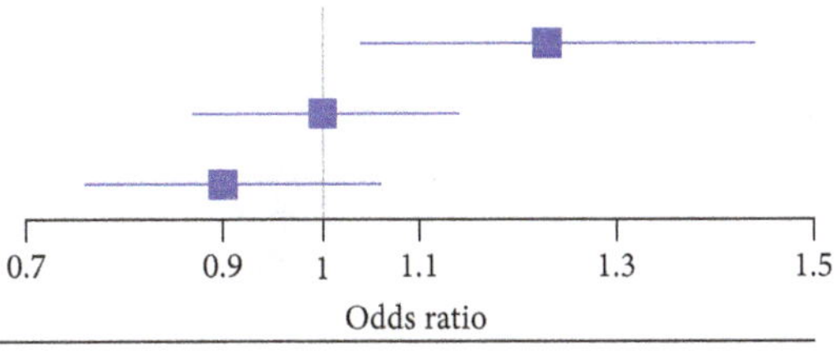

FIGURE 3: Multivariate logistic regression models for studying the relationship between BMI and acute kidney injury in hospitalised patients (total number of patients = 12,555; patients with acute kidney injury = 1606; patients with no acute kidney injury = 10,949). *Note.* BMI: body mass index; CI: confidence interval; OR: odds ratio. Adjusted variables in logistic regression models include age, gender, ethnicity, background diagnoses (cardiovascular disease, chronic kidney disease, diabetes mellitus, hepatobiliary disease, psychiatric illness, and gastrointestinal disease), primary diagnoses (infectious and parasitic diseases, neoplasm, diseases of the genitourinary system, diseases of the musculoskeletal system and connective tissue, and symptoms, signs, and ill-defined conditions), and procedures (otolaryngology related surgery, endoscopy, open laparotomy, and cardiology related percutaneous procedures).

also associated with an increased risk of AKI. The risk of AKI from infectious diseases was significantly higher for patients aged 55 years or older when compared to younger populations (OR for age 55–75: 2.35 [95% CI: 1.72–3.19]; OR for age > 75: 2.51 [95% CI: 1.90–3.30]). Patients that underwent procedures like endoscopy, open laparotomy, and surgeries related to otolaryngology showed a higher risk of AKI, while percutaneous cardiovascular procedures revealed the opposite. After adjusting the risk factors shown in Table 4 (age, gender, ethnicity, background diagnoses, primary diagnoses, and procedures), BMI of <18.5 kg/m^2 remained independently associated with the development of AKI in hospitalised patients (OR: 1.23 [95% CI: 1.04–1.44], $P = 0.014$), while overweight (BMI: 23–27.5 kg/m^2) and obese (BMI > 27.5 kg/m^2) patients did not show any significant associations (OR 1.00 for overweight [95% CI: 0.87–1.14]; OR 0.90 for obesity [95% CI: 0.76–1.06]; see Figure 3).

Subgroup analyses revealed a significant increase in the risk of AKI for patients aged >75 and those with BMI < 18.5 kg/m^2 (OR: 1.25 [95% CI: 1.01–1.56]), while the rest of the study population did not reveal similar findings (Figure 4). We also found that underweight patients who had recurrent admissions were predisposed to a higher risk of AKI (OR: 1.42 [95% CI: 1.09–1.84]; see Figure 5).

In order to distinguish the AKI risk among different age groups, we further tested the logistic model by adding interactions for age groups and BMI categories (i.e., addition of all possible combinations for individual age group *times* BMI categories, e.g., BMI < 18.5 kg/m^2 × age < 55 years). The possible interactions derived from all the crossovers were not statistically significant (Chi-square test = 5.58; $P = 0.47$), which implied that age was not an effect modifier for BMI and AKI.

To evaluate the relationship between AKI and BMI in a continuous manner, we built up RCS regression models based on 5 knots (i.e., 5%, 25%, 50%, 75%, and 95% percentiles of BMI) and 3 alternative prespecified knots (BMI = 18.5 kg/m^2, 23 kg/m^2, and 27.5 kg/m^2, same as cutoffs for BMI categorisation). RCS using 5 knots had a very similar

predicted probability of having AKI when compared with the primary logistic regression model as shown in Table 4 (correlation coefficient = 0.99, $P < 0.001$). RCS with the 3 prespecified knots' model also yielded a similar result (correlation coefficient = 1.0, $P < 0.001$). We repeated RCS using 5 knots with the addition of individual age group *times* BMI categories with crossover, again revealing negative interactions between age and BMI (Chi-square test = 13.18; $P = 0.11$). Figure 6 demonstrates the continuous relationship between BMI and the probability of having AKI stratified by age groups (adjusted with gender, ethnicity, background diagnoses, primary diagnoses, and procedures). The CIs of the odds ratio for the group of patients below 55 years of age do not overlap with those CIs for the group of patients >75 years old. This means that, compared to patients <55 years old, the effect of BMI on the occurrence of AKI is statistically significantly different from those patients >75 years old. We had a similar observation for patients aged 55–75 years whose BMI < 40. However, we were able to determine whether there is a significant difference in the effect of BMI on AKI between patients 55–75 years of age and patients >75 years of age due to their overlapped CIs. Overall, the adjusted RCS plot showed that, given the same BMI, different age groups had very similar differences in terms of the probability of developing AKI.

5. Discussion

5.1. Summary of Findings. This retrospective cohort study included 35,474 admissions to a general hospital serving a multiethnic population from January to December 2013. The incidence of AKI by KDIGO classification was 12.8%. We found that the overall risk of AKI was significantly higher in patients who were underweight (BMI < 18.5 kg/m^2) compared to normal BMI according to the WHO guidelines for Asians (18.5–23 kg/m^2). These findings were more prominent in the elderly population aged >75 who had repeated hospitalisation. However, multivariate analyses did not show any significant interaction between age group and BMI for the risk of developing AKI. The logistic regression and RCS

Variable	Age group	OR	95% CI	P value	
BMI group (reference: 18.5–23)					
<18.5	<55 years old	1.26	[0.75, 2.05]	0.37	
	55–75 years old	1.05	[0.78, 1.40]	0.73	
	>75 years old	1.25	[1.01, 1.56]	0.04	
23–27.5	<55 years old	1.26	[0.90, 1.78]	0.18	
	55–75 years old	0.91	[0.74, 1.12]	0.40	
	>75 years old	0.98	[0.79, 1.21]	0.83	
>27.5	<55 years old	0.94	[0.65, 1.36]	0.75	
	55–75 years old	0.83	[0.65, 1.05]	0.12	
	>75 years old	0.88	[0.64, 1.21]	0.45	

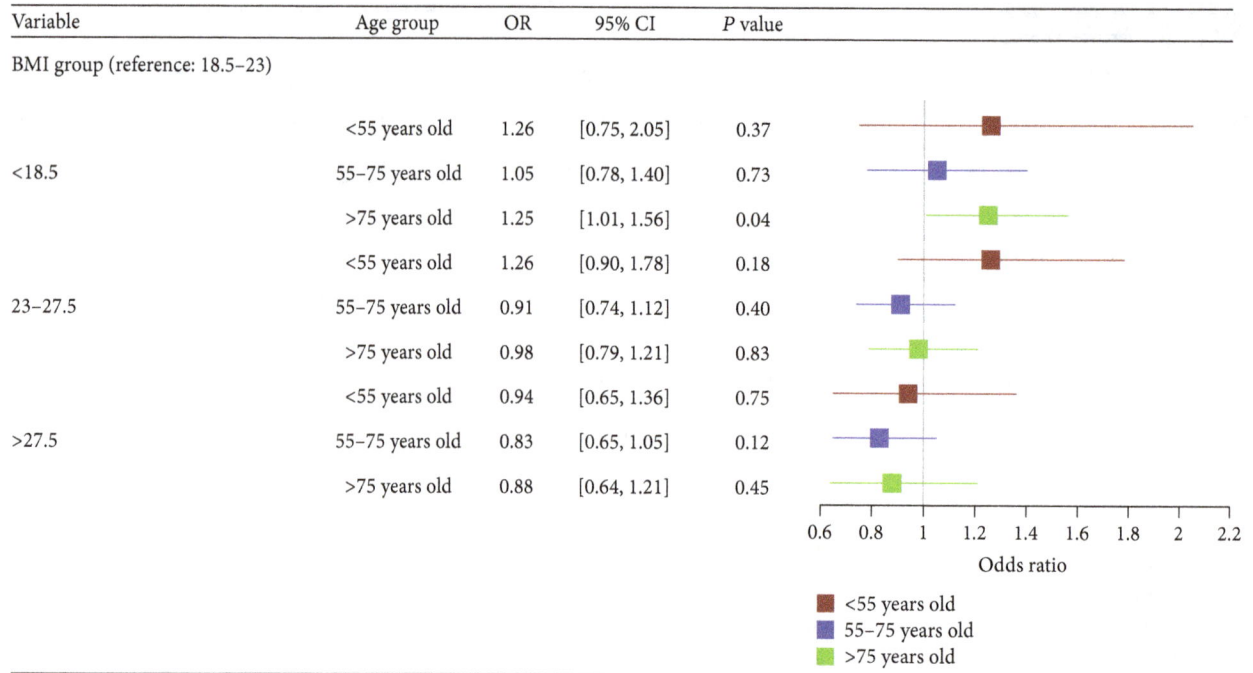

Legend: ■ <55 years old ■ 55–75 years old ■ >75 years old

FIGURE 4: Multivariate logistic regression models for studying the relationship between body mass index (BMI) and acute kidney injury (AKI) for different age groups of hospitalised patients (total number of patients under 55 years of age = 3960, where patients with AKI = 259; total number of patients aged 55–75 years = 4796, where patients with AKI = 681; total number of patients above 75 years old = 3799, where patients with AKI = 666). *Note.* BMI: body mass index; CI: confidence interval; OR: odds ratio. Adjusted variables in logistic regression models include age, gender, ethnicity, background diagnoses (cardiovascular disease, chronic kidney disease, diabetes mellitus, hepatobiliary disease, psychiatric illness, and gastrointestinal disease), primary diagnoses (infectious and parasitic diseases, neoplasm, diseases of the genitourinary system, diseases of the musculoskeletal system and connective tissue, and symptoms, signs, and ill-defined conditions), and procedures (otolaryngology related surgery, endoscopy, open laparotomy, and cardiology related percutaneous procedures).

Variable	Type of AKI admission	OR	95% CI	P value	
BMI group (reference: 18.5–23)					
<18.5	First	1.15	[0.95, 1.40]	0.14	
	Repeated	1.42	[1.09, 1.84]	0.009	
23–27.5	First	0.95	[0.80, 1.11]	0.50	
	Repeated	1.03	[0.82, 1.29]	0.80	
>27.5	First	0.89	[0.73, 1.08]	0.23	
	Repeated	0.85	[0.65, 1.12]	0.26	

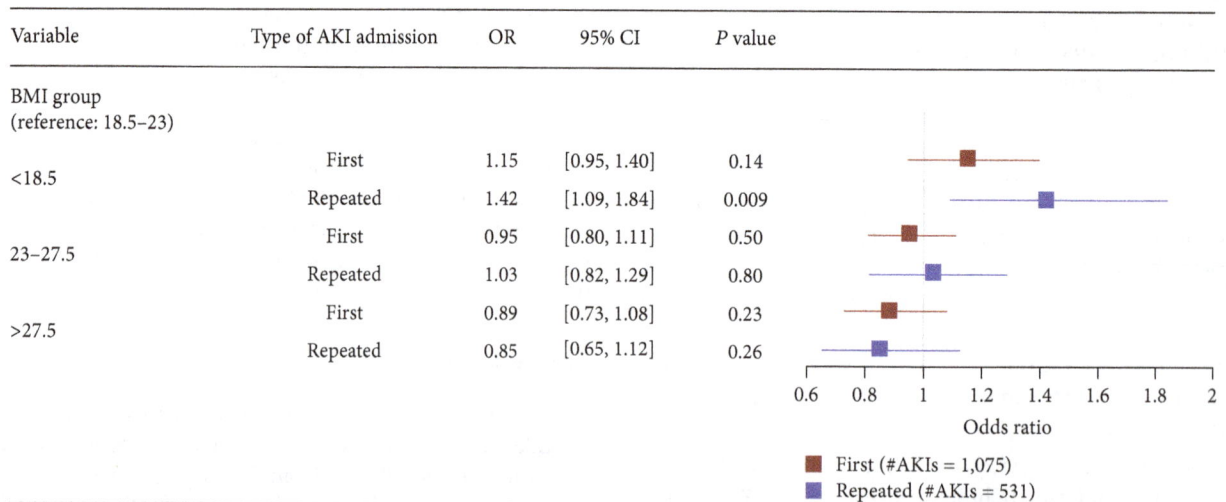

Legend: ■ First (#AKIs = 1,075) ■ Repeated (#AKIs = 531)

FIGURE 5: Multivariate logistic regression models for studying the relationship between BMI and acute kidney injury at their first (number of patients with acute kidney injury [#AKIs] = 1075) and repeated (number of patients with no acute kidney injury [#AKIs] = 531) admissions during the 12-month cohort period. *Note.* BMI: body mass index; CI: confidence interval; OR: odds ratio. Adjusted variables in logistic regression models include age, gender, ethnicity, background diagnoses (cardiovascular disease, chronic kidney disease, diabetes mellitus, hepatobiliary disease, psychiatric illness, and gastrointestinal disease), primary diagnoses (infectious and parasitic diseases, neoplasm, diseases of the genitourinary system, diseases of the musculoskeletal system and connective tissue, and symptoms, signs, and ill-defined conditions), and procedures (otolaryngology related surgery, endoscopy, open laparotomy, and cardiology related percutaneous procedures).

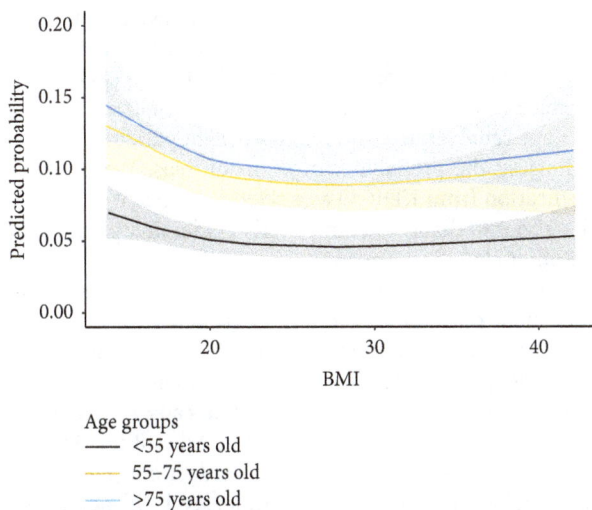

FIGURE 6: The nonlinear relation between continuous BMI and the probability of having AKI between different age groups by restricted cubic spline regression (total number of patients = 12,555; patients with acute kidney injury = 1606; patients with no acute kidney injury = 10,949). *Note.* BMI: body mass index; 95% confidence intervals (CIs) are denoted by a grey shadow. Adjusted variables in logistic regression models include age, gender, ethnicity, background diagnoses (cardiovascular disease, chronic kidney disease, diabetes mellitus, hepatobiliary disease, psychiatric illness, and gastrointestinal disease), primary diagnoses (infectious and parasitic diseases, neoplasm, diseases of the genitourinary system, diseases of the musculoskeletal system and connective tissue, and symptoms, signs, and ill-defined conditions), and procedures (otolaryngology related surgery, endoscopy, open laparotomy, and cardiology related percutaneous procedures).

analyses in addition to interactions between different age groups and BMI using categorised or continuous variables, respectively, did not affect the probability of developing AKI. The association between low BMI and AKI risk remained significant after adjusting for gender, comorbidities, primary diagnoses for respective hospital admissions, and procedures or surgical interventions, thus further highlighting the strength of this association.

5.2. Insights from Literature Review. Previous studies on the impact of BMI on AKI mainly focused on hospitalised surgical patients who underwent either cardiac [24] or noncardiac [4, 5, 25–27] surgery, or both medical and surgical patients with critical illnesses that required intensive care [6, 7, 28]. These studies consistently concluded the adverse effect of high BMI on the risk of AKI. The pathophysiologic pathway leading to AKI in obese surgical and critically ill patients was discussed in recent review articles [29–31]. The authors basically aligned with the observation on the adverse impact of high BMI on AKI, despite the physiological stress incurred during perioperative and postoperative periods together with hemodynamic instability when critically ill. In this study, we observed the reciprocal effect of BMI and AKI, where being underweight was associated with the risk of AKI.

This phenomenon is an interesting observation and makes one wonder whether multiethnic Asian hospitalised patients behave in a rather contradictory manner. In our study, we demonstrated several surgical interventions (endoscopy, cardiology related procedures, and open laparotomy) per se independently associated with the risk of AKI using the same logistic regression model involving BMI (Table 4). This observation parallels some studies whereas the effect of high BMI on AKI attenuated when concomitant risk factors were removed (e.g., CKD) [32] or accentuated when metabolic risk factors were inserted [25]. Thus, it remains unclear whether obesity is genuinely an independent risk factor for the development of AKI. Our study provides new insight into the relationship between BMI and AKI, whereby being underweight, rather than overweight, serves as an important yet undisclosed risk factor to kidney insult in hospitalised patients.

Information on the relationship between AKI and being underweight and likely malnourished was scarce [6, 33–35]. However, a paradoxical decrease in mortality and morbidity with an increase in BMI, referred to as the "obesity paradox," has been readily observed in patients with CKD [36–41], patients on long-term dialysis [42], and geriatric population [43]. As shown in Figure 6, among obese patients, there was a statistically nonsignificant increased probability of AKI. This is consistent with the result from a multicentre observational study in Austria with the lowest risk of developing AKI in patients with normal body weight (a "U" shaped curve) [6]. Similar findings on AKI and mortality were reported in Asian populations [10, 35]. The apparent knowledge gap in high BMI exerts protective or at best nondetrimental effects on AKI in hospitalised patients that could be explained by several mechanisms. The protective effect of obesity from inflammation (one of the most important pathophysiologies in AKI) is partially contributed generally by a higher level of lipoproteins in obese patients with endothelial protection from endotoxins in the renal vasculature [44]. On the other hand, underweight patients with chronic illnesses mimic the "protein energy wasting" status, whereby high background inflammatory burden and/or inflammatory response is/are triggered in reaction to acute illness during hospitalisation [45, 46]. It is well established that infection as one of the manifestations in acute illnesses is notorious for being the major risk factor for AKI in hospitalised patients [47]. Of note, during acute illnesses with high catabolic rate and increase in energy consumption, obese patients could optimise the utilisation of stored lipids through ketogenesis as an alternate energy source, alleviating the risk of organ injury [42, 48]. In our study, this association was stronger for patients aged 55 years or above, which is consistent with the previous studies, whereas older populations with lower energy reserve are susceptible to developing AKI [9, 49]. Given the independent association between AKI and BMI (adjusted with infective causes by the ICD code and interactions among different age groups), interplay among AKI, inflammation, and malnutrition that are triggered by noninfective processes should require elucidation in the future studies.

Subgroup analysis found that elderly patients (aged > 75) who were underweight incurred a higher risk of AKI compared to those with normal BMI. This echoed those findings from previous studies on elderly patients that use postoperative AKI or mortality as outcome measures [11, 26]. In the context of BMI measurement, particularly in the elderly population, where central obesity is the predominant type for overweight in Asians compared to the western population [12, 50], it is impossible to distinguish subcutaneous from visceral adipose tissue component by this simple calculation. Visceral adiposity is notorious and responsible for the development of metabolic syndrome and CKD; both predispose to the risk of AKI [25, 51]. Anthropometric assessments such as waist circumference and waist-to-hip ratio seem to reflect better as surrogates for the extent of visceral adipose mass [52]. However, BMI remains the preferred choice of measurement for obesity as it is simple to apply and easily accessible for routine practice in all hospitalised patients and large-scale studies as demonstrated in our study.

Another important clinical finding from our cohort is that recurrent admissions for underweight patients have been associated with the risk of developing AKI. Recent studies revealed the strong associations between AKI and hospital readmission, both in surgical and in nonsurgical patients [53, 54]. There are many reasons for underweight patients requiring repeated hospitalisation, partly linked to more complex interplay between comorbidities and risks of infection [55]. On the other hand, patients who had multiple hospitalisations within a short period of time might incur a significant impact on the nutritional status as well. The sequel of independent association between underweight and AKI from our study after adjusting for the variables provided insights for future studies to delineate the exact relationship between these two clinical entities.

5.3. Clinical Relevance to the New Findings. To apply the findings from our current study in clinical practice, we aim at first to generalise the measurement of BMI to all hospitalised patients instead of critically ill or surgical patients alone, since we can easily implement recording of body weight and height in routine nursing practice upon every hospital admission, same as blood pressure and temperature measurements. This could then further translate into a preventive strategy for the development of AKI before its actual occurrence with a subsequent timely intervention. While, in view of being an observational study, associations cannot be deemed causal in nature, the study allows us to identify underweight, particularly elderly population with a higher chance of readmission as a potentially high-risk group. This in turn allows us to take extra precautions in the management, such as dose adjustments in therapeutic drug administration and preventive measures when using contrast, and to maintain the hemodynamic stability in cardiovascular disease and sepsis; such events are commonly encountered in hospitalised individuals.

5.4. Strengths and Limitations. To the best of our knowledge, this is the first study providing the association between underweight and higher risk of developing AKI among hospitalised patients from a multiethnic Asian background. Moreover, this study included a significantly diverse spectrum of hospital presentations—only excluding pediatric, obstetric, end stage renal failure, and posttransplant patients—thereby minimising the probability of selection bias. We used AKI classification from KDIGO as a reference since it was shown to be a more reliable system in AKI epidemiological studies than other classifications [56].

Nonetheless, the intrinsic fallacies of this study, including recruitment of a cohort from a single centre and predominance of ethnicity, render generalisability to other ethnicity groups questionable. Its retrospective and observational nature, hence the establishment of a causal relationship between AKI and BMI, is impossible. Like other AKI epidemiological studies, we did not have data on urine output and also baseline plasma creatinine levels if not known previously. Furthermore, we only recruited patients who had creatinine measurements performed. This can lead to selection bias wherein those patients with short hospitalisation, who experienced self-limiting AKI, may have been missed from the analysis. We measured baseline creatinine in both inpatient and outpatient settings (for baseline creatinine), or derived baseline creatinine from the MDRD formula, whereby it may misclassify AKI particularly in the critical care settings [57], and its estimation may also become less reliable in obesity [14]. We also had insufficient data on the nutritional and functional status for our cohort, namely, albumin and acute inflammatory markers. Moreover, we do not have data for those patients who underwent hospitalisation prior to the study period (patients with AKI at the "first" admission shown in Figure 5 might be repeatedly admitted if we stretched the timeline of observation prior to the current study period). Malnourished patients are more likely to have readmissions that lead to potential bias in our study. All these factors may interfere with the actual incidence of AKI and subsequent analysis. Nevertheless, given the large sample size in this study and the substantial agreement from sensitivity analysis between baseline creatinine and those estimated by MDRD formula, the above effects, if any, would have negligible influences on the study outcomes.

6. Conclusions

In this single-centre study involving 12,555 multiethnic Asians, we found a significant association between being underweight and the risk of having AKI in acute care settings. Measuring BMI for all the admissions is straightforward. Using this novel risk factor to detect the population at risk in addition to the conventional factors is important for prevention, early identification, and targeted care to minimise AKI and subsequent progression to chronic kidney disease. Further studies that involve different populations are needed to establish a causal relationship between being underweight and this important and common clinical entity.

Ethical Approval

This study was approved by the National Health Group Domain Specific Review Board (DSRB) of Singapore.

Authors' Contributions

Allen Yan Lun Liu and Milind Nikam made contributions to the conception, design, and drafting of the manuscript. Jiexun Wang made contributions to the acquisition, statistical analysis, and interpretation of data. Boon Cheok Lai and Lee Ying Yeoh were involved in the interpretation of data, drafting of the manuscript, and revising it critically for important intellectual content. Allen Yan Lun Liu gave the final approval on the version to be published.

Acknowledgments

The authors are grateful to the Information Technology Department, Khoo Teck Puat Hospital, for extraction and acquisition of data from electronic record systems. This study had no bonding to any grants.

References

[1] N. Lameire, W. Van Biesen, and R. Vanholder, "The changing epidemiology of acute renal failure," *Nature Clinical Practice Nephrology*, vol. 2, no. 7, pp. 364–377, 2006.

[2] A. Khwaja, "KDIGO clinical practice guidelines for acute kidney injury," *Nephron Clinical Practice*, vol. 120, no. 4, pp. c179–c184, 2012.

[3] K. Kalantar-Zadeh, K. C. Abbott, A. K. Salahudeen et al., "Survival advantages of obesity in dialysis patients," *The American Journal of Clinical Nutrition*, vol. 81, no. 3, pp. 543–554, 2005.

[4] H. Myrvang, "Acute kidney injury: Obesity is associated with AKI after surgery via oxidative stress," *Nature Reviews Nephrology*, vol. 8, no. 8, p. 433, 2012.

[5] T. N. Weingarten, C. Gurrieri, J. M. McCaffrey et al., "Acute kidney injury following bariatric surgery," *Obesity Surgery*, vol. 23, no. 1, pp. 64–70, 2013.

[6] W. Druml, B. Metnitz, E. Schaden, P. Bauer, and P. G. H. Metnitz, "Impact of body mass on incidence and prognosis of acute kidney injury requiring renal replacement therapy," *Intensive Care Medicine*, vol. 36, no. 7, pp. 1221–1228, 2010.

[7] G. J. Soto, A. J. Frank, D. C. Christiani, and M. N. Gong, "Body mass index and acute kidney injury in the acute respiratory distress syndrome," *Critical Care Medicine*, vol. 40, no. 9, pp. 2601–2608, 2012.

[8] E. Gomes, R. Antunes, C. Dias, R. Arajo, and A. Costa-Pereira, "Acute kidney injury in severe trauma assessed by RIFLE criteria: A common feature without implications on mortality?" *Scandinavian Journal of Trauma, Resuscitation and Emergency Medicine*, vol. 18, no. 1, article no. 1, 2010.

[9] J. Wen, Q. Cheng, J. Zhao et al., "Hospital-acquired acute kidney injury in Chinese very elderly persons," *Journal of Nephrology*, vol. 26, no. 3, pp. 572–579, 2013.

[10] H.-H. Tsai, R.-F. Yen, C.-L. Lin, and C.-H. Kao, "Increased risk of dementia in patients hospitalized with acute kidney injury: A nationwide population-based cohort study," *PLoS ONE*, vol. 12, no. 2, Article ID e0171671, 2017.

[11] C.-T. Chao, V.-C. Wu, H.-B. Tsai et al., "Impact of body mass on outcomes of geriatric postoperative acute kidney injury patients," *Shock*, vol. 41, no. 5, pp. 400–405, 2014.

[12] WHO Expert Consultation, "Appropriate body-mass index for Asian populations and its implications for policy and intervention strategies," *The Lancet*, vol. 363, no. 9403, pp. 157–163, 2004.

[13] A. Misra, P. Chowbey, B. M. Makkar et al., "Consensus statement for diagnosis of obesity, abdominal obesity and the metabolic syndrome for Asian Indians and recommendations for physical activity, medical and surgical management," *Journal of the Association of Physicians of India*, vol. 57, pp. 163–170, 2009.

[14] J. C. Verhave, P. Fesler, J. Ribstein, G. Du Cailar, and A. Mimran, "Estimation of renal function in subjects with normal serum creatinine levels: Influence of age and body mass index," *American Journal of Kidney Diseases*, vol. 46, no. 2, pp. 233–241, 2005.

[15] J. R. Landis and G. G. Koch, "The measurement of observer agreement for categorical data," *Biometrics*, vol. 33, no. 1, pp. 159–174, 1977.

[16] D. G. Altman, *Practical Statistics for Medical Research*, Chapman and Hall, London, UK, 2006.

[17] E. D. Siew, S. K. Parr, K. Abdel-Kader et al., "Predictors of Recurrent AKI," *Journal of the American Society of Nephrology : JASN*, vol. 27, no. 4, pp. 1190–1200, 2016.

[18] F. Seccareccia, M. Lanti, A. Menotti, and M. Scanga, "Role of body mass index in the prediction of all cause mortality in over 62,000 men and women. The Italian RIFLE Pooling Project," *Journal of Epidemiology and Community Health*, vol. 52, no. 1, pp. 20–26, 1998.

[19] P. C. Austin and J. V. Tu, "Bootstrap methods for developing predictive models," *The American Statistician*, vol. 58, no. 2, pp. 131–137, 2004.

[20] R. Mehran, E. D. Aymong, E. Nikolsky et al., "A simple risk score for prediction of contrast-induced nephropathy after percutaneous coronary intervention: development and initial validation," *Journal of the American College of Cardiology*, vol. 44, no. 7, pp. 1393–1399, 2004.

[21] C. J. Stone, "[Generalized Additive Models]: Comment," *Statistical Science*, vol. 1, no. 3, pp. 312–314, 1986.

[22] S. Durrleman and R. Simon, "Flexible regression models with cubic splines," *Statistics in Medicine*, vol. 8, no. 5, pp. 551–561, 1989.

[23] S. W. Keith and D. B. Allison, "A free-knot spline modeling framework for piecewise linear logistic regression in complex samples with body mass index and mortality as an example," *Frontiers in Nutrition*, vol. 2014, 16 pages, 2014.

[24] F. T. Billings IV, M. Pretorius, J. S. Schildcrout et al., "Obesity and oxidative stress predict AKI after cardiac surgery," *Journal of the American Society of Nephrology*, vol. 23, no. 7, pp. 1221–1228, 2012.

[25] L. G. Glance, R. Wissler, D. B. Mukamel et al., "Perioperative outcomes among patients with the modified metabolic syndrome who are undergoing noncardiac surgery," *Anesthesiology*, vol. 113, no. 4, pp. 859–872, 2010.

[26] R. R. Kelz, C. E. Reinke, J. R. Zubizarreta et al., "Acute kidney injury, renal function, and the elderly obese surgical patient: A matched case-control study," *Annals of Surgery*, vol. 258, no. 2, pp. 359–363, 2013.

[27] A. B. Pedersen, H. Gammelager, J. Kahlert, H. T. Sørensen, and C. F. Christiansen, "Impact of body mass index on risk of acute kidney injury and mortality in elderly patients undergoing hip fracture surgery," *Osteoporosis International*, vol. 28, no. 3, pp. 1087–1097, 2017.

[28] I. D. Bucaloiu, R. M. Perkins, W. DiFilippo, T. Yahya, and E. Norfolk, "Acute kidney injury in the critically ill, morbidly obese patient: Diagnostic and therapeutic challenges in a unique patient population," *Critical Care Clinics*, vol. 26, no. 4, pp. 607–624, 2010.

[29] M. Suneja and A. B. Kumar, "Obesity and perioperative acute kidney injury: a focused review," *Journal of Critical Care*, vol. 29, no. 4, pp. e691–e696, 2014.

[30] M. Varrier and M. Ostermann, "Novel risk factors for acute kidney injury," *Current Opinion in Nephrology and Hypertension*, vol. 23, no. 6, pp. 560–569, 2014.

[31] H. Schiffl and S. M. Lang, "Obesity, acute kidney injury and outcome of critical illness," *International Urology and Nephrology*, vol. 49, no. 3, pp. 461–466, 2017.

[32] J. T. Mullen, D. W. Moorman, and D. L. Davenport, "The obesity paradox: body mass index and outcomes in patients undergoing nonbariatric general surgery," *Annals of Surgery*, vol. 250, no. 1, pp. 166–172, 2009.

[33] G. Le-Bert, O. Santana, A. M. Pineda, C. Zamora, G. A. Lamas, and J. Lamelas, "The obesity paradox in elderly obese patients undergoing coronary artery bypass surgery," *Interactive CardioVascular and Thoracic Surgery*, vol. 13, no. 2, pp. 124–127, 2011.

[34] S. C. Stamou, M. Nussbaum, R. M. Stiegel et al., "Effect of body mass index on outcomes after cardiac surgery: is there an obesity paradox?" *The Annals of Thoracic Surgery*, vol. 91, no. 1, pp. 42–47, 2011.

[35] H. Kim, J. Kim, C. Seo et al., "Body mass index is inversely associated with mortality in patients with acute kidney injury undergoing continuous renal replacement therapy," *Kidney Research and Clinical Practice*, vol. 36, no. 1, pp. 39–47, 2017.

[36] R. Agarwal, J. E. Bills, and R. P. Light, "Diagnosing obesity by body mass index in chronic kidney disease: an explanation for the 'obesity paradox?'," *Hypertension*, vol. 56, no. 5, pp. 893–900, 2010.

[37] S. Beddhu, "The body mass index paradox and an obesity, inflammation, and atherosclerosis syndrome in chronic kidney disease," *Seminars in Dialysis*, vol. 17, no. 3, pp. 229–232, 2004.

[38] S. Hafner, A. Hillenbrand, U. Knippschild, and P. Radermacher, "The obesity paradox and acute kidney injury: Beneficial effects of hyper-inflammation?" *Critical Care*, vol. 17, no. 6, article no. 1023, 2013.

[39] I. Valocikova, G. Valocik, B. Kristofova, and L. Druzbacka, "Obesity paradox and chronic kidney disease," *Bratislava Medical Journal*, vol. 112, no. 7, pp. 402–406, 2011.

[40] C. P. Kovesdy, J. E. Anderson, and K. Kalantar-Zadeh, "Paradoxical association between body mass index and mortality in men with CKD not yet on dialysis," *American Journal of Kidney Diseases*, vol. 49, no. 5, pp. 581–591, 2007.

[41] H. Kumakura, H. Kanai, M. Aizaki et al., "The influence of the obesity paradox and chronic kidney disease on long-term survival in a Japanese cohort with peripheral arterial disease," *Journal of Vascular Surgery*, vol. 52, no. 1, pp. 110–117, 2010.

[42] J. Park, S.-F. Ahmadi, E. Streja et al., "Obesity paradox in end-stage kidney disease patients," *Progress in Cardiovascular Diseases*, vol. 56, no. 4, pp. 415–425, 2014.

[43] S.-F. Ahmadi, E. Streja, G. Zahmatkesh et al., "Reverse Epidemiology of Traditional Cardiovascular Risk Factors in the Geriatric Population," *Journal of the American Medical Directors Association*, vol. 16, no. 11, pp. 933–939, 2015.

[44] P. Sleeman, N. N. Patel, H. Lin et al., "High fat feeding promotes obesity and renal inflammation and protects against post cardiopulmonary bypass acute kidney injury in swine," *Critical Care*, vol. 17, no. 5, article no. R262, 2013.

[45] K. Kalantar-Zadeh, T. A. Ikizler, G. Block, M. M. Avram, and J. D. Kopple, "Malnutrition-inflammation complex syndrome in dialysis patients: causes and consequences," *American Journal of Kidney Diseases*, vol. 42, no. 5, pp. 864–881, 2003.

[46] E. Fiaccadori, U. Maggiore, A. Cabassi, S. Morabito, G. Castellano, and G. Regolisti, "Nutritional Evaluation and Management of AKI Patients," *Journal of Renal Nutrition*, vol. 23, no. 3, pp. 255–258, 2013.

[47] D. C. Angus and T. van der Poll, "Severe sepsis and septic shock," *The New England Journal of Medicine*, vol. 369, no. 9, pp. 840–851, 2013.

[48] C. Goossens, M. B. Marques, S. Derde et al., "Premorbid obesity, but not nutrition, prevents critical illness-induced muscle wasting and weakness," *Journal of Cachexia, Sarcopenia and Muscle*, vol. 8, no. 1, pp. 89–101, 2017.

[49] A. Chronopoulos, D. N. Cruz, and C. Ronco, "Hospital-acquired acute kidney injury in the elderly," *Nature Reviews Nephrology*, vol. 6, no. 3, pp. 141–149, 2010.

[50] M. Deurenberg-Yap, S. K. Chew, and P. Deurenberg, "Elevated body fat percentage and cardiovascular risks at low body mass index levels among Singaporean Chinese, Malays and Indians," *Obesity Reviews*, vol. 3, no. 3, pp. 209–215, 2002.

[51] L. Chalmers, F. J. Kaskel, and O. Bamgbola, "The role of obesity and its bioclinical correlates in the progression of chronic kidney disease," *Advances in Chronic Kidney Disease*, vol. 13, no. 4, pp. 352–364, 2006.

[52] M. Ashwell, T. J. Cole, and A. K. Dixon, "Ratio of waist circumference to height is strong predictor of intra-abdominal fat," *British Medical Journal*, vol. 313, no. 7056, pp. 559-560, 1996.

[53] C. V. Thakar, P. J. Parikh, and Y. Liu, "Acute kidney injury (AKI) and risk of readmissions in patients with heart failure," *American Journal of Cardiology*, vol. 109, no. 10, pp. 1482–1486, 2012.

[54] S. Sawhney, A. Marks, N. Fluck, D. J. McLernon, G. J. Prescott, and C. Black, "Acute kidney injury as an independent risk factor for unplanned 90-day hospital readmissions," *BMC Nephrology*, vol. 18, no. 1, article no. 9, 2017.

[55] M. Gao, J. Sun, N. Young et al., "Impact of Body Mass Index on Outcomes in Cardiac Surgery," *Journal of Cardiothoracic and Vascular Anesthesia*, vol. 30, no. 5, pp. 1308–1316, 2016.

[56] T. Fujii, S. Uchino, M. Takinami, and R. Bellomo, "Validation of the kidney disease improving global outcomes criteria for AKI and comparison of three criteria in hospitalized patients," *Clinical Journal of the American Society of Nephrology*, vol. 9, no. 5, pp. 848–854, 2014.

[57] J. W. Pickering and Z. H. Endre, "Back-calculating baseline creatinine with MDRD misclassifies acute kidney injury in the intensive care unit," *Clinical Journal of the American Society of Nephrology*, vol. 5, no. 7, pp. 1165–1173, 2010.

27

Febuxostat Attenuates Renal Damage besides Exerting Hypouricemic Effect in Streptozotocin-Induced Diabetic Rats

Jianmin Ran,[1,2] **Gang Xu,**[1,2] **Huixuan Ma,**[1] **Hailing Xu,**[1] **Yan Liu,**[2,3] **Rongshao Tan,**[2] **Ping Zhu,**[1,2] **Jun Song,**[4] **and Gancheng Lao**[1,2]

[1]*Department of Endocrinology, Guangzhou Red Cross Hospital, Medical School of Jinan University, No. 396 Tong Fu Zhong Road, Guangzhou, China*
[2]*Guangzhou Institute of Disease-Oriented Nutritional Research, Guangzhou Red Cross Hospital, Medical School of Jinan University, No. 396 Tong Fu Zhong Road, Guangzhou, China*
[3]*Department of Nephrology, Guangzhou Red Cross Hospital, Medical School of Jinan University, No. 396 Tong Fu Zhong Road, Guangzhou, China*
[4]*Southern Medical University, No. 1023-1063 Southern Sha Tai Road, Guangzhou, China*

Correspondence should be addressed to Jianmin Ran; ranjm@msn.com

Academic Editor: Franca Anglani

Aim. In this study, we aimed to investigate the effects of febuxostat, a novel inhibitor of xanthine oxidase (XO), on renal damage in streptozotocin- (STZ-) induced diabetic rats. *Methods.* Diabetes was induced by the intraperitoneal injection of STZ in male Sprague-Dawley rats. Sham-injected rats served as controls. The control and diabetic rats were treated with and without febuxostat for 8 weeks, respectively. Fasting blood and 24-h urine samples were collected every 4 weeks. Rat livers were extracted for detecting gene expression, content, and bioactivity of XO. *Results.* Diabetic rats showed significantly increased serum uric acid (SUA), serum creatinine (SCr), and urea nitrogen (BUN) levels. Daily urinary albumin (UAE), uric acid (UUA), and creatinine (UCr) excretion were also significantly increased in these rats. In diabetic rats, at week 8, febuxostat decreased SUA by 18.9%, while UAA was increased by 52.0%. However, UCr and urinary urea nitrogen (UUN) levels remained unchanged, while SCr and BUN levels decreased by >30% in these rats. Although hepatic gene expression, content, and activity of XO increased significantly in diabetic rats, febuxostat only slightly decreased its content. *Conclusions.* Febuxostat significantly attenuated renal damage in STZ-induced diabetic rats in addition to exerting hypouricemic effect.

1. Introduction

Diabetic kidney disease (DKD) is the leading cause of end stage renal failure (ESRD) worldwide [1]. For many years, several mechanisms including renal hemodynamic alterations, renin-angiotensin-aldosterone system (RAAS) activation, inflammatory pathways, and reactive oxygen species (ROS) were widely studied in DKD, and various corresponding therapeutic agents have been developed [2]. However, DKD outcomes following administration of these therapeutic agents offered no promising improvement [1]. The underlying mechanisms and interventional targets of DKD should be essentially explored.

Several cohort and cross-sectional studies definitively established the relationship between hyperuricemia and the progress of DKD in either type 1 or type 2 diabetes [3–5]. Several clinical studies using hypouricemic agents such as allopurinol showed positive outcomes such as improving renal damage and postponing renal failure in patients with either diabetes or chronic kidney disease (CKD) [6]. Febuxostat (Fx) is a recently developed xanthine oxidase (XO) inhibitor, which has been definitively proved to be effective and safe for gout treatment [7]. XO is an enzyme that generates ROS by catalyzing the oxidation of hypoxanthine to xanthine and xanthine to uric acid. Some of the renal protective effects of Fx were clarified in animal models with

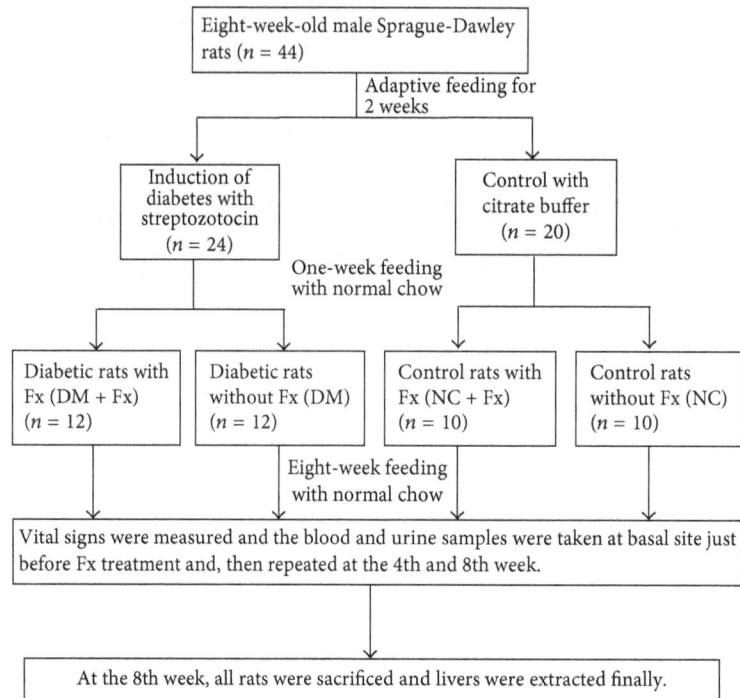

FIGURE 1: Schematic diagram of the animal experiment protocol. Fx: febuxostat. NC: the normal control group without Fx treatment; NC + Fx: the normal group with Fx treatment; DM: diabetic mellitus group without Fx treatment; DM + Fx: diabetic mellitus group with Fx treatment.

diabetes, such as db/db mice [8] and diabetic Zucker rats [9]. Despite these promising data, we noticed that the plasma uric acid (UA) levels in most studies were normal or even low because of the degradation of uricase, an enzyme that converts uric acid to allantoin, which is much more soluble than uric acid [10]. Alterations in UA metabolism were also seldom discussed in these papers. Suitable animal models characterized by both diabetes and hyperuricemia should be explored for researches in this field.

In our previous studies [11] on streptozotocin- (STZ-) induced diabetic rats, we found that serum UA concentration was significantly and permanently increased, which was accompanied by abnormalities in renal function, including increased serum creatinine (Scr) and albuminuria; enlarged glomeruli and tubular hyalinization were also prominent in these rats. Similar increase in UA concentration was seen in STZ-induced diabetic rats in other studies [12, 13]. Therefore, this rat model is more appropriate for researches on hyperuricemia in diabetic conditions. In the present study, we investigated the effects of Fx on renal injury in STZ-induced diabetic rats with the aim to search novel therapeutic method for DKD.

2. Materials and Methods

2.1. Animal Preparation. The overall animal experiment protocol is shown in Figure 1. Eight-week-old male Sprague-Dawley rats (Guangdong Medical Laboratory Animal Center, Foshan, China) weighing 200–220 g were adopted for this study. All rats were collectively housed (2 rats per cage)

and fed with standard rat chow for 2 weeks. For diabetes induction, the rats were intraperitoneally injected with STZ (dissolved in 50 mM citrate, pH = 4.2, Sigma, St Louis, USA) at a single dose of 65 mg/kg. Twenty-four rats with random blood glucose levels > 16.7 mmol/L at three different times were selected for the experiments. Twenty rats that served as controls were intraperitoneally injected with the same volume of citrate buffer.

2.2. Fx Treatment and Animal Experiments. After successful induction of diabetes for 2 weeks, the experimental diabetic and control rats were treated with Fx (Melone Pharmaceutical Co., Ltd, Dalian, China), which was dissolved in 0.5% carboxymethylcellulose sodium (CMC-Na, Fu Chen Chemical Reagents Factory, Tianjin, China), at a dose of 5 mg/kg/d via daily gavage for 8 weeks (Figure 1). The control rats were treated only with the same volume of CMC-Na. The rats were divided into 4 groups during this intervention period as follows: diabetic rats with (DM + Fx, $n = 12$) and without (DM, $n = 12$) Fx treatment, as well as normal control rats with (NC + Fx, $n = 10$) and without (NC, $n = 10$) Fx treatment.

Vital signs, including systolic blood pressure (SBP), diastolic blood pressure (DBP), and heart rate (HR) were recorded in fully conscious rats by using indirect tail-cuff equipment (LE5002, Harvard Apparatus, USA). After prewarming the rats for 20 min on a 37°C plate, the SBP, DBP, and HR of each rat were recorded.

Blood and urine samples were collected every 4 weeks at the baseline and at weeks 4 and 8, respectively. For urine sampling, the rats were individually housed in metabolic cages for 24 h; then, all urine samples were collected and volumetrically estimated. All rats were sacrificed after 8 weeks of Fx treatment, and the livers were removed for histologic, enzymatic, and genetic assays.

During the whole experiment, all rats were allowed free access to standard rat chow and water, and the room light was rotated at a 12-h light-dark cycle. On the morning of the experiment, foods were withdrawn 12 h before each operation. All animal experimental procedures were approved by the Ethnic Committee of Guangzhou Red Cross Hospital.

2.3. Biochemical Assays. The serum concentrations of glucose, triglyceride (TG), total cholesterol (TC), uric acid (SUA), urea nitrogen (BUN), and SCr were measured using the corresponding commercial kits on an automatic biochemical machine (ECHO, ECHO, Italy). The 24-h urine samples were collected and quantified. Urinary uric acid (UUA), urinary urea nitrogen (UUN), and urinary creatinine (UCr) were detected by the same automatic machine. Urinary albumin was determined by the standard bromocresol green method, and the 24 h amount of urinary albumin excretion (UAE) was then calculated.

2.4. Hepatic Content and Activity of XO. The hepatic content of XO was measured according to the previously described method [14]. Liver tissues weighing 0.25 g were mixed with 9 times the volume of purified water and homogenized. This mixture was centrifuged for 10 min at 3000 rpm, and the supernatant was separated. The XO concentration in the supernatant was measured by using the corresponding commercial ELISA kits (Huamei Bioengineer Ltd. Co, Wuhan, China).

For the measurement of hepatic XO activity, we determined the total protein content of the homogenate according to the Coomassie brilliant blue method [15] using a commercial reagent kit (Nanjing Jiancheng Bioengineering Institute, Nanjing, China). Substrate and buffers were added in the test and control reaction system (Nanjing Jiancheng Bioengineering Institute, Nanjing, China), respectively. The absorbance was measured at 530 nm after 20 min incubation at 37°C. Hepatic XO activity was calculated according to the absorbance difference and expressed as U/g protein.

2.5. Gene Expression. Hepatic gene expression of XO, the key enzyme for UA formation, was determined by real-time polymerase chain reaction (RT-PCR). Frozen tissues were homogenized and total RNA was extracted using a TRIzol kit (Invitrogen, CA, USA). RNA quality and quantity were assessed by automated capillary gel electrophoresis on a Bioanalyzer 2100 with RNA Nano LabChips (Agilent Technology, Tokyo, Japan). Then, total RNA (1 μg) was reversely transcribed using a cDNA synthesis kit (Promega, CA, USA) with random primers in a 20 μL PCR system according to the manufacturer's protocol. Quantitative PCR was performed by SYBR Green PCR Master Mix (Toyobo, Osaka, Japan) and ABI PRISM 7500 Sequence Detection System (Applied Biosystems Inc., CA, USA). Thermal cycling was carried out at 95°C for 15 min, followed by 40 cycles at 95°C for 15 s,

60°C for 15 s, and 72°C for 32 s. We used 18S rRNA as a housekeeping gene in RT-PCR. The specific primers were selected as follows: XO forward: 5'-GACAGGGTGTTTATGAAGCA-3', XO reverse: 5'-AACTCACTGCGCTCGTATAG-3'; 18S rRNA forward: 5'-CCTGGATACCGCAGCTAGGA-3', 18S rRNA reverse: 5'-GCGGCGCAATACGAATGCCCC-3'.

2.6. Statistical Analysis. The results are expressed as mean ± SD. One-way analysis of variance (ANOVA) and Mann–Whitney U test were selected for comparisons of differences between means and nonnormally distributed data differences, respectively. Statistical difference was accepted at $P < 0.05$.

3. Results

3.1. General Characteristics. Although the diabetic rats were more polyphagous and polydipsic than normal rats after induction of diabetes, Fx treatment reduced the daily food intake in diabetic rats at the 4th and 8th weeks (Figure 2, both $P < 0.05$). The daily water intake was not affected by Fx treatment in any rats. Diabetic rats lost their weight significantly, while the body weight of normal rats increased continuously during the whole experiment. In case of vital signs, the diabetic rats showed lower HR than normal rats at the 8th week ($P < 0.05$); SBP and DBP decreased in diabetic rats at this time point ($P < 0.05$). However, Fx did not exert any effects on these vital signs either in diabetic or normal rats.

3.2. Blood and Urine Biochemistry. The blood biochemical profile throughout the experiment is shown in Figure 3. After successful induction of diabetes, the fasting plasma glucose (FPG) in diabetic rats was maintained at very high levels during the experiment compared to that in normal rats (all $P < 0.05$). NC + Fx rats showed slightly higher plasma TG than the NC control group ($P < 0.05$), while the plasma TC level was comparable among all rat groups. In both diabetic and normal rats, Fx treatment did not alter the plasma glucose and lipid levels. SUA, SCr, and BUN levels increased significantly (all $P < 0.05$) in diabetic rats at the baseline. In diabetic rats, Fx treatment slightly decreased SUA by 18.9% at the 8th week ($P < 0.05$), while both SCr and BUN were significantly decreased to around 30.0% (both $P < 0.05$). SUA, SCr, and BUN were not affected by Fx treatment in normal rats (all $P > 0.05$).

Daily urinary excretions are depicted in Figure 4. UAE (at week 0, 149.42 ± 29.85 mg/d, 140.04 ± 30.11 mg/d, 8.89 ± 1.96 mg/d, and 10.52 ± 2.39 mg/d for DM, DM + Fx, NC, and NC + Fx group, resp.), UUA, UCr, and UUN remarkably increased in the diabetic rats (all $P < 0.05$ when DM was compared with NC group). Fx treatment significantly decreased the daily UAE level at the 4th (122.84 ± 32.65 mg/d for DM and 99.25 ± 31.25 mg/d for DM + Fx, $P < 0.05$) and 8th week (138.21 ± 22.57 mg/d for DM and 110.84 ± 29.18 mg/d for DM + Fx, $P < 0.05$) in diabetic rats. Notably, in diabetic rats, Fx treatment significantly increased UUA at the 4th and 8th weeks (both $P < 0.05$). In particular, at the

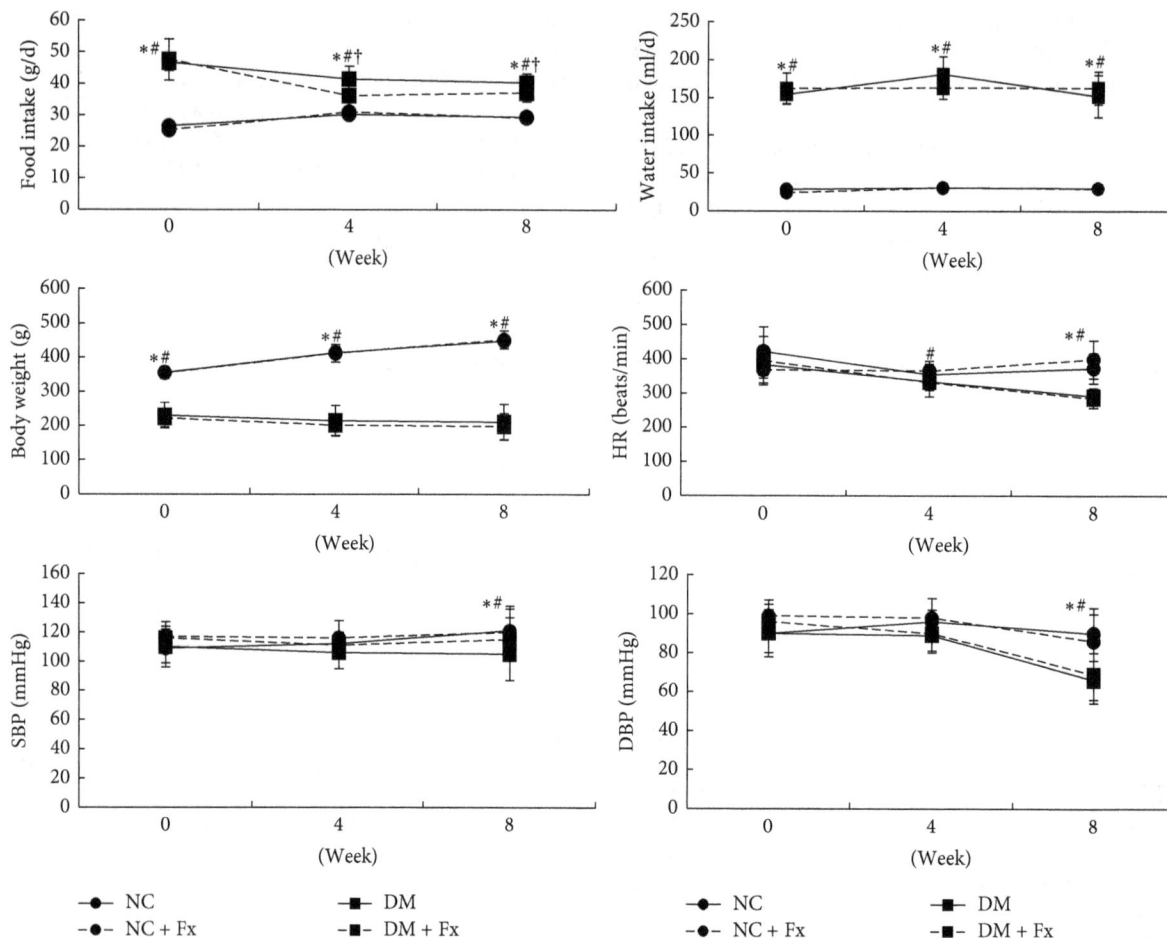

FIGURE 2: Time course of food intake, water intake, body weight, and main vital signs during the experiment after induction of diabetes. Heart rate (HR), systolic blood pressure (SBP), and diastolic blood pressure (DBP) were recorded by an indirect tail-cuff method. The circle with solid and dashed lines represents NC and NC + Fx groups, respectively, while the block symbol with solid and dashed lines shows data of DM and DM + Fx groups, respectively. Data are expressed as mean ± SD. Statistical significance ($P < 0.05$) was labeled as *, #, and † correspondingly, when the DM + Fx group was compared with NC, NC + Fx, and DM groups.

8th week, the daily UUA was significantly increased to 52.0% following Fx treatment. UCr and UUN were also increased after Fx treatment at the 4th week (both $P < 0.05$), but they were comparable at the 8th week (both $P > 0.05$). Fx did not change the aforementioned daily urinary excretions in normal rats during the experiment.

3.3. Hepatic Content, Activity, and Gene Expression of XO. The hepatic content of XO (125.59 ± 3.04 ng/mL for the DM group versus 59.94 ± 3.23 ng/mL for the CON group, $P < 0.05$) increased significantly in diabetic rats (Figure 5(a)). In addition, the enzymatic activity of XO (Figure 5(b)) increased significantly in diabetic rats compared to that in normal control rats (24.42 ± 2.95 U/g protein for the DM group versus 18.60 ± 2.16 U/g protein for the CON group, $P < 0.05$). Gene expression of XO showed the same trend as that of hepatic content and enzymatic activity (Figure 5(c)).

Fx treatment slightly decreased the hepatic XO content in diabetic rats (Figure 5(a), $P < 0.05$). Nevertheless, the treatment exerted no effects on hepatic enzymatic activity

and gene expression of XO in either diabetic or normal rats (Figures 5(b) and 5(c), all $P > 0.05$).

4. Discussion

Similar to our previous study [11], we found that STZ-induced diabetic rats developed high levels of SUA and renal damage, marked by elevated serum BUN, SCr, and daily UAE. Fx, a specific XO inhibitor, significantly reduced SUA and attenuated renal function without affecting the blood glucose, blood pressure, and lipid profile. These findings indicated that hyperuricemia and its related pathological processes could be an important and direct mechanism underlying renal damage in STZ-induced diabetic rats. Correspondingly, all therapies focusing on UA metabolism may retard the progression of diabetic renal injury [16].

It remains unclear how UA directly facilitates renal damage in diabetic patients and various diabetic animal models [17]. It is well known that RAAS triggers hemodynamic changes and inflammatory attacks; therefore, it plays pivotal

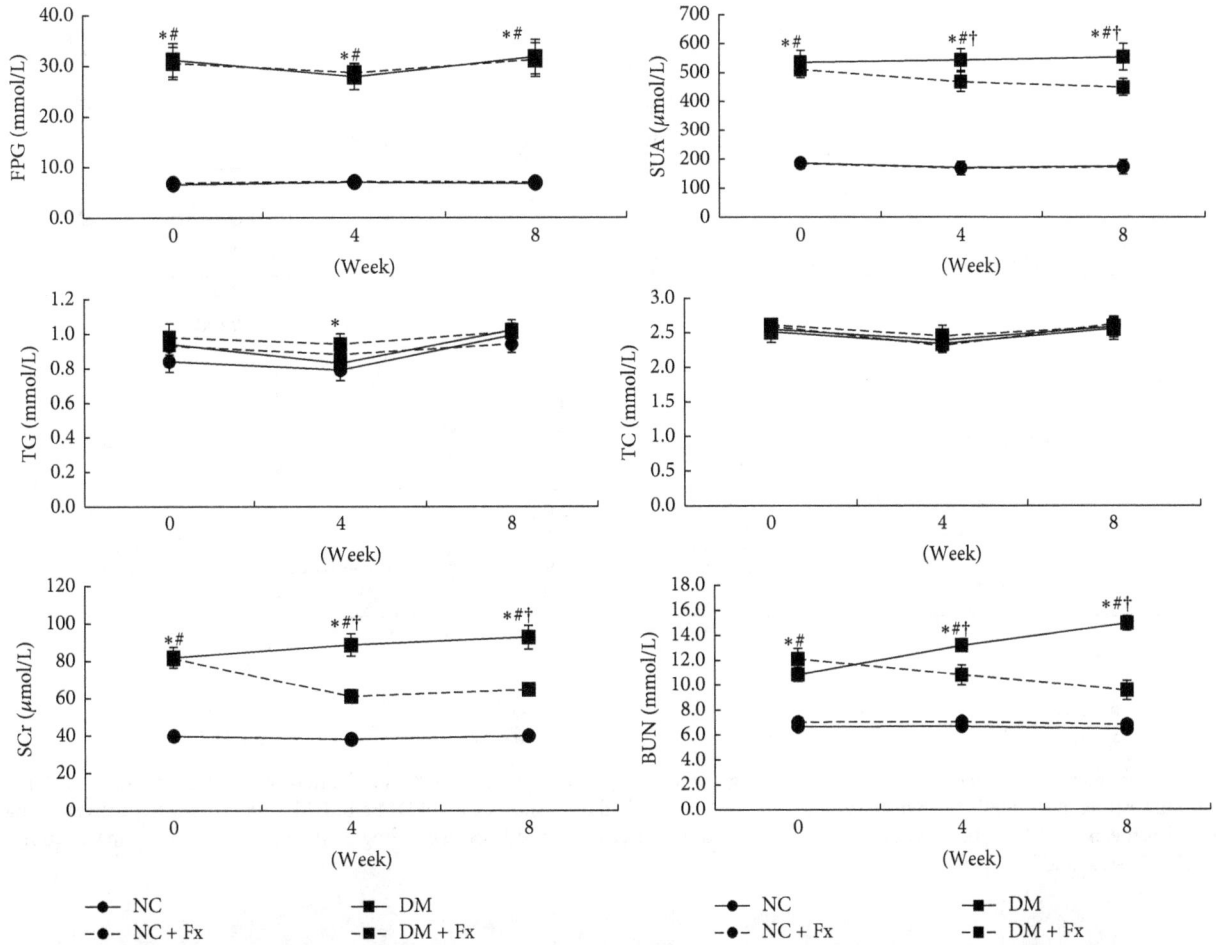

FIGURE 3: Time course of blood biochemical indices among the four rat groups. The circle with solid and dashed lines represents NC and NC + Fx groups, respectively, while the block symbol with solid and dashed lines shows data of DM and DM + Fx groups, respectively. Data are expressed as mean ± SD. Statistical significance ($P < 0.05$) was labeled as *, #, and † correspondingly, when the DM + Fx group was compared with NC, NC + Fx, and DM groups.

roles in DKD [18]. In vivo studies [19, 20] have demonstrated that UA may promote RAAS activity in CKD animal models. Several researches have reported links between UA metabolism and other proinflammatory pathways [21, 22]. Among them, the convincing one is that UA, as crystals causing cellular necrosis, can activate the inflammasome NLRP3, which consequently induces caspase-1 and its downstream cytokines including IL-1β and IL-18 [23, 24]. The latter two cytokines have been proved to be potentially expressed on tubular epithelial cells and may closely relate to UA-induced interstitial damage [25].

The present study showed that Fx significantly reduced SUA by 18% and attenuated renal damage. This result is consistent with that of several other animal and clinical studies. In diabetic db/db mice [26], Kosugi et al. found that tubulointerstitial injury is significantly attenuated by treatment with allopurinol, another XO inhibitor, for 8 weeks. Following Fx treatment, normalization of SUA and improvements in renal injury were also achieved in several diabetic models such as db/db mice [8, 27], Zucker diabetic rats [9], and STZ-induced diabetic rats [28]. Large-scale clinical trials

on the effects of lowering SUA on DKD progression are still scarce [29]. In a previous study in type 2 diabetic patients with DKD, daily UAE was significantly reduced after a 4-month intervention with allopurinol [30]. Recently, another study [31] showed that 3-year treatment with allopurinol in type 2 diabetic patients with asymptomatic hyperuricemia decreased UAE and SCr, while the glomerular filtration rate was increased. In the present study, daily UUN, UCr, and UUA increasing significantly after Fx treatment might be attributed to improved glomerular filtration; we regarded this as a novel finding if compared with other animal studies.

Compared with the above-mentioned animal researches, the most noticeable thing in our experiment is that Fx treatment decreased SUA to approximately 18% in diabetic rats, but in normal rats SUA was unchanged at the 8th week. Thus, SUA in DM + Fx group was still significantly higher than that in both NC and NC + Fx groups. According to previous studies, Fx at 5 mg/kg is a moderate dose for rats and mice [32]; however, we did not observe complete normalization of SUA when compared to that in few other studies involving SUA [33]. One reason for this

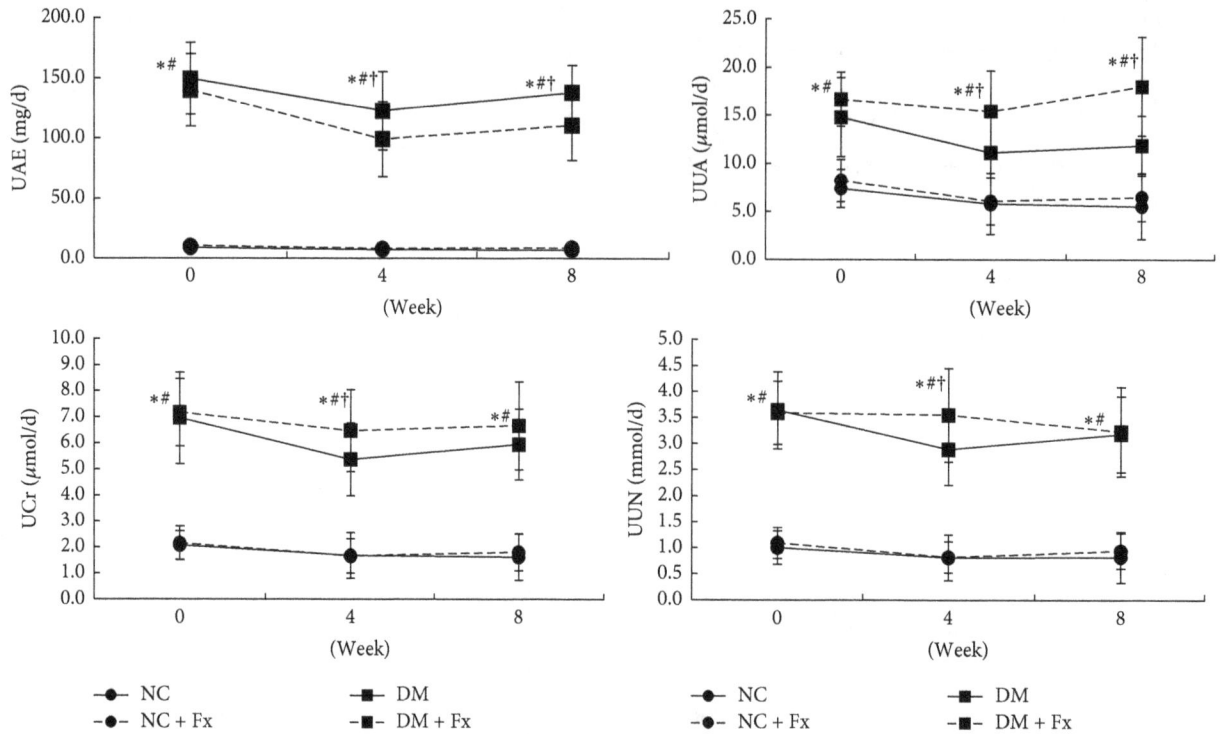

FIGURE 4: Time course of daily urinary excretions among the four rat groups. The circle with solid and dashed lines represents NC and NC + Fx groups, respectively, while the block symbol with solid and dashed lines shows data of DM and DM + Fx groups, respectively. Data are expressed as mean ± SD. Statistical significance ($P < 0.05$) was labeled as *, #, and † correspondingly, when the DM + Fx group was compared with NC, NC + Fx, and DM groups.

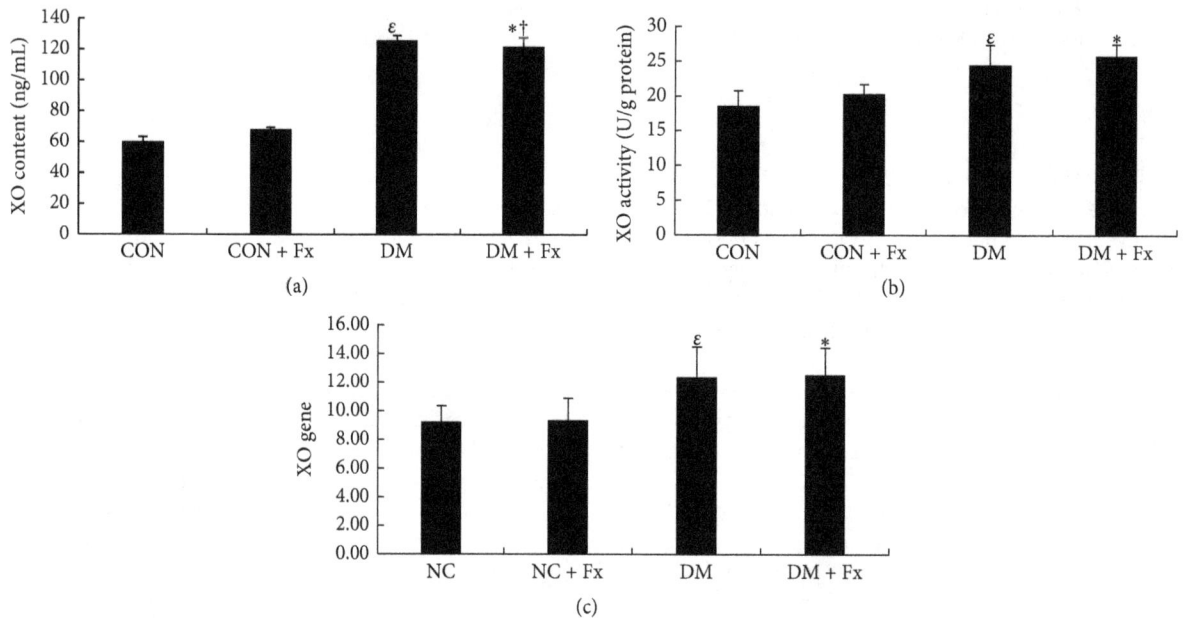

FIGURE 5: Hepatic content, activity, and gene expression of xanthine oxidase (XO). Hepatic content of XO (a) was expressed as its concentration in the supernatant of liver extract. Hepatic XO activity (b) was calculated according to the XO protein ratio and expressed as U/g protein. Relative gene expression (c) was determined by RT-PCR and shown in the graph as the amounts of initial template. Data are expressed as mean ± SD. $^{\varepsilon}P < 0.05$ when the DM group was compared with CON or CON + Fx group, $^{*}P < 0.05$ when DM + Fx group was compared with CON or CON + Fx, and † when compared with DM group, respectively.

might result from the relatively short-term intervention of Fx (only 8 weeks). Second, we speculate that STZ might aggravate UA metabolism by directly suppressing uricase to some extent, instead of promoting in vivo XO activity [34]. Significantly increased hepatic XO gene expression, content, and activity in diabetic rats were observed in our research, which were similar to those observed in several studies using other diabetic models, such as Zucker diabetic rats [9], Otsuka Long-Evans Tokushima fatty rats [35], and db/db mice [8]. We may conclude that diabetes itself rather than STZ activates XO, thereby promoting UA production in these rats [36]. This hypothesis can illustrate why Fx only slightly decreases SUA in STZ-induced diabetic rats when no hypoglycemic treatment is provided. Further studies are needed to elucidate the relationship between STZ and UA metabolism.

Despite the slight reduction of SUA, remarkable renal protective effects were observed in the diabetic rats. Daily UAE significantly decreased, and, more importantly, serum BUN and SCr decreased by more than 30% in these rats. Fx treatment should specifically target XO and this can inhibit in vivo UA production [9]. Hepatic content, activity, and gene expression were measured in our experiment. All these parameters were significantly increased in diabetic rats in agreement with the findings of other studies [8, 9, 35]. Nevertheless, exceptional results were observed in this study, including unchanged XO gene expression and activity and a slight decrease in hepatic XO content after Fx treatment in diabetic rats. Gene expression and activity of XO were unchanged which may result from the upregulating effects after the competitive inhibition by Fx. But anyway, Fx decreased SUA slightly and exerted minor effects on hepatic XO content. Simultaneously, Fx treatment did not make significant changes in body weight, blood pressure, and metabolic indices including blood glucose and lipid levels. These data throw light on mechanisms other than hypouricemic effect that may underlie the renal protective effects of Fx.

Several other researches explored the mechanisms involved in the attenuation of renal injury by Fx treatment. Sánchez-Lozada et al. found that Fx significantly reduced glomerular pressure and renal vasoconstriction in fructose-induced metabolic syndrome [33] and oxonic acid-induced hyperuricemic rat models [37]. Moreover, in STZ-induced diabetic rat models, Lee et al. [28] showed that Fx prevents renal damage mainly by ameliorating the inflammatory factors and oxidative stress, owing to its inhibitory effects on XO. In a recent study in Zucker diabetic rats, Komers et al. [9] examined the effect of Fx on oxidative stress. The simultaneous inhibition of profibrotic signaling by Fx might be another pivotal mechanism. We did not perform further experiments on glomerular structure and interstitial changes in our study. However, it is well known [38] that UA preferentially induces tubular damage. In our previous study, feeding the same diabetic rats with low protein diets decreased SUA and attenuated tubular injuries. In the present study, we noticed that daily UAE was increased after Fx

treatment in diabetic rats, which could not be appropriately explained by its direct pharmacological actions [39]. Unknown but important mechanisms of Fx on renal tubular damage should be investigated in future researches.

This study has several limitations. First, the morphologic alterations of glomerular and interstitial area after Fx treatment should be studied in a long-term experiment. Second, the renal hemodynamic parameters were not included in the study design, and these alterations may partly be responsible for the improvement of renal function in diabetic rats. Researches on the direct effects of UA on renal damage in diabetes have been initiated and more compromised data will be provided in the future.

5. Conclusions

Fx attenuated renal damage without any significant influence on glucose, blood pressure, and lipid levels in STZ-induced diabetic and hyperuricemic rats. The mild hypouricemic effects and actions of Fx on XO pave the way for researchers to explore other underlying mechanisms, especially in the tubules, besides its traditional targets.

Acknowledgments

The authors greatly thank all the staffs of Guangdong Medical Laboratory Animal Center for their excellent technical assistance in animal management and experiments. The study was supported by Guangzhou Science and Technology Project Fund (no. 201300000181, no. 2014Y2-00145, no. 2014Y2-00166, no. 14A33151295, and no. 2014J4100076), Guangzhou Scientific Fund for Clinical Study and Translational Medicine (no. 2014Y2-00549), and Guangdong Science and Technology Project Fund for Key Scientific Research Base (no. 2014B030303002).

References

[1] M. Afkarian, L. R. Zelnick, Y. N. Hall et al., "Clinical manifestations of kidney disease among US adults with diabetes, 1988–2014," *The Journal of the American Medical Association*, vol. 316, no. 6, pp. 602–610, 2016.

[2] N. Helou, A. Dwyer, M. Shaha, and A. Zanchi, "Multidisciplinary management of diabetic kidney disease: a systematic review and meta-analysis," *JBI Database of Systematic Reviews and Implementation Reports*, vol. 14, pp. 169–207, 2016.

[3] P. Hovind, P. Rossing, L. Tarnow, R. J. Johnson, and H. H. Parving, "Serum uric acid as a predictor for development of diabetic nephropathy in type 1 diabetes: an inception cohort study," *Diabetes*, vol. 58, pp. 1668–1671, 2009.

[4] Y. Hayashino, S. Okamura, S. Tsujii, and H. Ishii, "Association of serum uric acid levels with the risk of development or progression of albuminuria among Japanese patients with type 2 diabetes: a prospective cohort study [Diabetes Distress and Care Registry at Tenri (DDCRT 10)]," *Acta Diabetologica*, vol. 53, no. 4, pp. 599–607, 2016.

[5] Y.-H. Chang, C.-C. Lei, K.-C. Lin, D.-M. Chang, C.-H. Hsieh, and Y.-J. Lee, "Serum uric acid level as an indicator for CKD regression and progression in patients with type 2 diabetes mellitus—a 4.6-year cohort study," *Diabetes/Metabolism Research and Reviews*, vol. 32, pp. 557–564, 2016.

[6] C. Mende, "Management of chronic kidney disease: the relationship between serum uric acid and development of nephropathy," *Advances in Therapy*, vol. 32, no. 12, pp. 1177–1191, 2015.

[7] S. Li, H. Yang, Y. Guo et al., "Comparative efficacy and safety of urate-lowering therapy for the treatment of hyperuricemia: a systematic review and network meta-analysis," *Scientific Reports*, vol. 6, no. 1, Article ID 33082, 2016.

[8] T. Nakamura, T. Murase, M. Nampei et al., "Effects of topiroxostat and febuxostat on urinary albumin excretion and plasma xanthine oxidoreductase activity in db/db mice," *European Journal of Pharmacology*, vol. 780, pp. 224–231, 2016.

[9] R. Komers, B. Xu, J. Schneider, and T. T. Oyama, "Effects of xanthine oxidase inhibition with febuxostat on the development of nephropathy in experimental type 2 diabetes," *British Journal of Pharmacology*, vol. 173, pp. 2573–2588, 2016.

[10] J. T. Kratzer, M. A. Lanaspa, M. N. Murphy et al., "Evolutionary history and metabolic insights of ancient mammalian uricases," *Proceedings of the National Academy of Sciences of the United States of America*, vol. 111, no. 10, pp. 3763–3768, 2014.

[11] J. Ran, J. Ma, Y. Liu, R. Tan, H. Liu, and G. Lao, "Low protein diet inhibits uric acid synthesis and attenuates renal damage in streptozotocin-induced diabetic rats," *Journal of Diabetes Research*, vol. 2014, Article ID 287536, 2014.

[12] C. Wang, Y. Pan, Q.-Y. Zhang, F.-M. Wang, and L.-D. Kong, "Quercetin and allopurinol ameliorate kidney injury in STZ-treated rats with regulation of renal NLRP3 inflammasome activation and lipid accumulation," *PLoS ONE*, vol. 7, no. 6, Article ID e38285, 2012.

[13] D. S. Ibrahim and M. A. E. Abd El-Maksoud, "Effect of strawberry (Fragaria × ananassa) leaf extract on diabetic nephropathy in rats," *International Journal of Experimental Pathology*, vol. 96, no. 2, pp. 87–93, 2015.

[14] L. P. Peters and R. W. Teel, "Effect of high sucrose diet on liver enzyme content and activity and aflatoxin B1-induced mutagenesis," *In Vivo*, vol. 17, no. 2, pp. 205–210, 2003.

[15] Y. Jin and T. Manabe, "High-efficiency protein extraction from polyacrylamide gels for molecular mass measurement by matrix-assisted laser desorption/ionization-time of flight-mass spectrometry," *Electrophoresis*, vol. 26, no. 6, pp. 1019–1028, 2005.

[16] P. Hovind, P. Rossing, R. J. Johnson, and H.-H. Parving, "Serum uric acid as a new player in the development of diabetic nephropathy," *Journal of Renal Nutrition*, vol. 21, no. 1, pp. 124–127, 2011.

[17] P. Dousdampanis, K. Trigka, C. G. Musso, and C. Fourtounas, "Hyperuricemia and chronic kidney disease: an enigma yet to be solved," *Renal Failure*, vol. 36, no. 9, pp. 1351–1359, 2014.

[18] S. S. Roscioni, H. J. L. Heerspink, and D. De Zeeuw, "The effect of RAAS blockade on the progression of diabetic nephropathy," *Nature Reviews Nephrology*, vol. 10, no. 2, pp. 77–87, 2014.

[19] A. Eräranta, V. Kurra, A. M. Tahvanainen et al., "Oxonic acid-induced hyperuricemia elevates plasma aldosterone in experimental renal insufficiency," *Journal of Hypertension*, vol. 26, no. 8, pp. 1661–1668, 2008.

[20] D. B. Corry, P. Eslami, K. Yamamoto, M. D. Nyby, H. Makino, and M. L. Tuck, "Uric acid stimulates vascular smooth muscle cell proliferation and oxidative stress via the vascular renin-angiotensin system," *Journal of Hypertension*, vol. 26, no. 2, pp. 269–275, 2008.

[21] V. Filiopoulos, D. Hadjiyannakos, and D. Vlassopoulos, "New insights into uric acid effects on the progression and prognosis of chronic kidney disease," *Renal Failure*, vol. 34, no. 4, pp. 510–520, 2012.

[22] J. Wada and H. Makino, "Inflammation and the pathogenesis of diabetic nephropathy," *Clinical Science*, vol. 124, no. 3, pp. 139–152, 2013.

[23] Y. Qiu and L. Tang, "Roles of the NLRP3 inflammasome in the pathogenesis of diabetic nephropathy," *Pharmacological Research*, vol. 114, pp. 251–264, 2016.

[24] T. T. Braga, M. F. Forni, M. Correa-Costa et al., "Soluble uric acid activates the NLRP3 inflammasome," *Scientific Reports*, vol. 7, article 39884, 2017.

[25] S.-M. Kim, S.-H. Lee, Y.-G. Kim et al., "Hyperuricemia-induced NLRP3 activation of macrophages contributes to the progression of diabetic nephropathy," *American Journal of Physiology—Renal Physiology*, vol. 308, no. 9, pp. F993–F1003, 2015.

[26] T. Kosugi, T. Nakayama, M. Heinig et al., "Effect of lowering uric acid on renal disease in the type 2 diabetic db/db mice," *American Journal of Physiology—Renal Physiology*, vol. 297, no. 2, pp. F481–F488, 2009.

[27] A. Kushiyama, K. Tanaka, S. Hara, and S. Kawazu, "Linking uric acid metabolism to diabetic complications," *World Journal of Diabetes*, vol. 5, no. 6, pp. 787–795, 2014.

[28] H.-J. Lee, K. H. Jeong, Y. G. Kim et al., "Febuxostat ameliorates diabetic renal injury in a streptozotocin-induced diabetic rat model," *American Journal of Nephrology*, vol. 40, no. 1, pp. 56–63, 2014.

[29] D. M. Maahs, L. Caramori, D. Z. I. Cherney et al., "Uric acid lowering to prevent kidney function loss in diabetes: the preventing early renal function loss (PERL) allopurinol study," *Current Diabetes Reports*, vol. 13, no. 4, pp. 550–559, 2013.

[30] A. Momeni, S. Shahidi, S. Seirafian, S. Taheri, and S. Kheiri, "Effect of allopurinol in decreasing proteinuria in type 2 diabetic patients," *Iranian Journal of Kidney Diseases*, vol. 4, no. 2, pp. 128–132, 2010.

[31] P. Liu, Y. Chen, B. Wang, F. Zhang, D. Wang, and Y. Wang, "Allopurinol treatment improves renal function in patients with type 2 diabetes and asymptomatic hyperuricemia: 3-year randomized parallel-controlled study," *Clinical Endocrinology*, vol. 83, no. 4, pp. 475–482, 2015.

[32] B. Krishnamurthy, N. Rani, S. Bharti et al., "Febuxostat ameliorates doxorubicin-induced cardiotoxicity in rats," *Chemico-Biological Interactions*, vol. 237, pp. 96–103, 2015.

[33] L. G. Sánchez-Lozada, E. Tapia, P. Bautista-García et al., "Effects of febuxostat on metabolic and renal alterations in rats with fructose-induced metabolic syndrome," *American Journal of Physiology—Renal Physiology*, vol. 294, no. 4, pp. F710–F718, 2008.

[34] H. Osmundsen, B. Brodal, and R. Hovik, "A luminometric assay for peroxisomal β-oxidation. Effects of fasting and streptozotocin-diabetes on peroxisomal β-oxidation," *Biochemical Journal*, vol. 260, no. 1, pp. 215–220, 1989.

[35] I. J. Kim, Y. K. Kim, S. M. Son, K. W. Hong, and C. D. Kim, "Enhanced vascular production of superoxide in OLETF rat after the onset of hyperglycemia," *Diabetes Research and Clinical Practice*, vol. 60, no. 1, pp. 11–18, 2003.

[36] M. Banerjee and P. Vats, "Reactive metabolites and antioxidant gene polymorphisms in Type 2 diabetes mellitus," *Redox Biology*, vol. 2, no. 1, pp. 170–177, 2014.

[37] L. G. Sánchez-Lozada, E. Tapia, V. Soto et al., "Treatment with the xanthine oxidase inhibitor febuxostat lowers uric acid and alleviates systemic and glomerular hypertension in experimental hyperuricaemia," *Nephrology Dialysis Transplantation*, vol. 23, no. 4, pp. 1179–1185, 2008.

[38] S. A. Fathallah-Shaykh and M. T. Cramer, "Uric acid and the kidney," *Pediatric Nephrology*, vol. 29, no. 6, pp. 999–1008, 2014.

[39] B. Grabowski, R. Khosravan, J.-T. Wu, L. Vernillet, and C. Lademacher, "Effect of hydrochlorothiazide on the pharmacokinetics and pharmacodynamics of febuxostat, a non-purine selective inhibitor of xanthine oxidase," *British Journal of Clinical Pharmacology*, vol. 70, no. 1, pp. 57–64, 2010.

28

Renal Outcomes in Children with Operated Spina Bifida in Uganda

Helen J. Sims-Williams ⓘ,[1] Hugh P. Sims-Williams,[2]
Edith Mbabazi Kabachelor,[3] and Benjamin C. Warf[4]

[1]*Sheffield Kidney Institute, Sheffield Teaching Hospitals NHS Foundation Trust, Sheffield, UK*
[2]*Department of Neurosurgery, Sheffield Teaching Hospitals NHS Foundation Trust, Sheffield, UK*
[3]*CURE Children's Hospital of Uganda, Mbale, Uganda*
[4]*Department of Paediatric Neurosurgery, Boston Children's Hospital and Harvard Medical School, Boston, MA, USA*

Correspondence should be addressed to Helen J. Sims-Williams; helen.nye@cantab.net

Academic Editor: David B. Kershaw

Background. To describe the extent of renal disease in Ugandan children surviving at least ten years after spina bifida repair and to investigate risk factors for renal deterioration in this cohort. *Patients and Methods*. Children who had undergone spina bifida repair at CURE Children's Hospital of Uganda between 2000 and 2004 were invited to attend interview, physical examination, renal tract ultrasound, and a blood test (creatinine). Medical records were retrospectively reviewed. The following were considered evidence of renal damage: elevated creatinine, hypertension, and ultrasound findings of hydronephrosis, scarring, and discrepancy in renal size >1cm. Female sex, previous UTI, neurological level, mobility, detrusor leak point pressure, and adherence with clean intermittent catheterisation (CIC) were investigated for association with evidence of renal damage. *Results*. 65 of 68 children aged 10–14 completed the assessment. The majority (83%) reported incontinence. 17 children (26%) were performing CIC. One child had elevated creatinine. 25 children (38%) were hypertensive. There was a high prevalence of ultrasound abnormalities: hydronephrosis in 10 children (15%), scarring in 42 (64%), and >1cm size discrepancy in 28 (43%). No children with lesions at S1 or below had hydronephrosis (p = 0.025), but this group had comparable prevalence of renal size discrepancy, scarring, and hypertension to those children with higher lesions. *Conclusions*. Incontinence, ultrasound abnormalities, and hypertension are highly prevalent in a cohort of Ugandan children with spina bifida, including those with low neurological lesions. These findings support the early and universal initiation of CIC with anticholinergic therapy in a low-income setting.

1. Introduction

There are an estimated 37,000 children born with spina bifida every year in sub-Saharan Africa [1]. Although initial surgery can be life-saving, there is significant long-term morbidity and mortality associated with the condition, including renal complications. Chronic kidney disease (CKD) develops as a consequence of elevated detrusor pressures, vesicoureteric reflux, and recurrent urinary tract infections, leading to renal scarring [2, 3]. Additionally, urinary incontinence makes independence and socialisation more challenging and has been shown in some studies to negatively affect quality of life and self-esteem [4, 5]. In spite of the scale of the problem,

there have been no publications reporting long-term renal outcomes from a low-income setting.

Modern management of the neurogenic bladder has improved outcomes, most notably with the introduction of clean intermittent catheterisation (CIC) [6]. Urological surgery, dialysis, and transplantation are not available for the vast majority of children in sub-Saharan Africa. Prevention of CKD is therefore the only option, and, to this end, CIC with anticholinergics represents the mainstay of management.

Spina bifida repair has been performed at CURE Children's Hospital of Uganda (CCHU) since 2000. Ten-year survival of Ugandan children following repair of spina bifida has been reported elsewhere [7]. The aim of this cross-sectional study was to determine the extent of renal complications in surviving children. We also investigated predictors of poor renal outcomes to determine whether children at higher risk might be identified.

2. Patients and Methods

2.1. Study Design and Participants. Eligible patients were identified from the CCHU electronic database according to the following criteria: diagnosis of open spina bifida, presentation between December 2000 and December 2004, and age younger than six months at the time of primary operative closure. To facilitate home visits, the study area was restricted to 16 local districts [7].

Families of all patients recorded as alive were telephoned or visited at home by a research assistant. Surviving children were invited to attend CCHU on a specified date accompanied by a caregiver. They were offered reimbursement of travel costs, provision of meals, and overnight accommodation if required.

Ethical approval was granted by the Institutional Review Board of CCHU.

2.2. Management of Neurogenic Bladder. A basic cystometric test assessing detrusor leak point pressure (DLPP) was conducted shortly after spina bifida repair, or at the first follow-up visit. A DLPP greater than 40cm H_2O was considered to reflect a high risk bladder [8, 9]. Renal tract ultrasound scan was performed at the first follow-up appointment and on all subsequent visits.

The decision to commence CIC was based on the DLPP at initial cystometric evaluation, evidence of renal tract ultrasound abnormalities (predominantly hydronephrosis), and incontinence and its complications, such as pressure sores. Caregivers were trained in the technique of CIC, and a free supply of catheters and the anticholinergic oxybutynin (usually administered intravesically [10]) were provided by the International Federation for Spina Bifida and Hydrocephalus (IFSBH) to families at every visit.

2.3. Data Collection. The following information was obtained from the electronic database and clinical notes: results of cystometric testing; results of ultrasound scans; date of CIC initiation (and reason if given); documentation of urinary tract infections (UTI) with corresponding urine culture results; and comments relating to adherence with CIC. UTI was defined as "febrile or otherwise symptomatic with a positive urine culture" [11].

Informed consent was obtained from all caregivers, and children also completed an assent form. A translator was used in the majority of cases. Separate interviews were conducted with parent and child, covering a range of topics, including continence and CIC. Where there was disagreement between child and caregiver responses; for example, relating to continence, the "worst" response was selected.

Children underwent a physical assessment, including weight, height (where possible), and neurological examination to determine best motor level. Arm span was measured in all children using a tape measure, with the child's back against the wall and arms fully extended at right angles to the trunk. Values for height and arm span were recorded to the nearest millimetre. Height-for-age and BMI-for-age percentile for each child were calculated using *WHO AnthroPlus v1.0.4.*

Blood pressure was measured on the right arm with appropriate cuff selected according to the upper arm circumference. The first reading was taken after the child had been sitting quietly for at least five minutes. The second reading was taken later the same day, towards the end of the assessment, again after the child had been sitting quietly for five minutes.

The lowest values for systolic and diastolic blood pressure were retained and compared to internationally recognised normograms previously validated in Ugandan schoolchildren [12, 13]. Children were considered to be hypertensive if the lowest systolic and/or diastolic blood pressure result was at or above the 95th centile based on their sex, age, and height. Arm span was used as a proxy for height in all children.

Renal tract ultrasound scan was performed, reporting the maximum bipolar renal length, echogenicity, and dilation of the renal collecting system. A blood sample was taken to measure creatinine, and the Schwartz formula was applied to estimate glomerular filtration rate (GFR) [14].

2.4. Statistical Analysis. Since only one child had elevated serum creatinine, we studied markers of renal damage that might predict future development of excretory impairment: evidence of scarring, hydronephrosis, discrepancy in renal size >1cm, and presence of hypertension. All were treated as binary variables.

The following variables were investigated for an association with evidence of renal damage, according to previously published studies: female sex, previous UTI, neurological level (motor), mobility, elevated DLPP, and CIC adherence [3, 15–21]. These were all treated as binary variables. Regarding mobility, children were categorised as either unable to walk or able to walk (with or without walking aids). A DLPP >40cm H_2O is considered to predict an unsafe bladder, but some authors have used a threshold of >30cm H_2O [20, 21]; therefore we investigated both for associations with renal damage.

The Chi-Square test, and Fisher's exact test where appropriate, was used to compare relationships between categorical variables. All analyses were performed using SPSS (version 23 IBM Corp.).

3. Results

3.1. Patient Characteristics. Figure 1 outlines the process of patient identification and inclusion. Of 68 survivors, 66 attended CCHU for assessment. One child became distressed at the prospect of venepuncture and was therefore excluded, leaving 65 children aged 10-14 years in the final analysis.

A total of 13 children had visited the hospital within the last two years; the remainder had been lost to follow-up.

Patient characteristics are summarised in Table 1.

3.2. Management of Neurogenic Bladder. 55 children (85%) had undergone cystometric testing on at least one occasion.

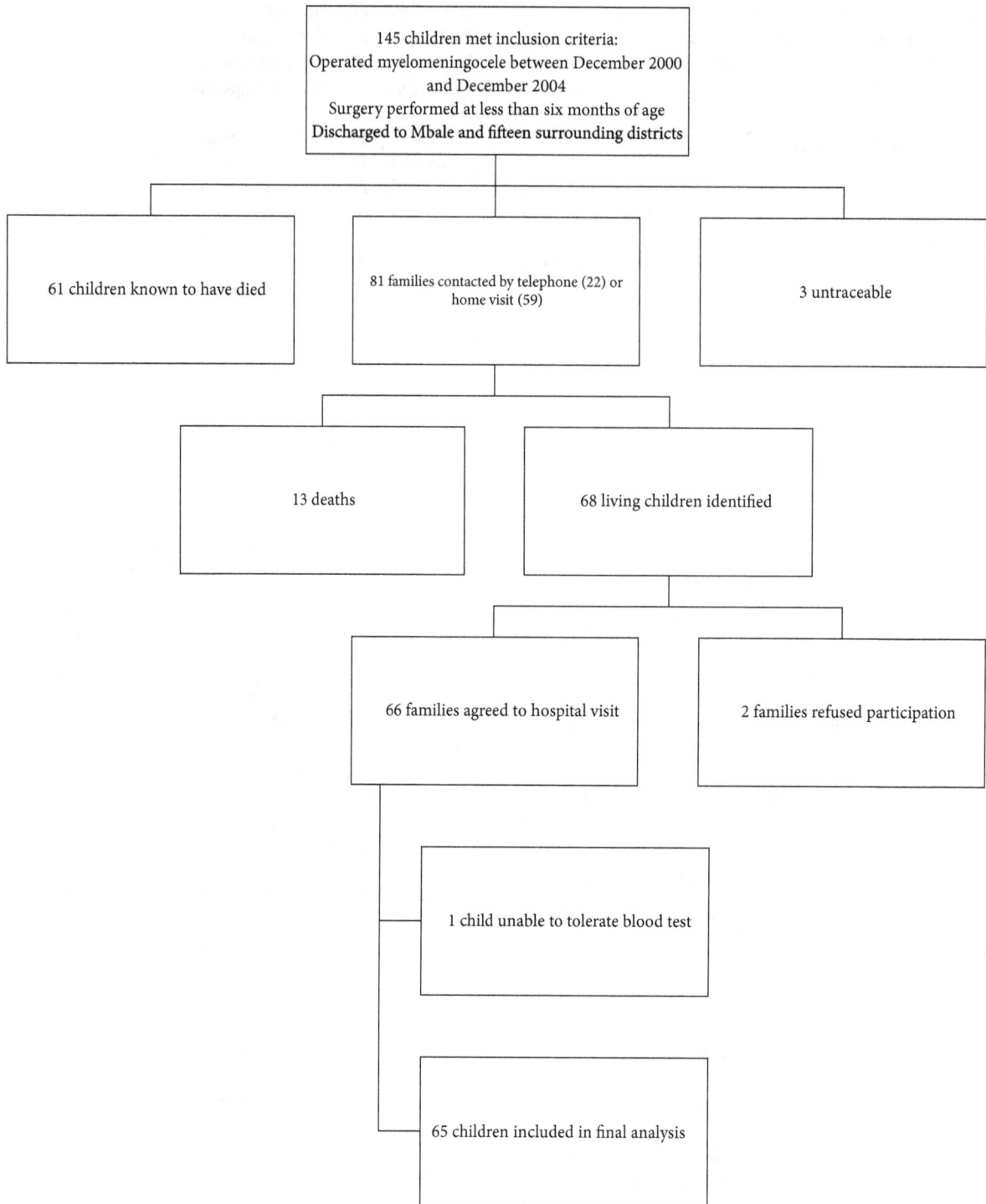

FIGURE 1: Flow diagram for patient inclusion.

Mean age at first testing was six months (range 0-45 months). The mean result for DLPP was 21cm H_2O (range 8-56cm H_2O). The mean DLPP among 24 females was 19.7cm H_2O and it was 21.9cm H_2O among 31 males (no significant difference). Four children had a DLPP greater than 40cm H_2O. Ten children had a DLPP greater than 30cm H_2O.

From notes review there was evidence of CIC training for parents of 60 children (92%) at a mean age of 36 months (range 0-99 months). For the five children in whom CIC was never initiated, one had a very low lesion, was continent, and underwent regular renal tract ultrasound scanning which was repeatedly normal. In the other four cases, notes review did

TABLE 1: Patient characteristics.

	Male (total 36) n (%)	Female (total 29) n (%)
Mean age at assessment (months)	141	146
Current motor level		
L2 and above	5 (14)	2 (7)
L3-L4	15 (42)	16 (55)
L5 and below	16 (44)	11 (38)
Mobility		
Able to walk (with or without aids)	20 (56)	15 (52)
Unable to walk	16 (44)	14 (48)
Detrusor leak point pressure (available for 55 children)		
Greater than 30cm H_2O	5 (14)	5 (17)
Greater than 40cm H_2O	3 (8)	1 (3)
Currently performing CIC		
Yes	7 (19)	10 (35)
No	29 (81)	19 (66)
Continence		
Always dry or mostly dry	3 (8)	8 (28)
Always wet or mostly wet	33 (92)	21 (72)
Previous symptomatic culture positive urinary tract infection		
None documented	17 (47)	12 (41)
At least one	19 (53)	17 (59)
Hypertension (based on height 50th centile)		
Yes	15 (42)	10 (35)
No	21 (58)	19 (66)
Renal scarring on ultrasound scan		
Normal size, shape and echogenicity of both kidneys	15 (42)	8 (28)
Echogenic grade 1 (at least one kidney)	12 (33)	10 (35)
Echogenic grade 2 (at least one kidney)	9 (25)	9 (31)
Echogenic grade 3 (at least one kidney)	0 (0)	2 (7)
Discrepancy in kidney size on ultrasound scan		
Less than 1cm	21 (58)	16 (55)
Greater than 1cm	15 (42)	13 (45)
Hydronephrosis on ultrasound scan		
Yes	5 (14)	5 (17)
No	31 (86)	24 (83)

not identify a deliberate decision, with three of the children defaulting from follow-up immediately or very soon after surgery.

At the time of this study, 17 children (26%) were undergoing CIC. Just over half (nine) were self-catheterising; CIC was performed by a caregiver in the remainder of cases. Intravesical oxybutynin was being used by six children. Of the 43 who had abandoned CIC, reasons given included running out of catheters, lack of time, and the child's distress (notably those in whom CIC had been initiated at an older age). Even among those who were performing CIC at the time of the study, notes review suggested that the majority had historically been inconsistent for similar reasons.

Only one child had undergone surgical intervention for neurogenic bladder: vesicostomy at the age of 13 months. Bladder repair and closure of suprapubic fistula were undertaken four years later.

3.3. Urinary Incontinence. 11 children (17%) were described as "always dry" or "mostly dry," while 54 (83%) were "always wet" or "mostly wet." There was a strong association between urinary continence and the practice of CIC: eight of 17 children (47%) performing CIC and three of 48 (6%) not performing CIC were dry or mostly dry ($p = 0.001$). All three children who were dry and not performing CIC had a motor level at S2 or lower. Boys were more likely than girls to be

TABLE 2: Frequency of hypertension. Hypertension was defined as lowest systolic and/or diastolic blood pressure at or above the 95th centile based on age and height.

	Frequency using arm span as proxy for height (%)	Frequency assuming height at 50th centile for age (%)
Hypertensive	28 (43)	25 (38)
Not hypertensive	37 (57)	40 (62)

incontinent of urine (92% versus 72%, $p = 0.05$), though CIC adherence between the two sexes was not significantly different.

3.4. Historical Urinary Tract Infections. From review of the medical records, 36 children (55%) had experienced at least one urinary tract infection (UTI); only eight children (12%) had two or more documented urinary tract infections.

3.5. Height and Weight. In 37 children (57%) it was not possible to measure height or recumbent length due to joint contractures, muscle weakness, or scoliosis. We therefore elected to use arm span as a proxy for height in all children. For the 28 children in whom values for both height and arm span were obtained, arm span overestimated height by a mean of 4% (range -2% to +13%). Only five children (8%) were at or above the 50th centile for height. 34 children (52%) were below the 1st centile for height. 15 children (23%) were at or above the 50th centile for BMI-for-age. 20 children (31%) were below the 1st centile for BMI-for-age.

3.6. Blood Pressure. 28 children were hypertensive (43%). Since our results suggested that arm span overestimated height in this group, this would tend to underestimate the severity of hypertension. However, since spina bifida is associated with short stature this might overestimate the prevalence of hypertension. Recategorising blood pressure based on an assumption of height at the 50th centile for age for all children, 25 children (38%) were considered to be hypertensive, Table 2.

3.7. Creatinine and Estimated GFR. Creatinine was below the limit of detection for the assay (0.05mg/dL) in 27 children. Nonambulant children were overrepresented in this group, with 21/30 (70%) having a very low creatinine, compared to 6/35 (17%) of children who were ambulant with or without walking aids ($p < 0.001$).

The median creatinine for the group was 0.2mg/dL. Only one child (aged 13 and weighing 13.2kg) had an elevated creatinine at 2 mg/dL (estimated GFR of 35 ml/min/1.73m^2). She had been identified as having a high risk bladder (DLPP 49cm H$_2$O) when she initially presented for surgical repair at the age of four months. Adherence with CIC had been variable, and she had been admitted to CCHU on five occasions with urosepsis.

3.8. Renal Tract Ultrasound. All children underwent an ultrasound scan of the renal tract during the study visit. There was evidence of mild or moderate hydronephrosis in ten children (15%); changes were bilateral in four.

In 42 children (64%) there was increased renal cortical echogenicity, in keeping with scarring. This was graded in severity: grade 1 (mild) in 22 (52%), grade 2 in 18 (43%), and grade 3 (severe) in two (5%). In most cases the changes were bilateral; in 15 children with asymmetrical abnormalities results were classified according to the more severely abnormal kidney.

A discrepancy in maximum bipolar length between left and right kidneys of greater than 1cm was documented in 28 children (43%).

3.9. Risk Factors for Renal Damage. None of the 20 children with a best motor level at S1 or below had hydronephrosis on renal tract ultrasound scan, compared to 22% (10/45) of those with higher motor levels (p = 0.025). However, there was no association between motor level and scarring, discrepancy in renal size, or hypertension. Neither was there any association between mobility and evidence of renal damage (scarring, hydronephrosis, discrepancy in renal size greater than 1 cm, and presence of hypertension).

Unexpectedly, children who were documented as having at least one UTI were less likely to be hypertensive (p = 0.049). Otherwise, there was no association between any other risk factors (female sex, history of UTI, elevated DLPP, and CIC adherence) and any of the outcome measures (Table 3).

4. Discussion

Individuals with spina bifida are at risk of CKD as a consequence of elevated detrusor pressures, vesicoureteric reflux, and recurrent urinary tract infections, leading to renal scarring. End-stage renal disease rarely develops in childhood [11, 22] but has been reported in low-income settings and has been attributed to suboptimal management, including lack of follow-up and failure to initiate CIC with anticholinergic therapy [23, 24].

In this study we evaluated renal outcomes in a cohort of 65 Ugandan children aged 10-14 who had undergone spina bifida repair before six months of age. Urological management was suboptimal, with poor attendance at follow-up and only 17 children (26%) continuing with CIC. Over half of the original cohort were no longer alive (74 of 142 children traced).

4.1. Evidence of Renal Damage. The pitfalls of creatinine measurement in individuals with spina bifida, most of whom have reduced muscle mass, are well-recognised [2, 11, 15]. Furthermore, many of these Ugandan children are likely to have been undernourished. In keeping with this, we found that creatinine was below the limit of detection for the assay

RISK FACTORS	Markers of renal damage			
	Hydronephrosis	Renal scarring	Kidney size discrepancy >1cm	Hypertension
Motor level				
L5 or above	**10/45**	30/45	20/45	18/45
S1 or below	**0/20**	12/20	8/20	7/20
	(p = 0.025)	(p = 0.60)	(p = 0.74)	(p = 0.70)
Mobility				
Unable to walk	7/30	19/30	12/30	13/30
Able to walk (with or without aids)	3/35	23/35	16/35	12/35
	(p = 0.17)	(p = 0.84)	(p = 0.64)	(p = 0.46)
Sex				
Female	5/29	21/29	13/29	10/29
Male	5/36	21/36	15/36	15/36
	(p = 0.74)	(p = 0.24)	(p = 0.80)	(p = 0.55)
Urinary tract infection				
At least one prior UTI	5/29	23/36	17/36	**10/36**
No documented UTI	5/36	19/29	11/29	**15/29**
	(p = 0.74)	(p = 0.89)	(p = 0.45)	**(p = 0.05)**
CIC adherence				
Never performed or abandoned CIC	6/48	30/48	22/48	18/48
Currently performing CIC	4/17	12/17	6/17	7/17
	(p = 0.43)	(p = 0.55)	(p = 0.45)	(p = 0.80)
Detrusor leak point pressure[#]				
DLPP >30	1/10	6/10	6/10	5/10
DLPP <30	8/45	31/45	18/45	17/45
	(p = 1.0)	(p = 0.71)	(p = 0.30)	(p = 0.50)

UTI = urinary tract infection; DLPP = detrusor leak point pressure; [#] DLPP results available for 55 children.

in 27 children (42%); the majority of these children were non-ambulant, suggesting higher lesion levels and consequently reduced muscle mass. Only one child had significant renal impairment defined by eGFR. Ultrasound revealed evidence of scarring in 64% of children and a size discrepancy of more than a centimetre between kidneys in 43%. These changes are consistent with irreversible cortical loss.

Ultrasound is thought to be adequately sensitive for detecting clinically significant renal parenchymal defects [22, 25]. Discrepancy in renal length detected on ultrasound has been found to correlate with abnormal dimercaptosuccinic acid (DMSA) findings in both adult and paediatric populations [26, 27].

In this cohort, 25 children were found to be hypertensive (38%) based on two readings during a single visit. Hypertension is well-recognised among children and young adults with spina bifida [28, 29] and is associated with progression of CKD, as in adults [2]. Treatment of hypertension in a low-income setting is challenging.

4.2. Risk Factors for Renal Damage. Many studies have investigated predictors of poor renal outcomes among patients with spina bifida in high-income countries. In the prospectively followed Cambridge cohort, 22 of 78 deaths (28%) at a mean age of 46 years were attributed to urological causes.

Deaths from urological causes occurred only in those with a sensory level of L1 or above, and there was only one urological death in those with motor level of L2 and below (neurological level assessed at birth) [3]. A cross-sectional study of 120 adults in the Netherlands found that ambulant patients (as opposed to wheelchair users) were unlikely to have unfavourable urodynamic findings [16].

The anatomical explanation for these findings is not obvious, bearing in mind that the innervation of the bladder and urethral sphincter extends as far as S2-S4 [30]. Certainly our results are not so reassuring. While none of the children with a low spinal lesion (motor level S1 and below) had hydronephrosis, there was no significant difference in the incidence of renal scarring, size discrepancy, or hypertension between this group and those with higher motor involvement. Furthermore, there was no correlation between ambulatory status and any of the markers of renal damage. Therefore, low neurological level should not lead to complacency in follow-up.

Our previously published survival study did identify an increased hazard of death among children with motor level L2 and above. Information relating to cause of death was available for 45/58 (78%) children. There was one death due to pyelonephritis (in a child aged 13 months with motor level L1) but no other urological causes were identified [7]. However it is most likely that parents would be unaware of the existence of CKD, and even end-stage renal failure, particularly since the majority of children were not attending follow-up.

Many studies have found an association between various urodynamic parameters and renal damage, though the predictive value of DLPP alone has not always been demonstrated [15, 17–20]. Elevated DLPP (using a cut-off of either >30cm H_2O or >40cm H_2O) measured at a mean age of six months was not found to be associated with renal scarring, kidney size discrepancy, hydronephrosis or hypertension in our cohort. More sophisticated urodynamic testing to formally describe the bladder pathology is not feasible in this setting; a decision to commence CIC based on DLPP results is inadequately sensitive and therefore unsafe.

In this cohort, children with a history of one or more urinary tract infections (UTIs) were less likely to be hypertensive. It is difficult to explain this finding. Some studies have found an association between UTIs during childhood and renal deterioration in later life [15]. Female sex has been identified as a risk factor for renal deterioration [17, 18], but we did not find this association in our relatively small cohort.

Delayed initiation of CIC, late referral, and poor adherence with treatment have all been associated with renal scarring, and the relationship with complex social circumstances has also been noted [17, 18, 20]. These issues are particularly relevant in our patient population and highlight the crucial need for education and support of families of a child with spina bifida.

4.3. Urinary Incontinence. Irrespective of renal tract damage and the development of CKD, urinary continence is an important goal of therapy for patients with neurogenic bladder. Incontinence has been reported to negatively affect quality of life and self-esteem [4, 5]. Two-thirds of patients can achieve social continence with CIC and anticholinergic medication [8], yet the majority of these children (83%) were described as "always wet" or "mostly wet."

The consequences of urinary incontinence will be amplified in a low-income setting, where the cost of nappies is prohibitive, and where laundry and personal care are more challenging. Indeed, we found that urinary incontinence was associated with poorer self-reported quality of life scores in this cohort of children [4]. This issue is also relevant to school attendance in Uganda [31].

4.4. Management of Neurogenic Bladder. The initiation of CIC for this cohort was not universal, prompted by elevated DLPP, abnormalities detected on follow-up ultrasound scans, or incontinence. Of 60 children in whom CIC was initiated, the majority had abandoned the practice. Even among the 17 who were performing CIC at the time of assessment, most had been erratic historically.

The relative merits of an expectant versus a proactive approach to the high risk bladder continue to be debated [8, 9, 22, 32]. An expectant approach requires frequent follow-up and close monitoring [33]. It also assumes that upper tract deterioration is reversible in all patients and does not address bladder compliance changes which may occur very early.

In a low-income setting, limited investigations are available and cost considerations significant. Attendance at long-term follow-up is generally poor. Urological surgery is unaffordable for the majority of families. Later institution of CIC can be difficult for the older child, and the family, to adapt to.

CCHU is one of a very small number of centres throughout Africa managing large numbers of children with spina bifida, supported by IFSBH. Current practice involves early institution of CIC (five times daily) with intravesical oxybutynin in all children following spina bifida repair. Subsequent treatment is tailored according to ultrasound findings and the development of safe urinary continence [22, 34]. While this is regarded as optimal medical management of the neurogenic bladder, outcomes from this cohort raise serious concerns about long-term adherence. In response to the findings of this study, a Spina Bifida Specialist Nurse was appointed in 2015, and the team expanded to include two nurses in 2017. We hope to demonstrate that a long-term relationship between families and an experienced member of staff, established during the first admission, will improve attendance at follow-up and adherence with treatment.

4.5. Limitations. Since this is a retrospective study, our findings are limited by the strong possibility of survival bias. We did not have complete information regarding cause of death, and in most cases we would expect the existence of CKD to be unknown, even if it contributed to or caused death. We did not reproduce findings from other studies in relation to risk factors for renal deterioration. This may, in part, be due to the relatively small size of the cohort.

We were unable to measure height in 57% of our subjects, and therefore we substituted arm span for all children. Arm span is frequently used to monitor growth in children with spina bifida, although the limitations of using it in place of height are well-recognised [35–37]. The study design did not allow for repeat measurements of blood pressure at follow-up visits as advised by international guidelines [12].

5. Conclusions

We have demonstrated that incontinence, ultrasound evidence of renal damage, and hypertension are highly prevalent in a cohort of Ugandan children surviving at least ten years after spina bifida repair, including those children with low neurological lesions (S1 and below) and previously normal DLPP. When treatments such as urological surgery, antihypertensive medication, dialysis, and transplantation are unavailable, prevention is of even greater importance.

Our findings support the early and universal initiation of CIC with anticholinergic therapy in this setting. Enabling families to persevere with this and supporting the transition to self-catheterisation should be a priority.

Disclosure

None of the funders had any involvement in study design, data collection, data analysis, manuscript preparation, or publication decisions.

Acknowledgments

The authors would like to acknowledge the assistance of Hellen Titin, Ezra Bamulikulwaki, Rebecca Muduwa, Moses Mukalu, Simon Omaset, and Melissa Kovacs in the conduct of this study. Dr. Helen J. Sims-Williams has been awarded the Thomas Watts Eden Paediatric Fellowship by the Royal College of Physicians (London). Patient follow-up was supported through Dr. Benjamin C. Warf's John D. and Catherine T. MacArthur Fellowship award.

References

[1] A. L. Albright, "Reflections on developing pediatric neurosurgery in Sub-Saharan Africa," *Journal of neurosurgery. Pediatrics*, vol. 18, no. 1, pp. 127–138, 2016.

[2] T. Müller, K. Arbeiter, and C. Aufricht, "Renal function in meningomyelocele: Risk factors, chronic renal failure, renal replacement therapy and transplantation," *Current Opinion in Urology*, vol. 12, no. 6, pp. 479–484, 2002.

[3] P. Oakeshott, F. Reid, A. Poulton, H. Markus, R. H. Whitaker, and G. M. Hunt, "Neurological level at birth predicts survival to the mid-40s and urological deaths in open spina bifida: a complete prospective cohort study," *Developmental Medicine & Child Neurology*, vol. 57, no. 7, pp. 634–638, 2015.

[4] H. J. Sims-Williams, H. P. Sims-Williams, E. Mbabazi Kabachelor, and B. C. Warf, "Quality of life among children with spina bifida in Uganda," *Archives of Disease in Childhood*, vol. 102, no. 11, pp. 1057–1061, 2017.

[5] C. Moore, B. A. Kogan, and A. Parekh, "Impact of urinary incontinence on self-concept in children with spina bifida," *The Journal of Urology*, vol. 171, no. 4, pp. 1659–1662, 2004.

[6] J. Lapides, A. C. Diokno, S. J. Silber, and B. S. Lowe, "Clean, intermittent self-catheterization in the treatment of urinary tract disease.," *The Journal of Urology*, vol. 107, no. 3, pp. 458–461, 1972.

[7] H. J. Sims-Williams, H. P. Sims-Williams, E. M. Kabachelor, J. Fotheringham, and B. C. Warf, "Ten-year survival of Ugandan infants after myelomeningocele closure," *Journal of Neurosurgery: Pediatrics*, vol. 19, no. 1, pp. 70–76, 2017.

[8] D. Frimberger, E. Cheng, and B. P. Kropp, "The Current Management of the Neurogenic Bladder in Children with Spina Bifida," *Pediatric Clinics of North America*, vol. 59, no. 4, pp. 757–767, 2012.

[9] S. B. Bauer, "Neurogenic bladder: etiology and assessment," *Pediatric Nephrology*, vol. 23, no. 4, pp. 541–551, 2008.

[10] G. Buyse, K. Waldeck, C. Verpoorten, H. Björk, P. Casaer, and K.-E. Andersson, "Intravesical oxybutynin for neurogenic bladder dysfunction: less systemic side effects due to reduced first pass metabolism," *The Journal of Urology*, vol. 160, part 1, no. 3, pp. 892–896, 1998.

[11] G. Filler, M. Gharib, S. Casier, P. Lödige, J. H. H. Ehrich, and S. Dave, "Prevention of chronic kidney disease in spina bifida," *International Urology and Nephrology*, vol. 44, no. 3, pp. 817–827, 2012.

[12] "National High Blood Pressure Education Program Working Group on High Blood Pressure in C, Adolescents (2004) The fourth report on the diagnosis, evaluation, and treatment of high blood pressure in children and adolescents," *Pediatrics*, vol. 114, Supplement 2, pp. 555–576, 2004.

[13] F. Kidy, D. Rutebarika, S. A. Lule et al., "Blood pressure in primary school children in Uganda: A cross-sectional survey," *BMC Public Health*, vol. 14, no. 1, 2014.

[14] G. J. Schwartz, G. B. Haycock, C. M. Edelmann Jr., and A. Spitzer, "A simple estimate of glomerular filtration rate in children derived from body length and plasma creatinine," *Pediatrics*, vol. 58, no. 2, pp. 259–263, 1976.

[15] P. W. Veenboer, J. L. H. R. Bosch, F. W. A. van Asbeck, and L. M. O. de Kort, "Upper and Lower Urinary Tract Outcomes in Adult Myelomeningocele Patients: A Systematic Review," *PLoS ONE*, vol. 7, no. 10, Article ID e48399, 2012.

[16] P. W. Veenboer, J. L. H. R. Bosch, P. F. W. M. Rosier et al., "Cross-sectional study of determinants of upper and lower urinary tract outcomes in adults with spinal dysraphism - New recommendations for urodynamic followup guidelines?" *The Journal of Urology*, vol. 192, no. 2, pp. 477–482, 2014.

[17] S. M. Delair, J. Eandi, M. J. White, T. Nguyen, A. R. Stone, and E. A. Kurzrock, "Renal cortical deterioration in children with spinal dysraphism: analysis of risk factors," *The Journal of Spinal Cord Medicine*, vol. 30, no. 1, pp. S30–S34, 2007.

[18] S. K. Ozel, Z. Dokumcu, C. Akyildiz, A. Avanoglu, and I. Ulman, "Factors affecting renal scar development in children with spina bifida," *Urologia Internationalis*, vol. 79, no. 2, pp. 133–136, 2007.

[19] E. A. Kurzrock and S. Polse, "Renal deterioration in myelodysplastic children: Urodynamic evaluation and clinical correlates," *The Journal of Urology*, vol. 159, no. 5, pp. 1657–1661, 1998.

[20] P. Wide, G. G. Mattsson, and S. Mattsson, "Renal preservation in children with neurogenic bladder-sphincter dysfunction followed in a national program," *Journal of Pediatric Urology*, vol. 8, no. 2, pp. 187–193, 2012.

[21] A. Jeruto, D. Poenaru, and R. Bransford, "Clean Intermittent Catheterization: Overview of Results in 194 Patients with Spina Bifida," *African Journal of Paediatric Surgery*, vol. 1, no. 1, pp. 20–23, 2004.

[22] P. Dik, A. J. Klijn, J. D. van Gool, C. C. E. de Jong-de Vos van Steenwijk, and T. P. V. M. de Jong, "Early start to therapy preserves kidney function in spina bifida patients," *European Urology*, vol. 49, no. 5, pp. 908–913, 2006.

[23] J. A. Kari, "Neuropathic bladder as a cause of chronic renal failure in children in developing countries," *Pediatric Nephrology*, vol. 21, no. 4, pp. 517–520, 2006.

[24] T. T. Mong Hiep, F. Janssen, K. Ismaili, D. Khai Minh, D. Vuong Kiet, and A. Robert, "Etiology and outcome of chronic renal failure in hospitalized children in Ho Chi Minh City, Vietnam," *Pediatric Nephrology*, vol. 23, no. 6, pp. 965–970, 2008.

[25] T. K. Levart, A. Kenig, J. J. Fettich, D. Ključevšek, G. Novljan, and R. B. Kenda, "Sensitivity of ultrasonography in detecting renal parenchymal defects in children," *Pediatric Nephrology*, vol. 17, no. 12, pp. 1059–1062, 2002.

[26] P. W. Veenboer, M. G. G. Hobbelink, J. L. H. Ruud Bosch et al., "Diagnostic accuracy of Tc-99m DMSA scintigraphy and renal ultrasonography for detecting renal scarring and relative

function in patients with spinal dysraphism," *Neurourology and Urodynamics*, vol. 34, no. 6, pp. 513–518, 2015.

[27] M. R. Khazaei, F. Mackie, A. R. Rosenberg, and G. Kainer, "Renal length discrepancy by ultrasound is a reliable predictor of an abnormal DMSA scan in children," *Pediatric Nephrology*, vol. 23, no. 1, pp. 99–105, 2008.

[28] L. Mazur, B. Lacy, and L. Wilsford, "The prevalence of hypertension in children with spina bifida," *Acta Paediatrica*, vol. 100, no. 8, pp. e80–e83, 2011.

[29] B. C. Stepanczuk, B. E. Dicianno, and T. S. Webb, "Young adults with Spina bifida may have higher occurrence of prehypertension and hypertension," *American Journal of Physical Medicine & Rehabilitation*, vol. 93, no. 3, pp. 200–206, 2014.

[30] C. J. Fowler, D. Griffiths, and W. C. de Groat, "The neural control of micturition," *Nature Reviews Neuroscience*, vol. 9, no. 6, pp. 453–466, 2008.

[31] F. Bannink, R. Idro, and G. V. Hove, "Teachers' and Parents' Perspectives on Inclusive Education for Children with Spina Bifida in Uganda," *Journal of Childhood & Developmental Disorders*, vol. 2, no. 2, 2016.

[32] B. Lee, N. Featherstone, P. Nagappan, L. McCarthy, and S. O'Toole, "British Association of Paediatric Urologists consensus statement on the management of the neuropathic bladder," *Journal of Pediatric Urology*, vol. 12, no. 2, pp. 76–87, 2016.

[33] C. V. Hopps and K. A. Kropp, "Preservation of renal function in children with myelomeningocele managed with basic newborn evaluation and close followup," *The Journal of Urology*, vol. 169, no. 1, pp. 305–308, 2003.

[34] T. P. V. M. Jong, R. Chrzan, A. J. Klijn, and P. Dik, "Treatment of the neurogenic bladder in spina bifida," *Pediatric Nephrology*, vol. 23, no. 6, pp. 889–896, 2008.

[35] D. B. Shurtleff, W. O. Walker, S. Duguay, D. Peterson, and D. Cardenas, "Obesity and myelomeningocele: Anthropometric measures," *The Journal of Spinal Cord Medicine*, vol. 33, no. 4, pp. 410–419, 2010.

[36] R. Trollmann, H. G. Dorr, D. Rotenstein, and D. Reigel, "Anthropomorphic measurements of patients with myelomeningocele [2]," *European Journal of Pediatrics*, vol. 155, no. 10, pp. 914-915, 1996.

[37] G. S. Liptak and A. El Samra, "Optimizing health care for children with spina bifida," *Developmental Disabilities Research Reviews*, vol. 16, no. 1, pp. 66–75, 2010.

29

Clinical Presentation, Outcomes, and Treatment of Membranous Nephropathy after Transplantation

Artur Q. B. da Silva (ID),[1] Taina V. de Sandes-Freitas (ID),[2] Juliana B. Mansur,[1] Jose Osmar Medicina-Pestana,[1] and Gianna Mastroianni-Kirsztajn (ID)[1]

[1]Federal University of São Paulo (UNIFESP), São Paulo, SP, Brazil
[2]Federal University of Ceará (UFC), Fortaleza, CE, Brazil

Correspondence should be addressed to Gianna Mastroianni-Kirsztajn; giannamk@uol.com.br

Academic Editor: Franca Anglani

There are scarce data about clinical presentation and outcomes of posttransplant membranous nephropathy (MN), and few reports include a large number of patients. This was a retrospective cohort including adult patients with posttransplant MN transplanted between 1983 and 2015 in a single center (n=41). Only patients with histological diagnosis of MN in kidney grafts were included. Clinical and laboratory presentation, histological findings, treatment, and outcomes were detailed. Patients were predominantly male (58.5%), with a mean age of 49.4 ± 13.2 years; 15 were considered as recurrent primary MN; 3 were class V lupus nephritis; 14 were considered as *de novo* cases, 7 secondary and 7 primary MN; and 9 cases were considered primary but it was not possible to distinguish between *de novo* MN and recurrence. Main clinical presentations were proteinuria (75.6%) and graft dysfunction (34.1%). Most patients with primary recurrent and *de novo* primary MN were submitted to changes in maintenance immunosuppressive regimen, but no standard strategy was identified; 31 patients presented partial or complete remission, and glomerulopathy appeared not to impact graft and patient survival.

1. Introduction

Membranous nephropathy (MN) is a common cause of nephrotic syndrome, and it is a prototype of autoimmune glomerular diseases [1]. In native kidneys, MN is more common in white men, adults in the fourth or fifth decade of life, and the elderly population [2]. It can be idiopathic in 70-80% of cases or secondary to infections (hepatitis B and C), drugs, neoplasia, systemic lupus erythematosus (SLE), and others [3]. Membranous nephropathy may occur in renal allografts as a recurrent or *de novo* disease [1]. Incidence of recurrent MN ranges from 10 to 45% and its impacts on transplants outcomes are controversial [4]. Recent findings in idiopathic MN suggest that in most patients the disease is caused by PLA2R autoantibodies. Such autoantibodies are involved in 50-60% of the cases of recurrent MN. Monitoring anti-PLA2R titers during follow-up helps to predict MN recurrence, and certain immunosuppressive treatments of anti-PLA2R positive patients may prevent recurrence [5, 6].

Nevertheless, this is not a marker that reveals the development of MN in all cases. It was already reported that some patients with anti-PLA2R antibodies at the time of transplantation would not develop MN recurrence [5, 7–9].

There are scarce data about clinical presentation and outcomes of posttransplant MN, and few reports include a large number of patients. Thus, all additional information about this glomerulopathy can be useful in patient management. This study aimed to describe clinical, laboratorial, and histological characteristics, as well as treatment and outcomes of patients with posttransplant MN in a high-volume transplant center.

2. Methods

2.1. Design and Population. This retrospective cohort included adult patients with posttransplant MN transplanted between 1983 and 2015 in a single center that performs about 900 transplants per year. Only patients with histological diagnosis (optical microscopy and immunofluorescence) of MN in kidney grafts were included. Patients were identified through biopsies database and/or were selected from those followed in the Glomerulopathies Section. Protocol biopsies are not routinely performed in the center. Data were obtained from medical records and electronic databases. The study protocol was approved by the local Ethics Committee (CAAE: 24309913.1.0000.5505).

2.2. Definitions. Proteinuria was defined as urinary protein excretion superior to 0.3 g per day in a 24-hour urine collection or 0.3g/g in protein-to-creatinine ratio (UPr/Cr) determined in a random urine specimen [10].

Renal function was assessed by serum creatinine (Cr) or by estimated glomerular filtration rate (eGFR) using 4-variable MDRD formula [11]. The last observation carried forward (LOCF) adjustment was used for missing GFR values, attributing 10 mL/min to patients who lost the graft and the last available value for those who died or lost follow-up. Baseline serum Cr was obtained by the average of last three measurements performed before posttransplant MN diagnosis. Graft dysfunction was defined as $\geq$ 50% or $\geq$ 0.3 mg/dL increase in baseline serum Cr confirmed in two different measurements.

Partial remission was defined as Cr stabilization in a value up to 25% above the baseline level associated with decrease of proteinuria by 50% or greater and <3.0 g/g when initial values were above 3.0 g/g. Complete remission was defined as serum Cr stabilization associated with proteinuria <0.3 g/g [12]. Spontaneous remission was defined as partial or complete remission without additional immunosuppressive treatment. All renal biopsies were processed according to standard techniques for light microscopy and immunofluorescence microscopy. Electron microscopy was not performed.

The immunosuppressive therapy was individualized according to our center protocols. Induction therapy, when indicated, consisted of anti-CD25 monoclonal antibodies or antithymocyte globulin; maintenance immunosuppression was based on calcineurin inhibitor (CNI, cyclosporine or tacrolimus) plus steroid and an antiproliferative drug (mycophenolate, azathioprine, or mTOR inhibitor).

2.3. Statistical Analysis. Categorical variables were expressed as frequency and percentages and compared using Chisquare or Fisher's exact test. Continuous variables were presented as mean and standard deviation (SD) and median when indicated; comparison between groups was performed using the Student's *t*-test. Survival analysis was obtained using the Kaplan-Meier method. Statistical analysis was performed using IBM SPSS® 22 Statistics software, and p value was considered significant when <5%.

3. Results

3.1. Demographics. Between 1983 and 2015, 12,643 kidney transplants (KT) were performed and 41 patients with posttransplant MN were identified. Patients were predominantly male (58.5%), with a mean age of 49.4 ± 13.2 years; 36.6% presented documented MN as chronic kidney disease etiology.

Most patients received kidneys from living donors (63.4%) with a mean age of 38.1 ± 16.3 years.

Most patients received no induction therapy (78.1%) and the initial maintenance immunosuppressive regimen was based on calcineurin inhibitor, steroid, and azathioprine in 56.1%, in accordance with the transplant center protocol during the study period. More detailed information about demographics is available in Table 1.

3.2. Clinical Presentation. Fifteen cases were considered as recurrent primary MN as patients have chronic kidney disease (CKD) due to biopsy-confirmed MN; 3 were class V lupus nephritis: 2 of this had previous diagnosis of lupus and 1 was classified as unknown etiology for CKD; 14 had defined causes for renal disease and were considered as *de novo* cases: 7 showed an underlying cause for posttransplant MN and were considered as secondary (brain, uterus, anus, thyroid, and prostate neoplasias, hepatitis C, and hepatitis B) and 7 were primary posttransplant MN; and 9 cases were considered primary but it was not possible to distinguish between *de novo* MN and recurrence, as patients had CKD for unknown or nonspecific chronic glomerulonephritis.

The most frequent initial manifestations of posttransplant MN were proteinuria (75.6%, 3.2 ± 1.2 g) and graft dysfunction (34.1%). Proteinuria > 0.3 g/day was observed at a median time of 40 months (ranging from 4 to 74) after KT. The mean levels of serum albumin and cholesterol were 3.4 ± 0.6g/dL and 198.8 ± 58.6 mg/dL, respectively. Compared to baseline values, eGFR decreased 26.8 ± 16.4% at diagnosis. Diagnostic allograft biopsy was performed 3.7 ± 2.5 months after the onset of proteinuria and a median time of 41 months (ranging from 12.3 to 87.8) after KT. MN stage 2 was the main histological presentation (60.9%), followed by stages 1 (24.4%) and 3 (14.7%) (Table 2).

3.3. Treatment. Patients with secondary posttransplant MN received renoprotection and treatment of underlying disease. Among patients with primary forms, 15 (45.5%) received angiotensin-converting enzyme inhibitors (ACEI) and/or angiotensin II receptor blockers (ARB). Maintenance immunosuppressive regimen was modified in 20 of the 33 patients (60.6%) with primary MN: 9 patients received high oral prednisone doses ($\geq$0.5mg/kg/day), with or without methylprednisolone pulse therapy; 4 patients were converted from azathioprine to mycophenolate; mTOR inhibitors were withdrawn in 3 patients, 2 of which were maintained temporarily on dual immunosuppressive regimen and 1 received mycophenolate instead; in 4 patients, modified Ponticelli regimen [14] was indicated, and antiproliferative drug was withdrawn. No patient received rituximab.

3.4. Outcomes. Fifteen patients had an apparently spontaneous remission. There were no significant differences between patients who presented spontaneous remission and those who did not remit or only remitted after immunosuppressive therapy concerning recipient age (47.6 ± 14.7 versus 50.4 ± 12.4 years old, p=0.514); donor source (living) (60 versus 65.4%, p=0.749); time since KT at diagnosis (36.8 ± 38.7 versus 62.9 ± 56 months, p=0.118); serum creatinine (1.7 ± 0.8

TABLE 1: Demographic characteristics of patients with posttransplant MN.

Variables	N = 41
Recipient gender – male, n(%)	24 (58.5)
Recipient age (years), mean ± DP	49.4 ± 13.2
Pretransplant dialysis, n(%)	40 (97.5)
Time on dialysis (months), mean ± DP	22.6 ± 24.1 (median = 16)
Etiology of end-stage renal disease, n(%)	
Membranous nephropathy	15 (36.6)
Lupus nephritis	2 (4.9)
Unknown	9 (22)
Chronic glomerulonephritis	5 (12.2)
Hypertension	5 (12.2)
Diabetes	2 (4.9)
Chronic pyelonephritis	1 (2.4)
Urological	1 (2.4)
Cortical necrosis	1 (2.4)
Panel reactive antibodies (%), mean ± DP	7.85 ± 22.6 (median = 0)
Donor source, n(%)	
Living	26 (63.4)
HLA identical	6 (14.6)
HLA haploidentical	16 (39)
HLA distinct	4 (9.8)
Deceased	15 (36.6)
Standard criteria donor	10 (24.4)
Expanded criteria donor[1]	5 (12.2)
Donor age (years), mean ± DP	38.1 ± 16.3
HLA mismatches, mean ± DP	2.3 ± 1.8
Cold ischemia time (hours), mean ± DP	25 ± 9
Induction therapy, n(%)	
None	32 (78.1)
Basiliximab	1 (2.4)
Thymoglobulin	8 (19.5)
Initial immunosuppressive regimen, n(%)	
CNI-PRED-AZA	23 (56.1)
CNI-PRED-MPA	14 (34.1)
CNI PRED-SRL	4 (9.8)

PRED: prednisone; CNI: calcineurin inhibitor; AZA: azathioprine; MPA: mycophenolic acid; SRL: sirolimus; HLA: human leukocyte antigens.
[1]United Network for Organ Sharing (UNOS) criteria [13].

versus 1.8 ± 1.5 mg/dL, p=0.835); proteinuria (3.5 ± 4.4 versus 2.9 ± 2.6 g, p=0.613); posttransplant MN category (recurrence) (48.4 versus 20%, p=0.152); or maintenance immunosuppression with mycophenolate (34.6 versus 33.3%, p=1.000).

Partial and complete remissions were observed in 25 (61%) and 11 (26.8%) patients, respectively, and occurred 358 ± 180 days after diagnosis (Table 3). Patients who presented partial or complete remissions were younger (46.8 ± 12.3 versus 57.3 ± 13.2, p=0.027), a higher proportion received living donor transplants (74.2 versus 30%, p=0.022), and a lower proportion was on mycophenolate (22.6 versus 70%, p=0.017) (Table 4).

One year after posttransplant MN diagnosis, proteinuria and serum creatinine were 2.6 ± 3 g/24h and 2.2 ± 1.1 mg/dL,

respectively. Adjusting for losses and deaths, mean eGFR was 34.2 ± 18.7 mL/min (Table 3). 1-, 3-, 5-, and 10-year patient survival was 97.5%, 94.7%, 88.3%, and 88.3%, respectively. Causes of death were infection (n=2), cardiovascular event (n=1), malignancy (n=1), and unknown (n=1). Death-censored graft survival at these periods was 95.1%, 86.9%, 86.9%, and 68.4%, respectively. Five of the 13 graft losses were attributed to posttransplant MN, and the remaining 8 cases were due to unspecific interstitial fibrosis and tubular atrophy.

As expected, one year after posttransplant MN diagnosis, patients who presented partial or complete remission showed lower serum creatinine (2.0 ± 1.0 versus 2.8 ± 1.3 mg/dL, p=0.049), higher eGFR (41.8 ± 18.9 versus 27.0 ± 12.9 mL/min, p=0.028), and lower proteinuria (1.5 ± 1.6 versus 6.1 ± 3.7 g, p<0.001). During the follow-up, there was a trend for a

TABLE 2: Clinical presentation of patients with posttransplant MN.

Variables	N = 41
Proteinuria > 0.3 g/g or g/24h, n(%)	31 (75.6)
Proteinuria[1] (g/g or g/24h), mean ± DP	3.2 ± 1.2
Time to onset of proteinuria > 0.3 g/g or g/24h (months), mean ± DP	49.5 ± 49.7 (median = 40)
Serum albumin[1] (g/dL), mean ± DP	3.4 ± 0.6
Serum total cholesterol[1] (mg/dL), mean ± DP	198.8 ± 58.6
Serum triglycerides[1] (mg/dL), mean ± DP	178.5 ± 78.7
Systolic blood pressure[1] (mmHg), mean ± DP	131 ± 7.8
Diastolic blood pressure[1] (mmHg), mean ± DP	82.2 ± 6.5
Graft dysfunction[1], n(%)	14 (34.1)
Serum creatinine[1] (mg/dL), mean ± DP	1.7 ± 0.6
eGFR[1] (mL/min/1.73m^2), mean ± DP	41.9 ± 14.3
eGFR decrease[1] (%), mean ± DP	26.8 ± 16.4
Time between proteinuria and graft biopsy (months), mean ± DP	3.7 ± 2.5
Time between KT and graft biopsy (months), mean ± DP	53.4 ± 51.5 (median = 41)
Histological stages of MN, n(%)	
Stage 1	10 (24.4)
Stage 2	25 (60.9)
Stage 3	6 (14.7)

eGFR: estimated glomerular filtration rate; KT: kidney transplant.
[1] At diagnosis.

TABLE 3: Posttransplant MN outcomes.

Variables	N = 41
Time on follow-up (months), mean ± DP	108.2 ± 52.8
Partial remission, n(%)	20 (48.78)
Complete remission, n(%)	11 (26.8)
Spontaneous remission, n(%)	15 (36.6)
Time to remission since diagnosis (days), mean ± DP	358 ± 180
Proteinuria (g/g or g/24h)[1], mean ± DP	2.6 ± 3 (median = 2)
Serum creatinine (mg/dL)[1], mean ± DP	2.2 ± 1.1
eGFR (mL/min/1.73m^2)[1], mean ± DP[1]	38.2 ± 19.5
eGFR - LOCF (mL/min/1.73m^2)[1], mean ± DP	34.2 ± 18.7

eGFR: estimated glomerular filtration rate; LOCF: last observation carried forward.
[1] 1 year after diagnosis.

lower rate of deaths in patients who remitted (6.5 versus 30%, p=0.083), but the rate of graft loss was similar (35.5 versus 50%, p=0.472).

4. Discussion

This study evaluated demography, clinical and histological presentation, treatment, and outcomes of a relatively large cohort of patients with posttransplant MN.

Unfortunately, a high proportion of patients did not have a confirmed diagnosis of chronic kidney disease (CKD) etiology (unknown and not defined chronic glomerulonephritis), which impairs the precise classification on recurrent and de novo cases. Besides, it is possible that some patients considered as having CKD due to hypertension actually have other underlying causes and that hypertension is secondary to renal disease.

More than a half of our cohort consisted of living donor transplants. This probably reflects the local practice in the early years of our transplant program, when living donor transplants were more common. The impact of the donor type on the risk of MN recurrence remains controversial [15].

Initial clinical and/or laboratorial presentation occurred late after KT and high proportion of patients presented nephrotic proteinuria, hypoalbuminemia, dyslipidemia, and graft dysfunction. Two patterns of MN recurrence were previously described [16]: "early recurrence" (within the first 6 months after KT), more common between living related donation, is generally oligosymptomatic, with mild proteinuria; on the other hand, "late recurrence" usually evolves with overt nephrotic syndrome. Since we did not perform protocol biopsies, even in the presence of isolated subnephrotic proteinuria, most of our cases were diagnosed in later stages. In this regard, we cannot rule out a higher

TABLE 4: Risk factors for posttransplant MN remission.

Variables	Partial or complete remission N=31	No remission N=10	p value
Recipient age (years old), mean ± DP	46.8 ± 12.3	57.3 ± 13.2	0.027
Time after KT at diagnosis (months), mean ± DP	54.6 ± 53.7	49.4 ± 46.4	0.782
Serum creatinine at diagnosis (mg/dL), mean ± DP	1.6 ± 0.7	2.1 ± 2.3	0.351
Proteinuria at diagnosis (g/24h or g/g), mean ± DP	2.9 ± 3.2	4.1 ± 3.5	0.337
Living donor, n(%)	23 (74.2)	3 (30)	0.022
RAAS blockade, n(%)	26 (83)	9 (90)	1.000
Change in maintenance IS after diagnosis, n(%)	16 (51)	4 (40)	0.719
Treatment with high dose steroids, n(%)	14 (45.2)	3 (30)	0.480
Treatment with Ponticelli scheme, n(%)	1 (3.2)	2 (20)	0.142

KT: kidney transplant; RAAS: *renin angiotensin aldosterone system.*

rate of subclinical MN recurrence in our patients, as renal biopsies were not always performed in the absence of overt proteinuria.

Regarding specific treatment, we observed a wide variety of approaches and a lack of standardization. This was probably due to the lack of a gold standard treatment for this glomerulopathy in KT recipients, who are already on immunosuppressive therapy. More recently, good results were described with the anti-CD20 rituximab for posttransplant MN treatment and prophylaxis. However, evidence is based on small sample size noncontrolled studies. Ideal dose and safety are important aspects to be evaluated [16–18]. Noteworthy, rituximab is not available or reimbursed by Brazilian government for this off-label clinical indication.

As expected and widely reported for MN on native kidneys and allografts, about one-third of patients presented spontaneous remission [17, 19] and the majority of patients had complete or partial remission. The impact of posttransplant MN on allograft survival remains controversial [4]. In fact, in our study graft and patient survival were similar to those previously reported by our center [20–22].

Although the sample did not allow robust conclusions, we observed that remission rates were more frequent in younger recipients receiving living donor kidneys. Higher remission rates in younger patients were previously reported by studies on native kidneys [23]. However, to the best of our knowledge, there are no previous reports linking remission rates and donor source.

This study has some limitations that should be pointed out: (a) it is a single center, retrospective study, including patients transplanted in different decades; (b) it was not possible to estimate posttransplant MN incidence, since there was not a systematic recording or database for glomerular diseases in our center; (c) we did not assessed the antibodies against phospholipase A2 receptors (PLA2R) and thrombospondin type I domain-containing 7A (THSD7A), whose presence and intensity are related to recurrence; and (d) C4d

was not routinely performed on graft biopsies. As strengths, this is a relatively large sample size, considering the low prevalence of the disease. Besides, the detailed description of diagnosis and treatment adds important information about the clinical management of such patients.

In summary late onset proteinuria, hypoalbuminemia, hypercholesterolemia, and graft dysfunction were the main clinical manifestations of posttransplant MN. RAAS blockade was common and there was not a standard treatment. The course was benign, with high proportion of remission rates and no impact on survival.

Disclosure

The data of this article has been presented as a poster at 54th ERA-EDTA Congress and it was published as abstract in *Nephrology Dialysis Transplantation*, Volume 32, Issue suppl_3, 1 May 2017, Pages iii503, https://doi.org/10.1093/ndt/gfx165.MP205.

Acknowledgments

The authors are especially grateful to Professor Marcello Fabiano de Franco (*in memoriam*) for his invaluable contribution to Renal Pathology in Brazil. Artur Q. B. da Silva was supported by a CNPq grant during this study.

References

[1] P. A. Carmo, G. Mastroianni-Kirsztajn, W. B. Carmo, M. F. Franco, and M. G. Bastos, "Histopathological findings in elderly patients," *Jornal Brasileiro de Nefrologia*, vol. 32, no. 3, pp. 282–287, 2010.

[2] J. K. J. Deegens and J. F. M. Wetzels, "Membranous nephropathy in the older adult: Epidemiology, diagnosis and management," *Drugs & Aging*, vol. 24, no. 9, pp. 717–732, 2007.

[3] R. J. Glassock, "The pathogenesis of idiopathic membranous nephropathy: a 50-year odyssey," *American Journal of Kidney Diseases*, vol. 56, no. 1, pp. 157–167, 2010.

[4] F. G. Cosio and D. C. Cattran, "Recent advances in our understanding of recurrent primary glomerulonephritis after kidney transplantation," *Kidney International*, vol. 91, no. 2, pp. 304–314, 2017.

[5] A. Kattah, R. Ayalon, L. H. Beck Jr. et al., "Anti-phospholipase A$_2$ receptor antibodies in recurrent membranous nephropathy," *American Journal of Transplantation*, vol. 15, no. 5, pp. 1349–1359, 2015.

[6] B. Seitz-Polski, C. Payré, D. Ambrosetti et al., "Prediction of membranous nephropathy recurrence after transplantation by monitoring of anti-PLA2R1 (M-type phospholipase A2 receptor) autoantibodies: A case series of 15 patients," *Nephrology Dialysis Transplantation*, vol. 29, no. 12, pp. 2334–2342, 2014.

[7] R. Stahl, E. Hoxha, and K. Fechner, "PLA2R autoantibodies and recurrent membranous nephropathy after transplantation," *The New England Journal of Medicine*, vol. 363, no. 5, pp. 496–498, 2010.

[8] L. F. Quintana, M. Blasco, M. Seras et al., "Antiphospholipase A2 receptor antibody levels predict the risk of posttransplantation recurrence of membranous nephropathy," *Transplantation*, vol. 99, no. 8, pp. 1709–1714, 2015.

[9] H. Debiec, L. Martin, C. Jouanneau et al., "Autoantibodies specific for the phospholipase A 2 receptor in recurrent and de novo membranous nephropathy," *American Journal of Transplantation*, vol. 11, no. 10, pp. 2144–2152, 2011.

[10] M.-P. M. Mayayo, M. Martinez Alonso, J. M. Valdivielso Revilla, and E. Fernández-Giráldez, "A new gender-specific formula to estimate 24-hour urine protein from protein to creatinine ratio," *Nephron*, vol. 133, no. 4, pp. 232–238, 2016.

[11] L. Czyżewski, J. Wyzgał, E. Czyżewska et al., "Performance of the MDRD, CKD-EPI, and cockcroft-gault formulas in relation to nutritional status in stable renal transplant recipients," *Transplantation Proceedings*, vol. 48, no. 5, pp. 1494–1497, 2016.

[12] B. Seitz-Polski, G. Lambeau, and V. Esnault, "Membranous nephropathy: Pathophysiology and history," *Nephrol Ther*, vol. 13, 1, pp. S75–S81, 2017.

[13] U.S. Health Resources and Services Administration United Network for Organ Sharing, "Policies and rationale for transplantation of organs for foreign nationals and exportation of organs outside the United States; general notice," *Fed Regist*, vol. 53, pp. 8977-8978, 1988.

[14] C. Ponticelli, P. Zucchelli, P. Passerini et al., "A 10-year follow-up of a randomized study with methylprednisolone and chlorambucil in membranous nephropathy," *Kidney International*, vol. 48, no. 5, pp. 1600–1604, 1995.

[15] G. Moroni, B. Gallelli, S. Quaglini et al., "Long-term outcome of renal transplantation in patients with idiopathic membranous glomerulonephritis (MN)," *Nephrology Dialysis Transplantation*, vol. 25, no. 10, pp. 3408–3415, 2010.

[16] B. Sprangers, G. I. Lefkowitz, S. D. Cohen et al., "Beneficial effect of rituximab in the treatment of recurrent idiopathic membranous nephropathy after kidney transplantation," *Clinical Journal of the American Society of Nephrology*, vol. 5, no. 5, pp. 790–797, 2010.

[17] A. Grupper, L. D. Cornell, F. C. Fervenza, L. H. Beck, E. Lorenz, and F. G. Cosio, "Recurrent membranous nephropathy after kidney transplantation: treatment and long-term implications," *Transplantation*, vol. 100, no. 12, pp. 2710–2716, 2016.

[18] Z. M. El-Zoghby, J. P. Grande, M. G. Fraile, S. M. Norby, F. C. Fervenza, and F. G. Cosio, "Recurrent idiopathic membranous nephropathy: early diagnosis by protocol biopsies and treatment with anti-CD20 monoclonal antibodies," *American Journal of Transplantation*, vol. 9, no. 12, pp. 2800–2807, 2009.

[19] T. S. Dabade, J. P. Grande, S. M. Norby, F. C. Fervenza, and F. G. Cosio, "Recurrent idiopathic membranous nephropathy after kidney transplantation: A surveillance biopsy study," *American Journal of Transplantation*, vol. 8, no. 6, pp. 1318–1322, 2008.

[20] J. O. Medina-Pestana, N. Z. Galante, H. Tedesco-Silva Jr. et al., "Kidney transplantation in Brazil and its geographic disparity," *Jornal Brasileiro de Nefrologia*, vol. 33, no. 4, pp. 472–484, 2011.

[21] J. Medina Pestana, "Excellence and efficiency through a structured large scale approach: the hospital do rim in São Paulo, Brazil," *Transplantation*, vol. 101, no. 8, pp. 1735–1738, 2017.

[22] D. B. Cordeiro Cabral, T. V. de Sandes-Freitas, J. O. Medina-Pestana, and G. Mastroianni-Kirsztajn, "Clinical features, treatment and prognostic factors of post-transplant immunoglobulin a nephropathy," *Annals of Transplantation*, vol. 23, pp. 166–175, 2018.

[23] N. Polanco, E. Gutiérrez, F. Rivera et al., "Spontaneous remission of nephrotic syndrome in membranous nephropathy with chronic renal impairment," *Nephrology Dialysis Transplantation*, vol. 27, no. 1, pp. 231–234, 2012.

30

High Serum Alkaline Phosphatase, Hypercalcaemia, Race, and Mortality in South African Maintenance Haemodialysis Patients

Bala Waziri, Raquel Duarte, and Saraladevi Naicker

Department of Internal Medicine, Faculty of Health Sciences, University of the Witwatersrand, Johannesburg, South Africa

Correspondence should be addressed to Bala Waziri; balawaziri@gmail.com

Academic Editor: Jaime Uribarri

Objective. To determine the association between serum total alkaline phosphatase (TAP) and mortality in African maintenance haemodialysis patients (MHD). *Patients and Methods.* The study enrolled a total of 213 patients on MHD from two dialysis centers in Johannesburg between January 2009 and March 2016. Patients were categorized into a low TAP group ($\leq$112 U/L) versus a high TAP group (>112 U/L) based on a median TAP of 112 U/L. *Results.* During the follow-up period of 7 years, there were 55 (25.8%) deaths. After adjusting for cofounders such as age, other markers of bone disorder, and comorbidity (diabetes mellitus), patients in the high TAP group had significantly higher risk of death compared to patients in the low TAP group (hazard ratio, 2.50; 95% CI 1.24–5.01, $P = 0.01$). Similarly, serum calcium >2.75 mmol/L was associated with increased risk of death compared to patients within levels of 2.10–2.37 mmol/L (HR 6.34, 95% CI 1.40–28.76; $P = 0.02$). The HR for death in white patients compared to black patients was 6.88; 95% CI 1.82–25.88; $P = 0.004$. *Conclusion.* High levels of serum alkaline phosphatase, hypercalcaemia, and white race are associated with increased risk of death in MHD patients.

1. Introduction

Prior to the availability of commercial intact parathyroid hormone (PTH) assays, serum total alkaline phosphatase (TAP) measurements were used as one of the surrogate markers of high bone turnover that was utilized in the management of chronic kidney disease mineral and bone disorder (CKD-MBD) [1]. Subsequently, in 2003 the Kidney Disease Outcome Quality Initiative (KDOQI) guidelines on CKD-MBD made no recommendations regarding the use of alkaline phosphatase and this has made it a less preferred marker to PTH. However, in 2009 the Kidney Disease Improving Global Outcomes (KDIGO) guidelines recommended measurement of TAP every 12 months in CKD 4-5D [2] and more recently evidence continued to emerge on the importance of higher levels of alkaline phosphatase in the pathogenesis of vascular calcification via hydrolysis of pyrophosphate which is a potent inhibitor of vascular calcification [3–5]. This was further supported by a study that showed elevated levels of alkaline phosphatase, independent of PTH, calcium, or phosphorus as predictor of coronary artery calcification in haemodialysis patients [6]. Interestingly, in a recent secondary analysis

of the handling erythropoietin resistance with oxypentifylline (HERO) trial, high levels of alkaline phosphatase were also associated with erythropoietin stimulating agent hyporesponsiveness [7]. These findings may likely explain the unclear pathophysiologic link between high serum alkaline phosphatase and mortality in haemodialysis patients [6].

Although the role of racial disparities in adverse clinical outcomes remains controversial and inconclusive, some studies have demonstrated survival benefits attributable to race in patients undergoing MHD [8, 9]. In addition, the impact of these biochemical abnormalities have been shown to differ across race and thus the need for race specific target values for these markers of mineral bone disorder [10, 11].

Therefore, the aim of this study was to determine if there is a link between high serum alkaline phosphatase and mortality in African MHD patients.

2. Patients and Methods

This study was a retrospective review of patients undergoing MHD from two dialysis centers in Johannesburg between

January 2009 and March 2016. A total of 213 patients aged ≥ 18 years with available baseline line variables of interest were included. Exclusion criteria included patients with missing important data for analysis, being on dialysis for less than three months, having active or chronic liver disease, and having malignancies. In addition, we excluded Indian and mixed races to allow for a proper comparison between black and white patients. Retrieved data included patients' demographic characteristics, blood pressure measurements, duration on haemodialysis, comorbid disease, and medication history related to CKD-MBD. Determination of race was based on self-report by the participants.

Patients were categorized into the low TAP group (≤112 U/L) versus the high TAP group (>112 U/L) based on median TAP level of 112 U/L. Secondary analysis involved exploring the relationship between race, other markers of mineral bone disorder, and primary outcome. In line with a previous study [12] total calcium levels were categorized into four categories with the KDOQI target range as the reference category. Based on the KDIGO CKD-MBD guidelines, PTH was divided into three categories.

The primary outcome of this study was death and events other than death were censored and this included kidney transplantation, loss to follow-up, or still undergoing haemodialysis at the end of the study.

2.1. Laboratory Measurements.

Patients' baseline biochemical parameters (within the first three months of initiating dialysis) were assessed. Most of the biochemical markers were measured monthly except for quarterly PTH. Plasma intact PTH was measured by an electrochemiluminescence immunoassay (ECLIA) run on a Cobas 6000 autoanalyzer (Roche Diagnostics, Mannheim, Germany; reference range 10–65 pg/mL). Serum 25-OH vitamin D was measured by a chemiluminescent microparticle immunoassay (CMIA) technique run on the ARCHITECT C8000 autoanalyzer (Abbott Laboratories, Abbott Park, IL, US). Reference ranges are as follows: <10 ng/mL as severe deficiency, 10–29 ng/mL as moderate deficiency, 30–100 ng/mL as sufficiency, and >100 ng/mL as toxic.

Serum calcium, phosphate, and alkaline phosphatase were measured using the ARCHITECT C8000 autoanalyzer (Abbot Laboratories, Abbott Park, IL, US). The corrected calcium was determined using the formula: corrected calcium (mmol/L) = calcium measured (mmol/L) + 0.02 [40-albumin (g/L)]. Total alkaline phosphatase reference range is 53–128 U/L.

Plasma albumin was measured by colorimetric (bromocresol green) method on a Cobas 6000 autoanalyzer (Roche Diagnostics, Mannheim, Germany; reference range 35–52 g/L).

Other biochemical parameters were determined using routine laboratory techniques.

Blood samples were generally collected predialysis at midweek with the exception of the postdialysis serum urea for kinetic modeling.

Calculation of normalized protein catabolic rate was based on the formula [13], nPCR = $(0.136 \times F) + 0.251$, where $F = $ Kt/V $\times$ ([predialysis BUN + postdialysis BUN] $\div$ 2).

2.2. Statistical Analyses.

Pearson's or Fisher's exact test was utilized for proportion comparisons. Continuous variables are presented as means ± standard deviations or median and interquartile range (IQR) as appropriate. Associations between serum alkaline phosphatase and other biochemical parameters were assessed by multiple linear regression analyses. The Cox proportional model was used to determine the crude and adjusted hazard ratios of death for different categories of serum alkaline phosphatase, calcium, PTH, phosphate, 25-OH vitamin D, and white versus black patients. Patients' demographic and baseline characteristics were compared between the low and high total alkaline phosphatase groups as well as white versus black patients, using an independent t-test and Mann–Whitney U test for normally distributed and nonnormally distributed variables, respectively. One-way ANOVA and Kruskal-Wallis tests were used to compare normally and nonnormally distributed continuous variables across categories of serum calcium.

A P value of less than 0.05 was considered statistically significant at the 95% confidence interval. All analyses were performed using STATA version 12 (STATA Corp., TX, USA).

3. Results

The study included two hundred and thirteen patients (137 men, 76 women) undergoing MHD. The mean (±SD) of age, median dialysis vintage, and mean Kt/V were 54.5 ± 15.6 years, 24 months (IQR, 12–48), and 1.44 ± 0.3, respectively. The majority of the patients were on three times weekly, 4 hr sessions of haemodialysis. Most of the patients were dialyzed with a dialysate calcium concentration of 1.50 mmol/L, which is usually modified based on serum levels of calcium. The blood and dialysis flow rates are generally 300–400 mls/min and 500 mls/min, respectively. However, these values varied according to patient's blood pressure and haemodynamic state. A native arteriovenous fistula was used in more than half of the study population (60.6%). Almost all patients (93.0%) were on ESAs.

Table 1 shows the comparisons of baseline clinical characteristics between patients in high TAP and low TAP groups. The low alkaline phosphatase group had significantly higher mean age than the high TAP group. Other parameters were comparable between the groups. For the management of CKD-MBD, 76.9% of the patients were on calcium carbonate and 64.3% on alfacalcidol with a similar distribution of drug usage across the groups. The study population included 120 (56.3%) black and 93 (43.7%) white patients. The mean age, hemoglobin concentration, albumin, and phosphate levels were significantly higher in white compared to black patients. 56 (26.3%) of the study population had diabetes and the proportion was higher in black patients (30.0% versus 21.5%, $P = 0.02$) (Table 2).

The characteristics of the patients across different categories of serum calcium levels are shown in Table 3. Patients

TABLE 1: Comparisons of baseline characteristics between patients in high TAP and low TAP groups.

Characteristic	All ($N = 213$)	TAP $\leq$ 112 ($n = 98$)	TAP $>$ 112 ($n = 115$)	P value
Age (years)	54.53 ± 15.62	57.3 ± 15.5	51.1 ± 15.1	0.008
Female, n (%)	76 (35.7%)	35 (35.7%)	41 (35.7%)	0.25
Diabetes, n (%)	56 (26.3%)	27 (27.6%)	29 (25.2%)	0.76
Weight (Kg)	71 ± 9.6	70 ± 9.5	69 ± 9.6	0.53
BMI (Kg/m^2)	24.7 ± 0.9	24.9 ± 1.0	24.5 ± 1.6	0.83
Dialysis vintage (months)	24 (12–48)	36 (12–60)	36 (12–48)	0.55
Systolic Bp (mmHg)	134 ± 21.8	135.5 ± 19.6	133.5 ± 24.4	0.38
Diastolic Bp (mmHg)	72.0 ± 13.73	70.7 ± 12.0	74.1 ± 13.8	0.86
Haemoglobin (g/dL)	10.3 ± 2.0	10.2 ± 1.9	9.9 ± 2.1	0.10
Potassium (mmol/L)	4.62 ± 0.8	4.6 ± 0.9	4.6 ± 0.8	0.55
Calcium (mmol/L)	2.25 ± 0.14	2.32 ± 0.30	2.34 ± 0.29	0.58
Corrected calcium (mmol/L)	2.40 ± 0.25	2.50 ± 0.22	2.50 ± 0.21	0.42
iPTH (pg/mL)	307 (148–656)	246 (137–527)	325 (152–693)	0.09
Phosphate (mmol/L)	1.59 ± 0.6	1.60 ± 0.6	1.40 ± 0.6	0.07
25-OH vitamin D (ng/mL)	21.16 ± 10.71	20.4 ± 8.8	22.2 ± 12.9	0.83
Alkaline phosphatase (U/L)	112 (74–163)	74 (62–96)	163 (130–223)	<0.001
Albumin (g/L)	31.9 ± 6.0	32.6 ± 5.4	30.3 ± 6.5	0.98
Type of vascular access				
Arteriovenous fistula	129 (60.6%)	65 (66.3%)	64 (55.7%)	0.23
Graft	39 (18.3%)	23 (23.5%)	26 (22.6%)	0.88
Catheter	45 (21.1%)	21 (21.4%)	24 (20.9%)	0.97
Alanine transaminase (U/L)	21.1 ± 8.9	17.6 ± 8.7	22.9 ± 8.8	0.20
Kt/V	1.44 ± 0.28	1.4 ± 0.3	1.4 ± 0.2	0.72
n PCR (g/kg/day)	1.10 ± 0.24	1.02 ± 0.30	1.08 ± 0.27	0.56
T. cholesterol (mmol/L)	4.18 ± 0.91	4.3 ± 0.9	4.1 ± 0.9	0.14
Medications				
Calcium carbonate, n (%)	163 (76.5%)	77 (78.6%)	86 (74.7%)	0.74
Alfacalcidol, n (%)	137 (64.3%)	61 (62.2%)	76 (66.1%)	0.55
ESA n (%)	198 (93.0%)	94 (95.9)	104 (90.4%)	0.50
ESA dose (U/week)	13373 ± 4205	13714 ± 4768	12957 ± 3457	0.53

Continuous variables are presented as means ± standard deviations or median (interquartile range) and categorical data as frequencies (percentages), BP = blood pressure, i PTH = intact parathyroid hormone, TAP = total alkaline phosphatase, ESA = erythropoietin stimulating agent, n PCR = normalized protein catabolic rate, and BMI = body mass index.

in the highest category of calcium levels had significantly lower mean serum creatinine, and a few of them were on calcium carbonate and alfacalcidol. No significant differences were found in other parameters of the patients across the serum calcium categories. The overall mean dialysate calcium was 1.65 ± 0.24 mmol/L and patients with higher levels of calcium are more likely to be dialyzed with lower dialysate calcium concentration. To further explore our practice pattern regarding treatment of hypercalcaemia, available data revealed that only 5 patients in the highest category of calcium had undergone a parathyroidectomy while the majority of them were dialyzed with 1.25 mmol/L of dialysate calcium concentration and had their calcium carbonate and alfacalcidol discontinued.

During a follow-up period of 7 years there were 57 (26.8%) deaths. After adjusting for cofounders such as age, other markers of bone disorder (calcium, phosphate, and PTH), serum alanine transaminase, 25-OH vitamin D, and comorbidity (diabetes mellitus), patients in the high TAP group had a significantly higher risk of death compared to patients in the low TAP group (hazard ratio, 2.5; 95% CI 1.24–5.01, log rank $P = 0.01$).

Patients in the highest category of corrected calcium (>2.75 mmol/L) had more than a sixfold increased risk of death compared to patients with normal calcium (HR 6.34, 95% CI 1.40–28.76; $P = 0.02$). Similarly, we found a significant association between race and mortality, in which white patients had an accentuated six fold increase in adjusted hazard ratio for death compared to black patients (HR 6.88, 95% CI 1.82–25.88; $P = 0.004$) (Table 4). Figures 1, 2, and 3 show Kaplan Meir Survival curves for TAP, race, and calcium levels, respectively.

Univariate linear regression analysis revealed a significant association between TAP and age ($r^2 = 0.04$, $P = 0.008$), corrected calcium ($r^2 = 0.03$, $P = 0.04$), and PTH ($r^2 = 0.04$, $P = 0.006$). In multivariate regression analyses PTH

TABLE 2: Baseline characteristics of study population by race.

Parameters	All ($n = 213$)	Black ($n = 120$)	White ($n = 93$)	P value
Age (years)	54.53 ± 15.62	51.0 ± 14.6	58.7 ± 15.9	<0.001
Haemoglobin (g/dL)	10.3 ± 2.00	9.9 ± 1.98	10.7 ± 1.94	0.004
Systolic Bp (mmHg)	134 ± 21.8	130 ± 20.3	139 ± 22.8	0.98
PTH (pg/mL)	307 (148–656)	327 (137–658)	290 (149–618)	0.97
Calcium (mmol/L)	2.28 ± 0.22	2.26 ± 0.22	2.30 ± 0.21	0.94
Phosphate (mmol/L)	1.59 ± 0.56	1.49 ± 0.57	1.71 ± 0.53	0.004
Albumin (g/L)	31.9 ± 6.0	30.8 ± 6.5	33.04 ± 5.5	0.03
25(OH) vitamin D (ng/mL)	21.16 ± 10.71	20.57 ± 9.79	21.80 ± 11.67	0.77
TAP (U/L)	112 (74–163)	110 (75–151)	115 (71–164)	0.33
T. cholesterol (mmol/L)	4.2 ± 0.8	4.0 ± 0.9	4.1 ± 0.9	0.05
Diabetes, n (%)	56 (26.3%)	36 (30.0%)	20 (21.5%)	0.02
Male, n (%)	137 (64.3%)	72 (60.0%)	65 (69.9%)	0.07
Kt/V	1.44 ± 0.3	1.41 ± 0.3	1.46 ± 0.30	0.40

Continuous variables are presented as means ± standard deviations or median (interquartile range) and categorical data as frequencies (percentages). BP = blood pressure, TAP = total alkaline phosphatase, and PTH = parathyroid hormone.

TABLE 3: Patient characteristics by serum calcium categories.

Parameters	<2.10 mmol/L ($n = 31$)	2.10–2.37 mmol/L ($n = 92$)	2.38–2.75 mmol/L ($n = 57$)	>2.75 mmol/L ($n = 33$)	P-value
Age (years)	50.9 ± 15.0	52.9 ± 15.0	58.3 ± 16.4	56.5 ± 26.1	0.09
Systolic Bp (mmHg)	130.9 ± 18.6	138.8 ± 21.5	139.8 ± 30.7	138.9 ± 21.5	0.18
Diastolic Bp (mmHg)	71.2 ± 15.3	71.7 ± 11.2	76.4 ± 18.9	71.2 ± 11.1	0.38
Haemoglobin (g/dL)	10.8 ± 2.4	10.2 ± 1.9	10.1 ± 1.9	8.15 ± 1.9	0.20
Albumin g/L	32.0 ± 5.2	32.7 ± 6.0	30.5 ± 6.6	29.5 ± 5.0	0.26
T.chol (mmol/L)	4.3 ± 1.0	4.2 ± 0.9	4.2 ± 0.9	4.1 ± 0.9	0.97
25-OH vitamin D (ng/mL)	22.8 ± 9.1	22.0 ± 10.4	18.1 ± 8.1	15.8 ± 3.5	0.11
PTH (pg/mL)	568.8 ± 334.8	458.64 ± 424.4	366.2 ± 405.1	254.0 ± 103.2	0.01
Phosphate (mmol/L)	1.5 ± 0.6	1.6 ± 0.6	1.5 ± 0.5	1.6 ± 0.5	0.66
Creatinine(μmol/L)	822.5 ± 261.0	734.4 ± 283.2	592.5 ± 245.5	489.5 ± 355.7	0.002
Kt/V	1.4 ± 0.2	1.5 ± 0.3	1.4 ± 0.3	1.4 ± 0.4	0.33
Dialysis vintage (months)	31.3 ± 23.0	34.2 ± 23.0	30.9 ± 21.1	30.0 ± 8.9	0.80
Dialysate calcium (mmol/L)	1.65 ± 0.24	1.63 ± 0.14	1.63 ± 0.14	1.54 ± 0.24	0.50
DM, n	13	15	17	11	0.40
Medications					
Calcium carbonate n (%)	30 (96.8%)	79 (85.7%)	41 (71.9%)	13 (39.4%)	<0.001
Alfacalcidol n (%)	28 (90.3%)	63 (68.4%)	35 (61.4%)	11 (33.3%)	<0.001

Continuous variables are presented as means ± standard deviations or median (interquartile range) and categorical data as frequencies (percentages). BP = blood pressure, PTH = parathyroid hormone, P values derived by one-way ANOVA, and Kruskal-Wallis tests for continuous variables and Chi-squared for categorical variables. Serum categories based on KDOQI reference range.

and calcium remained significantly correlated with TAP, $P =$ 0.006 and 0.04, respectively.

4. Discussion

Several studies from Europe, America, and Asia have consistently shown a linear relationship between high serum alkaline phosphate and mortality in the haemodialysis population [14–17], while results relating to other markers of mineral metabolism revealed nonlinear (U or J patterns) associations

[12, 18, 19]. Such data relating to the impact of markers of CKD-MBD on mortality in African MHD patients are lacking. In this present study, higher levels of TAP, hypercalcaemia, and white race were associated with increased risk of death. These findings are consistent with other large studies where higher levels of TAP were independently associated with higher risk of mortality [14, 17].

Interestingly, this association was also reported in CKD patients as well as in the general population [20, 21]. The National Health and Nutrition Examination Survey (NHANES) data revealed an independent association

TABLE 4: Crude and adjusted hazard ratio (95% CI) of primary outcome by baseline characteristics.

Parameter	Crude HR	95% CI	P	Adjusted HR	95% CI	P
TAP > 112 U/L	2.20	1.12–4.32	0.02	2.50	1.24–5.01	0.01
Calcium (mmol/L)						
<2.10	0.66	0.32–1.35	0.26	0.97	0.22–4.26	0.97
≥2.10–≤2.37	1.00	Reference				
>2.37–≤2.75	2.31	1.20–4.44	0.02	1.54	0.57–4.18	0.39
>2.75	6.82	1.55–30.1	0.01	6.34	1.40–28.76	0.02
PTH (pg/mL)						
<130	1.00	Reference				
≥130–≤585	1.26	0.57–2.79	0.56	2.77	0.61–12.58	0.19
≥585	1.05	0.44–2.49	0.92	2.22	0.42–11.65	0.35
Phosphate > 1.50 mmol/L	1.09	0.61–1.95	0.77	1.43	0.47-4.40	0.53
25 OH vitamin D ≤ 30 ng/mL	2.21	0.66–7.35	0.19	1.07	0.23–4.79	0.92
White race	1.69	0.95–3.04	0.08	6.88	1.82–25.88	0.004

HR = hazard ratio, CI = confidence interval, TAP = total alkaline phosphate, and PTH intact parathyroid hormone. Adjusted for age, phosphate, calcium, PTH, TAP, diabetes, systolic BP, 25-OH vitamin D, alanine transaminase and albumin, and serum calcium categories based on KDOQI reference range.

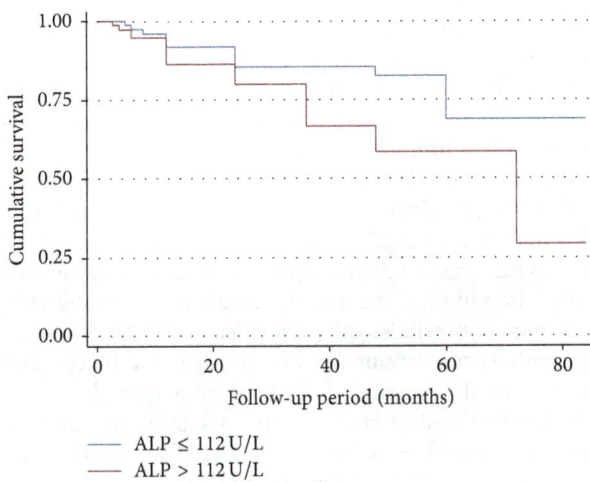

FIGURE 1: Kaplan Meier curve comparing patients in the high alkaline phosphatase to low alkaline phosphatase group ($P = 0.01$).

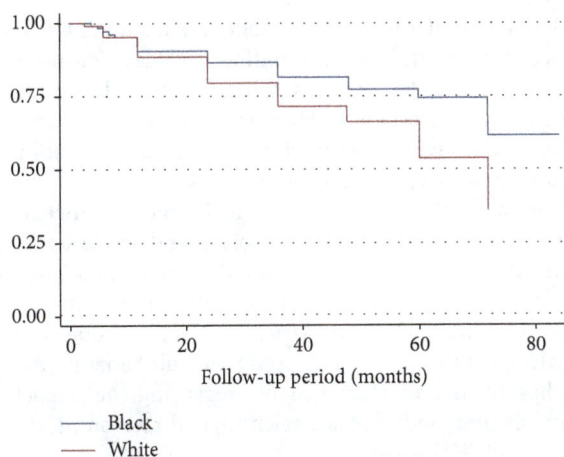

FIGURE 2: Kaplan Meier survival curve between black and white ($P = 0.004$).

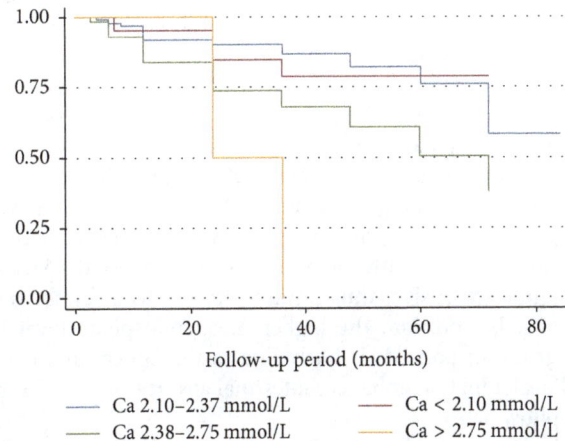

FIGURE 3: Kaplan Meier survival curves for different categories of calcium ($P = 0.02$). Calcium categories based on KDOQI reference range.

between elevated levels of TAP and mortality in the general population [21]. This further supports the notion that TAP is more than a marker of high bone turnover and may be a reliable predictor of mortality.

The mechanisms for this association have been linked to enhanced vascular calcification by high levels of serum TAP through hydrolysis of pyrophosphate or activation of apatite crystal formation [22]. In addition to vascular calcification, elevated levels of TAP have been associated with high C reactive protein, insulin resistance, and 25-OH vitamin D deficiency [23–26]. In contrast to our study, we found no significant difference in the mean levels of 25-OH vitamin D between patients with high TAP and low TAP.

Despite the variations in the cut-off points for defining hypercalcaemia by various studies, hypercalcaemia has been consistently associated with increased risk for mortality in haemodialysis patients [12, 18, 27]. Consistent with our finding, a linear relation was observed between higher calcium categories and increased risk of death [12, 18]. In a large global representation of HD patients including the three phases of the dialysis outcomes and practice patterns study (DOPPSI, II and III) with 25,588 HD patients, calcium levels greater than 10.0 mg/dL (>2.5 mmol/L) were significantly associated with greater risk of all cause and cardiovascular mortality in both baseline and time dependent models [27]. The reasons for this consistent association could be linked to acceleration of arterial calcification by hypercalcaemia [28, 29]. Besides vascular calcification, high levels of calcium, but not high PTH, have been associated with poor mental health in MHD patients [30]. In contrast, studies relating to hypocalcaemia and risk of death have yielded contradictory reports. Lowrie and Lew [31] were the first to establish the association of increased mortality with calcium levels <9.0 mg in over 12,000 HD patients, while in another large study from the US involving 40, 538 HD patients, the mortality risk with low serum calcium levels was attenuated after adjusting for confounding variables [18]. In the dialysis outcomes and practice patterns study [32], serum calcium levels < 7.8 mg were associated with lower mortality risk. In agreement with DOPPS, we found a similar trend, though not statistically significant, with serum calcium levels below 2.12 mmol/L.

Hypercalcaemia is an undesirable effect associated with the use of calcium based phosphate binders and vitamin D analogues in controlling secondary hyperparathyroidism. This may likely have accounted for the lower levels of PTH seen in our category of patients with calcium levels above 2.75 mmol/L. Although cinacalcet which is one of the newer drugs that effectively lowers PTH without raising serum calcium levels recently became available in South Africa, it is quite expensive, thus limiting its use to a few of our patients. In addition, the higher mean phosphate level in this group of patients is likely due to the concomitant use of alfacalcidol that enhances intestinal absorption of calcium and phosphate.

A notable finding in the current study is that white patients have a poor survival rate compared to black patients. This finding is consistent with recent emerging data from the USA that reported better survival in black patients compared with white patients on MHD [10]. The reasons underlying this racial survival benefit remain unclear, and several studies have proposed explanations for the better survival of black MHD patients compared to whites. A large US observational study reported that the widely perceived survival advantage for black dialysis patients applies only to older adults, with a reversal of the higher risk of death in the younger age group (<50 years) [33]. This is contrary to several studies including the current study, where the risk persisted after adjusting for the significantly higher mean age in the white patients [34, 35]. Indeed, the better survival in black patients persisted in a study that comprehensively adjusted for demographics and dialysis modality among several other cofounding variables [34].

Another important observation we made in this study was that white patients had significantly higher levels of serum albumin. We expected this to give white patients a survival benefit. However, the reason for this reversal could likely be explained by a finding from a previous study where

markers of worse nutritional status (hypoalbuminemia) or smaller muscle mass and increased body fat in African American patients correlated less strongly with mortality than in whites [36]. Additionally, studies have criticized the use of serum albumin in CKD patients as a marker of nutritional status as inappropriate [37, 38]. In fact, the hazard ratio becomes accentuated after adjusting for serum albumin suggesting that the effect of race on mortality is likely to be through other mechanisms besides nutritional status.

In line with previous studies [33, 39], black patients had higher median intact PTH though this was not statistically significant. Some studies have reported survival benefit with active vitamin D therapy and that black patients are more likely to receive active vitamin agents due to higher PTH compared to white patients [40, 41]. However, it is unlikely that treatment with vitamin D alone may explain the racial survival paradox that has existed for several years. Additionally, reports relating to PTH levels have been controversial and studies are divided on which levels are associated with increased mortality. Similar to earlier [17, 18, 42] and more recent studies [10, 43], we did not find significant association of mortality with severe hyperparathyroidism. On the other hand, studies that have shown significant associations are not unified on what levels of PTH are associated with increased mortality. Therefore, randomized control trials are needed to show the effect of treatment on PTH levels that are associated with favorable clinical outcomes.

Our findings should be considered in the context of the following limitations. Firstly, the retrospective nature of this study could not allow us to make causal associations between markers of mineral bone disease and study outcome (death). In addition, the use of a single baseline laboratory measurement precludes the performance of time dependent Cox analysis to account for variations in the biochemical markers on the impact of death over a period of time. However, few studies have shown no significant difference between the baseline and time dependent Cox analysis [12].

Secondly, the relatively small sample size precludes generalizability of our findings to African HD patients. Thus, there is a need for multicentre studies in Africa, to provide robust data on this important clinical entity (CKD-MBD) in African HD patients.

Thirdly, similar to several observational studies we could not account for residual confounding variables. For instance, aside from diabetes mellitus, other comorbid conditions could not be ascertained. However, part of the exclusion criteria was to avoid patients with some coexisting conditions that are known as potential confounders.

The strengths of this study lie in the heterogeneous nature of our study population (black and white patients) in an African setting which has allowed comparisons of data not only for Black Africans with Black Americans, but also between whites in Africa and USA/Europe. To our knowledge, this is the first study in Sub-Saharan Africa that has given important insights regarding the impact of serum alkaline phosphatase, calcium, and race on mortality in African MHD patients.

In summary, high TAP, hypercalcaemia, and white race are associated with increased risk of death in MHD patients, thus, reaffirming the need to pay more attention to the two modifiable risk factors (calcium and TAP) in the management of CKD-MBD.

Ethical Approval

All procedures performed in this study were in accordance with the ethical standards of the institutional and/or national research committee and with the 1964 Helsinki Declaration and its later amendments or comparable ethical standards. The research protocol was approved by the Health Research and Ethics committee (HREC) of the University of the Witwatersrand; clearance certificate number is M141016.

Acknowledgments

This study was partly supported by grants from the AstraZeneca Research Trust and the National Kidney Foundation of South Africa (NKFSA) ADCOCK INGRAM research grant.

References

[1] W. L. Lau and K. Kalantar-Zadeh, "Towards the revival of alkaline phosphatase for the management of bone disease, mortality and hip fractures," *Nephrology Dialysis Transplantation*, vol. 29, no. 8, pp. 1450–1452, 2014.

[2] Kidney Disease: Improving Global Outcomes (KDIGO) CKD-MBD Work Group, "KDIGO clinical practice guideline for the diagnosis, evaluation, prevention, and treatment of chronic kidney disease–mineral and bone disorder (CKD–MBD)," *Kidney International*, vol. 76, supplement 113, pp. S1–S130, 2009.

[3] K. A. Lomashvili, P. Garg, S. Narisawa, J. L. Millan, and W. C. O'Neill, "Upregulation of alkaline phosphatase and pyrophosphate hydrolysis: potential mechanism for uremic vascular calcification," *Kidney International*, vol. 73, no. 9, pp. 1024–1030, 2008.

[4] W. C. O'Neill, "Pyrophosphate, alkaline phosphatase, and vascular calcification," *Circulation Research*, vol. 99, no. 2, article e2, 2006.

[5] M. K. Sigrist, M. W. Taal, P. Bungay, and C. W. McIntyre, "Progressive vascular calcification over 2 years is associated with arterial stiffening and increased mortality in patients with stages 4 and 5 chronic kidney disease," *Clinical Journal of the American Society of Nephrology*, vol. 2, no. 6, pp. 1241–1248, 2007.

[6] R. Shantouf, C. P. Kovesdy, Y. Kim et al., "Association of serum alkaline phosphatase with coronary artery calcification in maintenance hemodialysis patients," *Clinical Journal of the American Society of Nephrology*, vol. 4, no. 6, pp. 1106–1114, 2009.

[7] S. V. Badve, L. Zhang, J. S. Coombes et al., "Association between serum alkaline phosphatase and primary resistance to erythropoiesis stimulating agents in chronic kidney disease: a secondary analysis of the HERO trial," *Canadian Journal of Kidney Health and Disease*, vol. 2, no. 33, 2015.

[8] K. C. Norris, K. Kalantar-Zadeh, and J. D. Kopple, "The role of race in survival among patients undergoing dialysis," *Nephrology News & Issues*, vol. 25, no. 13, pp. 13–16, 2011.

[9] G. Yan, K. C. Norris, A. J. Yu et al., "The relationship of age, race, and ethnicity with survival in dialysis patients," *Clinical Journal of the American Society of Nephrology*, vol. 8, no. 6, pp. 953–961, 2013.

[10] J. J. Scialla, R. S. Parekh, J. A. Eustace et al., "Race, mineral homeostasis and mortality in patients with end-stage renal disease on dialysis," *American Journal of Nephrology*, vol. 42, no. 1, pp. 25–34, 2015.

[11] C. Robinson-Cohen, A. N. Hoofnagle, J. H. Ix et al., "Racial differences in the association of serum 25-hydroxyvitamin D concentration with coronary heart disease events," *The Journal of the American Medical Association*, vol. 310, no. 2, pp. 179–188, 2013.

[12] J. Floege, J. Kim, E. Ireland et al., "Serum iPTH, calcium and phosphate, and the risk of mortality in a European haemodialysis population," *Nephrology Dialysis Transplantation*, vol. 26, no. 6, pp. 1948–1955, 2011.

[13] B. O. Lightfoot, R. J. Caruana, L. L. Mulloy, and M. E. Fincher, "Simple formula for calculating normalized protein catabolic rate (NPCR) in haemodialysis (HD) patients (abstract)," *Journal of the American Society of Nephrology*, vol. 4, p. 363, 1993.

[14] M. J. Blayney, R. L. Pisoni, J. L. Bragg-Gresham et al., "High alkaline phosphatase levels in hemodialysis patients are associated with higher risk of hospitalization and death," *Kidney International*, vol. 74, no. 5, pp. 655–663, 2008.

[15] J. Beige, R. Wendt, M. Girndt, K.-H. Queck, R. Fiedler, and P. Jehle, "Association of serum alkaline phosphatase with mortality in non-selected european patients with ckd5d: an observational, three-centre survival analysis," *BMJ Open*, vol. 4, no. 2, Article ID e004275, 2014.

[16] D. L. Regidor, C. P. Kovesdy, R. Mehrotra et al., "Serum alkaline phosphatase predicts mortality among maintenance hemodialysis patients," *Journal of the American Society of Nephrology*, vol. 19, no. 11, pp. 2193–2203, 2008.

[17] K. Kalantar-Zadeh, N. Kuwae, D. L. Regidor et al., "Survival predictability of time-varying indicators of bone disease in maintenance hemodialysis patients," *Kidney International*, vol. 70, no. 4, pp. 771–780, 2006.

[18] G. A. Block, P. S. Klassen, J. M. Lazarus, N. Ofsthun, E. G. Lowrie, and G. M. Chertow, "Mineral metabolism, mortality, and morbidity in maintenance hemodialysis," *Journal of the American Society of Nephrology*, vol. 15, no. 8, pp. 2208–2218, 2004.

[19] J. Cunningham and J. Silver, "CKD-MBD: comfort in the trough of the U," *Nephrology Dialysis Transplantation*, vol. 26, no. 6, pp. 1764–1766, 2011.

[20] S. Beddhu, X. Ma, B. Baird, A. K. Cheung, and T. Greene, "Serum alkaline phosphatase and mortality in African Americans with chronic kidney disease," *Clinical Journal of the American Society of Nephrology*, vol. 4, no. 11, pp. 1805–1810, 2009.

[21] M. Tonelli, G. Curhan, M. Pfeffer et al., "Relation between alkaline phosphatase, serum phosphate, and all-cause or cardiovascular mortality," *Circulation*, vol. 120, no. 18, pp. 1784–1792, 2009.

[22] M. Schoppet and C. M. Shanahan, "Role for alkaline phosphatase as an inducer of vascular calcification in renal failure?" *Kidney International*, vol. 73, no. 9, pp. 989–991, 2008.

[23] B. M. Y. Cheung, K. L. Ong, R. V. Cheung et al., "Association between plasma alkaline phosphatase and C-reactive protein in Hong Kong Chinese," *Clinical Chemistry and Laboratory Medicine*, vol. 46, no. 4, pp. 523–527, 2008.

[24] A. J. G. Hanley, K. Williams, A. Festa, L. E. Wagenknecht, R. B. D'Agostino Jr., and S. M. Haffner, "Liver markers and development of the metabolic syndrome: the insulin resistance atherosclerosis study," *Diabetes*, vol. 54, no. 11, pp. 3140–3147, 2005.

[25] J. R. Chaudhuri, K. R. Mridula, A. Anamika et al., "Deficiency of 25-hydroxyvitamin d and dyslipidemia in Indian subjects," *Journal of Lipids*, vol. 2013, Article ID 623420, 7 pages, 2013.

[26] P. Lips, T. Duong, A. Oleksik et al., "A global study of vitamin D status and parathyroid function in postmenopausal women with osteoporosis: baseline data from the multiple outcomes of raloxifene evaluation clinical trial," *The Journal of Clinical Endocrinology & Metabolism*, vol. 86, no. 3, pp. 1212–1221, 2001.

[27] F. Tentori, M. J. Blayney, J. M. Albert et al., "Mortality risk for dialysis patients with different levels of serum calcium, phosphorus, and PTH: The Dialysis Outcomes and Practice Patterns Study (DOPPS)," *American Journal of Kidney Diseases*, vol. 52, no. 3, pp. 519–530, 2008.

[28] G. M. London, S. J. Marchais, A. P. Guérin, P. Boutouyrie, F. Métivier, and M.-C. de Vernejoul, "Association of bone activity, calcium load, aortic stiffness, and calcifications in ESRD," *Journal of the American Society of Nephrology*, vol. 19, no. 9, pp. 1827–1835, 2008.

[29] M. Noordzij, E. M. Cranenburg, L. F. Engelsman et al., "Progression of aortic calcification is associated with disorders of mineral metabolism and mortality in chronic dialysis patients," *Nephrology Dialysis Transplantation*, vol. 26, no. 5, pp. 1662–1669, 2011.

[30] M. Tanaka, S. Yamazaki, Y. Hayashino et al., "Hypercalcaemia is associated with poor mental health in haemodialysis patients: results from Japan DOPPS," *Nephrology Dialysis Transplantation*, vol. 22, no. 6, pp. 1658–1664, 2007.

[31] E. G. Lowrie and N. L. Lew, "Death risk in hemodialysis patients: the predictive value of commonly measured variables and an evaluation of death rate differences between facilities," *American Journal of Kidney Diseases*, vol. 15, no. 5, pp. 458–482, 1990.

[32] E. W. Young, J. M. Albert, S. Satayathum et al., "Predictors and consequences of altered mineral metabolism: the Dialysis Outcomes and Practice Patterns Study," *Kidney International*, vol. 67, no. 3, pp. 1179–1187, 2005.

[33] L. M. Kucirka, M. E. Grams, J. Lessler et al., "Association of race and age with survival among patients undergoing dialysis," *The Journal of the American Medical Association*, vol. 306, no. 6, pp. 620–626, 2011.

[34] E. Streja, C. P. Kovesdy, M. Z. Molnar et al., "Role of nutritional status and inflammation in higher survival of African American and hispanic hemodialysis patients," *American Journal of Kidney Diseases*, vol. 57, no. 6, pp. 883–893, 2011.

[35] D. C. Crews, S. M. Sozio, Y. Liu, J. Coresh, and N. R. Powe, "Inflammation and the paradox of racial differences in dialysis survival," *Journal of the American Society of Nephrology*, vol. 22, no. 12, pp. 2279–2286, 2011.

[36] U. Feroze, N. Noori, C. P. Kovesdy et al., "Quality-of-life and mortality in hemodialysis patients: roles of race and nutritional status," *Clinical Journal of the American Society of Nephrology*, vol. 6, no. 5, pp. 1100–1111, 2011.

[37] A. N. Friedman and S. Z. Fadem, "Reassessment of albumin as a nutritional marker in kidney disease," *Journal of the American Society of Nephrology*, vol. 21, no. 2, pp. 223–230, 2010.

[38] W. E. Mitch, "Malnutrition: a frequent misdiagnosis for hemodialysis patients," *The Journal of Clinical Investigation*, vol. 110, no. 4, pp. 437–439, 2002.

[39] O. M. Gutiérrez, W. R. Farwell, D. Kermah, and E. N. Taylor, "Racial differences in the relationship between vitamin D, bone mineral density, and parathyroid hormone in the National Health and Nutrition Examination Survey," *Osteoporosis International*, vol. 22, no. 6, pp. 1745–1753, 2011.

[40] M. Wolf, J. Betancourt, Y. Chang et al., "Impact of activated vitamin D and race on survival among hemodialysis patients," *Journal of the American Society of Nephrology*, vol. 19, no. 7, pp. 1379–1388, 2008.

[41] M. L. Melamed, J. A. Eustace, L. Plantinga et al., "Changes in serum calcium, phosphate, and PTH and the risk of death in incident dialysis patients: a longitudinal study," *Kidney International*, vol. 70, no. 2, pp. 351–357, 2006.

[42] R. Wald, M. J. Sarnak, H. Tighiouart et al., "Disordered mineral metabolism in hemodialysis patients: an analysis of cumulative effects in the hemodialysis (HEMO) Study," *American Journal of Kidney Diseases*, vol. 52, no. 3, pp. 531–540, 2008.

[43] M. Fukagawa, R. Kido, H. Komaba et al., "Abnormal mineral metabolism and mortality in hemodialysis patients with secondary hyperparathyroidism: evidence from marginal structural models used to adjust for time-dependent confounding," *American Journal of Kidney Diseases*, vol. 63, no. 6, pp. 979–987, 2014.

Permissions

List of Contributors

Andrew S. Allegretti, Guillermo Ortiz, Julia Wenger, Joseph J. Deferio, Joshua Wibecan, Sahir Kalim and Ravi I. Thadhani
Division of Nephrology, Department of Medicine, Massachusetts General Hospital, Boston, MA 02114, USA

Hector Tamez
Division of Cardiology, Department of Medicine, Beth Israel Deaconess Medical Center, Boston, MA 02114, USA

Raymond T. Chung,
Liver Center and Gastrointestinal Division, Department of Medicine, Massachusetts General Hospital, Boston, MA 02114, USA

S. Ananth Karumanchi
Division of Nephrology, Department of Medicine, Beth Israel Deaconess Medical Center, Boston, MA 02215, USA

Shatha Hussain Ali and Ban A. Abdulmajeed
College of Medicine, Al-Nahrain University, Baghdad, Iraq

Rasha Kasim Mohammed
Al-Imamein Al-Kadhimein Medical City, Baghdad, Iraq

Hussein Ali Saheb
College of Pharmacy, University of Al Qadisiyah, Diwaniyah, Iraq

Bancha Satirapoj, Anan Promrattanakun, Ouppatham Supasyndh and Panbuppa Choovichian
Division of Nephrology, Department of Medicine, Phramongkutklao Hospital and College of Medicine, Bangkok 10400, Thailand

Roberto José Barone, María Inés Cámpora, Nélida Susana Gimenez, Liliana Ramirez, Sergio Alberto Panese and Mónica Santopietro
Peritoneal Dialysis Program, Hurlingham RenalTherapy Services, 1431 Buenos Aires, Argentina

Hernán Trimarchi, Matías Paulero, Tatiana Rengel, Mariano Forrester, Fernando Lombi, Vanesa Pomeranz and Romina Iriarte
Nephrology Service, Hospital Brit´anico de Buenos Aires, Buenos Aires, Argentina

Romina Canzonieri, Amalia Schiel, Aníbal Stern and Alexis Muryan
Central Laboratory, Hospital Brit´anico de Buenos Aires, Buenos Aires, Argentina

Juan Politei
Neurology Department, Laboratorio de Neuroqu´ımica Dr. Nestor Chamoles, Buenos Aires, Argentina

Cristian Costales-Collaguazo and Elsa Zotta
IFIBIO Houssay, CONICET, Physiopathology, Pharmacy and Biochemistry Faculty, Universidad de Buenos Aires, Buenos Aires, Argentina

Lara Valiño-Rivas
IIS-Fundaci´on Jimenez Diaz, School of Medicine, UAM, Madrid, Spain

Alberto Ortiz and María Dolores Sanchez-Niño
IIS-Fundaci´on Jimenez Diaz, School of Medicine, UAM, Madrid, Spain
REDINREN, Madrid, Spain

Boon Wee Teo, Ping Tyug Loh, Qi Chun Toh, Hui Xu and Evan J. C. Lee
Department of Medicine, Yong Loo Lin School of Medicine, National University of Singapore, 1E Kent Ridge Road, Level 10 NUHS Tower Block, Singapore 119228

Weng Kin Wong
National University Health System, Singapore 119228

Peh Joo Ho and Kwok Pui Choi
Department of Statistics and Applied Probability, Faculty of Science, National University of Singapore, Singapore 119228

Sharon Saw
Department of Laboratory Medicine, National University Health System, Singapore 119228

Titus Lau
Department of Medicine, National University Health System, Singapore 119228

Sunil Sethi
Department of Pathology, Yong Loo Lin School of Medicine, National University of Singapore, Singapore 119228

Mattie Feasel Wolf
Emory University School of Medicine, 2015 Uppergate Drive NE, Atlanta, GA 30322, USA

Chia-shi Wang and Larry A. Greenbaum
Emory University School of Medicine, 2015 Uppergate Drive NE, Atlanta, GA 30322, USA
Children's Healthcare of Atlanta, 1677 Tullie Circle, Atlanta, GA 30329, USA

Jia Yan, Robert Palmer and James Bost
Children's Healthcare of Atlanta, 1677 Tullie Circle, Atlanta, GA 30329, USA

Sara Querido
Department of Nephrology Centro Hospitalar do Médio Tejo, Avenida Xanana Gusmão, Apartado 45, 2350-754 Torres Novas, Portugal

Patrícia Quadros Branco, Elisabete Costa, Sara Pereira, Maria Augusta Gaspar and José Diogo Barata
Department of Nephrology, Centro Hospitalar de Lisboa Ocidental, Carnaxide, Portugal

Alexandra Douglas, Dev Jegatheesan, Linh Pham, Sonny Huynh and Dwarakanathan Ranganathan
Royal Brisbane andWomen's Hospital, Herston, Brisbane, QLD, Australia

Charan Bale
Royal Brisbane andWomen's Hospital, Herston, Brisbane, QLD, Australia
Dr. D. Y. PatilMedical College, Pune, India

Atul Mulay
Dr. D. Y. PatilMedical College, Pune, India

Takeo Edamatsu, Ayako Fujieda, Atsuko Ezawa and Yoshiharu Itoh
Pharmaceutical Division, Kureha Corporation, 3-26-2 Hyakunin-cho, Shinjuku-ku, Tokyo 169-8503, Japan

Hassan Izzedine
Department of Nephrology, Pitie-Salpetriere Hospital, 75013 Paris, France
Department of Nephrology, Monceau Park International Clinic, 75017 Paris, France

Yafa Falush
Institute of Nephrology, Schneider Children's Medical Center of Israel, 49202 Petah Tikva, Israel

Daniella Levy Erez, Irit Krause, Amit Dagan, Roxana Cleper and Miriam Davidovits
Institute of Nephrology, Schneider Children's Medical Center of Israel, 49202 Petah Tikva, Israel
Sackler Faculty of Medicine, Tel Aviv University, 6997801 Tel Aviv, Israel

Daniel Bia and Yanina Zócalo
Physiology Department, School of Medicine, CUiiDARTE, Republic University, 11800 Montevideo, Uruguay

Cintia Galli
National Council of Technical and Scientific Research (CONICET), C1033AAJ Buenos Aires, Argentina
Technological National University, C1179AAQ Buenos Aires, Argentina

Edmundo I. Cabrera Fischer
National Council of Technical and Scientific Research (CONICET), C1033AAJ Buenos Aires, Argentina
Technological National University, C1179AAQ Buenos Aires, Argentina
Favaloro University, Solis, C1093AAS Buenos Aires, Argentina

Ricardo L. Armentano
Technological National University, C1179AAQ Buenos Aires, Argentina
Favaloro University, Solis, C1093AAS Buenos Aires, Argentina

Rodolfo Valtuille
Fresenius FME Burzaco, B1852FZD Buenos Aires, Argentina

Sandra A. Wray
Favaloro University, Solis, C1093AAS Buenos Aires, Argentina

Shahrzad Shahidi
Isfahan Kidney Disease Research Center, Isfahan University of Medical Sciences, Isfahan, Iran

Marziyeh Hoseinbalam and Bijan Iraj
Isfahan Endocrine andMetabolismResearch Center, Isfahan University of Medical Sciences, Isfahan, Iran

Mojtaba Akbari
Department of Epidemiology, School of Health and Nutrition, Shiraz University of Medical Sciences, Shiraz, Iran

Jacques Ducros and Henri Merault
Centre de Dialyse AUDRA, Hôpital RICOU, Pointe-á-Pitre, Guadeloupe, France
Service de Néphrologie, Centre Hospitalier Universitaire, Guadeloupe, France

Lydia Foucan
Centre de Dialyse AUDRA, Hôpital RICOU, Pointe-á-Pitre, Guadeloupe, France
Equipe de Recherche Epidémiologie Clinique et Médecine sur le Risque Cardio Métabolique, ECM/LAMIA, EA 4540, Université des Antilles, Centre Hospitalier Universitaire, Guadeloupe, France

Laurent Larifla
Service de Cardiologie, Centre Hospitalier Universitaire, Guadeloupe, France
Equipe de Recherche Epidémiologie Clinique et Médecine sur le Risque Cardio Métabolique, ECM/ LAMIA, EA 4540, Universit´e des Antilles, Centre Hospitalier Universitaire, Guadeloupe, France

Jose Jayme Galvão De Lima, Luis Henrique W. Gowdak and Luiz Aparecido Bortolotto
Heart Institute (InCor), Hospital das Clínicas, University of São Paulo Medical School, 05403-000 São Paulo, SP, Brazil

Henrique Cotchi Simbo Muela
Heart Institute (InCor), Hospital das Clínicas, University of São Paulo Medical School, 05403-000 São Paulo, SP, Brazil
Faculty of Medicine, Agostinho Neto University, Luanda, Angola

Flávio J. de Paula
Renal Transplant Unit, Urology, Hospital das Clínicas, University of São Paulo Medical School, 05403 000 São Paulo, SP, Brazil

Ludimila D'Avila e Silva Allemand, Otávio Toledo Nóbrega, Joel Paulo Russomano Veiga and Einstein Francisco Camargos
Universidade de Brasília (UnB), Brasília, DF, Brazil

Juliane Pena Lauar
Centro Brasiliense de Nefrologia, Brasília, DF, Brazil

Rajit A. Gilhotra, Beverly T. Rodrigues, Venkat N. Vangaveti and Usman H. Malabu
School of Medicine and Dentistry, James Cook University, Townsville, QLD 4811, Australia

Sinee Disthabanchong
Division of Nephrology, Department ofMedicine, Faculty ofMedicine, Ramathibodi Hospital, Mahidol University, Bangkok, Thailand

Saeed Yadranji Aghdam
Reynolds Institute on Aging, Room No. 4151, 629 Jack Stephens Drive, Little Rock, AR 72205, USA
Department of Geriatrics, University of Arkansas for Medical Sciences, Little Rock, AR, USA

Ali Mahmoudpour
Norgen Biotek Corp., 3430 Schmon Parkway, Thorold, ON, Canada L2V 4Y6

Benjamin A. Derman
Section of Hematology/Oncology, University of Chicago, 5841 S.Maryland Ave, M/C 2115, Chicago, IL 60637, USA

Jochen Reiser
Department of Medicine, Rush University Medical Center, Chicago, IL, USA

Sanjib Basu and Agne Paner
Division of Hematology/Oncology, Rush University Medical Center, Chicago, IL, USA

Randa I. Farah
Department of Internal Medicine, School of Medicine, University of Jordan, Amman, Jordan

L. Y. Wong
Chronic Disease Epidemiology, Population Health, National Healthcare Group, Singapore

M. P. H. S. Toh
Chronic Disease Epidemiology, Population Health, National Healthcare Group, Singapore
Population Health, National Healthcare Group, Singapore

A. S. T. Liew and W. T. Weng
Renal Medicine, Tan Tock Seng Hospital, Singapore

C. K. Lim
Clinical Services, National Healthcare Group Polyclinics, Singapore

A. Vathsala
Nephrology, National University Hospital, Singapore

Temesgen Fiseha and Zemenu Tamir
Department of Clinical Laboratory Science, College of Medicine and Health Sciences, Wollo University, Dessie, Ethiopia

Elani Streja, Ting-Yan Chan, Janet Lee, Melissa Soohoo and Connie M. Rhee
Harold Simmons Center for Kidney Disease Research and Epidemiology, School of Medicine, University of California, Irvine, Orange, CA, USA

Jongha Park
Harold Simmons Center for Kidney Disease Research and Epidemiology, School of Medicine, University of California, Irvine, Orange, CA, USA
Division of Nephrology, Ulsan University Hospital, University of Ulsan College of Medicine, Ulsan, Republic of Korea

Kamyar Kalantar-Zadeh
Harold Simmons Center for Kidney Disease Research and Epidemiology, School of Medicine, University of California, Irvine, Orange, CA, USA
Department of Epidemiology, UCLA Fielding School of Public Health, Los Angeles, CA, USA

Division of Nephrology and Hypertension, School of Medicine, University of California, Irvine, Orange, CA, USA

Onyebuchi A. Arah
Department of Epidemiology, UCLA Fielding School of Public Health, Los Angeles, CA, USA

Allen Yan Lun Liu, Boon Cheok Lai and Lee Ying Yeoh
Division of Renal Medicine, Department of General Medicine, Khoo Teck Puat Hospital, Singapore

Jiexun Wang
Clinical ResearchUnit, Khoo Teck Puat Hospital, Singapore

Milind Nikam
Fresenius Medical Care Pte. Ltd., Singapore

Huixuan Ma and Hailing Xu
Department of Endocrinology, Guangzhou Red Cross Hospital, Medical School of Jinan University, No. 396 Tong Fu Zhong Road, Guangzhou, China

Jianmin Ran, Gang Xu, Ping Zhu and Gancheng Lao
Department of Endocrinology, Guangzhou Red Cross Hospital, Medical School of Jinan University, No. 396 Tong Fu Zhong Road, Guangzhou, China
Guangzhou Institute of Disease-Oriented Nutritional Research, Guangzhou Red Cross Hospital, Medical School of Jinan University, No. 396 Tong Fu Zhong Road, Guangzhou, China

Rongshao Tan
Guangzhou Institute of Disease-Oriented Nutritional Research, Guangzhou Red Cross Hospital, Medical School of Jinan University, No. 396 Tong Fu Zhong Road, Guangzhou, China

Yan Liu
Guangzhou Institute of Disease-Oriented Nutritional Research, Guangzhou Red Cross Hospital, Medical School of Jinan University, No. 396 Tong Fu Zhong Road, Guangzhou, China
Department of Nephrology, Guangzhou Red Cross Hospital, Medical School of Jinan University, No. 396 Tong Fu Zhong Road, Guangzhou, China

Jun Song
SouthernMedical University, No. 1023-1063 Southern Sha Tai Road, Guangzhou, China

Helen J. Sims-Williams
Sheffield Kidney Institute, Sheffield Teaching Hospitals NHS Foundation Trust, Sheffield, UK

Hugh P. Sims-Williams
Department of Neurosurgery, Sheffield Teaching Hospitals NHS Foundation Trust, Sheffield, UK

Edith Mbabazi Kabachelor
CURE Children's Hospital of Uganda, Mbale, Uganda

Benjamin C. Warf
Department of Paediatric Neurosurgery, Boston Children's Hospital and Harvard Medical School, Boston, MA, USA

Artur Q. B. da Silva, Juliana B. Mansur, Jose Osmar Medicina-Pestana and Gianna Mastroianni-Kirsztajn
Federal University of São Paulo (UNIFESP), São Paulo, SP, Brazil

Taina V. de Sandes-Freitas
Federal University of Ceará (UFC), Fortaleza, CE, Brazil

Bala Waziri, Raquel Duarte and Saraladevi Naicker
Department of Internal Medicine, Faculty of Health Sciences, University of the Witwatersrand, Johannesburg, South Africa

Index